GENETIC TOXICOLOGY
An Agricultural Perspective

BASIC LIFE SCIENCES

Alexander Hollaender, General Editor

Associated Universities, Inc.
Washington, D.C.

A Continuation Order Plan is available for this series. A continuation order will bring delivery of each new volume immediately upon publication. Volumes are billed only upon actual shipment. For further information please contact the publisher.

GENETIC TOXICOLOGY
An Agricultural Perspective

Edited by
RAYMOND A. FLECK
University of California, Davis
Davis, California

and

ALEXANDER HOLLAENDER
Associated Universities, Inc.
Washington, D.C.

SPRINGER SCIENCE+BUSINESS MEDIA, LLC

Library of Congress Cataloging in Publication Data

Main entry under title:

Genetic toxicology.

(Basic life sciences; v. 21)
"Proceedings of a symposium on Genetic Toxicology: an Agricultural Perspective, held
November 1 – 5, 1981, at the University of California, Davis, California"—T.p. verso.
Includes bibliographical references and index.
1. Pollution—Toxicology—Congresses. 2. Pesticides—Toxicology—Congresses. 3. Chem-
ical mutagenesis—Congresses. 4. Veterinary toxicology—Congresses. I. Fleck, Raymond A.,
1927 – 	. II. Hollaender, Alexander, 1898 – 	. III. Series.
RA566.G44 1982 		363.1'79 				82-16476
ISBN 978-1-4684-4354-7 		ISBN 978-1-4684-4352-3 (eBook)
DOI 10.1007/978-1-4684-4352-3

Proceedings of a symposium on Genetic Toxicology: An Agricultural Perspective, held
November 1 – 5, 1981, at the University of California, Davis, California

© 1982 Springer Science+Business Media New York
Originally published by Plenum Press, New York in 1982
Softcover reprint of the hardcover 1st edition 1982

FOREWORD

To meet the needs of an ever-growing world population for food and fiber, agriculture uses an arsenal of chemicals to control insects, weeds and other pests that compete with man in the agricultural arena. In addition to their intended effect, many of these biologically active materials affect non-target organisms including man himself. There is concern about the resulting occupational exposure of those who work in agriculture and the environmental health of those who live in rural areas. Unintended side effects from the use of agricultural chemicals are further complicated by the dispersal of these substances well beyond the area of immediate use, through food chains, atmospheric transport, irrigation runoff, percolation to and diffusion through ground-water, sometimes giving rise to public health and environmental problems at a distance from the place of application.

In addition to toxic substances introduced into the agro-ecosystem by man, one must be concerned about naturally occurring agents including mycotoxins, plant poisons, infective biological agents and the levels of certain heavy metals. The formation of toxic substances, many of them mutagenic, during cooking and other processing of food is a related problem.

While acute effects are more immediate and somewhat readily discerned, chronic and genetic effects tend to be more obscure and sometimes surface in a crisis situation long after substantial damage has been sustained. Genotoxicity assays and epidemiological studies play increasing roles in predicting and evaluating long-term effects of low-level exposure to toxic materials. The sensitivity and specificity of such assays and studies need to be appreciated so that real problems are not overlooked and non-problems are not mistaken for real ones. The improvement of genotoxicity assays, the identification of those with the greatest value in various situations, and the extrapolation of their results to man are subjects of earnest dialog.

Society's growing awareness and readiness to protect itself and future generations, as well as the environment, are manifest in

laws and regulations. But using scientific studies and test
results in risk assessment is an inexact science, as is the
weighing of benefits against costs.

These issues were discussed at a symposium on the Davis campus
of the University of California in November 1981. We are indebted
to many persons who made the symposium possible: the program
planning committee, speakers, chairmen, panelists, participants,
and those who handled arrangements. Financial support was provided
by the Atlantic Richfield Foundation, the College of Agricultural
and Environmental Sciences of the University of California at
Davis, and by a number of federal agencies: the U.S. Department of
Agriculture, the National Institute of Environmental Health
Sciences, the Environmental Protection Agency and the Department of
Energy.

Timely publication of these proceedings was made possible by
the diligence of Dr. Alexander Hollaender, the authors, Claire
Wilson of the Council of Research Planning in Biological Sciences,
Leslie Schmidt of Plenum Publishing Corporation, and John Woolcott
of the Department of Environmental Toxicology at UC Davis.

Raymond A. Fleck
Food Protection & Toxicology Center
University of California at Davis

Scientific Advisory Committee:

Raymond A. Fleck, Food Protection and Toxicology Center, University
of California, Davis, CA; Richard Hill, U.S. Environmental Protec-
tion Agency, Washington, D.C.; Alexander Hollaender (Chairman),
Associated Universities, Inc., Washington, D.C.; Gordon W. Newell,
National Academy of Sciences, Washington, D.C.; Verne A. Ray, Pfizer,
Inc., Groton, CT; Gerald G. Still, U.S. Department of Agriculture,
Washington, D.C.; Raymond C. Valentine, University of California,
Davis, CA; Michael D. Waters, U.S. Environmental Protection Agency,
Research Triangle Park, N.C.; and Avril Woodhead, Biology Department,
Brookhaven National Laboratory, Upton, LI, NY.

CONTENTS

WELCOMING COMMENTS

Charles E. Hess

College of Agricultural and Environmental Sciences
University of California
Davis, California 95616

It is an honor and highly appropriate to have a conference
dealing with Genetic Toxicology: An Agricultural Perspective on
the Davis Campus of the University of California. The Campus
started in 1909 as the College Farm to provide agriculture students
from Berkeley with some practical experience. In 1922, the Bache-
lor of Science in Agriculture was offered. The Campus has grown to
have an outstanding School of Veterinary Medicine, College of
Letters and Science, College of Engineering, School of Medicine,
School of Law, and a School of Administration. Since those early
beginnings, the College of Agriculture and Environmental Sciences
has grown to be one of the largest in the United States with 4700
undergraduate and 1000 graduate students, and is part of the
largest experiment station in the United States.

It is also located in a state that has the largest U. S. agricultural enterprise with a 14 billion dollar farm gate value and
supplying the United States with over 25 percent of its fruits and
vegetables. Some 25 percent of California products are shipped
overseas.

So what we do in California affects the nation and many parts
of the world both directly through the export of food and fiber and
indirectly through the export of ideas and technology.

As you know, part of that technology includes the use of
chemicals -- chemicals which control insects, disease, and weeds
and others which stimulate and regulate growth. Without these compounds, agriculture would not be as productive and there would be
considerable losses between harvest of crops and use by the
consumer.

But, we now know through more sophisticated analytical
techniques and equipment that the chemicals we use or their
metabolites become part of the food chain. We also know that some
of these compounds have subtle effects upon the genome which may
not be readily apparent. We have also learned that there are
naturally-occurring substances such as heavy metals, mycotoxins,
and toxins from poisonous plants which can also be genotoxic. It
is therefore highly appropriate that this conference be held in one
of the important agricultural colleges in the United States and in
a state where agriculture is its number one industry. Since our
products and ideas reach throughout the nation -- yes, even the
world -- we have a responsibility that they are safe, not only from
immediate toxic effects, but also from the subtle and long-term
effects of genetic toxicity.

We appreciate the work you are doing and for coming to this
symposium to share your research ideas and results. With this
information, we can work to make our food and fiber and our
technology even safer for the consumer and the environment.

INTRODUCTION AND OVERVIEW

CHAIRMAN'S COMMENTS

Michael D. Waters

Genetic Toxicology Division
U.S. Environmental Protection Agency
Research Triangle Park, NC 27711

Modern agriculture is highly dependent upon the use of chemical and biological agents to produce the food and fiber needed to sustain human and animal life. Agricultural science has successfully produced many valuable products and has, for the large part, adopted appropriate measures to ensure their efficacy and safety. Indeed, it is essential that efficacy and safety be considered simultaneously. Since many agricultural products are by their very nature toxic, it is important that their use be restricted to situations where appropriate benefits accrue and where relative safety can be maintained. It is also important to recognize that nothing is completely safe; nor is it possible to achieve desired benefits without incurring some risks.

Our concern in this conference is with a particular kind of biological activity for which the relative risks are, at best, difficult to assess. Genetically mediated toxic effects do not necessarily parallel general toxicity and may be unrelated to the desired biological properties of an agricultural agent.

The challenge then, is to detect genetic activity and to accurately assess its potential hazard to man and to the ecosystem. This first session should provide the perspective to enable us to address that challenge.

OVERVIEW OF GENETIC TOXICOLOGY

George R. Hoffmann

Department of Biology
College of the Holy Cross
Worcester, Massachusetts 01610

INTRODUCTION

The field of genetic toxicology exists because of the concern
that environmental agents can cause genetic damage in man and
thereby have an adverse effect on human health. Genetic toxicologists are concerned about effects both in germ cells and in
somatic cells. An increase in the incidence of mutational events
in human eggs or sperms could lead to an increase in the incidence
of genetic disease and disability in future generations. In contrast, effects in somatic cells do not pose a threat to future
generations, because they are not genetically transmitted beyond
the individual in which they occur. The lack of transmissibility
to progeny does not mean that genetic damage in somatic cells makes
no contribution to the human disease burden. Rather, there is good
reason to believe that mutations in somatic cells play an important
part in the initiation of cancers (76). In fact, the great
majority of chemicals that are known to cause cancer in laboratory
animals or man also cause mutational events in one or more
organisms in which they have been tested.

Genetic toxicology therefore has two major aspects. The first
concerns the effects of mutagenesis on future generations. It
encompasses efforts to identify agents that can cause mutations in
human germ cells and to assess the risks that they pose. The other
aspect of genetic toxicology, which has its roots in the correlation
between mutagenesis and carcinogenesis, is the use of laboratory
mutation tests as predictive indicators of carcinogenesis.

To provide an overview of genetic toxicology, I shall first
trace its historic origins in genetics, then discuss its

implications for human health, and conclude with a synopsis of its
status as a subdiscipline of toxicology.

Historic Origins of Genetic Toxicology

At the turn of the century, the principles of inheritance,
which had been discovered by Gregor Mendel some 35 years earlier,
were rediscovered by Hugo de Vries, Carl Correns, and Erich von
Tschermak-Seysenegg. The rediscovery led to an explosion of
activity in genetic research. This activity made use of spontaneously occurring mutants that were found in wild and laboratory
populations of organisms.

A major event in the history of genetics was the discovery in
1927 that ionizing radiation can cause an increase in the rate at
which mutations occur. Specifically, Hermann J. Muller (55) demonstrated that X-rays induce sex-linked recessive lethal mutations in
the fruit fly, Drosophila melanogaster. X-rays were thus the first
known mutagen. The following year, L. R. Stadler (75) extended
Muller's result by reporting the mutagenicity of ionizing radiation
in barley, and within a few years the mutagenicity of ultraviolet
light had also been reported (6). There was some speculation at
the time that chemicals might also be capable of inducing mutations. A few reports of chemical mutagenesis were published before
1940, but they were not definitive demonstrations of mutation induction. The first unequivocal evidence of chemical mutagensis was
obtained in Scotland during World War II, when Charlotte Auerbach
and J. M. Robson demonstrated that mustard gas was mutagenic in
fruit flies; because of wartime censorship, the results were not
published until after the war (10-12). At about the same time, F.
Oehlkers (56) in Germany and I. A. Rapoport (63) in the Soviet
Union independently found that several other chemicals induce chromosome aberrations and gene mutations, respectively. An expansion
of research on chemical mutagenesis soon followed. Within a few
years, a rather large number of chemicals had been shown to be
mutagenic, and among these were several that were effective
mutagens at low doses at which they exhibited no other pronounced
toxic effects.

Early interest in chemical mutagens centered around their use
in basic genetic research; there was also some interest in the possibility of using mutagens to introduce useful genetic variations into
organisms of industrial and agricultural importance. It was not
long, however, before a darker side to chemical mutagenesis
surfaced. By the 1950's and early 1960's, H. J. Muller, Alfred Bar-
thelmess, Charlotte Auerbach, Joshua Lederberg, Alexander Hollaender, and others had already voiced concern that environmental mutagens might cause irreversible genetic damage in man.

The era of environmental mutagenesis thus began with the
recognition that mutagens may pose a risk for human health. The
risk seemed especially insidious because the consequences of
exposure to mutagens may not be evident until long after exposure
has occurred and the damage is already done. The thrust in
environmental mutagenesis therefore became the development of means
for identifying mutagens and minimizing human exposure to them.

Implications of Mutagenesis for Human Health

The major classes of mutational change are gene mutations,
which are modifications in the structure of DNA of individual
genes; chromosome aberrations, in which segments of chromosomes
containing many genes are deleted, duplicated, or rearranged; and
alterations in chromosome number. All three types of genetic
alterations are known to be inducible by mutagens in experimental
organisms, and all have implications for human health. Together,
they make a considerable contribution to the total burden of human
disease.

It is estimated that more than 6% (19, 39) of all live-born
infants suffer from genetic defects or malformations. A large
proportion of the genetic disease burden is ascribable to gene
mutations that are already present in the population. There is no
reason to believe, however, that environmental mutagens cannot
increase the frequency of these mutations and thereby lead to increases in the incidence of genetic diseases. Alterations in chromosome structure and number also contribute to the genetic disease
burden, in that about 0.6% of live-born infants have chromosomal
abnormalitites (19,39), most of which are associated with defined
syndromes. For example, the relatively common disorder Down's
syndrome, which is caused by the presence of an extra copy of chromosome #21, affects approximately 0.1% of newborn infants (39). In
addition to the causation of genetic diseases, chromosomal
abnormalities contribute to human suffering through prenatal
deaths. It has been estimated that 6% of stillbirths and 50% of
the spontaneous abortions that are detected between weeks 8 and 20
of pregnancy are chromosomally abnormal (39). Unfortunately, the
magnitude of the contribution of environmental mutagens to the
burden of disease, disability, and fetal deaths is unknown.

Gene mutations can be categorized on several bases, among
which are the molecular mechanism of mutation induction and the
pattern of inheritance of the characteristic that the gene determines. With respect to molecular mechanisms, the two major types
of gene mutations are base-pair substitutions and frameshift mutations. In a base-pair substitution, one base pair in DNA (e.g.,
adenine-thymine) is replaced by another (e.g., guanine-cytosine or
thymine-adenine). Such a change in base sequence in DNA often
leads to a change in the amino acid sequence in the protein that is

encoded by the gene. If the altered protein functions differently
from the original protein, the difference is reflected in the characteristics of the mutant relative to those of the nonmutant.

In a frameshift mutation, there is an addition or a deletion
of one or a few base pairs in the structure of DNA. Because the
sequence of base pairs in DNA is interpreted in living organisms as
a code that is read three base pairs at a time, a frameshift mutation alters all of the code words after the point at which a base
pair is added or deleted. The amino acid sequence of the gene
product (i.e., protein) is therefore grossly altered and in many
cases is incomplete, because the newly generated sequence of bases
is apt to contain a code word that specifies no amino acid at
all. Frameshift mutations thereby result in nonfunctional gene
products. The mutant, which lacks the function of that gene product, differs from the nonmutant by whatever characteristics are
conferred by that missing gene function in the complex physiology
of the organism.

My reason for discussing base-pair substitutions and frameshift mutations is that mutagens may exhibit specificity for particular mechanisms of mutagenesis. Acridine mustards, for example,
induce predominantly frameshift mutations (9), whereas some other
mutagens, like diethyl sulfate, preferentially induce base-pair
substitutions (37). Still other mutagens, like ultraviolet light,
induce a mixture of alterations (46). Because base-pair substitutions and frameshift mutations both lead to altered or missing gene
products with potentially deleterious effects, the capacity to
detect agents that induce either of these types of mutation is
important for protecting people from mutagen exposures.

With respect to patterns of inheritance, gene mutations can be
classified as dominant or recessive. A recessive mutation is one
that is expressed only when inherited from both parents (i.e., when
homozygous). Expression therefore requires that the gene of
maternal origin and that of paternal origin for a given characteristic both be of the mutant type. In contrast, only a single
copy of a dominant gene is required for its expression. Although
molecular mechanisms of mutagenesis and dominance are not totally
unrelated, both base-pair substitutions and frameshift mutations
can be either dominant or recessive in expression.

Both dominant and recessive gene mutations have implications
for human health. More than 1,000 disorders that are inherited as
recessive mutations are known, familiar examples being albinism and
cystic fibrosis. It has been estimated that about 5% of hospital-
ized children in major medical centers have conditions that are
related to recessive mutations (22). The great majority of such
mutations are likely to be inherited from previous generations
rather than being new mutations. Dominant mutations, however, are

also important for disease burden, and it is likely that new mutations make a larger contribution to the incidence of dominant disorders than to that of recessive disorders. In this respect,
recessive genes on the X-chromosome would be expected to be more
like dominant genes, in that only a single copy of a mutation is
required for its expression in males. The total incidence of disorders that are ascribable to dominant and X-linked mutations has
been estimated to be about 1% of live births (19). Unfortunately,
it is not yet possible to estimate the impact of chemically induced
mutation on the incidence of either dominant or recessive genetic
disease.

The induction of dominant mutations constitutes a greater
concern for human genetic welfare in the foreseeable future than
does the induction of recessive mutations (except X-linked mutations), because many generations would be required for the new
recessive mutations to be expressed. Dominant mutations, which
need be present only singly for expression, would be expressed in
the first generation after their occurrence.

A complicating factor in interpreting the effects of dominant
mutations versus recessive mutations is that many "recessive" mutations seem not to be recessive in the strictest sense, but rather
are expressed to a very limited extent even when present singly
(i.e., in heterozygotes). For example, people with the recessive
diseases xeroderma pigmentosum and ataxia telangiectasia have,
among other symptoms, a greatly elevated risk of cancer. It has
been reported that these patients' relatives, who do not have the
diseases, nevertheless have a cancer incidence somewhat higher than
that of the general population (78, 79). Apparently, a single copy
of the recessive genes has a slight deleterious effect. Data from
experimental organisms similarly suggest that recessive mutations
are often expressed to a slight extent in heterozygotes. Therefore, even for the next few generations, we cannot ignore recessive
mutations, but must be concerned about their minor effects in
heterozygotes. Fortunately, mutagens are not expected to be
specific for the induction of either dominant or recessive
mutations, and protecting against mutagenesis would therefore be
likely to protect against the induction of both types of mutations.

Sources of Relevant Data in Genetic Toxicology

Most areas of toxicology rely on laboratory data for the identification and assessment of hazards. Frequently there are also
data from human exposures that corroborate or lend credibility to
the experimental data. In genetic toxicology, however, data on
mutagenesis in human germ cells are essentially nonexistent and
even data for somatic cells in vivo are quite limited.

One might expect that the incidence of dominant diseases could be monitored as an indication of genetic damage in man. Monitoring for such diseases, called the "sentinel phenotypes" approach, is not, however, a very sensitive indicator of changes in mutation rates (77). Individual genetic diseases are rare and their diagnosis is not always unequivocal. The approach would require monitoring very large populations, and it could be difficult to ascribe any increases in the incidence of the sentinel phenotypes to an ultimate cause. Detecting electrophoretic protein variants in the offspring of a study population would similarly be unsuitable for routine use in environmental mutagenesis. Although these approaches can make a valuable contribution to our knowledge of human mutation frequencies, they are not readily applicable to the monitoring of defined human populations of limited size for evidence of mutagenesis. Because of these limitations, no mutagen has yet been shown unequivocally to induce heritable alterations in human germ cells.

Before leaving this topic, I should note that several promising methods for human mutational monitoring are under development. Gene mutations (5), chromosome aberrations (30), and sister chromatid exchanges (60) can be detected in human somatic cells. The presence of mutagens in human urine can be detected with microbial tests (89). Morphological abnormalities in human sperm (88) and cytochemical evidence for the presence of two Y-chromosomes in human sperm (43) have also been used as indicators of mutagen exposure.

Although recent developments in human monitoring are encouraging, the data base is very limited, and important problems remain to be resolved. Applying epidemiologic methods to genetic toxicology is an important area of study, but doing so is not simple. The exposed populations are often small; the patterns of exposure are frequently complex and involve many confounding variables; and the doses are variable and not readily measured. Because of the paucity of information from human populations, genetic toxicology relies heavily on laboratory tests--perhaps more heavily than other fields of toxicology, where data for human exposures are often better.

Reliance on laboratory tests necessitates a dependence on the validity of extrapolation from one species to another. Fortunately, the justification for extrapolating among species, even across broad phylogenetic lines, is stronger in genetic toxicology than in most other areas of toxicologic study. The conceptual basis for such extrapolations lies in DNA being the hereditary material in all organisms from bacteria to mammals. Chemicals that interact with DNA in ways that cause mutation in one species are likely to be mutagenic in other species as well. Although this generalization cannot be interpreted rigidly, because of differences among species in routes of chemical exposure, metabolism and pharmacologic disposition of toxicants, and repair of genetic damage, it nevertheless has enough merit to be useful in the identification of genetic hazards.

Experimental data in comparative mutagenesis also provide support for extrapolation among species. Most agents that are mutagenic in one species or test system can also be detected as mutagens in other species and assays (23, 38). The carcinogenesis literature also provides a link between laboratory mutagenicity data and human health. Most evidence regarding mechanisms of chemical carcinogenesis suggests that mutational events are involved in the initiation of cancer (76). Strong correlations have been reported, moreover, between the carcinogenicity of chemicals in experimental mammals and their mutagenicity in short-term tests (13,17, 51, 52, 62). Even pessimistic estimates of the capacity of mutagenicity tests to differentiate between carcinogens and noncarcinogens reveal correlations that are strong enough to permit use in the preliminary screening of chemicals to identify carcinogens (64).

Short-term mutagenicity tests are of interest not only as predictive tools for carcinogenicity but also for mutagenicity per se. Because of complicating factors, including metabolism, pharmacologic disposition, and repair, one cannot expect to project results from short-term tests to mammalian germ cells without errors; for example, diethylnitrosamine and several other chemicals that induce mutations in short-term tests are nonmutagenic in tests for mutations in mammalian germ cells (67, 68). Nevertheless, agents that are mutagenic in short-term tests are more likely to be mutagenic in man than those that are not. In the absence of mammalian genetic data, the suspicion that a given agent is a human mutagen is enhanced if the short-term test results are supported by data, such as alkylation of testicular DNA or induction of morphological sperm abnormalities, that show that the agent affects germinal tissue in whole mammals.

In attempting to project short-term test results to intact mammals, one is faced with complex problems in relating dosages in submammalian systems to mammalian exposures. There are marked differences in routes of exposure, uptake, metabolism, toxicity, and units of measurement among organisms and test systems. A variety of mechanisms have been used in attempting to relate exposure levels to germ-cell dose and to standardize or compare results from diverse organisms and test systems. These approaches include correcting for DNA content in various organisms (3,35), relating chemical exposures to equivalent radiation exposures (25, 26, 28), and using molecular dosimetry in which chemical adducts in DNA are measured directly (1,2,47,48). Despite considerable effort, our current capacity to relate mutagenesis data from short-term tests to whole mammals and particularly to genetic risks in man are still quite primitive.

Test Systems in Genetic Toxicology

Test systems have been developed for the detection of a diversity of genetic effects in a wide range of experimental organisms and cell types. There is a growing data base on chemical mutagenesis in assay systems in bacteria, fungi, mammalian cells in culture, vascular plants, insects, and intact mammals. The files of the Environmental Mutagen Information Center (EMIC) in Oak Ridge, Tennessee, reveal that there are at least 35,000 publications that concern genetic effects of at least 11,500 different chemicals.

Table 1 lists some of the major test systems used in genetic toxicology. A detailed discussion of the characteristics of mutagenicity tests is beyond the scope of this overview of genetic toxicology; I would, however, like to discuss some general features of tests and identify some of the major advantages and limitations of particular types of tests.

A widely used means of detecting mutations in microorganisms is the selection of revertants in auxotrophic strains. An auxotroph is an organism that has a nutritional requirement in addition to the requirements of wild-type strains of that species. For example, strains of E. coli that have a mutation in one of the genes that code for enzymes involved in the synthesis of tryptophan require tryptophan to grow and are said to be tryptophan auxotrophs. If bacteria of a tryptophan auxotrophic strain are plated in petri dishes of medium without tryptophan, only those bacteria that contain a mutation, called a reversion, that corrects the defect of the original mutation are able to grow. By counting colonies of bacteria in such strains, one can calculate a revertant frequency; similarly one can compare revertant frequencies in untreated bacteria and in chemically treated bacteria as a means of detecting mutagenic chemicals.

Reversion tests in microorganisms have been conducted since the early days of chemical mutagenesis, when many carcinogens were first found to be mutagenic in microbial tests. A problem in firmly establishing the correlation between mutagenicity and carcinogenicity was that mutagenic effects of certain classes of potent carcinogens, notably the nitrosamines and polynuclear aromatic hydrocarbons, could not be detected in microbial tests. The explanation for this apparent lack of correlation is that these compounds are mutagenic and carcinogenic only after they are modified in mammalian metabolism. Such chemicals that require metabolic activation to be mutagenic are called promutagens.

A major advance in mutagenicity testing was Heinrich Malling's demonstration that homogenates of mammalian tissues can be used to activate promutagens in vitro. Specifically, Malling (50) showed that dimethylnitrosamine, which was not mutagenic itself in micro-

organisms, could be detected as a mutagen in bacteria if the microorganisms were simultaneously exposed to the chemical and a
postmitochondrial supernatant from mouse liver. Shortly
thereafter, Bruce Ames and his co-workers showed that a variety of
carcinogens, including polynuclear aromatic hydrocarbons, could
similarly be detected as mutagens when activated by rat liver or
human liver extracts (7). The rat liver metabolic activation
system, frequently called an S9 (i.e., 9000 x g supernatant) mix,
is now a standard part of microbial mutagenicity testing (8).

The most widely used of all mutagenicity tests is the
Salmonella/mammalian microsome test developed by Bruce Ames and his
colleagues at the University of California in Berkeley (8). This
test, also called the Ames test, detects the reversion of histidine
auxotrophic strains of Salmonella typhimurium. It includes strains
for the detection of both base-pair substitution and frameshift
mutations and is capable of detecting a wide variety of mutagens
and promutagens. In addition to the Ames test, a number of other
tests in bacteria and fungi use reversion of auxotrophs as a means
of detecting mutations.

Another strategy that has been used in microbial mutagenicity
testing is the detection of drug-resistant mutants. For example,
mutants that are resistant to the toxic effects of 8-azaguanine
have been studied in a variety of microorganisms. Drug resistance
has also been exploited as a means of detecting mutations in
mammalian cells in culture, and several important mammalian cell
test systems are based on this principle. Detection of resistance
to 6-thioguanine and other purine analogues, trifluorothymidine and
other pyrimidine analogues, and ouabain are the most frequently
employed tests in mammalian cell cultures. Although the reversion
of auxotrophs and the detection of drug-resistant mutants are the
most commonly used strategies for mutation detection in short-term
tests, other methods also exist. For example, mutations that are
distinguished by altered colony color have been used in many
studies of mutagenesis in fungi. Besides tests for gene mutations,
tests have been developed in fungi for the study of mutagen-induced
mitotic recombination and aneuploidy, and mammalian cell cultures
are widely used to study chromosome aberrations and sister chromatid exchanges.

Drosophila tests permit the detection of a variety of genetic
changes, including gene mutations, chromosome aberrations, and
changes in chromosome number. The Drosophila sex-linked recessive
lethal test, which detects gene mutations and small deletions, is a
relatively simple, whole animal test for which there is a rather
extensive data base. Tests in vascular plants also permit the
study of both gene mutations and cytogenetic damage. A promising
recent use of plant assays is in situ monitoring for environmental
mutagens, including mutagen detection under field conditions.

Table 1. Test Systems in Genetic Toxicology

Test Systems	Effects Measured	Selected References
Bacterial reversion tests (e.g., the Ames Salmonella/mammalian microsome test and the E. coli WP2 reversion system)	Reversion of auxotrophs by base-pair substitutions or frameshift mutations	Ames, McCann, and Yamasaki, 1975 Brusick et al., 1980 Hollstein et al., 1979 McCann et al., 1975
Bacterial drug-resistance tests (e.g., 8-azaguanine-resistance in Salmonella)	Gene mutations (i.e., forward mutations) that confer resistance to an inhibitory chemical	Hollstein et al., 1979 Skopek et al., 1978
Bacterial repair tests (e.g., the E. coli polA test and the B. subtilis rec assay)	Greater killing of strains that are deficient in the repair of DNA damage than in repair-proficient strains	Hollstein et al., 1979 Kada et al., 1980 Rosenkranz and Leifer, 1980
Bacterial inductests (e.g., induction of prophage λ in E. coli)	Induction of lysis in bacterial strains that harbor quiescent (i.e., lysogenic) bacteriophages	Heinemann, 1971 Hollstein et al., 1979 Moreau et al., 1976
Forward mutation tests in fungi (e.g., red adenine mutants in Neurospora or yeasts)	Gene mutations and small deletions (e.g., mutations in genes that code for enzymes involved in purine biosynthesis are detected as red colonies in white strains or vice versa)	deSerres and Malling, 1971 Hollstein et al., 1979 Mortimer and Manney, 1971
Reversion tests in fungi (e.g., reversion of auxotrophs in Neurospora or yeasts)	Reversion of auxotrophic mutations by base-pair substitutions or frameshift mutations	Hollstein et al., 1979 Mortimer and Manney, 1971 Ong, 1978

Table 1. Continued

Test Systems	Effects Measured	Selected References
Recombinogenicity in yeasts (e.g., strains D3, D4, D5, and D7 of Saccharomyces cerevisiae)	Mitotic crossing over and mitotic gene conversion	Hollstein et al., 1979; Zimmermann, 1973, 1975; Zimmermann et al., 1975
Aneuploidy tests in fungi (e.g., strain D6 in Saccharomyces and Griffiths' test in Neurospora)	Aneuploidy in mitotic cells and meiotic nondisjunction	Griffiths, 1979; Parry et al., 1979; Parry and Zimmermann, 1976
Drug-resistance in mammalian cells (e.g., thymidine kinase mutants in mouse lymphoma cells; hypoxanthine-guanine phosphoribo-syltransferase mutants in Chinese hamster cells or human cells)	Gene mutations (i.e., forward mutations) that confer resistance to inhibitory chemicals (e.g., trifluorothymidine or 6-thioguanine)	Bartsch et al., 1980; Clive et al., 1979; Hollstein et al., 1979; Thilly et al., 1980
Mammalian cell cytogenetic tests (e.g., cytogenetic analysis of Chinese hamster cells or human cells grown in vitro)	Chromosomal aberrations and sister chromatid exchanges	Evans, 1976; Hollstein et al., 1979; Perry, 1980; Wolff, 1977
Repair assays in mammalian cells (e.g., unscheduled DNA synthesis tests in rat hepatocytes or human fibroblasts)	DNA synthesis associated with repair of genetic damage	Hollstein et al., 1979; San and Stich, 1975; Williams, 1977, 1980
Vascular plant mutation tests (e.g., the Tradescantia stamen hair test, the waxy locus test in maize, and chlorophyll mutation tests)	Gene mutations	Conger and Carabia, 1977; Ehrenberg, 1971; Plewa and Wagner, 1981; Schairer et al., 1978; Underbrink et al., 1973

Table 1. Continued

Test Systems	Effects Measured	Selected References
Vascular plant cytogenetic tests (e.g., analysis of mitotic cells in root tips or shoot tips; analysis of meiotic cells in microsporocytes)	Chromosomal aberrations	Grant, 1978 Kihlman, 1971, 1977 Ma, 1981
Drosophila sex-linked recessive lethal test	Gene mutations and small deletions	Abrahamson and Lewis, 1971 Vogel and Sobels, 1976 Würgler et al., 1977
Drosophila tests for chromosomal alterations (e.g., heritable translocation tests; sex-chromosome loss test)	Chromosome breakage, rearrangements, and loss	Abrahamson and Lewis, 1971 Vogel and Sobels, 1976 Würgler et al., 1977
Mammalian cytogenetic tests (e.g., cytogenetic analysis of rodent bone marrow, lymphocytes, or spermatocytes; micronucleus test)	Chromosomal aberrations and sister chromatid exchanges	Brewen and Preston, 1978 Hollstein et al., 1979 Jenssen and Ramel, 1980 Perry, 1980 Wolff, 1977
Mouse or rat dominant lethal tests	Deaths of fetuses sired by treated male animals; indirect evidence of chromosome damage	Bateman and Epstein, 1971 Russell and Matter, 1980
Mouse sperm abnormality test	Morphologically abnormal sperm	Topham, 1980 Wyrobek and Bruce, 1978
Mouse somatic-cell specific-locus test (i.e. mouse spot test)	Mutations in defined genes in somatic cells	Fahrig, 1978 Russell and Matter, 1980

Table 1. Continued

Test Systems	Effects Measured	Selected References
Mouse aneuploidy test	Sex-chromosome loss due to chromosome breakage and nondisjunction	Russell, 1976 Russell and Matter, 1980
Mouse heritable translocation test	Chromosome rearrangements in mammalian germ cells	Generoso et al., 1980 Russell and Matter, 1980
Mouse skeletal mutation test	Skeletal abnormalities in progeny of treated males; evidence of mutational damage	Selby and Selby, 1977
Mouse germ-cell specific-locus mutation tests (e.g., morphological specific locus test; electrophoretic specific locus test)	Gene mutations and/or deletions in defined genes in germ cells	Johnson and Lewis, 1981 Russell et al., 1979 Russell and Matter, 1980

A variety of tests have been developed for the detection of gene mutations and chromosomal alterations in the germ cells and somatic cells of intact mammals, especially mice. Because of their obvious relevance for man, mammalian tests occupy a position of particular importance in genetic toxicology; several of the major test systems in mammals are listed in Table 1.

Considerations in Mutagenicity Testing

To be useful, a short-term test should predict an effect in man. For example, a perfect short-term carcinogenicity test would respond to all carcinogenic chemicals and be unresponsive to all noncarcinogens. In real tests, however, some carcinogens escape detection and are commonly called "false negatives" in that test; noncarcinogens that are positive in the test are often referred to as "false positives."

Two important characteristics of a test system for carcinogens are its sensitivity and its specificity (21, 73). "Sensitivity" refers to the proportion of carcinogens that are positive in the test, and "specificity" refers to the proportion of noncarcinogens that are negative. False negatives reduce the sensitivity of a test, and false positives reduce its specificity. A useful test combines a high sensitivity with a high specificity. The serious-ness of deficiencies in either sensitivity or specificity depends on the intended use of the test in making decisions, because the consequences of false positives and false negatives are different at different stages in the safety evaluation of chemicals. As tests are refined and their validation becomes more complete, it may become possible to devise testing strategies that use tests in combinations to optimize their strengths and minimize their inadequacies with respect to either sensitivity or specificity.

The distribution of chemicals among chemical classes can af-fect test performance, because tests differ in their effectiveness of detection of different classes of mutagens and carcinogens. In test validation, chemicals should therefore be selected from a broad range of chemical classes. It is also important in test validation that both potent mutagens and weak mutagens be included among the agents tested.

Typically, a large proportion of the chemicals studied in validating test systems are carcinogens, whereas the proportion of carcinogens encountered in actual testing situations is lower. As the proportion of carcinogens among the chemicals tested is reduced, the proportion of false positives among all positives becomes larger. This problem is inherent in testing and demon-strates that specificity is an important attribute of a test; it suggests, furthermore, that one should only accept with reserva-tions the common viewpoint that false negatives are a much more important inadequacy in a test than false positives.

The terms "false positive," "false negative," and "validation" have meaning only in comparison to the "true" properties of the agents in question. In many cases these properties are not known with certainty, and it is therefore likely that some "false positives" are actually positives for which the point of reference is incorrectly classified. For example, a weak carcinogen that is considered noncarcinogenic because of inadequate carcinogenicity data would incorrectly be interpreted as a "false positive" if it were positive in a short-term test.

In discussing test validation, reference is frequently made to carcinogenesis. In contrast to its use with respect to carcinogenesis, the term "validation" has little meaning for mutagenesis per se, because the data base on the induction of gene mutations in whole mammals is very limited. With respect to mutagenesis, one can therefore only consider concordance among tests but not "validation" in a strict sense.

Microbial tests are used in genetic toxicology because they can be performed quickly and inexpensively. Large numbers of chemicals can therefore be screened in microorganisms. Many microbial tests successfully predict effects in mammals, offer an extensive data base for comparative purposes, and permit refined genetic characterization of the induced alterations. The primary limitations of microbial tests lie in the fact that the test organisms are phylogenetically distant from man. Microbial tests cannot account for all aspects of exposure and dosimetry in mammals or for differences between germ cells and somatic cells in sensitivity to mutagenesis. The capabilities of metabolic activation systems that are used with short-term tests cannot be assumed to be identical to metabolism in intact animals. Differences in repair processes may also cause differences in mutational responses in different organisms.

Presumed relevance for human health is greater in assay systems that use indicator organisms or cells that are higher in the phylogenetic hierarchy. Assays in cultured mammalian cells, for example, offer a eukaryotic cellular organization that may respond to mutagenesis more as human cells would in vivo that do prokaryotic bacterial cells. Tests in Drosophila offer the increased relevance of a whole animal system that has germ cell stages that are analogous to mammalian germ cell stages. A problem in genetic toxicology testing is that such gains in relevance for man are accompanied by increases in the cost of the tests and the time required to perform them.

In mammalian tests, the problems of relating experimental exposures in the test organism to human exposures are lessened, but the difficult issue of extrapolation from high doses and acute exposures to low doses and chronic exposures must still be considered. It should be noted, moreover, that genetic tests in whole mammals tend to be costly and time consuming; consequently, they cannot be applied as readily as microbial tests to screening large numbers of chemicals. Identifying mutagens and assessing the risks that they pose therefore require the application of a variety of short-term tests that are able to detect a broad spectrum of mutational events and tests in whole mammals for the detailed study of important compounds.

The problem posed by mutagenic chemicals in the environment is extremely complex; and our capabilities in certain aspects of genetic toxicology, such as genetic risk assessment, can only be regarded as primitive. Nevertheless, there have been important advances in basic mutation research and progress in the development and refinement of genetic toxicology tests. Environmental mutagenesis is gradually being incorporated into the mainstream of toxicology, and analysis for mutagenicity is becoming part of the standard toxicologic evaluation of chemicals. The problem of environmental mutagens will not be easily resolved, but the progress that has already taken place suggests a basis for optimism that at least some mutational hazards for man can be avoided or minimized.

REFERENCES

1. Aaron, C. S. and W. R. Lee, Molecular dosimetry of the mutagen ethyl methanesulfonate in Drosophila melanogaster spermatozoa: Linear relation of DNA alkylation per sperm cell (dose) to sex-linked recessive lethals, Mutation Res. 49, 27-44 (1978).
2. Aaron, C. S., A. A. Van Zeeland, G. R. Mohn, A. T. Natarajan, A. G. A. C. Knaap, A. D. Tates, and B. W. Glickman, Molecular dosimetry of the chemical mutagen ethyl methanesulfonate: Quantitative comparison of mutation induction in Escherichia coli, V79 Chinese hamster cells and L5178Y mouse lymphoma cells, and some cytological results in vitro and in vivo, Mutation Res. 69, 201-216 (1980).
3. Abrahamson, S., M. A. Bender, A. D. Conger, and S. Wolff, Uniformity of radiation-induced mutation rates among different species, Nature 245, 460-462 (1973).
4. Abrahamson, S. and E. B. Lewis, The detection of mutations in Drosophila melanogaster, in: Chemical Mutagens: Principles and Methods for Their Detection, Vol. 2 (A. Hollaender, ed.), pp. 461-487, Plenum Press, New York (1971).
5. Albertini, R. J., Drug-resistant lymphocytes in man as indicators of somatic cell mutation, Teratogenesis, Carcinogenesis, and Mutagenesis 1, 25-48 (1980).
6. Altenburg, E., The artificial production of mutations by ultraviolet light, Amer. Naturalist 68, 491-507 (1934).

7. Ames, B. N., W. E. Durston, E. Yamasaki, and F. D. Lee, Car-
    cinogens are mutagens: A simple test system combining liver
    homogenates for activation and bacteria for detection, Proc.
    Natl. Acad. Sci. U.S.A. 70, 2281-2285 (1973).

8. Ames, B. N., J. McCann, and E. Yamasaki, Methods for detecting
    carcinogens and mutagens with the Salmonella/mammalian-micro-
    some mutagenicity test, Mutation Res. 31: 347-364 (1975).

9. Ames, B. N. and H. J. Whitfield, Jr., Frameshift mutagenesis
    in Salmonella, Cold Spring Harbor Symp. Quant. Biol. 31, 221-
    225 (1966).

10. Auerbach, C., History of research on chemical mutagenesis,
    in: Chemical Mutagens: Principles and Methods for Their
    Detection, Vol. 3 (A. Hollaender, ed.), pp. 1-19, Plenum
    Press, New York (1973).

11. Auerbach, C. and J. M. Robson, Chemical production of muta-
    tions, Nature 157, 302 (1946).

12. Auerbach, C. and J. M. Robson, The production of mutations by
    chemical substances, Proc. Roy. Soc. Edinburgh (B) 62, 271-283
    (1947).

13. Bartsch, H., C. Malaveille, A.-M. Camus, G. Martel-Planche, G.
    Brun, A. Hautefeuille, N. Sabadie, A. Barbin, T. Kuroki, C.
    Drevon, C. Piccoli, and R. Montesano, Validation and compara-
    tive studies on 180 chemicals with S. typhimurium strains and
    V79 Chinese hamster cells in the presence of various
    metabolizing systems, Mutation Res. 76, 1-50 (1980).

14. Bateman, A. J. and S. S. Epstein, Dominant lethal mutations in
    mammals, in: Chemical Mutagens: Principles and Methods for
    Their Detection, Vol. 2 (A. Hollaender, ed.), pp. 541-568,
    Plenum Press, New York (1971).

15. Brewen, J. G. and R. J. Preston, Analysis of chromosome aber-
    rations in mammalian germ cells, in: Chemical Mutagens:
    Principles and Methods for Their Detection, Vol. 5 (A.
    Hollaender and F. J. deSerres, eds.), pp. 127-150, Plenum
    Press, New York (1978).

16. Brusick, D. J., V. F. Simmon, H. S. Rosenkranz, V. A. Ray, and
    R. S. Stafford, An evaluation of the Escherichia coli WP2 and
    WP2uvrA reverse mutation assay, Mutation Res. 76, 169-190
    (1980).

17. Campbell, T. C., Chemical carcinogens and human risk assess-
    ment, Fed. Proc. 39, 2467-2484 (1980).

18. Clive, D., K. O. Johnson, J. F. S. Spector, A. G. Batson, and
    M. M. M. Brown, Validation and characterization of the
    L5178Y/TK+/- mouse lymphoma mutagen assay system, Mutation
    Res. 59, 61-108 (1979).

19. Committee on the Biological Effects of Ionizing Radiations,
    The Effects on Populations of Exposure to Low Levels of Ioni-
    zing Radiation, National Academy Press, Washington (1980).

20. Conger, B. V. and J. V. Carabia, Mutagenic effectiveness and
    efficiency of sodium azide versus ethyl methanesulfonate in
    maize: Induction of somatic mutations at the yg_2 locus by

treatment of seeds differing in metabolic state and cell population, Mutation Res. 46, 285-296 (1977).

21. Cooper, J. A., R. Saracci, and P. Cole, Describing the
    validity of carcinogen screening tests, Brit. J. Cancer 39,
    87-89 (1979).

22. Department of Health, Education and Welfare Committee to Co-
    ordinate Toxicology and Related Programs, Subcommittee on
    Environmental Mutagenesis, Approaches to Determining the Muta-
    genic Properties of Chemicals: Risk to Future Generations, J.
    Environ. Pathol. Toxicol. 1, 301-352 (1977).

23. deSerres, F. J. and J. Ashby (eds.), Evaluation of Short-Term
    Tests for Carcinogens: Report of the International Col-
    laborative Program, Elsevier/North Holland, Amsterdam (1981).

24. deSerres, F. J. and H. V. Malling, Measurement of recessive
    lethal damage over the entire genome and at two specific loci
    in the ad-3 region of a two-component heterokaryon of Neu-
    rospora crassa, in: Chemical Mutagens: Principles and
    Methods for Their Detection, Vol. 2 (A. Hollaender, ed.), pp.
    311-342, Plenum Press, New York (1971).

25. Drake, J. W. and other members of Committee 17 appointed by
    the Council of the Environmental Mutagen Society, Environmen-
    tal mutagenic hazards, Science 187, 503-514 (1975).

26. Ehling, U. H., Evaluation of genetic hazards in man from radi-
    ation and chemical mutagens, in: Radiobiological Equivalents
    of Chemical Pollutants, pp. 71-81, International Atomic Energy
    Agency (1980).

27. Ehrenberg, L., Higher Plants, in: Chemical Mutagens:
    Principles and Methods for Their Detection, Vol. 2 (A. Hol-
    laender, ed.), pp. 365-386, Plenum Press, New York (1971).

28. Ehrenberg, L., Risk assessment of ethylene oxide and other
    compounds, in: Banbury Report 1, Assessing Chemical
    Mutagens: The Risk to Humans (V. K. McElheny and S. Abraham-
    son, eds.), pp. 157-190, Cold Spring Harbor Laboratory (1979).

29. Evans, H. J., Cytological methods for detecting chemical muta-
    gens, in: Chemical Mutagens: Principles and Methods for
    Their Detection, Vol. 4 (A. Hollaender, ed.), 1-29, Plenum
    Press, New York (1976).

30. Evans, H. J. and D. C. Lloyd (eds.), Mutagen-Induced Chromo-
    some Damage in Man, Yale University Press, New Haven, 355
    pp. (1978).

31. Fahrig, R., The mammalian spot test: A sensitive in vivo
    method for the detection of genetic alterations in somatic
    cells of mice, in: Chemical Mutagens: Principles and Methods
    for Their Detection, Vol. 5 (A. Hollaender and F. J. deSerres,
    eds.), pp. 151-176, Plenum Press, New York (1978).

32. Generoso, W. M., J. B. Bishop, D. G. Gosslee, G. W. Newell,
    C.-J. Sheu, and E. von Halle, Heritable translocation test in
    mice, Mutation Res. 76 191-215 (1980).

33. Grant, W. F., Chromosome aberrations in plants as a monitoring
    system, Environ. Health Perspect. 27, 37-43 (1978).

34. Griffiths, A. J. F., Neurospora prototroph selection system for studying aneuploid production, Environ. Health Perspect. 31, 75-80 (1979).

35. Heddle, J. A. and K. Athanasiou, Mutation rate, genome size and their relation to the rec concept, Nature 258, 359-361 (1975).

36. Heinemann, B., Prophage induction in lysogenic bacteria as a method of detecting potential mutagenic, carcinogenic, car-cinostatic, and teratogenic agents, in: Chemical Mutagens: Principles and Methods for Their Detection, Vol. 1 (A. Hollaender, ed.), pp. 235-266, Plenum Press, New York (1971).

37. Hoffmann, G. R., Genetic effects of dimethyl sulfate, diethyl sulfate, and related compounds, Mutation Res. 75, 63-129 (1980).

38. Hollstein, M., J. McCann, F. A. Angelosanto, and W. W. Nichols, Short-term tests for carcinogens and mutagens, Mutation Res. 65, 133-226 (1979).

39. Hook, E. B., Human teratogenic and mutagenic markers in moni-toring about point sources of pollution, Environ. Res. 25, 178-203 (1981).

40. Jenssen, D. and C. Ramel, The micronucleus test as part of a short-term mutagenicity test program for the prediction of carcinogenicity evaluated by 143 agents tested, Mutation Res. 75, 191-202 (1980).

41. Johnson, F. M. and S. E. Lewis, Electrophoretically detected germinal mutations induced in the mouse by ethylnitrosourea, Proc. Natl. Acad. Sci. U.S.A. 78, 3138-3141 (1981).

42. Kada, T., K. Hirano, and Y. Shirasu, Screening of environmen-tal chemical mutagens by the rec-assay system with Bacillus subtilis, in: Chemical Mutagens: Principles and Methods for Their Detection, Vol. 6 (F. J. deSerres and A. Hollaender, eds.), pp. 149-173, Plenum Press, New York (1980).

43. Kapp, R. W., Jr., Detection of aneuploidy in human sperm, Environ. Health Perspect. 31, 27-31 (1979).

44. Kihlman, B. A., Root tips for studying the effects of chemi-cals on chromosomes, in: Chemical Mutagens: Principles and Methods for Their Detection, Vol. 2 (A. Hollaender, ed.), pp. 489-514, Plenum Press, New York (1971).

45. Kihlman, B. A., Root tips of Vicia faba for the study of the induction of chromosome aberrations, in: Handbook of Muta-genicity Test Procedures (B. J. Kilbey, M. Legator, W. Nichols, and C. Ramel, eds.), pp. 389-400, Elsevier/North Holland, Amsterdam (1977).

46. Kilbey, B. J., F. J. deSerres, and H. V. Malling, Identifica-tion of the genetic alteration at the molecular level of ultraviolet light-induced ad-3B mutants in Neurospora crassa, Mutation Res. 12, 47-56 (1971).

47. Lee, W. R., Dosimetry of alkylating agents, in: Banbury Report 1, Assessing Chemical Mutagens: The Risk to Humans (V. K. McElheny and S. Abrahamson, eds.), pp. 191-200, Cold Spring Harbor Laboratory (1979).

48. Lee, W. R., Dosimetry of chemical mutagens in eukaryote germ
     cells, in: Chemical Mutagens: Principles and Methods for
     Their Detection, Vol. 5 (A. Hollaender and F. J. deSerres,
     eds.), pp. 177-202, Plenum Press, New York (1978).
49. Ma, T.-H., Tradescantia micronucleus bioassay and pollen tube
     chromatid aberration test for in situ monitoring and mutagen
     screening, Environ. Health Perspect. 37, 85-90 (1981).
50. Malling, H. V., Dimethylnitrosamines: Formation of mutagenic
     compounds by interaction with mouse liver microsomes, Mutation
     Res. 13, 425-429 (1971).
51. McCann, J. and B. N. Ames, The Salmonella/microsome mutagen-
     icity test: Predictive value for animal carcinogenicity,
     in: Mutagenesis: Advances in Modern Toxicology, Vol. 5 (W.
     G. Flamm and M. A. Mehlman, eds.), pp. 87-108, Hemisphere
     Publishing Co. (Wiley), Washington, D.C. (1978).
52. McCann, J., E. Choi, E. Yamasaki, and B. N. Ames, Detection of
     carcinogens as mutagens in the Salmonella/microsome test:
     Assay of 300 chemicals, Proc. Natl. Acad. Sci. U.S.A. 72,
     5135-5139 (1975).
53. Moreau, P., A. Bailone, and R. Devoret, Prophage λ induction
     in Escherichia coli K12 envA uvrB: A highly sensitive test
     for potential carcinogens, Proc. Natl. Acad. Sci. U.S.A. 73,
     3700-3704 (1976).
54. Mortimer, R. K. and T. R. Manney, Mutation induction in yeast,
     in: Chemical Mutagens: Principles and Methods for Their
     Detection, Vol. 1 (A. Hollaender, ed.), pp. 289-310, Plenum
     Press, New York (1971).
55. Muller, H. J., Artificial transmutation of the gene, Science
     66, 84-87 (1927).
56. Oehlkers, F. Die Auslosung von Chromosomenmutationsen in der
     Meiosis durch Einwirkung von Chemikalien, Z. Ind. Abst. u.
     Vererbungsl. 81, 313-341 (1943).
57. T.-M. Ong, Use of the spot, plate and suspension test systems
     for the detection of the mutagenicity of environmental agents
     and chemical carcinogens in Neurospora crassa, Mutation Res.
     53, 297-308 (1978).
58. Parry, J. M., D. Sharp, and E. M. Parry, Detection of mitotic
     and meiotic aneuploidy in the yeast Saccharomyces cerevisiae,
     Environ. Health Perspect. 31, 97-111 (1979).
59. Parry, J. M. and F. K. Zimmermann, The detection of monosomic
     colonies produced by mitotic chromosome non-disjunction in the
     yeast Saccharomyces cerevisiae, Mutation Res. 36, 49-66
     (1976).
60. Perry, P. E. Chemical mutagens and sister-chromatid exchange,
     in: Chemical Mutagens: Principles and Methods for Their
     Detection, Vol. 6 (F. J. deSerres and A. Hollaender, eds.),
     pp. 1-39, Plenum Press, New York (1980).
61. Plewa, M. J. and E. D. Wagner, Germinal cell mutagenesis in
     specially designed maize genotypes, Environ. Health Perspect.
     37, 61 (1981).

62. Purchase, I. F. H., E. Longstaff, J. Ashby, J. A. Styles, D. Anderson, P. S. Lefevre and F. R. Westwood, An evaluation of 6 short-term tests for detecting organic chemical carcinogens, Brit. J. Cancer 37, 873-959 (1978).

63. Rapoport, I. A., Carbonyl compounds and the chemical mechanism of mutations, C. R. (Dokl.) Acad. Sci. U.R.S.S., N.S. 54, 65-67 (1946).

64. Rinkus, S. J. and M. S. Legator, Chemical characterization of 465 known or suspected carcinogens and their correlation with mutagenic activity in the Salmonella typhimurium system, Cancer Res. 39, 3289-3318 (1979).

65. Rosenkranz, H. S. and Z. Leifer, Determining the DNA-modifying activity of chemicals using DNA-polymerase-deficient Escherichia coli, in: Chemical Mutagens: Principles and Methods for Their Detection, Vol. 6 (F. J. deSerres and A. Hollaender, eds.), pp. 109-147, Plenum Press, New York (1980).

66. Russell, L. B., Numerical sex-chromosome anomalies in mammals: Their spontaneous occurrence and use in mutagenesis studies, in: Chemical Mutagens: Principles and Methods for Their Detection, Vol. 4 (A. Hollaender, ed.), pp. 55-91, Plenum Press, New York (1976).

67. Russell, W. L. and E. M. Kelly, Ineffectiveness of diethylnitrosamine in the induction of specific-locus mutations in mice, Genetics 91, s109-s110 (1979).

68. Russell, W. L., E. M. Kelly, P. R. Hunsicker, J. W. Bangham, S. C. Maddux, and E. L. Phipps, Specific-locus test shows ethylnitrosourea to be the most potent mutagen in the mouse, Proc. Natl. Acad. Sci. U.S.A. 76, 5818-5819 (1979).

69. Russell, L. B. and B. E. Matter, Whole-mammal mutagenicity tests: Evaluation of five methods, Mutation Res. 75, 279-302 (1980).

70. San, R. H. C. and H. F. Stich, DNA repair synthesis of cultured human cells as a rapid bioassay for chemical carcinogens, Int. J. Cancer 16, 284-291 (1975).

71. Schairer, L. A., J. Van't Hof, C. G. Hayes, R. M. Burton, and F. J. deSerres, Exploratory monitoring of air pollutants for mutagenicity activity with the Tradescantia stamen hair system, Environ. Health Perspect. 27, 51-60 (1978).

72. Selby, P. B. and P. R. Selby, Gamma-ray-induced dominant mutations that cause skeletal abnormalities in mice, Mutation Res. 43, 357-375 (1977).

73. Shelby, M. D. and I. F. H. Purchase, Assay systems and criteria for their comparisons, in: Evaluation of Short-Term Tests for Carcinogens: Report of the International Collaborative Program, (F. J. deSerres and J. Ashby, eds.), pp. 16-20, Elsevier/North Holland, Amsterdam (1981).

74. Skopek, T. R., H. L. Liber, D. A. Kaden, and W. G. Thilly, Relative sensitivities of forward and reverse mutation assays in Salmonella typhimurium, Proc. Natl. Acad. Sci. U.S.A. 75, 4465-4469 (1978).

75. Stadler, L. R., Genetic effects of X-rays in maize, Proc. Natl. Acad. Sci. U.S.A. 14, 69-75 (1928).

76. Straus, D. S., Somatic mutation, cellular differentiation, and cancer causation, J. Natl. Cancer Inst. 67, 233-241 (1981).

77. Sutton, H. E., The impact of induced mutations on human populations, Mutation Res. 33, 17-24 (1975).

78. Swift, M. and C. Chase, Cancer in families with xeroderma pigmentosum, J. Natl. Cancer Inst. 62, 1415-1421 (1979).

79. Swift, M., L. Sholman, M. Perry, and C. Chase, Malignant neoplasms in the families of patients with ataxia-telangiectasia, Cancer Res. 36, 209-215 (1976).

80. Thilly, W. G., J. G. DeLuca, E. E. Furth, H. Hoppe IV, D. A. Kaden, J. J. Krolewski, H. L. Liber, T. R. Skopek, S. A. Slapikoff, R. J. Tizard, and B. W. Penman, Gene-locus mutation assays in diploid human lymphoblast lines, in: Chemical Mutagens: Principles and Methods for Their Detection, Vol. 6 (F. J. deSerres and A. Hollaender, eds.), pp. 331-364, Plenum Press, New York (1980).

81. Topham, J. C., Do induced sperm-head abnormalities in mice specifically identify mammalian mutagens rather than carcinogens?, Mutation Res. 74, 379-387 (1980).

82. Underbrink, A. G., L. A. Schairer, and A. H. Sparrow, Tradescantia stamen hairs: A radiobiological test system applicable to chemical mutagenesis, in: Chemical Mutagens: Principles and Methods for Their Detection, Vol. 3 (A. Hollaender, ed.), pp. 171-207, Plenum Press, New York (1973).

83. Vogel, E. and F. H. Sobels, The function of Drosophila in genetic toxicology testing, in: Chemical Mutagens: Principles and Methods for Their Detection, Vol. 4 (A. Hollaender, ed.), pp. 93-142, Plenum Press, New York (1976).

84. Williams, G. M., Detection of chemical carcinogens by unscheduled DNA synthesis in rat liver primary cell cultures, Cancer Res. 37, 1845-1851 (1977).

85. Williams, G. M., The detection of chemical mutagens/carcinogens by DNA repair and mutagenesis in liver cultures, in: Chemical Mutagens: Principles and Methods for Their Detection, Vol. 6 (F. J. deSerres and A. Hollaender, eds.), pp. 61-79, Plenum Press, New York (1980).

86. Wolff, S., Sister chromatid exchange, Ann. Rev. Genet. 11, 183-201 (1977).

87. Würgler, F. E., F. H. Sobels, and E. Vogel, Drosophila as assay system for detecting genetic changes, in: Handbook of Mutagenicity Test Procedures (B. J. Kilbey, M. Legator, W. Nichols, and C. Ramel, eds.), pp. 335-373, Elsevier/North Holland, Amsterdam (1977).

88. Wyrobek, A. J. and W. R. Bruce, The induction of sperm-shape abnormalities in mice and humans, in: Chemical Mutagens: Principles and Methods for Their Detection, Vol. 5 (A. Hollaender and F. J. deSerres, eds.), pp. 257-285, Plenum Press, New York (1978).

89. Yamasaki, E. and B. N. Ames, Concentration of mutagens from urine by absorption with the nonpolar resin XAD-2: Cigarette smokers have mutagenic urine, Proc. Natl. Acad. Sci. U.S.A. 74, 3555-3559 (1977).

90. Zimmermann, F. K., A yeast strain for visual screening for the two reciprocal products of mitotic crossing over, Mutation Res. 21, 263-269 (1973).

91. Zimmermann, F. K., Procedures used in the induction of mitotic recombination and mutation in the yeast Saccharomyces cerevisiae, Mutation Res. 31, 71-86 (1975).

92. Zimmermann, F. K., R. Kern, and H. Rasenberger, A yeast strain for simultaneous detection of induced mitotic crossing over, mitotic gene conversion and reverse mutation, Mutation Res. 28, 381-388 (1975).

INTRODUCTION TO AN INTERNATIONAL SYMPOSIUM ON GENETIC TOXICOLOGY -

AN AGRICULTURAL PERSPECTIVE

Gerald G. Still

Science and Education
U. S. Department of Agriculture
Beltsville, MD 20705

Man and his agriculture have moved through 12,000 years of
history together. Today most people, with their new found freedom
from the soil, have forgotten the basic relationship which binds us
-- a relationship that allows freedom but not independence. Food
is the only indispensable product that man produces, and it makes
us totally dependent on the land and our farmers.

Man's success in his effort to provide food and fiber of
acceptable quality has been achieved through a complete system of
interdependent parts including fertilizers, high yielding varieties, cropping systems, irrigation, mechanization, and agricultural
chemicals. One measure of this success can be seen in the yield of
corn (maize) in the USA. Data show a relatively constant yield per
acre from 1880 to 1940; however, from 1940 to present there has
been a continued, almost explosive, increase in productivity in
corn in this country. From 1880 to 1940 the average yields were 20
to 30 Bu/A; the average corn yield for 1979 was 108 Bu/A. The
average rate of corn yield increase, averaged for approximately 8
million acres from 1950 through 1979, was 2.33 Bu/A/year, and the
trend line is continuing upward. In fact, I was talking with a
Nebraska corn farmer the other day, and he told me that in the
1920s and 30s their farm's corn yields were 20 to 25 Bu/A. This
year (1981) with irrigation, using modern technology and management, the same farm yielded 150 Bu/A.

The list of such successes is very long. Hundreds of examples
of the breakthroughs in fertilizers, high-yielding varieties, soil
management systems, irrigation methods, mechanization, and agricultural chemicals could be cited. The USDA Agricultural Research
Service (Federal research), the Cooperative State Research Service

(State experiment stations), and the private research sector are
responsible for these successes. Without any one of these three
institutions, the others would not have been able to deliver the
technology and material that have resulted in these unprecedented
agricultural advances.

Another measure of U. S. agricultural success is in the number
of persons who receive their sustenance from a single farm
worker. In 1820, one American farmer supplied food, feed, and
fiber to support 3.8 fellow citizens. In 1940, one farmer
supported 10.3 people. By 1978, one farmer supported 46.5
nonagricultural Americans. This has, however, resulted in a lack
of awareness and understanding of the problems associated with food
and fiber production by a large segment of the population.

There is a lack of the public's appreciation for the cost-
benefit relationships between application of technology, increasing
productivity, low cost food and fiber, food safety, and environmental quality. The appearance of even one apple maggot in a
polyethelene pack of apples, will induce cries of anger at the
local grocery store. In terms of productivity, we are dealing not
only with quantity but also in quality and safety.

When we consider the vast growth in productivity in American
agriculture, we are really only addressing the last 40 years -- an
extremely short period of time within the span of human
agricultural endeavor. As we consider the question of genetic
toxicology in relation to the agricultural ecosystem and
agriculture's products, it is well to keep in mind other rapid
changes. We must also consider the change in the demands of the
consuming public; change in the assessment of levels of food
quality and safety; the requirements to meet market demands both
from the standpoint of the farmer, an independent entrepreneur, and
from his clients -- the agribusiness industry, the food industry,
the people of this country, and indeed, an ever-growing segment of
the world population.

Demands placed on the quality of the finished product by the
consumer today are far greater than those of 40 years ago. These
demands undoubtedly have resulted in reduced hazards from naturally
occurring contaminants such as aflatoxin, plant and insect debris,
and so on. But questions are now being raised about possible residues from other sources in the agricultural production process.
Within the scope of genetic toxicants, the following are all potentials for consideration: fertilizers, crop protectants and regulators, insecticides, nematocides, herbicides, flowering stimulators,
abscission stimulators, materials to induce resistance to plant
stress, insect growth regulators, and natural biological resistance
factors which are bred into plants to help them withstand pathogens
and insects. These important production tools have been under

development and application in American agriculture at an
increasing rate over the last 30 years. However, this activity has
not been pursued in a vacuum, but rather has had increasing scrutiny and regulation. The Food and Drug Administration and the
Environmental Protection Agency (which took over part of this responsibility from the USDA) have responsibility in this area. Each
of these institutions has specific, relevant, and statutory authorities. These institutions are represented in this symposium, and
there are many here who are far more able to discuss their history
and present roles than I.

From the agricultural perspective, however, we must at all
times carefully assess and test the balance between the various
factors of the equation--increased productivity, the economics of
that productivity, the safety of the technology on the environment,
on workers, and on the consumers of the products. This balancing
process is evolving and we are seeking an equilibrium. There have
been and there will continue to be differences of opinion as to
where the balance between the extremes of opinions should be. It
is incumbent upon the scientific community and those institutions
that deal with social policy making to continue this balancing
process. Our goal must be to sustain or increase productivity in
concert with society's demands to meet its perceived value of the
various components of the equation.

Let's look at one class of agricultural chemicals where such
balance appears to be evolving. Insecticides have had a positive
impact upon productivity. Until the last few years, many of those
materials were highly toxic, had a broad spectrum of biological
activity, and had long persistance in the environment. The new
materials that have been and are being produced and considered for
production are materials that are site-specific, have short half-
lives, and whose environmental degradation products are of low
toxicity.

I personally worked on such a material a number of years
ago. It was a chitin inhibitor which is labeled for use as an
insecticide. (Chitin is part of certain insects' hard outer
covering.) The material was specifically chemically optimized and
designed, first, to inhibit the biosynthesis of chitin; second, to
have a long environmental half-life on plant leaves; third, to have
a very short half-life in soils; and fourth, to have a very low
mammalian toxicity. When comparing the agricultural or environmental toxicology of this compound with the first and second generation of insecticides, we see that we have moved a great distance
toward insecticides that better meet the criteria for the cost-
benefit relationship. With appropriate market incentives, the
trend in agricultural chemicals will be more and more in favor of
these types of materials. This will move agriculture away from the
use of the older materials which, in part, have been responsible

for the explosive increase in productivity in the last 30 years,
but by which has resulted an environmental cost that was considered
unacceptable by segments of our society.

One of the success stories in agricultural productivity has
been the development of high-yielding varieties. In most cases,
these varieties possess natural resistance to pathogens and other
threats. The question has been raised concerning the chemical
toxicity of these naturally occurring plant protection materials.

Scientists speculate that there is widespread occurrence of
natural chemical toxins in plant materials. In fact, there are
many who speculate that these natural chemical toxins placed a
severe restriction on primitive man's use of vegetable foods. They
regard the discovery of fire for cooking as a major evolutionary
step that paved the way for both the agricultural revolution and
the population explosion. Artifacts of tools for hunting date back
over 3.5 million years. There is no widespread evidence of cooking
until about 40,000 years ago, and then these artifacts appear on
the scene in profusion. Cooking destroys vegetable toxins, helping
humans to thrive in a hostile environment. Clearly, natural chemical toxins have been a major tool in increasing plant productivity. As the cost-benefit relationships are weighed, it is also
necessary to realize that we have and will continue to develop
detoxification mechanisms.

Let me further illustrate this point. It has been claimed
that one serving of turnips naturally contains 100 times as much
malignant goiterogenic activity as one serving of cranberries contaminated with aminotriazole. This natural toxin was isolated in
pure form, injected at high doses into experimental animals, and
was shown to cause cancer. However, when experimental animals were
fed whole turnips, no cancer was induced. Detoxification or lack
of bioavailability, or both, are responsible for this phenomenon.
Herein lies the essence of the argument. Synthetically or
naturally synthesized toxins used in the agro-ecosystem are environmentally degraded or detoxified. If they are not, institutional
restrictions will bar their entry into the food production system.

It is therefore part of this agricultural perspective that
when we assess genetic toxicology we recognize that by practice--
such as cooking--or by the action of the human biological system,
the capability to overcome these toxic challenges is enormous.
Biological detoxification capacity will be discussed in some detail
in other presentations before this symposium.

There are a number of pests that as part of their natural
foraging habits or their genesis in plant tissues or in the soil,
open portals for infection or carry infection themselves. A prime
example of this is the bacterium, _Aspergillus flavis_, which pro-

duces the mycotoxin called aflatoxin, a confirmed potent animal
carcinogen. Aflatoxin occurs in pest infested food and feed crops
in the field. It subsequently enters into the human food chain
directly (for example, in nuts) or indirectly through animal feed
and into milk and eggs for human consumption.

Such a situation calls for determining which pest control
tools should be used, and assessing the risk of using them versus
the risk of not using them in light of the ultimate goal—safe
food. This situation actually occurred in 1979 in Arizona. A pest
infestation in cotton—most importantly of pink·boll worm—resulted
in aflatoxin contamination of cottonseed meal fed to milk cows, and
thus in contamination of milk. Aflatoxin levels were shown to rise
sharply in fields where pink boll worm infestation levels exceeded
1 to 2 percent in July and August. Arizona, like most Cotton Belt
States, has ongoing integrated pest management programs for cotton
insect control. But in this emergency situation, the decision had
to be made to adjust the integrated pest management program and use
chemical pesticides for control. The decisive factor was that with
the previous program, it was the practice to allow a 10 to 15 percent infestation of pink boll worms before applying chemical pest
control measures. It therefore became obvious that increased chemical control of the pest was required to keep the infestation level
at or below 1 to 2 percent, thereby assuring the safety and whole-
someness of the animal feed and ultimately the food for human
consumption.

This leads me to the next point. We must control disease and
insect depredations not only so that food is safe and wholesome,
but also because such damage defeats the productivity gains that
would otherwise be possible. Dr. Warren C. Shaw, USDA, has pointed
out that, "Pests cause losses in agricultural production of crops,
livestock, forest, and aquatic resources estimated at 30 percent of
their sale value."

It is incongruous to discuss and move on research to enhance
future productivity without simultaneously addressing these most
serious and massive deterrents to productivity. What value has
increased photosynthetic efficiency if the major site of photosyn-
thesis—the leaves—is damaged by disease or insects? What value
is nitrogen fixation transferred to nonleguminous plants, or the
development of drought resistance, if the plant roots are not protected against nematodes, soil insects, and pathogens? Genetically
diverse pest resistance that is effective during the fruiting stage
of a plant is never realized when the seed or seedlings are
destroyed or damaged by soil-borne pests. Agricultural scientists
have the competence to successfully address this massive program,
but more change is necessary in the societal attitudes that currently constrain the full use of our plant protection technology.
We must strive to achieve a balance, as I stressed earlier, between
productivity goals and society's demands and perceptions.

The impact of societal attitudes on genetic toxicology is
highly important. It is a consideration that has been and will
continue to be a component in the decision making process. Technological advances and their benefits--increased productivity--have
and must continue to be balanced in the cost-benefit relationship. The cost must include not only the economic considerations
but also the toxicological considerations; negative effects on
nontarget organisms; residues of the original material or toxic
byproducts in the food chain; the problem of acute effects and
chronic genetic effects; the epidemiology and genotoxicity of these
materials at long-term, low-level exposure to people and the environment. All of these considerations must have high priority,
and they must be in balance with the rest of the social economic
equation.

From the agricultural perspective, we must recognize where we
were, where we are, and what the demands upon this system will be
in the future. All indicators point to and indeed demand that we
not only sustain our agricultural productivity, but increase it to
meet increasing world needs. In order to meet that challenge,
continual vigilance and continued rational balancing will be necessary in our approach to the decision making process, so that the
equilibrium we seek will be gained in a timely and reasonable
fashion.

DISCUSSION

Q. I was interested in your thesis that men may be able to develop
   detoxification mechanisms that will lessen the hazards of natural or man-made toxins.

A. STILL: As described in the text of this speech, man has
   historically developed a number of processes that resulted in
   detoxification of natural plant toxins. For example, heating
   (cooking) or indeed the addition of various condiments such as
   shift in pH using vinegar. As far as alterations in man's
   biological detoxification processes, this is, of course, a
   scenario which I suspect is not realistic to consider under
   these conditions. There is no question that mammalian systems
   have many protective mechanisms, such as the example used in
   the speech with turnips.

Q. You gave an estimate that 30 percent of the dollar value of our
   crops is lost to pests. How has this fraction changed with
   time from 1900 to present?

A. STILL: I do not have the literature base with me to address
   this in actual figures; however, it is my assumption that the
   percentage was much greater in 1900. With plant protection

during the production phase of agriculture, this has decreased
steadily since 1940 with a simultaneous increase in quality of
the products. An example would be the quality of soft fruit in
the markets available prior to 1940 and at present.

Q. SUGIMURA: What were the active components responsible for the
goiterogenic activity found in turnips?

A. STILL: There are two main components, the strongest being 5-
vinyl-2-thioloxazolidone. The predominant member of the second
weak group is methylsulfonylpropyl-isothiocyanate. For more
detailed information see the National Academy of Science publication "Toxicants Occuring in Foods", first edition, 1966.

HEALTH RISKS AND EXPOSURE

William M. Upholt

525 East Indian Spring Drive
Silver Spring, Maryland 20901

It is somewhat of a truism to say that without exposure no
toxic chemical can cause adverse health effects. Over four hundred
years ago, Paracelsus(1) said words to the effect that "dosage
alone determines toxicity." Thus, no matter how toxic a chemical
may be, its potential risk to humans (or to the environment) is
controlled by potential exposure. The confidence in the fact that
it is possible to use a substance while controlling exposure to it
has led to the claim that even the most toxic substance can be used
safely. Our problem, then, in discussing "Health Risks and
Exposure" is one of determining how much exposure to a particular
substance can be tolerated and how can exposure be restricted to
that level or below.

The first question, then, is what level of exposure can be
tolerated? This, of course, depends upon two major factors--what
level of risk of adverse health effects is acceptable and what
level of exposure assures that that level of risk will not be
exceeded.

The determination of what level of risk is acceptable must be
a judgemental one. Since, in the absence of a demonstrated
population threshold, a zero risk is obtainable only by eliminating
all possibility of exposure, the question can be restated as how
much risk can be tolerated in order to enjoy the benefits of the
use of the substance in question. This, in turn, will depend upon
how much it costs (in both direct and indirect costs) to reduce
that risk further. Since the indirect costs (which may include
health, esthetic, and others as well as economic costs) may be very
difficult to identify as well as to quantify, and since they often
accrue to individuals who receive no apparent benefit from the use

of the substance, this question often becomes very complex and must
be asked in the framework of social acceptability or governmental
regulations.

In order to make a rational decision as to what level of risk
is acceptable, some information is needed as to the level of risk
that is associated with a given level of exposure. Thus, the
determination of the relationship between level of exposure and
risk of adverse effect is critical to rational decision-making.
Furthermore, techniques of measuring those levels of exposure as
well as methods of controlling levels of exposure are important to
implementation of such decisions.

The relationship between the level of exposure and risk of
adverse effect in humans has commonly been estimated by the use of
experimental animals to which measured dosages of the toxic
substance are administered. The nature of the adverse effects can
thus be determined as well as the proportion of those exposed at a
given dosage which show an adverse effect within a stated time
period. The route of exposure, the vehicle (or carrier) of the
toxicant, the age, sex, and condition of the animal, the length of
exposure, the delay after exposure (if any), and the methods used
for detecting adverse effects are all important to describing the
relationship. Normally, there should be control animals, some of
which should receive none of the toxicant.

There are numerous ways of describing the relationship of
effects to dosage as revealed by such tests, but perhaps the most
common is to express the results in a graph with the dosage (or
some function of it) on the abscissa and the number of animals
showing the identified effect on the ordinate (often in terms of
percentage test animals, sometimes in probability units or
probits). The resulting curve is then used to estimate the degree
of risk (fraction of population expected to show the effect) at any
particular dosage under the experimental conditions.

The complications involved in converting such an estimate of
risk to animals under experimental conditions into an estimate of
risk to humans under usual conditions of exposure are much too
complex to even describe in this paper. Rather, I will concentrate
on some of the problems involved in attempting to extrapolate from
the experimental dosages (always relatively high) to the dosages
associated with the risks that might be considered as acceptable to
humans. The most important aspect of this is that it most commonly
involves extrapolation to dosages considerably lower than those
that produced the adverse effect experimentally.

This is not always true, however, particularly if there are
available good epidemiologic data from human exposure to the
toxicant, whether due to occupation, accident, controlled tests, or

simply natural exposure. For example, such data has shown that
exposure to fluorides, comparable to over one part per million in
drinking water, produces fluorosis, or mottled enamel of the
teeth. It has also shown that significantly less than the
equivalent of one part per million results in excessive dental
caries. Thus, there is good data to justify a decision to allow
exposure to fluorides to a level equivalent to one part per million
in drinking water.

Of course, in addition to the fact that the apparently
acceptable risk level for fluorides is high enough to be within the
experimental range, this decision is aided by the fact that the
dosage/adverse response curve for fluorides reached a minimum
response at a dosage level below which adverse effects increased
instead of continuing to decrease. Similarly shaped curves may
also occur with vitamins and other substances that are essential at
low dosages and toxic at higher dosages. (Whether this represents
a true toxicity threshold or alternatively the intersection of two
curves describing different effects of fluorides is unimportant to
this discussion.)

Another problem of continuing debate among toxicologists is
whether or not the dose/response curve ever reaches a dosage (other
than zero) so low that no adverse effect can be expected. This is
commonly believed to be true for many types of toxic effects even
though the exact dosage or threshold which is the maximum at which
no adverse effect occurs can not be determined accurately with the
relatively small numbers of experimental animals tested at each
dosage. If such a point were accurately determined it would be a
great temptation to tell the regulators that zero risk is
attainable by keeping exposure below that threshold and thus any
higher level of exposure and of risk has to be avoided or justified
by strong evidence of resultant benefits.

This assumption has been the basis of many regulatory
decisions in the past in spite of the fact that the "no-adverse-
effect" dosage cannot be determined accurately with small numbers
of animals. To compensate for this fact, a "safety factor" has
commonly been suggested. In fact, another safety factor has
usually been required to compensate for the unknown difference in
susceptibility between humans and the experimental species.

The lack of either adequate experimental evidence as to the
exact "no-adverse-effect" level or accepted theoretical models to
show exactly at what dosage this point should occur has prompted
the use of a number of judgemental terms to justify action in the
face of such uncertainty. "Without appreciable risk," "practical
certainty," and "negligible" are terms that have been used to
encourage regulatory agencies to set "acceptable risks" based upon
the assumption of a true but unproven "no-adverse-effect" level and

to call them "safe" levels. No doubt such judgemental advice from scientists and other experts has been useful to regulatory agencies, but it has also encouraged them to avoid adequate consideration of costs in making their decisions.

With the growing concern of scientists and the public with potentially carcinogenic chemicals, a theory has been advocated that carcinogenesis (and presumably mutagenesis and teratogenesis) are self-supporting processes such that once the process has been initiated (possibly by a single molecule) it progresses to its full expression as an adverse effect without the need for additional stimulation by the chemical agent. On this basis, it was claimed that there is no true "no-adverse-effect" level of exposure short of zero exposure. Thus, they rejected the judgemental terms described above to suggest zero risk and recommended instead the use of the Delaney clause. In an effort to solve this problem experimentally, at least one study has exposed enough experimental animals to low enough dosages of a known carcinogen (in the experimental species used) to establish the point at which only one percent of the exposed animals would show the induced cancer (2). It was hoped that this would throw light on the shape of the dosage/response curve at these very low dosages. Apparently, it has not settled the question but (among other things) has stimulated increased interest in a different method of estimating risk; i.e., estimating the time to tumor (or death from cancer) as a function of dosage.

It appears that there is still no single widely acceptable, mathematical model for estimating risk of adverse effect at a series of very low levels that would permit a balancing of decreased risk (achieved by lowering exposure) against increased societal costs. Nevertheless, there is a growing body of qualitative evidence that might permit a useful description of relative potency between various toxicants and even provide some suggestion of the potential increase in risk resulting from allowing a small increment in exposure. Certainly it is also possible to describe the adverse effects that may be expected as a result of very low exposures and the sequelae if exposure is increased or prolonged. Such descriptive and qualitative data should be of great value to a regulatory agency that wants to make modern chemicals available for reasonable uses without increasing too greatly the risk of adverse effects. If this is true, then it is clearly desirable to improve methods of measuring exposure and preventing unnecessary exposure.

Efforts to measure exposure of humans to a variety of toxic chemicals must take into consideration the route of exposure and their rates of absorption as well as the progress of the toxicant from the entry portal to the target tissue and the metabolic changes en route. Early efforts in occupational health put

considerable emphasis on inhalation exposure and resulted in
standards based largely on air concentration in the work place.
Factors such as particle size and its relationship both to
inhalation and to retention in the lungs were important in
establishing acceptable air concentrations. Dermal exposure was of
primary interest in those toxicants that had a direct effect upon
the skin and those few that rapidly penetrated the skin. Oral
exposure was of concern both through accidental (or purposeful)
swallowing of a toxicant and from the standpoint of food additives
and contaminants. Injection has never been of great concern except
in terms of drugs, whether taken purposely or by mistake.

There are problems with measuring exposure by each of these
routes. For each case the direct measure at the portal may be most
useful both for determining the relative exposure by each route and
also for measuring the effectiveness of preventive measures. On
the other hand, the determination of the total exposure can often
be done more accurately by measures such as determining the blood
level or urinary excretion at various times after exposure. For
some toxicants, measure of storage in fat or other tissues by
biopsy may be useful (though somewhat drastic) but may not reflect
the true level of exposure of the susceptible tissue at any given
point in time.

All of these measurement techniques are difficult to apply to
large populations. To do that requires some sort of restricted
sampling design that accounts for the many individual variations in
exposure in any large population. Once effective measurement
techniques have been established, they can also be used to estimate
effectiveness of exposure restriction efforts by comparing two or
more populations appropriately.

Exposure through the environment (air, water, soil, and food
chain) is always difficult to measure but it could be estimated by
methods designed to measure total exposure and then subtracting
therefrom any known direct exposure. Effects on other organisms in
the environment are not covered in this paper.

Finally, if the judgement of what is an acceptable level of
risk is to be based upon a consideration of one or more possible
regulatory alternatives, then it is necessary to devise methods of
reducing exposures significantly without increasing societal costs
too much. For this purpose, it is desirable to know which portals
of entry are most important in the case of a given toxicant. Then
the alternatives can be selected with these portals in mind.
Formulation and method of application, handling, or use can affect
particle size and so they offer approaches to reduce, selectively,
exposure by respiratory or dermal routes. Use of solvents in
formulations can affect rate of penetration through the skin.
Similarly, protective devices should be designed with the route of

principal exposure in mind. Even prohibition of certain uses of
chemical may be a selective method of reducing exposure. Of
course, the effectiveness of any technique designed to reduce
exposure should be assessed by measuring the actual exposure
following such techniques and comparing that with the level found
without using the technique. In this way, the decision-makers can
be given reasonable descriptions not only of the hazards but also
of the levels of risk associated with various alternative
regulatory plans. Perhaps of equal importance would be the
estimate of the increment in exposure and thus of the increment of
risk between various potential regulatory alternatives.

In the final analysis, the success or failure of any effort to
assure that risk of adverse effect does not exceed a judgementally
determined "acceptable risk," must involve careful epidemiologic
studies of populations at risk both with and without the
restrictive measures. This can be very difficult and expensive,
especially if the adverse effect is long delayed in becoming
manifest or if the effect is common in populations that are not
exposed to the substance in question. Thus, in many cases, it may
be more satisfactory to assess the sucess or failure of a hazard
control program by means of measuring exposure rather than the
effects.

In conclusion, it is clear that estimation and restriction of
exposure to a toxic substance may be just as important as
toxicological assessment of hazard. Moreover, it may be fraught
with as many technological problems as the toxicological
assessment. Consequently, I would suggest that regulatory
decision-makers should demand as good evidence of competency and
quality in the exposure information they consider as they now
demand in toxicological information. If I may be permitted to
paraphrase Paracelsus, I would say that to the extent exposure
controls dosage, "exposure alone determines toxicity."

REFERENCES

1. Paracelsus' Drey Bücher, Cologne, 1564, as quoted (and
    translated) by Wayland J. Hayes, Jr. in Toxicology of
    Pesticides 1975. Williams & Wilkins, Baltimore.
2. In 1971, the Food and Drug Administration and the
    Environmental Protection Agency of the U.S. Government
    established a National Center for Toxicologic Research at
    Jefferson, Arkansas, specifically to explore the effects of
    known carcinogens at the very low levels of exposure needed to
    produce tumors in one percent of exposed animals and to
    explore other aspects of toxicology of especial importance to
    regulatory agencies. It required nearly a decade and many
    thousands of experimental mice to complete the "ED01"
    experiment. A number of conferences have been conducted

during 1979 to 1981, by various scientific groups to discuss
the results of this massive experiment.

DISCUSSION

Q.   EL-SEBAE: I still recall your call for global guidelines for
the protection of the environment by standardization of
toxicological requirements for registration and handling of
pesticides. This started more than five years ago. Is there
any progress along this line through UN agencies such as
UNESCO, MAB or UNEP agencies?

A.   UPHOLT: I believe the need for a "global strategy" to guide
pest control and the use of pesticides is as great today as it
was in 1976 when I suggested it through the Man and the
Biosphere (MAB) Program of UNESCO. Development of such a
strategy would require full cooperation of both the World
Health Organization and the Food and Agricultural Organization
as well as the United Nations Environmental Program. The WHO
and FAO felt (I believe) that their program of seeking
harmonization of requirements for pesticide registration
demanded a higher priority for their limited resources than
did the proposed "global strategy." The Man and the Biosphere
Program is co-sponsoring a group of studies on how various
countries throughout the world perceive the risks associated
with pests as well as pesticides. These studies in some 12 or
more countries, mostly in the Southern hemisphere, may form a
good basis for a "global strategy" should the latter be
undertaken sometime in the future.

Q.   What are the background exposures or other sources of cancer?

A.   UPHOLT: In most cases people will be exposed to numerous
carcinogens. In fact most of us are probably exposed to
enough carcinogens that we will eventually succumb to cancer
if we do not die of something else sooner. Given this
situation, I believe we should simply measure the incremental
exposure and thus estimate the incremental risk of cancer.
Such incremental risks may well avoid the problems of
extrapolating to very low levels of exposure and thus should
be more accurate than estimates that assume the chemical in
question to be the only carcinogen involved.

Q.   ZIMMERMAN: A related problem is the determination of risk of
a particular single compound when, in fact, we are trying to
assess the total risk to an individual, which is perhaps the
sum of hundreds of these single compounds. Thus, we cannot
consider a safe or acceptable level of one substance, without
considering all of the other agents which are within our

control and for which we are trying to estimate risk. The incremental risk increase of a single compound may indeed be small in comparison with the risk due to those agents beyond our control, but the sum of risks, plus any synergistic interactions may be far from negligible. How would you deal with these difficulties?

A.   UPHOLT: It is true that the contribution of one single compound to the total risk to an individual is apt to be quite small. By the same token the benefit in terms of reducing risk to the individual (or to a population for that matter) or regulating that single compound is equally small and may not justify the sacrifice of the use of that single compound. Nevertheless each chemical must be considered by itself unless several compounds are sufficiently similar to be considered together. The fact is that no regulation or combination of regulations (including "banning" of some chemicals) can assure safety in any absolute sense. In the real world we must consider each significant chemical or similar group of chemicals one at a time to decide whether a proposed regulation will increase safety sufficiently to justify taking the regulatory action. In summation, such regulatory actions may indeed significantly reduce total risk (though not eliminate it).

Q.   MENDELSOHN: Can you comment about another aspect of your incremental approach? I refer to the effect of background cancer rates. Cancer deaths are common. Incremental exposure to carcinogens will give incremental cancer deaths. But no one knows which death is incremental; hence a regulated increment will lead to the risk of someone being responsible for all cancers of a given type--as being pressed today by the U.S. Congress.

A.   UPHOLT: I can see no rationale for considering a person (or corporation) responsible for specific cases of cancer unless the cancer is of a rare type associated very clearly with a specific carcinogen. Even in such cases the causal relationship can be demonstrated only with a detectible increase in incidence associated with exposure to the chemical in question. In this case, it is the increment in cases that permits the association between the chemical and the cancer cases.

My opinion is that no person (or corporation) should be held liable for any cancer caused by the use of a chemical carcinogen if that use has been considered by the appropriate regulatory agency and the risks of cancer considered justified by the resultant societal benefit. The exception would be if gross negligence was involved in the use. Of course, the regulatory decision might be challenged for sufficient reason.

APPROACHES TO THE GENETIC SAFETY EVALUTION OF AGRICULTURAL

CHEMICALS

Verne A. Ray

Medical Research Laboratories
Pfizer, Inc.
Groton, Connecticut 06340

INTRODUCTION

The utility of information acquired from the application of genetic tests to the safety evaluation of agricultural chemicals such as animal drugs or pesticides, involves the same considerations that are used for other environmental substances. Data from a battery of short-term tests composed primarily of in vitro models are used to indicate the potential for certain types of irreversible toxicity. Reproducibly positive results in a suitably selected group of assays, properly performed, indicates the compound under study is a potential mutagen and/or a potential carcinogen. Further studies in mammals are required to determine if this potential is expressed as heritable genetic change or as carcinogenicity. It must be stressed that meaningful evaluations are dependent on a group of assays in a screening phase because no single assay can perform the safety evaluation function adequately. Both gene mutation and chromosomal-level effects must be evaluated. Further, there is a need for comparative test information which gives perspective to any single test result and provides the genetic toxicologist the means to evaluate the toxic potential of the chemical. Also, the absence of an extensive data base across the spectrum of chemical classes makes a degree of redundancy in assay application necessary.

Test Battery Selection

The selection of a suitable battery of assays has been and continues to be under study by several national and international groups. A battery which has been identified by the DHSS Committee on Mutagenicity of Chemicals in Food Consumer Products and the

45

Environment (U. K.) (1981) for screening chemicals for mutagenic properties has four components.

1. "A test designed to demonstrate the induction of point mutations in established bacterial test systems such as Salmonella typhimurium, Escherichia coli or Bacillus subtilis. The tests should be conducted with and without the use of appropriate metabolic activation systems.

2. A test designed to demonstrate the production of chromosome damage in appropriate mammalian cells grown in vitro with and without the use of appropriate metabolic activation systems.

3. The induction of mutations in mammalian cells grown in vitro.

                              or

    Tests designed to induce recessive lethals in Drosophila.

4. A test designed to demonstrate the induction of chromosomal damage in the intact animal using either the micronucleus test or, preferably, the metaphase analysis of bone marrow or other proliferative cells.

                              or

    The induction of germ cell damage as demonstrated by the dominant-lethal test in the rat or mouse."

It was the opinion of the committee that the recommended basic package screening procedure should detect, if fully and properly exploited, the great majority of the potential mutagens among the chemicals entering the human environment. Any further improvement at the screening level was seen as entailing an expenditure of effort out of all proportion to the value of the additional information that might be gained.

The Food Safety Council Scientific Committee (1980) devised a system for approaching the estimation of risk offered by the ingestion of any component of food. The system is applicable to normal ingredients, an additive, an environmental contaminant, a natural toxicant, a pesticide, a packaging constituent which transfers to food or any other substance which is likely to be found in food. The system consists of a series of assessments including genetic toxicology. The genetic assessment is approached following definition of test material, exposure and acute toxicity. A safety decision tree positions genetic toxicology and metabolism studies as concurrently performed parts of the decision network. The committee felt that the emphasis given to these two components "not only reflects recent progress in methodology and understanding, but also makes possible a more systematic and reassuring way of making safety decisions without lifetime feeding." They also felt that "a safety decision system that does not offer this possibility ignores one of the major problems of the day."

The purposes of the Genetic Toxicology Assessment are:

(1)   To provide a qualitative indication of presence or absence of mutagenic or potential carcinogenic activity.

(2)   If the battery of tests indicates mutagenic activity, to determine the nature of genetic changes.

(3)   To provide guidance in risk assessment and quantitation of human risk.

(4)   To provide test procedures in support of metabolism studies for detecting and characterizing biologically active metabolites and tracing their separation and purification.

There are six assays identified to be used in the primary genetic assessment.

1.   Assay for induction of point mutations in microbial cell systems incorporating in vitro activating systems.

2.   Assay for induction of point mutations in cultured mammalian cells incorporating a mammalian activating system.

3.   Assay for induction of chromosomal changes in vitro in cultured mammalian cells.

4.   Tests for induction of chromosomal changes in vivo by cytogenetic analysis of metaphase figures or use of the micronucleus test.

5.   Testing of body fluids of treated mammals using microbial indicator systems.

6.   Assay for cell transformation using appropriate in vitro cultured mammalian or human cell lines.

These two batteries, one by the DHSS and the other by the Food Safety Council Scientific Committee are listed to emphasize the

growing consensus among genetic toxicologists who have to make
decisions on the selection of tests for safety evaluation
purposes. Efforts of other groups such as the EPA, Gene-Tox
Scientific Assessment Panel (49) could be listed and it is
recognized that different approaches to screening can be applied
depending upon the needs addressed and number of substances to be
evaluated. Under some circumstances a tier or sequential approach
would be advocated. However, even under these circumstances, assay
selection is focusing on a few assays which time and experience are
documenting as the most useful.

The FDA has proposed (Fed. Regis. 44 #55, 17070-17114. (1979))
that a small group of mutagenicity assays be used in determining
the potential toxicological activity of edible tissue residues from
drug treated animals. This determination is part of a threshold
assessment to determine if a compound or its metabolites require
long term carcinogenicity studies. The battery of assays tests the
ability of the compound(s) to induce point mutations in two test
systems that have been demonstrated to have a high correlation
between detected mutagens and positive results in in vivo carcinogenesis bioassays. Systems which have shown this correlation include point mutations in bacteria, point mutations in the x-linked
recessive lethal test in Drosophila, and point mutations in
mammalian cells in culture. Unscheduled DNA repair synthesis in
mammalian cells in culture should also be included in the battery. Three of the four assays mentioned in this document are for
gene mutation and have been identified in other batteries for detecting compounds with carcinogenic potential. The UDS assay result depends on a demonstrable biological endpoint in another assay
such as mutation, in vitro transformation or carcinogenicity to be
utilized in a hazard evaluation context.

In a recent validation study of bacterial and mammalian mutagenicity tests utilizing 180 chemicals, Bartsch et al. (5) noted
that of 26 carcinogens tested in Salmonella and V79 Chinese hamster
assays, 25 were detected as mutagens when the results from both
tests were combined. Purchase et al. (45) evaluated 6 short-term
tests for detecting chemical carcinogens utilizing 120 compounds.
They reported a battery composed of the Ames Salmonella assay and
in vitro transformation (BHK21) detected 56 out of 58
carcinogens. The compounds missed were dimethylstilbestrol and
vinyl chloride. These two assays combined also declared 6 compounds as positive which had negative carcinogenicity results.

A minimal or core group of assays for the detection of mutagenic and carcinogenic potential of chemicals has been under investigation at Pfizer for the past 4 years. Components of this
battery are as follows: (1) Bacterial point mutation assay with
four strains of Salmonella typhimurium; (1a) assay of urine from
mice treated with test chemical on Salmonella strains; (2)

mammalian cell point mutation assay with mouse lymphoma (L5178Y);
(3) cytogenetic analysis in vivo with rat or mouse bone marrow
cells; (4) a cytogenetic assay in human lymphocytes in vitro with
mitotic indices as an indicator for dose selection; and (5)
transformation in hamster embryo cells in vitro, Ray, V. A. (46).
Wherein comparative data exist, a subgroup of this battery composed
of the Syrian hamster embryo clonal assay for in vitro
transformation, the Ames Salmonella assay and the mouse lymphoma
(L5178Y) or Chinese hamster ovary cell gene mutation assays has
shown considerable promise as a valuable group of tests for
assessing the carcinogenic potential of chemicals. It should be
stated that although the Ames Salmonella and mouse lymphoma or
Chinese hamster ovary cell assays may be performed routinely, the
Syrian hamster embryo assay is difficult to develop to a point
where routine application is feasible. A computerized selection of
compounds within a data base of 517 substances on which comparative
results were available is shown in Table 1. Of the 61 compounds
listed, 51 showed agreement between rodent carcinogenicity
determinations and the battery of 3 assays. A positive agreement
here means a positive result in one or more of the short-term tests
and the rodent bioassay. Agreement on negative compounds means
negative in all 3 short-term tests and the rodent bioassays. This
group of 61 compounds contained 42 carcinogens (68.8%), 14 noncarcinogens (23.3%) and 5 indeterminate substances (8.2%).

   Of the remaining 10 compounds one substance, phenobarbital,
was negative in the short-term tests but had a declaration of positive in rodent bioassays. Another, methylcarbamate, was negative
in short-term tests but indeterminate in rodent bioassays. The
remaining 8 compounds that are positive in short-term tests can be
divided on the basis of carcinogenicity results into two groups;
positive and indeterminate. The four compounds whose carcinogenicity is indeterminate are as follows:

	COMPOUND	STT RESULT
1.	Acridine orange	SHE(+),Sal(+),ML(+)
2.	Hycanthone	SHE(+),Sal(+),ML(+),CHO(+)
3.	Phenylenediamine, M	SHE(+),Sal(+),ML(+)
4.	Succinic anhydride	SHE(+),Sal(?),ML(N)

The remaining four compounds that have negative carcinogenicity
determinations but are positive in the short-term tests are:

	COMPOUND	STT RESULT
1.	Benzo(e)pyrene	SHE(+),Sal(+),ML(+),CHO(+)
2.	Epoxybutane, 1,2	SHE(+),Sal(+),ML(+)
3.	Methotrexate	SHE(-),Sal(-),ML(+),W
4.	Phenylenediamine, 4 Nitro 0	SHE(+),Sal(+),ML(+)

Table 1. Comparative Test Results for Selected Compounds

COMPOUND	ANIM	IVT	AMES	MMC	REFERENCES			
ACETONE	–	N	–	N	31	41	31	1
ACETOXY-2-AAF,N	+	P	P	P	31	41	31	1
ACETYLAMINOFLUORENE,2	+	P	+	+	31	41	31	9
ACETYLAMINOFLUORENE,4	–	N	?	–	31	44	31	9
ACRIDINE ORANGE	I	P	+	+	31	40	31	1
AF-2	+	P	P	P	31	42	31	9
AFLATOXIN B1	R	P	+	P	24	41	31	15
AMINOAZOBENZENE,4	R	P	+	+	22	41	31	3
AMINOFLUORENE,2	+	P	+	+	31	41	31	3
ANILINE	R	N	–	+	33	44	31	1
ANTHRACENE	–	N	–	–	31	41	31	1
AURAMINE	B	+	+	–	17	41	31	1
BENZ(A)ANTHRACENE	M	P	+	+	18	41	31	1
BENZO(A)PYRENE	B	P	+	+	18	41	31	9
BENZO(E)PYRENE	–	+	+	+	18	41	31	9
BERYLLIUM SULFATE	R	P	+	P	17	41	47	16
BROMODEOXYURIDINE,5	–	N	–	?	41	41	13	6
CADMIUM CHLORIDE	B	P	?	P	25	7	30	16
CAFFEINE	–	N	–	N	31	44	31	1
CAPROLACTONE,E	–	N	–	N	31	41	31	9
CYCLOPHOSPHAMIDE	B	P	+	+	23	44	31	9
DIAMINOANISOLE,2,4	B	N	+	P	32	40	4	39
DIETHYL NITROSAMINE	B	+	+	+	17	41	31	9
DIETHYLSTILBESTROL	B	P	?	P	20	44	31	9
DIMETHYL CARBAMYLCHLORIDE	M	P	P	+	26	41	31	3
DIMETHYL NITROSAMINE	B	P	+	+	17	41	31	9
DIMETHYL SULFOXIDE	–	N	–	N	31	41	31	1
DIMETHYL-B(A)A,7,12	+	P	+	+	31	41	31	16
DIPHENYL NITROSAMINE	R	P	–	–	36	41	31	9
EPOXYBUTANE,1,2-	–	P	P	P	31	43	31	1
ETHANOL	–	N	–	N	31	41	31	1
ETHYL METHANESULFONATE	B	P	P	P	21	44	31	9
GLYCIDALDEHYDE	B	P	+	+	25	41	31	3
HYCANTHONE METHANESULFONATE	I	P	P	P	27	17	31	9
HYDRAZINE	B	P	+	N	19	41	31	1
HYDROXY-2-AAF,N	+	P	+	P	31	41	31	16
LEAD ACETATE	B	P	–	N	17	41	47	2
METHANOL	–	N	–	N	41	41	53	1
METHOTREXATE	–	N	–	P	34	41	47	9
METHYL CARBAMATE	I	N	–	–	26	43	31	3
METHYL IODIDE	R	P	P	P	28	41	31	9
METHYL METHANESULFONATE	B	P	P	P	21	8	31	9
METHYLCHOLANTHRENE,3	+	P	+	+	31	41	31	1
MNNG	B	P	P	P	19	41	31	9
NATULAN	+	P	–	P	35	41	31	9
NICKEL CHLORIDE/SULFATE	+	+	+	P	41	41	41	2
NITRITE,SODIUM	+	N	+	–	31	40	31	16
NITRO-O-PHENYLENEDIAMINE,4	–	P	+	P	37	43	11	39
NITRO-P-PHENYLENEDIAMINE,2	M	P	+	P	29	43	11	40
NITROBIPHENYL,4	+	P	P	+	19	41	31	3
NITROQUINOLINE-1-OXIDE,4	+	P	P	P	31	41	31	1
NITROSOETHYLUREA,N	B	P	P	P	17	41	31	16
PHENOBARBITAL,SODIUM	B	N	–	N	27	44	31	1
PHENYLENEDIAMINE,M-	I	P	+	P	29	43	4	39

Table 1.   Continued

COMPOUND	ANIMT	IVT	AMES	MC	REFERENCES			
PROPIOLACTONE,BETA	B	+	P	P	19	44	31	9
PYRENE	-	N	-	-	31	41	31	1
SACCHARIN	R	N	-	P	38	38	38	9
SUCCINIC ANHYDRIDE	I	P	?	N	28	41	31	9
THIOACETAMIDE	B	P	-	-	21	41	31	3
URACIL MUSTARD	B	P	P	P	23	43	31	9
URETHANE	B	+	-	-	21	41	31	3

Animal Carcinogenicity Assays
- M, R and B - Positive in mouse, rat or both.
- I - Indeterminate

In Vitro Transformation and Mutagenicity Assays
- + and - indicates positive or negative with metabolic
  activation.
- P and N indicates positive or negative without metabolic
  activation.

It is interesting to note that of the four compounds declared
positive in short-term tests and indeterminate in carcinogenicity
assays, three out of the four were positive in all three short-term
tests. Three of the four compounds which had declarations of negative in rodent bioassays were also positive in all three short-term
tests.

The overall performance of the three test battery on compounds
that were designated as carcinogenic or non-carcinogenic was 51
detected correctly out of 56 compounds, or 91 percent. The detection rate of carcinogens was 41 out of 42 compounds, or 97.9 percent. Ten out of 14 non-carcinogens were labelled correctly by STT
for a 71.4% rate. Because of the high sensitivity of these three
assays for detecting carcinogenic potential, a negative result
appears to be highly significant and of considerable value in the
safety evaluation process.

Although the number of compounds is relatively small on which
comparative data in all three short-term tests and carcinogenicity
are available, it does indicate that emphasis should be given to
this small battery in screening and collaborative studies.
Further, when a battery of tests declares a substance as mutagenic
and capable of producing in vitro transformation, its toxic potential has to be regarded with more than a modicum of concern. At

the very least, additional documentations of this type are needed
to establish confidence in the utility of short-term tests as
indicators of carcinogenic potential and to serve as a focus for
re-examination of rodent bioassays as the ultimate indicator of
carcinogenicity declarations in toxicology.

Utility of Genetic Toxicology Information

The role of genetic toxicology in the safety evaluation process is to identify mutagenic and carcinogenic potential of chemicals, to evaluate the spectrum of effects and to give an indication
of potency relative to known compounds. If data from compounds of
similar structure are available, such comparisons may be instructive.

The subsequent hazard evaluation and risk assessment of genotoxic compounds is enhanced by this knowledge which provides for
informed utility of a genotoxic substance where need or benefit is
established and no suitable non-genotoxic substitute is available. Levels of exposure, environmental persistence and degree of
food or water contamination which result from utility of pesticides
or other agricultural chemicals are evaluations which superimpose
on this knowledge. The genetic toxicology evaluation thus provides
an early measure of certain types of toxicity which cannot be
acquired in any other way than long-term animal exposures and gives
perspective to the hazard evaluation and risk assessment process.

REFERENCES

1. Amacher, D. E., S. C. Paillet, G. Turner, V. A. Ray, and D. S.
    Salsburg. Point mutations at the thymidine kinase locus in
    L5178Y mouse lymphoma cells. II. Test validation and inter-
    pretation. Mutation res. 72, 447-474 (1980).
2. Amacher, D. E. and S. C. Paillet, Induction of trifluorothy-
    midine-resistant mutants by metal ions in L5178Y/TK$^{+/-}$
    cells. Mutation Res. 78,279-288 (1980).
3. Amacher, D. E. and G. N. Turner. Mutagenic activity of car-
    cinogens and noncarcinogens in the L5178T/TK$^{+/-}$ cell/liver
    supernatant mutation assay. Mutation Res. (in press) (1981).
4. Ames, B. N., H. O. Kammen, and E. Yamasaki, Hair dyes are
    mutagenic: Identification of a variety of mutagenic ingre-
    dients. Prod. Nat. Acad. Sci. USA 72, 2423-2427 (1975).
5. Bartsch, H., C. Malaveille, A.-M. Camus, G. Martel-Planche, G.
    Breen, A. Hautefeuille, N. Sabadie, A. Barbin, T. Kuroki, C.
    Drevon, C. Piscoli and R. Montesano, Bacterial and mammalian
    mutagenicity tests: Validation and comparative studies on 180
    chemicals. IARC Scientific Publications No. 27, 179-241
    (1980).

6. Burki, H. J., BUDR and fluorescent light-induced mutagenesis in synchronous Chinese hamster cells in vitro. Rad. Res. 70, 650 (1977).

7. Casto, B. C., W. J. Pieczynski, R. L. Nelson, and J. A. Dipaolo. In vitro transformation and enhancement of viral transformation with metals. Proc. Amer. Ass. Can. Res. 17, 12 (1976).

8. Casto, B. C., N. Janosko, and J. A. Dipaolo, Development of a focus assay model for transformation of hamster cells in vitro by chemical carcinogens. Can. Res. 37, 3508-3515 (1977).

9. Clive, D., K. O. Johnson, J. F. S. Spector, A. G. Batson and M. M. Brown. Validation and characterization of the L5178Y/TK$^{+/-}$ mouse lymphoma mutagen assay system. Mutation Res. 59, 61-108 (1979).

10. Guidelines for the Testing of Chemicals for Mutagenicity. Report of Committee on Mutagenicity of Chemicals in Food, Consumer Products and the Environment, P. E. Polani, Chairman, DHSS Report No. 24. Her Majesty's Stationery Office, London (1981).

11. Dunkel, V. C. Mutagenic activity of chemicals previously tested for carcinogenicity in the National Cancer Institute bioassay program, in: Molecular and Cellular Aspects of Car-cinogen Screening Tests. (R. Montesano, H. Bartsch, L. Toma-tis, W. Davis, eds.) IARC Scientific Publications #27, International Agency for Research on Cancer, Lyon, 1980.

12. Proposed System for Food Safety Assessment. Final Report of the Scientific Committee of the Food Safety Council. V. O. Wodicka, Chairman. Food Safety Council, 1725 K. Street, N.W., Washington, DC 2006 (1980).

13. Heddle, J. A. and W. R. Bruce, Comparison of tests for muta-genicity or carcinogenicity using assays for sperm abnormali-ties, formation of micronuclei, mutations in Salmonella, in: Origins of Human Cancer. Book C. Human Risk. Assessment (H. H. Hiatt, J. D. Watson, J. A. Wi, eds.) Cold Spring Harbor Laboratory, Cold Spring Harbor, New York (1977).

14. Hetrick, F. H. and W. L. Kos, Transformation of cell cultures as a parameter for detecting potential carcinogenicity of antischistosomal drugs. J. Toxicol. Environ. Health 1, 323-327 (1975).

15. Hollstein, M. and J. McCann, Short-term tests for carcinogens and mutagens. Mutation Res. 65, 133-226 (1979).

16. Hsie, A. W., J. O'Neill, San-Sebastian, Jr., D. B. Couch, P. A. Brimer, W. N. C. Sun., J. C. Fuscoe, N. L. Forbes, R. Machanoff, J. C. Riddle, and M. H. Hsie. Quantitative mamma-lian cell genetic toxicology: Study of the cytotoxicity and mutagenicity of seventy individual environmental agents re-lated to energy technologies and the subfractions of a crude synthetic oil in the CHO/HGPRT system. Report: EPA-600/9-78-027 PP. 293-315 (1978).

17. IARC Monographs on the Evaluation of the Carcinogenic Risk of
     Chemicals to Man: Some Inorganic Substances, Chlorinated
     Hydrocarbons, Aromatic Amines, N-Nitroso Compounds and Natural
     Products, Volume 1, 1972.
18. IARC Monographs on the Evaluation of the Carcinogenic Risk of
     Chemicals to Man: Certain Polycyclic Aromatic Hydrocarbons
     and Heterocyclic Compounds, Volume 3, 1973.
19. IARC Monographs on the Evaluation of the Carcinogenic Risk of
     Chemicals to Man: Some Aromatic Amines, Hydrazine Related
     Substances, N-Nitroso Compounds and Miscellaneous Alkylating
     Agents, Volume 4, June 1973.
20. IARC Monographs on the Evaluation of the Carcinogenic Risk of
     Chemicals to Man: Sex Hormones, Volume 6, February, 1974.
21. IARC Monographs on the Evaluation of the Carcinogenic Risk of
     Chemicals to Man: Some Anti-Thyroid and Related Substance,
     Volume 7, 1974.
22. IARC Monographs on the Evaluation of the Carcinogenic Risk of
     Chemicals to Man: Some Aromatic Azo Compounds, Volume 8,
     1975.
23. IARC Monographs on the Evaluation of the Carcinogenic Risk of
     Chemicals to Man: Some Aziridines, N-, S and O Mustard and
     Selenium, Volume 9, April, 1975.
24. IARC Monographs on the Evaluation of the Carcinogenic Risk of
     Chemicals to Man: Some Naturally Occurring Substances, Volume
     10, 1976.
25. IARC Monographs on the Evaluation of the Carcinogenic Risk of
     Chemicals to Man: Cadmium, Nickel, some Epoxides, Miscel-
     laneous Industrial Chemicals and General Considerations on
     Volatile Anesthetics, Volume 11, February, 1976.
26. IARC Monographs on the Evaluation of the Carcinogenic Risk of
     Chemicals to Man: Some Carbamates, Thiocarbamates and Carba-
     zides, Volume 12, 1976.
27. IARC Monographs on the Evaluation of the Carcinogenic Risk of
     Chemicals to Man: Some Miscellaneous Pharmaceutical Sub-
     stances, Volume 13, 1977.
28. IARC Monographs on the Evaluation of the Carcinogenic Risk of
     Chemicals to Man: Some Fumigants, the Herbicides 2,4,5-T,
     Chlorinated Dibenzodioxins and Miscellaneous Industrial Chem-
     icals, Volume 15, February, 1977.
29. IARC Monographs on the Evaluation of the Carcinogenic Risk of
     Chemicals to Man: Some Aromatic Amines and Related Nitro
     Compounds - Hair Dyes, Coloring Agents and Miscellaneous
     Industrial Chemicals, Volume 16, 1978.
30. Kalina, L. M., G. N. Polukhina, and L. I. Lukasheva, Salmon-
     ella typhimurium: Test system for indication of mutagenic
     activity of environmental hazards. I. Detection mutagenic
     effect of heavy metals salts using in vivo and in vitro assays
     without metabolic activation. Genetika 13, 1089-1092 (1977).

31. McCann, J., E. Choi, E. Yamasaki and B. N. Ames. Detection of
     carcinogens as mutagens in the Salmonella microsome test:
     Assay of 300 chemicals. Proc. Nat. Acad. Sci. USA 72, 5135-
     5139 (1975).

32. NCI Bioassay of 2,4-diaminoanisole sulfate for possible car-
     cinogenicity. Technical Report Series NCI-CG-TR-84.

33. NCI Bioassay of Aniline Hydrochloride for Possible Carcino-
     genicity. Technical Report Series NCI-CG-TR-130.

34. NCI Bioassay of Selected Cancer Chemotherapeutic Agents of
     Possible Carcinogenicity. DHEW Publication No (NIH) 78-1329.

35. NCI Bioassay of Procarbazine (Natulan) for Possible carcino-
     genicity. Technical Report Series NCI-CG-TR-19.

36. NCI Bioassay of N-Nitrosodiphenylamine for Possible Carcino-
     genicity. Technical Report Series NCI-CG-TR-164.

37. NCI Bioassay of 4-Nitro-O-Phenylenediamine for Possible Car-
     cinogenicity. Technical Report Series NCI-CG-TR-180.

38. OTC Cancer Testing Technology and Saccharin. Office of Tech-
     nology Assessment (OTA) Report 1977 #052-003-00471-2, U. S.
     Gov't Printing Office, Washington, DC 20402.

39. Palmer, K. A., A. Denunzio and S. J. Green. The mutagenic
     assay of some hair dye components using the thymidine kinase
     locus of L5178Y mouse lymphoma cells. J. Environ. Path. Toxi-
     col. 1, 87-91 (1977).

40. Pienta, R. J. Personal communication.

41. Pienta, R. J., J. A. Poiley, and W. B. Lebherz, III. Morpho-
     logical transformation of early passage golden Syrian hamster
     embryo cells derived from cryopreserved primary cultures: A
     reliable in vitro bioassay for identifying diverse carcino-
     gens. Int. J. Cancer 19, 642-655 (1977).

42. Pienta, R. J., W. B. Lebherz, III, and S. Takayama. Malignant
     transformation of cryopreserved early passage Syrian golden
     hamster cells by 2-(2-furyl)-3-(5-nitro-2-furyl)acrylamide
     (AF-2). Cancer Lett. 5, 245-251 (1978).

43. Pienta, R. J. In vitro transformation of cultured cells.
     Presentation at Symposium No. 12 Bioassay Systems for Carcino-
     gens at the XIIth International Cancer Congress, Buenos Aires,
     Argentina, October 6, 1978.

44. Purchase, I. F. H., E. Longstaff, J. Ashby, J. A. Styles, D.
     Anderson, P. A. Lefevre and F. R. Westwood. An evaluation of
     6 short-term tests for detecting organic chemical carcino-
     gens. Br. J. Cancer 37, 873-903 (1978).

45. Purchase, I. F. H., E. Longstaff, J. Ashbey, J. A. Styles, D.
     Anderson, P. A. Lefevre, and F. R. Westwood. Evaluation of
     six short-term tests for detecting organic chemical carcino-
     gens and recommendations for their use. Nature 264, 624-627
     (1976).

46. Ray, V. A. Application of microbial and mammalian cells to
     the assessment of mutagenicity. Pharmacological Review 30,
     537-546 (1979).

56   VERNE A. RAY

47. Simmon, V. F., K. Kauhanen, and R. G. Tardiff. Mutagenic
    activity of chemicals identified in drinking water. Dev.
    Toxicol. Environ. Sci. 2, 249-258 (1977).
48. Simmon, V. R. *In vitro* mutagenicity assays of chemical car-
    cinogens and related compounds with *Salmonella typhimurium*. J.
    Natl. Cancer. Inst. 63, 893-899 (1979).
49. Waters, M. D. and A. Auletta. The Gene-Tox Program: Genetic
    Activity Evaluation. J. Chem. Inform. Computer Sci. 35-38
    (1981).

BASES FOR CONCERN

CHAIRMAN'S COMMENTS

Nemat O. Borhani

Department of Community Health
University of California
Davis, California 95616

Welcome to the first session of the afternoon of this symposium on Genetic Toxicology: An Agricultural Perspective. Three excellent topics on urban and rural patterns of cancer incidence, cancer risks associated with agriculture, and extrapolation of mutagenicity testing to man will be presented during this session by a panel of distinguished investigators. All these, in one way or another, deal with application of epidemiological tools in our scientific endeavors in this field. As an epidemiologist, I would like to make a few remarks for a brief introduction.

I am sure the contributions of epidemiology to the development of ideas for future medical research and improvement of health in general needs no emphasis. This issue is no longer the subject for heated debate that it once was. The medical literature is replete with excellent examples of epidemiological research which has been of value at all levels of health and social services. Despite this apparent success, which perhaps was most evident in the late 19th century, due to the classic work of prominent investigators such as Snow, Farr and Chadwick, there is today a serious challenge facing epidemiologists; that is, to directly take the results of epidemiological findings into account when making policy decisions that affect the industry, including agriculture, the consumer, and the society as a whole.

The topic of this symposium is an excellent example of such a complexity that the scientists, the agricultural industry, the farmers, and the people as a whole face with regard to the toxic agents used in the agro-ecosystem.

In terms of genetic-toxicology, especially from an
agricultural point of view, we deal with that particular branch of
epidemiology which is concerned with the study of the interaction
of environmental and gentic determinants of health of the
population. The methods used to study this interaction are
different from those of "traditional" epidemiology (1).

For example, it is one of the concerns of the agricultural
industry that pesticides, used frequently in modern agriculture,
are potential hazards to health. That is, residues of these
pesticides in food and water supplies may have potent adverse
effects such as carcinogenicity, teratogenicity, and
mutagenicity. To understand this important perspective we must
appreciate the special meanings that epidemiologists attribute to
the word "environment" and "carcinogenesis." On the one hand the
epidemiologist's perspective of carcinogenesis is, at best,
empirical. On the other hand, the word "environment" to an
epidemiologist refers to any influence other than that of the
genetic material inherited from an individual's parents (2). This
distinction is important to consider because to an epidemiologist
the concept of environmental exposure ranges widely in its
specificity. When we describe the association between a disease
and a given occupation, we do indeed use a combination of many
factors loosely defined as the "occupation" (e.g., farmer). To be
sure, such a distinction may be more important in theory than in
practice. Nevertheless, it is a distinction that must be borne in
mind.

To illustrate this point I would like to review, briefly--to
set the stage, if you will--my understanding of the pesticides used
in modern agriculture and their potential hazards to health. There
are, as you know, three generations of pesticides. The first
generation, used prior to 1945, included naturally occurring
organics and inorganic compounds such as copper, zinc, and
arsenates. The second generation began with the use of synthetic
organics, with the advent of DDT and other organochlorine
pesticides (OCP). Problems with insect resistance and other
recognized environmental hazards associated with the use of these
agents led to a reduction, over the years, in the production, and
use, of organochlorine pesticides (OCP) and an increase in the
production, and use, of other classes of synthetic organic
pesticides such as organophosphates (OP). The third generation of
pesticides includes the newly developed integrated pest control
management systems. The latter which is still in its infancy
requires more epidemiological studies. On the other hand, there
seems to be ample epidemiological and toxicological evidence on the
potential hazards of the second generation of pesticides, namely
organochlorine pesticides (OCP) and the organophosphates (OP).
Unfortunately this evidence does not appear to be conclusive, at
least with regard to direct human evidence on the carcinogenicity

of organochlorine pesticides (OCP). For example, the 1974
monograph of the International Agency for Research on Cancer (IARC)
concluded that "...no reported epidemiologic studies justify any
conclusions, which in some instances have been drawn, as to their
noncarcinogenicity..." (3). Other investigators, however, feel
that the number of workers at risk and the duration of risk in
published studies have been adequate to draw a valid inference as
to the claim of noncarcinogenicity (4).

The increased use of organophosphate pesticides which, in
recent years, replaced the less toxic but more persistent
chlorinated hydrocarbons such as DDT, has resulted in a new class
of occupational hazards for the agricultural industry. It is
generally accepted that such a hazard occurs from prolonged worker
contact with organophosphate residues on crop foliage.
Intoxication is usually manifested by nervous system dysfunction
due to phosphorylation and inactivation of cholinesterase (CHE) by
these pesticides.

Recently my colleagues and I participated in an
interdisciplinary project conducted by the Department of Community
Health, School of Medicine, the Department of Environmental
Toxicology, Agricultural Engineering and the Agricultural Extension
Service of the University of California at Davis to determine
whether any physiolocial effects occurred from organophosphate
(Guthion) residue exposure among normal agricultural field labor
population. We monitored whole blood cholinesterase (CHE)
activity, urinary dialkylphosphate excretion and reflex activity.
Also, we measured Guthion residue levels on the foliage and
correlated the foliage residue levels with the observed exposure
response (5). In terms of cholinesterase activity (CHE), 13 of 16
thinners and all 3 foremen studied showed a continuous decline in
their whole blood cholinesterase activity, as compared to
baseline. Of the 72 recorded day-to-day changes in cholinesterase
activity, 13 showed a decrease of more than 10% of which 4 were
more than 15%. I must emphasize, however, that although one worker
showed a consistent decrease in CHE activity, reaching an
impressive 30% decline at the end of the work week, daily changes
in CHE activity among workers were quite erratic and fluctuated
widely. Thus, the interpretation of our findings with respect to
any logical inference to the potential hazards of organophosphate
pesticides is very difficult, if not impossible, especially since
physical examination of these workers before and after the exposure
period revealed an absence of any clincial sign of organophosphate
intoxication, even though group mean dialkylphophate excretion
levels provided a semi-quantitative indication of exposure to
Guthion.

It is terribly important, therefore, to appreciate the
timeliness of today's symposium so that we can examine the status

of our knowledge and identify the types of studies that are needed
to answer so many burning questions in this important field.

REFERENCES

1.   Schull, W. J. and Weiss, K. M., Genetic Epidemiology, Four
     Strategies: Epidemiologic Review, Vol. II, pp 1-18, 1980.
2.   Maclure, K. M. and MacMahon B., An Epidemiologic Perspectives
     of Environmental Carcinogenesis: Epidemiologic Review,
     Vol. II, pp. 19-48, 1980.
3.   IARC: Some Organochlorine Pesticides Monograph, Vol. V, 1974.
4.   Epstein, S. S., The Carcinogenicity of Organochlorine
     Pesticides, in: Origins of Human Cancer. Hiatt, Watson and
     Winston, (eds.) Cold Sspring Harbor Laboratory, Book A, pp.
     243-265, 1977.
5.   Kraus, J. F., Richards, D. M., Borhani, N. O., Mull, R.,
     Kilgore, W., and Winterlin, W., Physiological Responses to
     Organophosphate Residue in Field Workers. Archives of
     Environmental Contamination and Toxicology, Vol. V, pp. 471-
     485, 1977.

PATTERNS IN URBAN AND RURAL CANCER INCIDENCE

Roger R. Connelly

Biometry Branch
National Cancer Institute
Bethesda, MD

INTRODUCTION

The Third National Cancer Survey (TNCS) was a project of the Biometry Branch of the National Cancer Institute conducted during the 3-year period 1969-71 in seven metropolitan areas and the two states of Iowa and Colorado. The primary objective was to provide detailed information on the incidence of cancer in the United States. The findings of the survey by sex, race, age, and geographic area of the patient and by anatomic site and histologic type of the cancer have been published (1). The primary purpose of this report is to present the results of additional analyses of the TNCS data from Iowa and Colorado for urban and rural cancer patterns. Comparisons with earlier and more recent data on the incidence of cancer in urban and rural areas of Iowa are also made for selected primary sites.

MATERIAL

Iowa and Colorado Cases Diagnosed During 1969-71

There were 27,418 primary invasive cancers diagnosed among Iowa residents and 16,128 diagnosed among Colorado residents during the 3-year period 1969-71. These totals do not include a few cancer patients of unknown sex or age, any in situ carcinomas, or any nonmelanoma skin cancers. Cases without microscopically confirmed diagnoses (13.0% in Iowa and 7.4% in Colorado) were included. For further details on the material as obtained through the operation of the TNCS, see the Introduction in (1).

Iowa Cases Diagnosed during 1950

An earlier cancer morbidity survey in Iowa (2) provided urban-rural finding for 1950 which can be compared to the Iowa results for 1969-71. The earlier survey included all skin cancers while only skin melanomas were included in the TNCS. To make comparisons between surveys for all sites combined more comparable, all skin cancers were excluded from both sets of data.

Iowa Cases Diagnosed During 1973-78

Iowa is a participant in the Surveillance, Epidemiology, and End Results (SEER) program, a continuing project of the Biometry Branch which was initiated in 1972 (3). Data comparable to that collected during the TNCS from 62,724 cancer cases diagnosed among Iowa residents during the years 1973-78 were available for analysis.

METHODS OF ANALYSIS

Urban - Rural Classification

The Bureau of the Census defines the urban population of the country as all persons living in urbanized areas and in places of 2,500 inhabitants of more outside urbanized areas; persons not classified as urban constitute the rural population. The residential information available for each Iowa and Colorado cancer case diagnosed during 1969-71 was scrutinized and the Census definition of urban and rural residence was followed in classifying cases.

Cases residing in or near small towns (less than 2,500 inhabitants) were classifed as rural residents. Cases from larger towns with detailed street-address information such as house number and street name were classified as urban residents if their address indicated they resided inside the boundry of an urbanized area or a place of 2,500 or more inhabitants outside an urbanized area. Census tract maps for each urbanized area and street maps for all places with 10,000 or more inhabitants (and some smaller places) were utilized. Cases with a street address such as "rural route", "RFD", or "star route" were arbitrarily classified as rural residents. For those with a street address of "general delivery" or "P. O. Box", additional residential information was sought from death certificates, city directories, and telephone directories; cases for which no additonal residential information was obtained (196 or 0.7% of Iowa cases, 172 or 1.1% of Colorado cases) were arbitrarily classified as urban residents.

Each urbanized area (seven in Iowa and four in Colorado) contained sufficient inhabitants to warrant separate analysis. For

urban residents living outside urbanized areas, subgroups were
formed on the basis of size-of-place. Subgroups of the rural
population were formed by considering the concentration of farmers
among the rural residents of each county. Within each state, the
counties were ranked according to the ratio of farm to nonfarm
residents among the rural residents of each county as enumerated in
the 1970 Census. Based on this ratio, counties were grouped into
five strata of about equal rural population size and analyses were
performed for each of the five strata.

     For Iowa cases diagnosed during 1973-78, the only residential
information routinely coded was county of residence. This was
utilized to form pseudo urban-rural subgroups. Of Iowa's 99
counties, 18 were completely rural (no place of 2,500 or more
people) but they contained only 17% of the total rural population
(1970 Census). These 18 counties were therefore combined with 31
mostly rural counties (largest place of size 2,500 to 5,000).
Residents of these 49 counties encompassed 43% of the State's rural
population and only 8% of the urban population. Analyses for
residents of these 49 'rural' counties were compared to those for
residents of seven counties containing the seven urbanized areas
(termed 'urban' counties) and the remaining 43 'suburban'
counties. Similar subgroups of the TNCS data were formed so that
comparisons could be made over 3 time periods, 1969-71, 1973-75,
and 1976-78.

Analytic Methods

     Average annual cancer incidence rates per 100,000 population
for urban and rural residents were calculated by primary site, sex
and age. Race was not included as an analytic variable since few
cases were other than white. Incidence rates adjusted to the age
distribution of the population of the United States in 1970 were
calculated by the direct method. Rates adjusted to the 1950
standard population were also calculated for use in comparisons
were earlier data which were already adjusted to that standard.

     The relative risk is used to measure the strength of the
association of cancer incidence with urban-rural residence. The
relative risk is defined as the cancer incidence rate for urban
residents divided by the rate for rural residents of the same sex
and age. To test the hypothesis that a relative risk equals one, a
chi-square test with one degree of freedom based on a Poisson model
was carried out (4,5). Exact tests were performed when there were
no rural cases (6). Relative risks summarized over several or all
age strata were calculated using a noniterative maximum likelihood
method for small Poisson probabilities (7) and associated chi-
square tests for heterogeneity of age-specific relative risks were
performed (7). This summary relative risk for all ages combined
seldom varied appreciably from the ratio of urban to rural age-
adjusted incidence rates, a frequently used summary statistic.

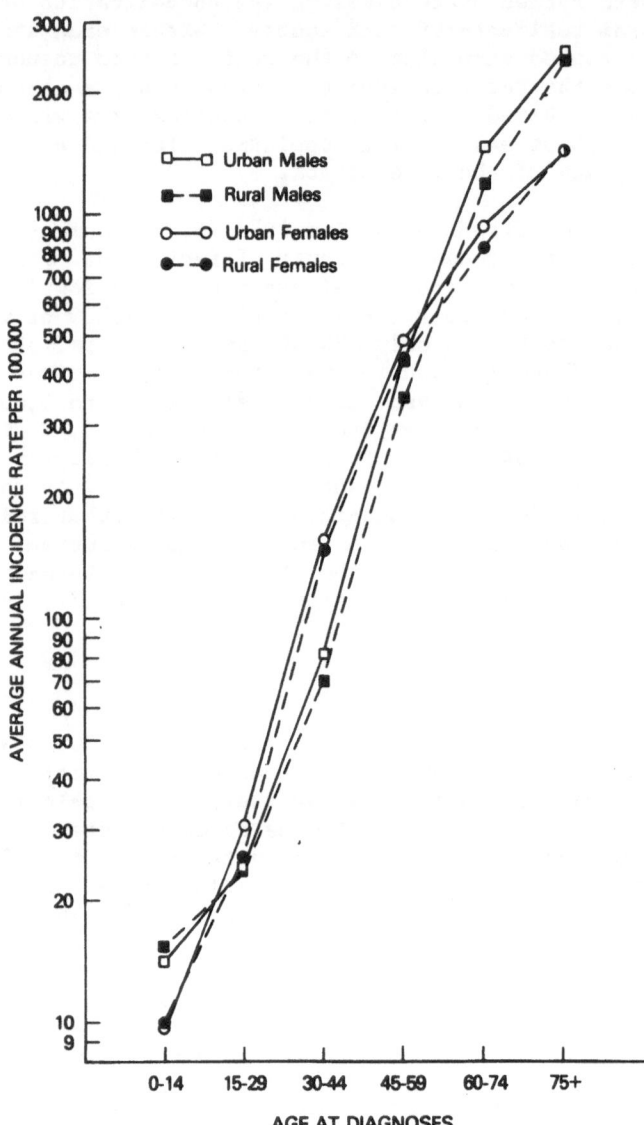

Fig. 1.   Average annual age-specific incidence rates per 100,000 for
          cancer (all sites combined excluding nonmelanoma skin cancer)
          among urban and rural residents of Iowa by sex during 1969-
          71.

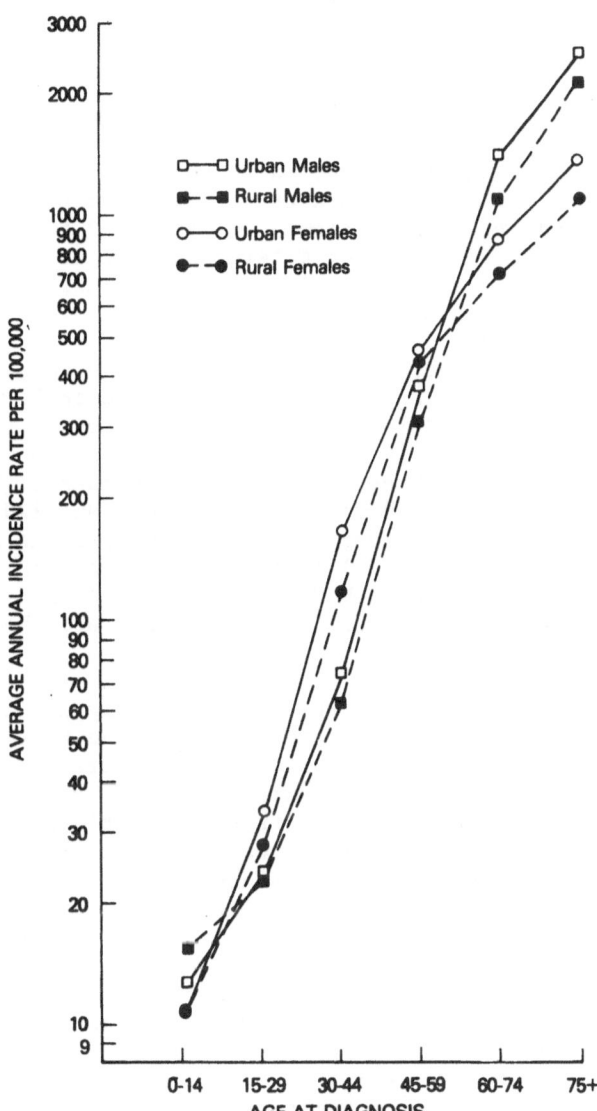

Fig. 2. Average annual age-specific incidence rates per 100,000 for cancer (all sites combined excluding nonmelanoma skin cancer) among urban and rural residents of Colorado by sex during 1969-71.

For tests of monotomic trends in incidence rates over time, the Mantel-Haenszel statistic modified for Poisson probabilities was used (4,5).

RESULTS

Urban-Rural Relative Risks for Cancer, 1969-71

Sex and age-specific incidence rates for cancer (all sites combined excluding nonmelanoma skin cancer) among urban and rural residents are shown in Figure 1 (Iowa) and Figure 2 (Colorado). Age and sex are obviously stronger determinants of cancer incidence rates than urban-rural residence. An urban-rural differential is apparent, however, with urban rates usually exceeding rural rates. Differences are minimal at the extremes of the age range in Iowa and rural rates are actually higher than urban rates among young males in both states and among young females in Iowa. Age-specific relative risks (ratios of urban to rural rates for 5-year age groups) among women are sufficiently homogeneous to warrent use of the summary relative risk over the entire age range. These summary relative risks of 1.19 for Colorado women and 1.07 for Iowa women are significantly different from 1.00. Comparable figures for men are 1.22 (Colorado) and 1.17 (Iowa) but there is significant heterogeneity in risk with age among men and these overall figures, while statistically significant, are therefore of dubious summary value.

Summary relative risks are appropriate descriptors of the finding by primary site of cancer since none of the tests for heterogeneity of age-specific relative risks was statistically significant. Variation in summary relative risks by detailed primary site and site groups is illustrated in Table 1 where the findings for Iowa men and women are presented. Similar detailed primary site analyses for Colorado residents are not shown but the findings in both states for the major sites of cancer and selected other sites are presented in Table 2 (men) and Table 3 (women).

As shown in Table 2, summary relative risks (all ages) were significantly elevated for three major cancer sites among Iowa and Colorado men: 1) lung, bronchus and trachea; 2) colon exluding rectum; and 3) bladder. For one less common cancer site, the esophagus, and for one group of related sites, those of the buccal cavity and pharynx (excluding lip), relative risks were also significantly elevated among men in both states. The risk for prostate cancer, a major site, was significantly high among urban men in Colorado but not among men in Iowa. Relative risks for larynx cancer were high among men in both states although statistical significance was obtained only in Iowa. Increased risks for rural residents (summary relative risks significantly less than one) were encountered infrequently: 1) for lip cancer in

Table 1. Urban and Rural Incidence Rates and Relative Risks for Cancer by Primary Site and Sex; Iowa, 1969-71

Primary Site	Males					Females				
	Number of Cases		Age-adjusted Incidence Rate		Summary Relative Risk†	Number of Cases		Age-adjusted Incidence Rate		Summary Relative Risk†
	Urban	Rural	Urban	Rural		Urban	Rural	Urban	Rural	
All Sites	7759	6102	343.5	293.3	1.17**	8089	5468	267.8	247.3	1.07**
Buccal Cav. & Pharynx	360	325	16.2	15.9	1.02	154		5.2	3.1	1.57**
Lip	115	170	5.1	8.2	0.63**	5	4	0.1	0.2	0.90
Tongue	42	30	1.9	1.5	1.30	33	17	1.0	0.7	1.37
Salivary Gland	22	29	1.0	1.5	0.67	27	19	1.0	0.9	1.01
Gum & Mouth	88	41	4.0	2.1	1.97**	53	16	1.8	0.4	2.42**
Nasopharynx	11	14	0.5	0.7	0.72	12	0	0.4	0.0	oo**
Tonsil	24	16	1.1	0.8	1.41	13	0	0.5	0.0	oo**
Other Pharynx	58	25	2.6	1.2	2.20**	11	6	0.4	0.3	1.38
Digestive System	2023	1669	89.4	79.4	1.12**	2162	1451	64.8	60.5	1.08
Esophagus	100	66	4.5	3.1	1.42*	33	16	1.1	0.7	1.50
Stomach	282	273	12.3	12.8	0.95	215	148	5.8	5.9	1.06
Small Intestine	37	32	1.5	1.5	1.05	37	18	1.2	1.2	1.00
Colon excl. Rectum	780	648	34.4	31.0	1.11*	1116	731	33.7	30.9	1.09
Transverse Colon	105	95	4.7	4.6	1.02	166	119	5.1	5.1	1.00
Descending Colon	77	51	3.4	2.5	1.39	80	49	2.5	2.2	1.18
Sigmoid Colon	321	247	14.2	11.8	1.21*	333	206	10.5	9.1	1.17
Cecum	110	105	4.8	5.0	0.97	237	146	6.8	5.8	1.13
Appendix	4	3	0.2	0.2	1.06	6	5	0.2	0.2	0.85
Ascending Colon	88	70	3.9	3.4	1.16	161	104	4.7	4.3	1.09
Large Int., NOS	75	77	3.3	3.6	0.90	133	102	3.9	4.1	0.91
Rectum & Recto. Jct.	401	334	17.8	15.9	1.12	353	251	10.8	10.6	1.00
Rectosigmoid Jct.	100	88	4.5	4.2	1.06	99	72	3.1	3.1	0.99
Rectum	301	246	13.4	11.7	1.14	254	179	7.7	7.5	1.01
Liver	54	31	2.4	1.5	1.59*	38	34	1.2	1.4	0.78
Gallbladder	28	19	1.2	0.9	1.39	69	59	2.0	2.5	0.83
Other Biliary	36	23	1.6	1.1	1.45	29	17	0.9	0.6	1.19
Pancreas	270	216	11.9	10.3	1.16	217	144	6.2	5.8	1.06
Retroper., Omen., Mes.	20	18	0.9	0.8	0.98	22	10	0.6	0.4	1.60
Other Digestive Syst.	15	9	0.6	0.8	0.76	33	23	1.0	0.9	1.01
Respiratory System	1814	1189	81.7	57.3	1.43**	373	189	13.0	8.4	1.46**
Larynx	188	108	8.6	5.3	1.63**	18	4	0.7	0.2	3.39*
Lung, Bronc. & Trachea	1595	1062	71.8	51.0	1.41**	342	171	11.9	7.7	1.48**
Other Respiratory Syst.	31	19	1.4	1.0	1.46	13	14	0.4	0.6	0.65
Bones & Joints	16	18	0.7	0.9	0.75	20	12	0.8	0.6	1.19
Soft Tissues	44	34	1.9	1.7	1.10	45	34	1.5	1.7	0.94
Melanomas of Skin	81	72	3.6	3.8	0.97	82	59	3.0	3.0	0.99
Breast	16	8	0.7	0.4	1.84	2163	1508	74.2	69.9	1.06
Female Genital System						1602	1117	57.6	53.9	1.06
Cervix Uteri						478	282	18.2	14.6	1.25**
Corpus Uteri						527	400	18.7	18.9	0.99
Uterus, NOS						88	75	3.5	3.5	0.87
Ovary						428	296	15.1	14.1	1.07
Vagina						16	11	0.5	0.5	1.05
Vulva						52	42	1.5	1.7	0.86
Other Fem. Gen. Syst.						13	11	0.4	0.6	0.84

Table 1. Continued

Site										
Male Genital System	1447	1245	62.7	58.5	1.07					
Prostate	1334	1169	57.7	54.2	1.06					
Testis	84	57	3.7	3.4	1.07					
Penis	27	15	1.2	0.7	1.68					
Other Male Gen. Syst.	2	4	0.1	0.2	0.47					
Urinary System	769	590	34.1	28.2	1.21**	326	200	10.1	8.3	1.16
Bladder	540	417	23.8	19.8	1.20**	202	105	6.0	4.1	1.35*
Kidney & Renal Pelvis	200	162	9.0	7.8	1.13	110	88	3.6	3.9	0.91
Other Urinary Syst.	29	11	1.3	0.5	2.44**	14	7	0.4	0.3	1.42
Eye & Orbit	15	15	0.7	0.7	0.87	18	16	0.7	0.8	0.84
Brain & Other Nerv. Syst.	129	88	5.8	4.4	1.26	95	93	3.3	3.5	0.76
Brain	120	82	5.4	4.4	1.28	89	87	3.3	4.5	0.75
Other Nervous Syst.	9	6	0.4	0.3		6	6	0.2	0.3	0.77
Endocrine System	52	32	2.3	1.7	1.37	108	75	4.0	4.2	1.00
Thyroid	45	21	2.0	1.1	1.83*	100	70	3.7	3.9	0.98
Other Endocrine System	7	11	0.3	0.6	0.53	8	5	0.3	0.3	1.23
Lymphomas	285	252	12.6	12.8	0.97	255	192	8.6	9.1	0.94
Lympho & Retic. Sarc.	137	123	6.1	6.1	1.00	133	109	4.4	4.8	0.88
Hodgkin's Disease	95	76	4.2	4.1	0.99	74	51	2.6	2.8	0.96
Other Lymphomas	53	53	2.4	2.7	0.88	48	32	1.5	1.5	1.08
Multiple Myeloma	95	69	4.2	3.2	1.29	98	63	3.0	2.7	1.12
Leukemia	319	306	13.9	15.1	0.93	265	190	8.2	8.1	0.98
Unknown Primary Site	294	190	13.0	9.0	1.43**	323	198	9.7	8.2	1.16

† * (**) = significantly different from 1.00 at $p < 0.05$ (0.01).

Table 2. Urban-Rural Relative Risks for Selected Primary Sites of Cancer by Age; Males, Iowa and Colorado, 1969-71

Primary Site and State	Number of Cases Urban	Rural	Age-adjusted Inc. Rate Urban	Rural	Summary Relative Risk[†] All Ages	00-24	25-34	35-44	45-54	55-64	65+
All Sites:											
Iowa	7,759	6,102	343.5	293.3	1.17**	0.85	1.34	1.16	1.23**	1.30**	1.13**
Colorado	6,340	1,759	325.6	267.9	1.22**	0.79	2.04**	1.06	1.11	1.40**	1.20**
Buccal Cav. (excl. Lip):											
Iowa	245	155	11.1	7.7	1.46**	--	--	1.35	1.40	1.68**	1.37*
Colorado	188	36	9.4	5.4	1.75**	--	--	0.88	1.40	2.74**	1.58
Lip:											
Iowa	115	170	5.1	8.2	0.63**	--	--	0.56	0.45*	0.51**	0.76
Colorado	85	32	4.3	4.8	0.91	--	--	--	0.30**	1.37	0.81
Esophagus:											
Iowa	100	66	4.3	3.1	1.42*	--	--	--	3.01*	1.87**	1.03
Colorado	78	13	4.0	2.0	2.05*	--	--	--	3.93	2.36	1.54
Stomach:											
Iowa	282	273	12.3	12.8	0.95	--	--	--	0.93	1.09	0.92
Colorado	228	78	11.9	12.1	1.00	--	--	--	1.37	1.56	0.87
Colon excl. Rectum:											
Iowa	780	648	34.4	31.0	1.11*	--	--	1.09	1.04	1.29**	1.09
Colorado	561	128	29.4	19.7	1.49**	--	--	0.76	0.99	1.96**	1.54**
Rectum & Recto. Juct.:											
Iowa	401	334	17.8	15.9	1.12	--	--	1.19	1.42	1.18	1.05
Colorado	254	78	13.1	11.9	1.11	--	--	1.03	1.27	1.20	1.03
Pancreas:											
Iowa	270	216	11.9	10.3	1.16	--	--	--	1.04	1.56*	1.12
Colorado	220	76	11.5	11.5	1.00	--	--	--	1.50	0.76	1.04
Larynx:											
Iowa	188	108	8.6	5.3	1.63*	--	--	--	0.87	1.95**	1.90**
Colorado	137	33	6.9	4.8	1.42	--	--	--	1.09	1.99**	1.48
Lung, Bron. & Trachea:											
Iowa	1,595	1,062	71.8	51.0	1.41**	--	1.42	1.20	1.45**	1.44**	1.40**
Colorado	1,105	325	57.4	48.4	1.18**	--	--	1.15	1.05	1.16	1.23*
Prostate:											
Iowa	1,334	1,169	57.7	54.2	1.06	--	--	--	0.67	1.23	1.05
Colorado	1,343	379	73.2	59.8	1.22**	--	--	--	0.83	1.34*	1.22**
Bladder:											
Iowa	540	417	23.8	19.8	1.20**	--	--	1.03	1.26	1.42*	1.14
Colorado	503	133	26.3	20.6	1.29**	--	--	3.10	1.08	1.57**	1.20
Kidney & Renal Pelvis:											
Iowa	200	162	9.0	7.8	1.13	--	--	0.89	1.40	1.12	1.07
Colorado	170	53	8.6	7.9	1.09	--	--	--	1.62	1.78	0.90
Brain:											
Iowa	120	82	5.4	4.4	1.26	1.36	--	0.72	0.74	1.31	2.19**
Colorado	107	28	4.9	4.0	1.21	0.63	--	0.69	1.19	4.36*	1.33
Lymphomas:											
Iowa	235	252	12.6	12.8	0.97	1.27	1.34	1.76	1.16	0.85	0.83
Colorado	222	61	10.1	9.2	1.13	0.49	1.03	0.77	1.24	1.58	0.91
Leukemia:											
Iowa	319	306	13.9	15.1	0.93	0.53**	0.80	1.17	0.98	1.22	0.97
Colorado	231	75	11.2	11.2	0.99	0.64	--	0.88	0.90	0.71	1.35

[†] Summary Relative Risk

* (**) = significantly different from 1.00 at p < 0.05 (0.01); -- = not shown if based on < 10 cases.

Table 3. Urban-Rural Relative Risks for Selected Primary Sites of Cancer by Age; Females, Iowa and Colorado, 1969-71

Primary Site and State	Number of Cases		Age-adjusted Inc. Rate		Summary Relative Risk [†]						
	Urban	Rural	Urban	Rural	All Ages	00-24	25-34	35-44	45-54	55-64	65+
All Sites:											
Iowa	8,089	5,468	267.8	247.3	1.07**	1.01	1.20	1.05	1.12**	1.14**	1.03
Colorado	6,590	1,439	256.8	216.6	1.19**	1.11	1.31	1.35**	1.10	1.16*	1.21**
Buccal Cav. (excl. Lip):											
Iowa	149	67	5.1	2.9	1.61**	--	--	--	2.03	2.82**	1.21
Colorado	116	22	4.6	3.3	1.38	--	--	--	0.84	2.30	1.25
Stomach:											
Iowa	215	148	5.8	5.9	1.00	--	--	--	0.61	1.12	1.03
Colorado	147	31	5.4	4.8	1.15	--	--	--	0.39	1.18	1.23
Colon excl. Rectum:											
Iowa	1,116	731	33.7	30.9	1.09	--	--	0.91	1.07	1.02	1.12
Colorado	866	150	27.0	23.0	1.18	--	--	1.16	1.34	0.97	1.22
Rectum & Recto. Juct.:											
Iowa	353	251	10.8	10.6	1.00	--	--	1.07	0.97	1.15	0.97
Colorado	202	51	7.7	7.8	0.99	--	--	0.63	0.70	1.77	0.90
Pancreas:											
Iowa	217	144	6.2	5.8	1.06	--	--	--	2.09	0.82	1.04
Colorado	199	46	7.7	7.0	1.09	--	--	--	0.74	1.04	1.23
Lung, Bron. & Trachea:											
Iowa	342	171	11.9	7.7	1.48**	--	--	1.14	1.44	1.92**	1.28
Colorado	287	62	11.4	9.4	1.22	--	--	1.76	1.00	1.04	1.66*
Breast:											
Iowa	2,163	1508	74.2	69.9	1.06	--	1.50	1.17	1.07	1.05	1.02
Colorado	1,904	403	75.5	60.1	1.26*	--	1.35	1.58**	1.20	1.10	1.30**
Cervix Uteri:											
Iowa	478	282	18.2	14.6	1.25**	3.02	1.05	1.15	1.25	1.50*	1.23
Colorado	340	89	13.2	13.1	1.01	--	0.84	1.18	0.79	1.32	1.05
Corpus Uteri:											
Iowa	527	400	18.7	18.9	0.99	--	--	0.89	1.04	1.01	0.98
Colorado	466	104	19.2	15.7	1.22	--	--	1.76	1.26	1.11	1.24
Ovary:											
Iowa	428	296	15.1	14.1	1.07	0.85	3.49*	1.18	0.86	1.07	1.12
Colorado	365	87	14.4	13.0	1.11	1.11	1.35	0.79	1.05	1.73*	0.93
Bladder:											
Iowa	202	105	6.0	4.1	1.35*	--	--	--	4.35*	2.15*	1.13
Colorado	160	31	6.1	4.8	1.28	--	--	--	0.95	1.22	1.31
Kidney & Renal Pelvis:											
Iowa	110	88	3.6	3.9	0.91	1.27	--	--	0.99	1.00	0.84
Colorado	97	21	3.8	3.2	1.19	--	--	--	1.03	0.84	1.16
Brain:											
Iowa	89	87	3.3	4.5	0.75	0.49**	1.07	0.57	0.60	0.67	1.23
Colorado	92	19	3.6	2.8	1.32	∞ **	--	0.28	0.79	1.62	0.95
Lymphomas:											
Iowa	255	192	8.6	9.1	0.94	1.26	0.70	0.94	1.19	0.89	0.89
Colorado	195	39	7.5	5.9	1.28	1.56	1.94	0.84	2.24	1.36	1.08
Leukemia:											
Iowa	265	190	8.2	8.1	0.98	1.47	--	0.87	2.09	0.91	0.90
Colorado	223	50	8.5	7.5	1.13	0.98	0.64	2.79	0.97	1.34	1.19

[†] = Summary Relative Risk

* (**) = significantly different from 1.00 at p < 0.05 (0.01); -- = not shown if based on < 10 cases.

Iowa (all ages) and in Colorado at ages 45-54; and 2) for leukemia in Iowa at ages under 25.

Among women (Table 3), significantly elevated summary relative risks (all ages) were observed in Iowa for the following cancers: 1) cervix uteri; 2) lung, bronchus and trachea; 3) bladder; and 4) buccal cavity and pharynx (excluding lip). Only for breast cancer was the risk for urban women in Colorado significantly elevated. The only increased risk among rural residents was for brain cancer at ages under 25 in Iowa. In direct constrast, 30 urban residents and no rural residents of this age in Colorado developed brain cancer during the years 1969-71.

For some sites of cancer, incidence rates for Iowa and Colorado residents were much lower than rates for residents of the other seven metropolitan areas that participated in the Third National Cancer Survey (1). This was usually due to the low rates among rural residents of these states (Tables 2 and 3). Differences in rates among residents of large cities in Iowa and Colorado compared to residents of small cities in these states are also of interest. Incidence rates for subgroups of the urban population in Iowa and Colorado and, for comparison purposes, rates for the other TNCS participants, are presented for selected primary sites in Figures 3 to 11.

For each primary site, the average annual age-adjusted (1970 standard) incidence rates for white males (M) and females (F) in the entire Third National Cancer Survey (TNCS) are shown by the first two bars (one bar for sex-specific analyses). Within the TNCS bars, the rates for each of the nine areas that participated in the survey are shown as points with only rates for Iowa (IA) and Colorado (CO) specifically identified. Iowa and then Colorado rates are shown for three residence subgroups: urban, inside urbanized areas (IUA); urban, outside urbanized areas (OUA); and rural. Within the 'Urban IUA' bars, the rates for the seven urbanized areas in Iowa [Des Moines (DM), Cedar Rapids (CR), Davenport (DA), Waterloo (WA), Sioux City (SC), Council Bluffs (CB), and Dubuque (DU)] and the four in Colorado [Denver (DE), Colorado Springs (CS), Pueblo (PU), and Boulder (BO)] are shown as points with high rate urbanized areas specifically identified. Few pronounced trends in rates by size-of-place were observed for urban residents living outside urbanized areas so no specific points are presented within the 'Urban OUA' bars. Within the 'Rural' bars, the rates for each strata formed on the basis of the farm/nonfarm ratios are shown as points with only the two strata having the highest concentration of farmers (F) specifically identified.

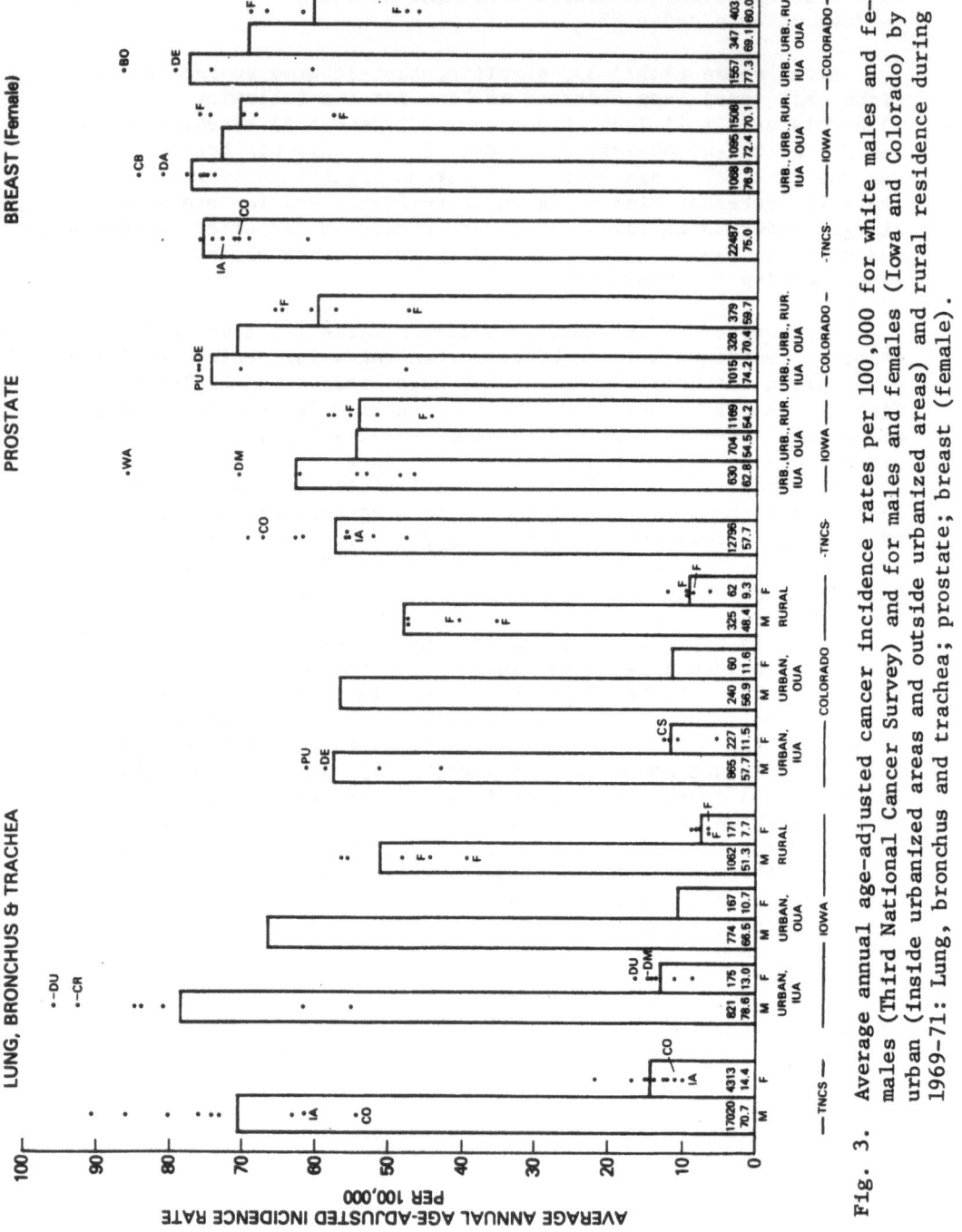

Fig. 3. Average annual age-adjusted cancer incidence rates per 100,000 for white males and females (Third National Cancer Survey) and for males and females (Iowa and Colorado) by
urban (inside urbanized areas and outside urbanized areas) and rural residence during
1969-71: Lung, bronchus and trachea; prostate; breast (female).

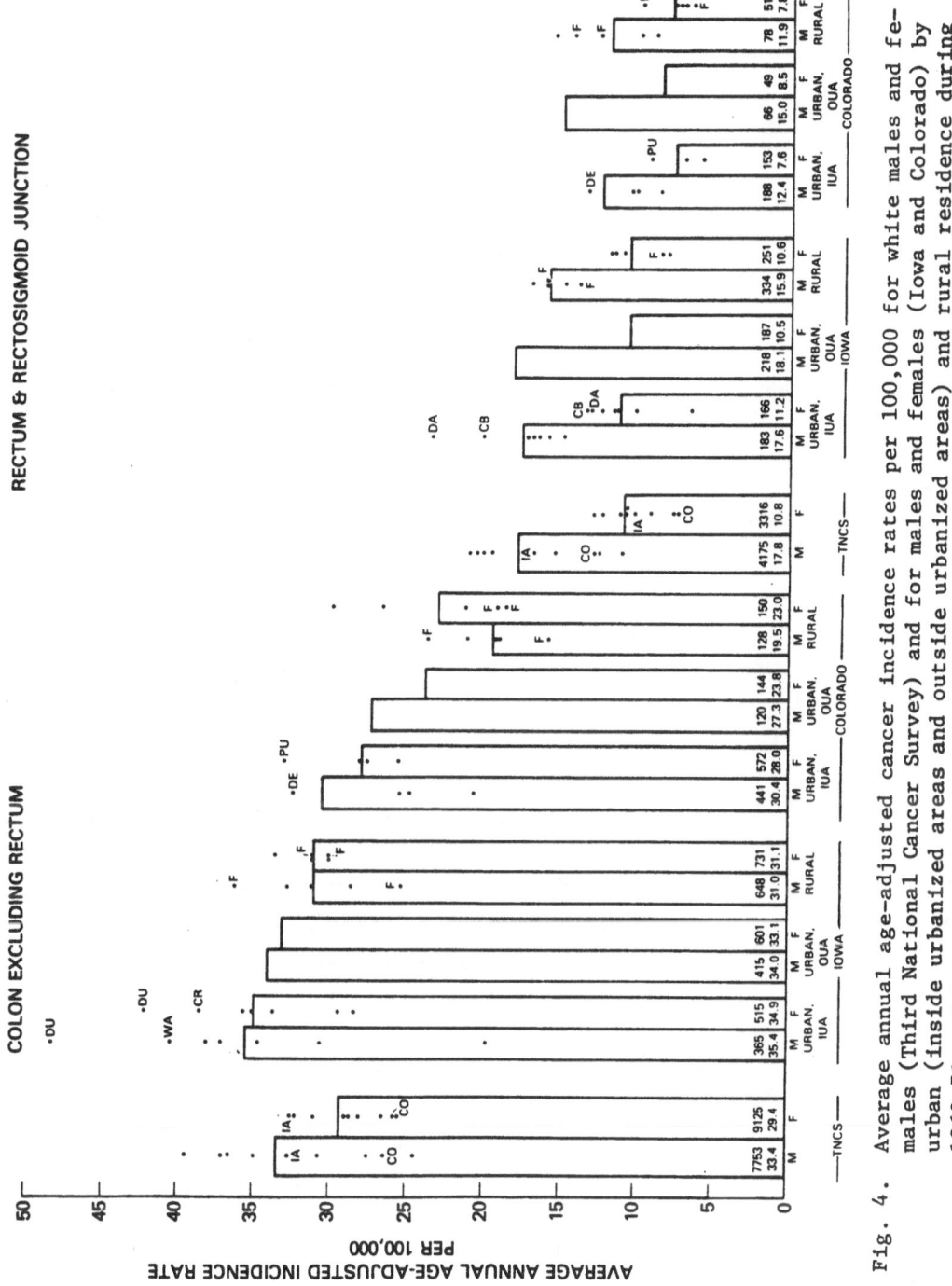

Fig. 4. Average annual age-adjusted cancer incidence rates per 100,000 for white males and females (Third National Cancer Survey) and for males and females (Iowa and Colorado) by urban (inside urbanized areas and outside urbanized areas) and rural residence during 1969-71: Colon, excluding rectum; rectum and rectosigmoid junction.

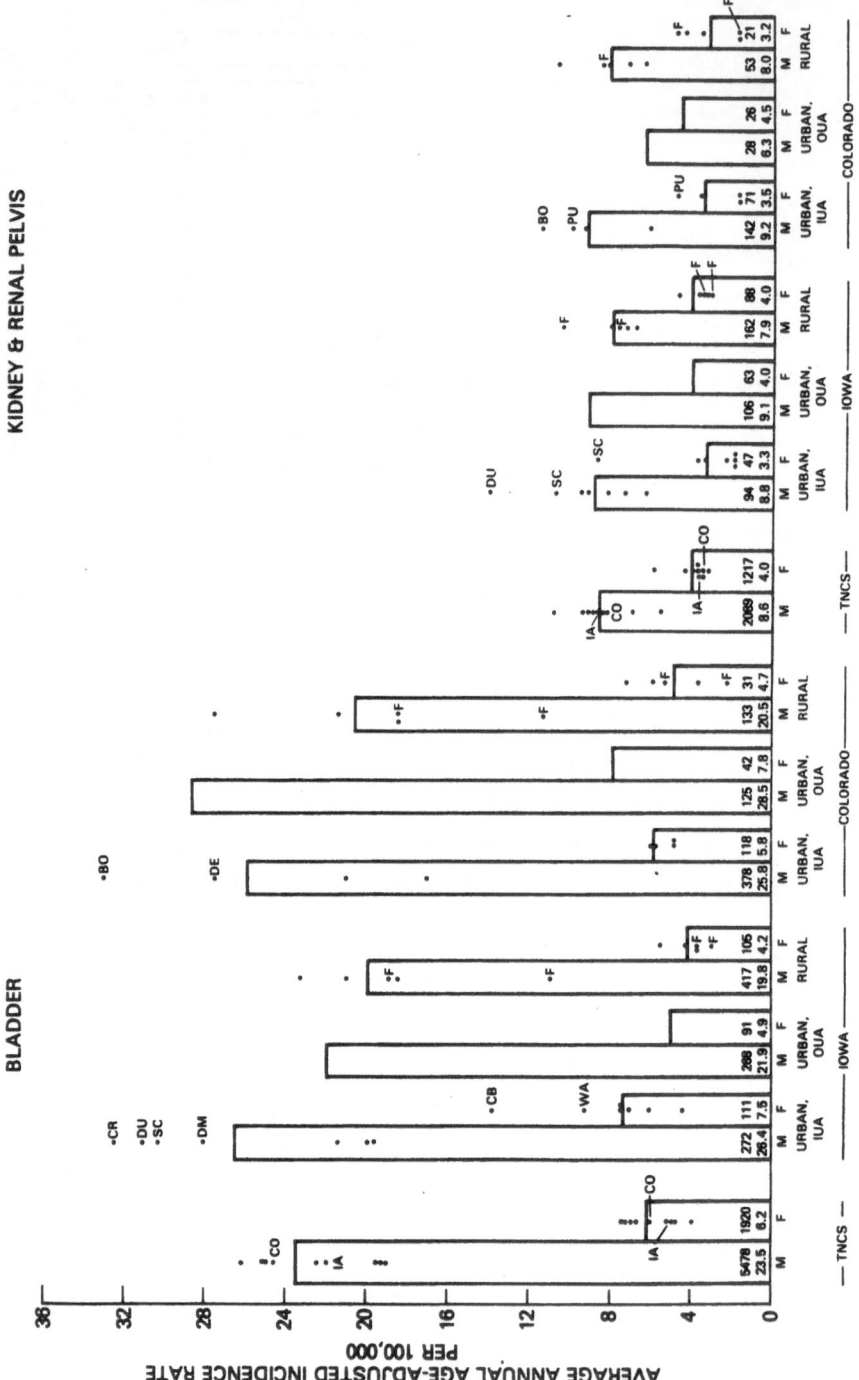

Fig. 5. Average annual age-adjusted cancer incidence rates per 100,000 for white males and females (Third National Cancer Survey) and for males and females (Iowa and Colorado) by
urban (inside urbanized areas and outside urbanized areas) and rural residence during
1969-71: Bladder; kidney and renal pelvis.

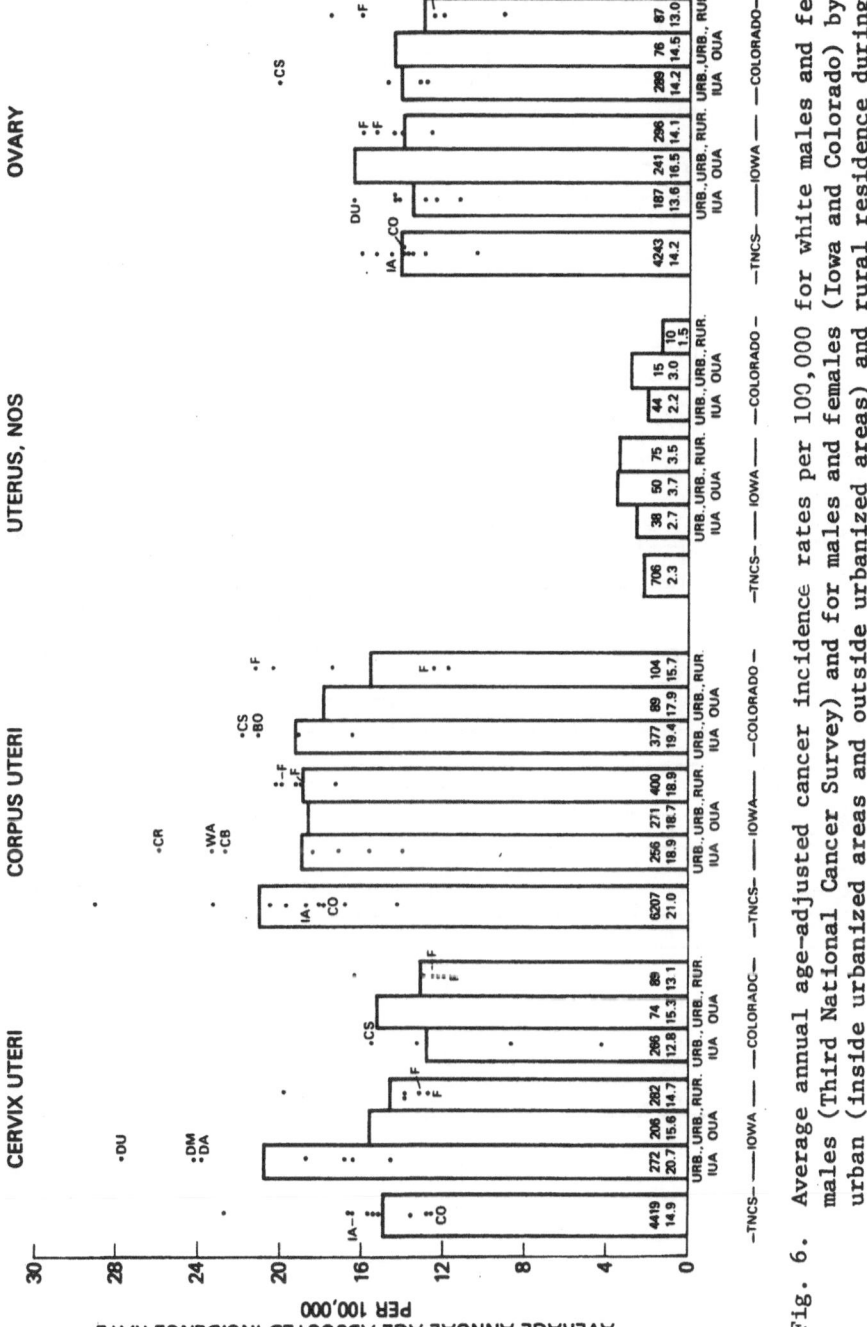

Fig. 6. Average annual age-adjusted cancer incidence rates per 100,000 for white males and females (Third National Cancer Survey) and for males and females (Iowa and Colorado) by urban (inside urbanized areas and outside urbanized areas) and rural residence during 1969-71: Cervix uteri; corpus uteri; uterus, not otherwise specified; ovary.

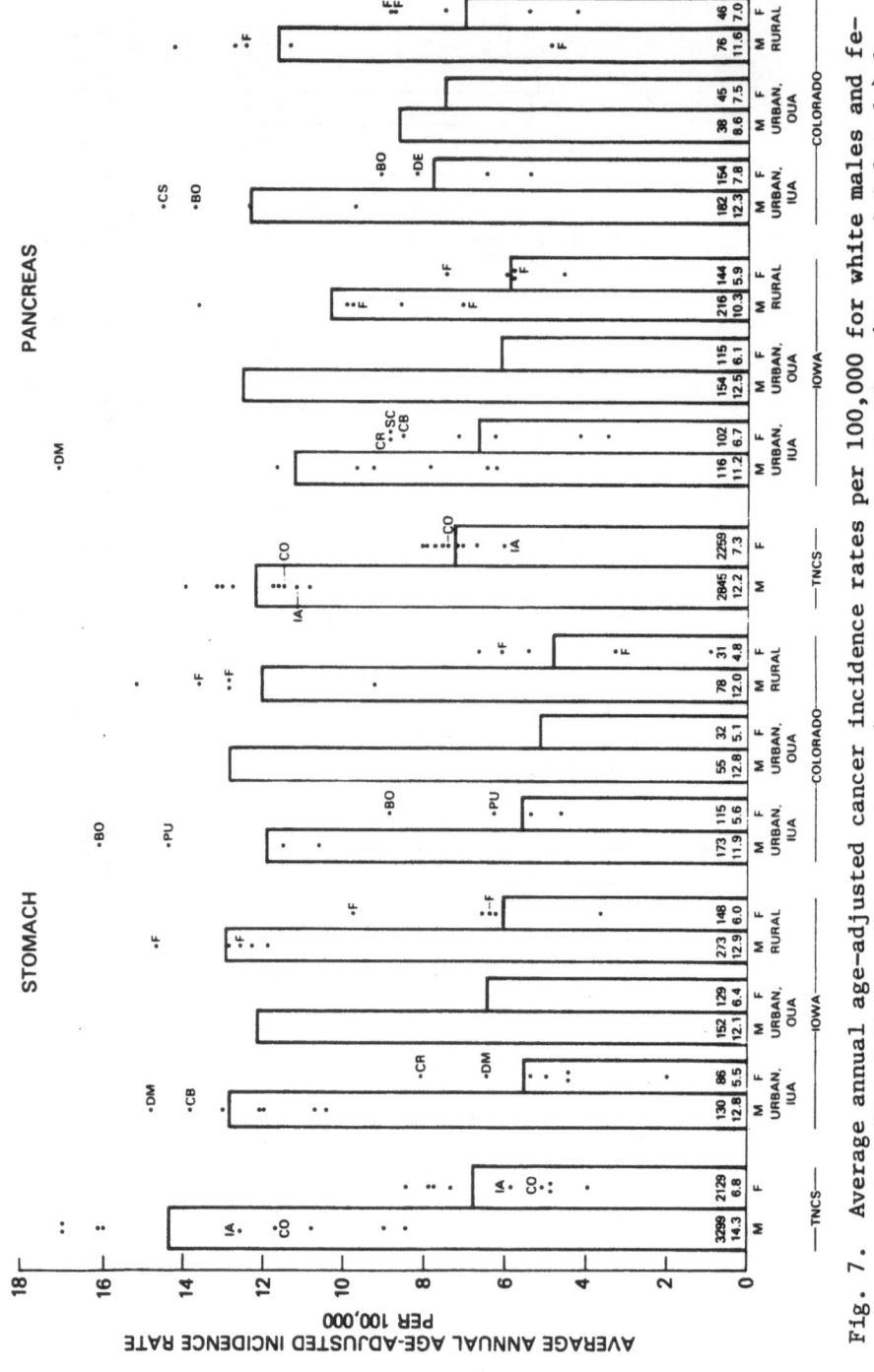

Fig. 7. Average annual age-adjusted cancer incidence rates per 100,000 for white males and females (Third National Cancer Survey) and for males and females (Iowa and Colorado) by
urban (inside urbanized areas and outside urbanized areas) and rural residence during
1969-71: Stomach; pancreas.

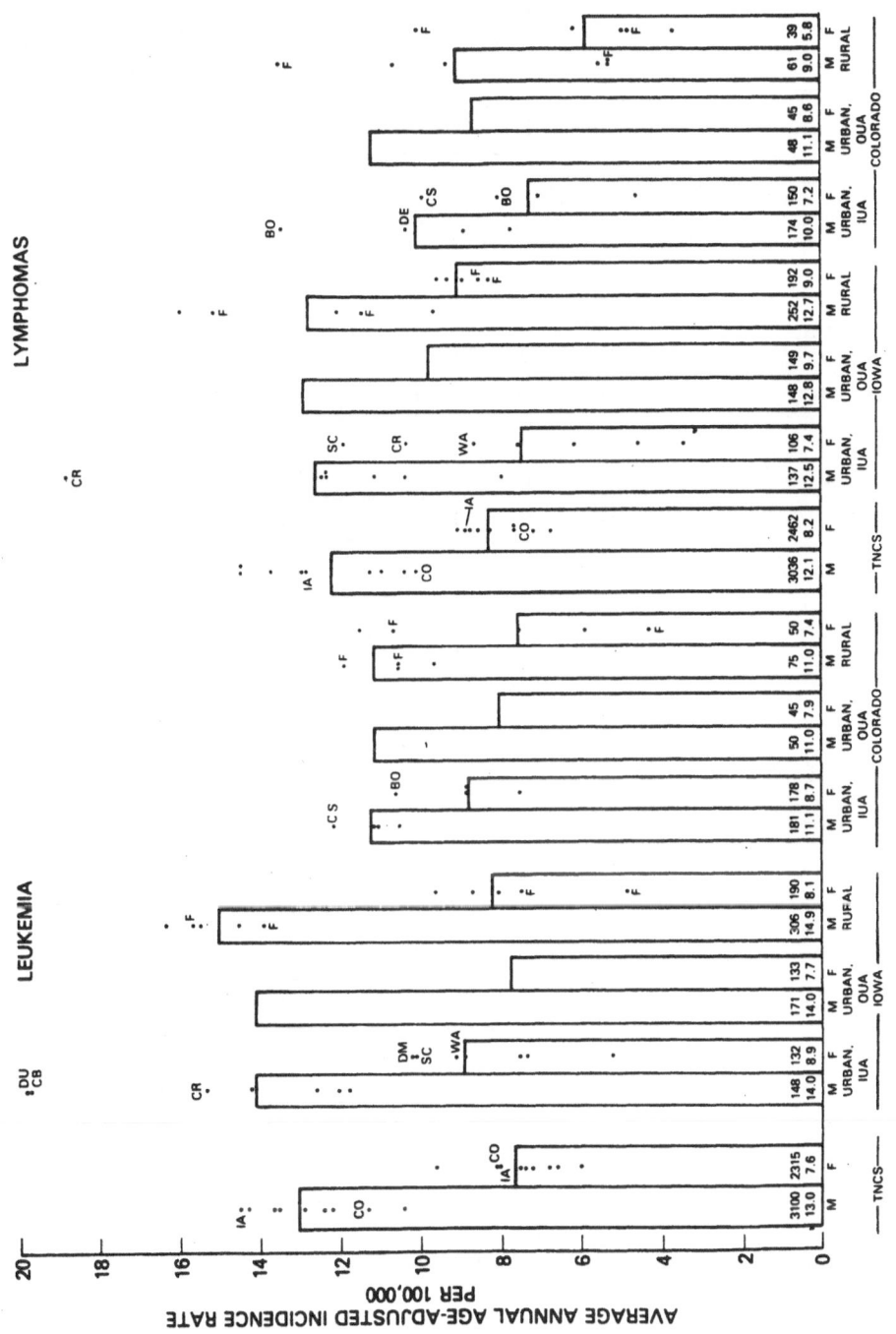

Fig. 8. Average annual age-adjusted cancer incidence rates per 100,000 for white males and females (Third National Cancer Survey) and for males and females (Iowa and Colorado) by
urban (inside urbanized areas and outside urbanized areas) and rural residence during
1969-71: Leukemia; lymphoma.

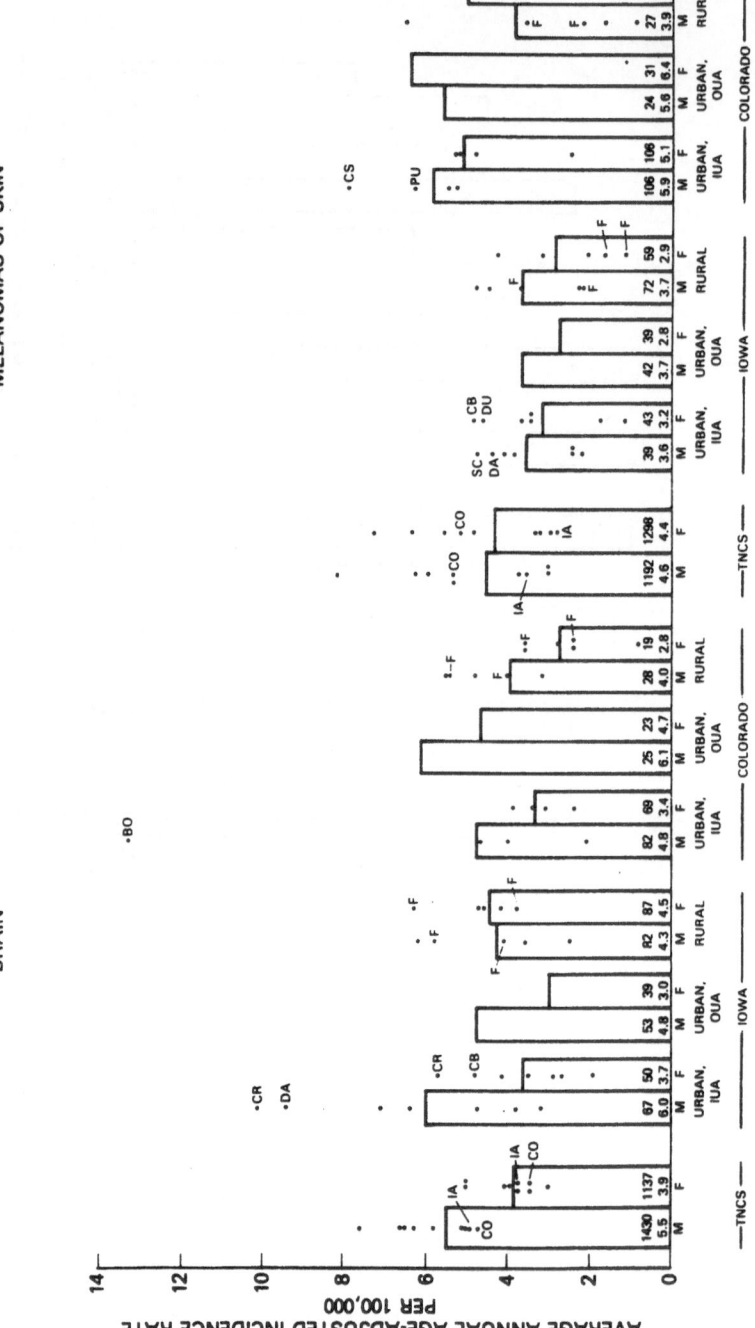

Fig. 9. Average annual age-adjusted cancer incidence rates per 100,000 for white males and females (Third National Cancer Survey) and for males and females (Iowa and Colorado) by
urban (inside urbanized areas and outside urbanized areas) and rural residence during
1969-71: Brain; melanomas of skin.

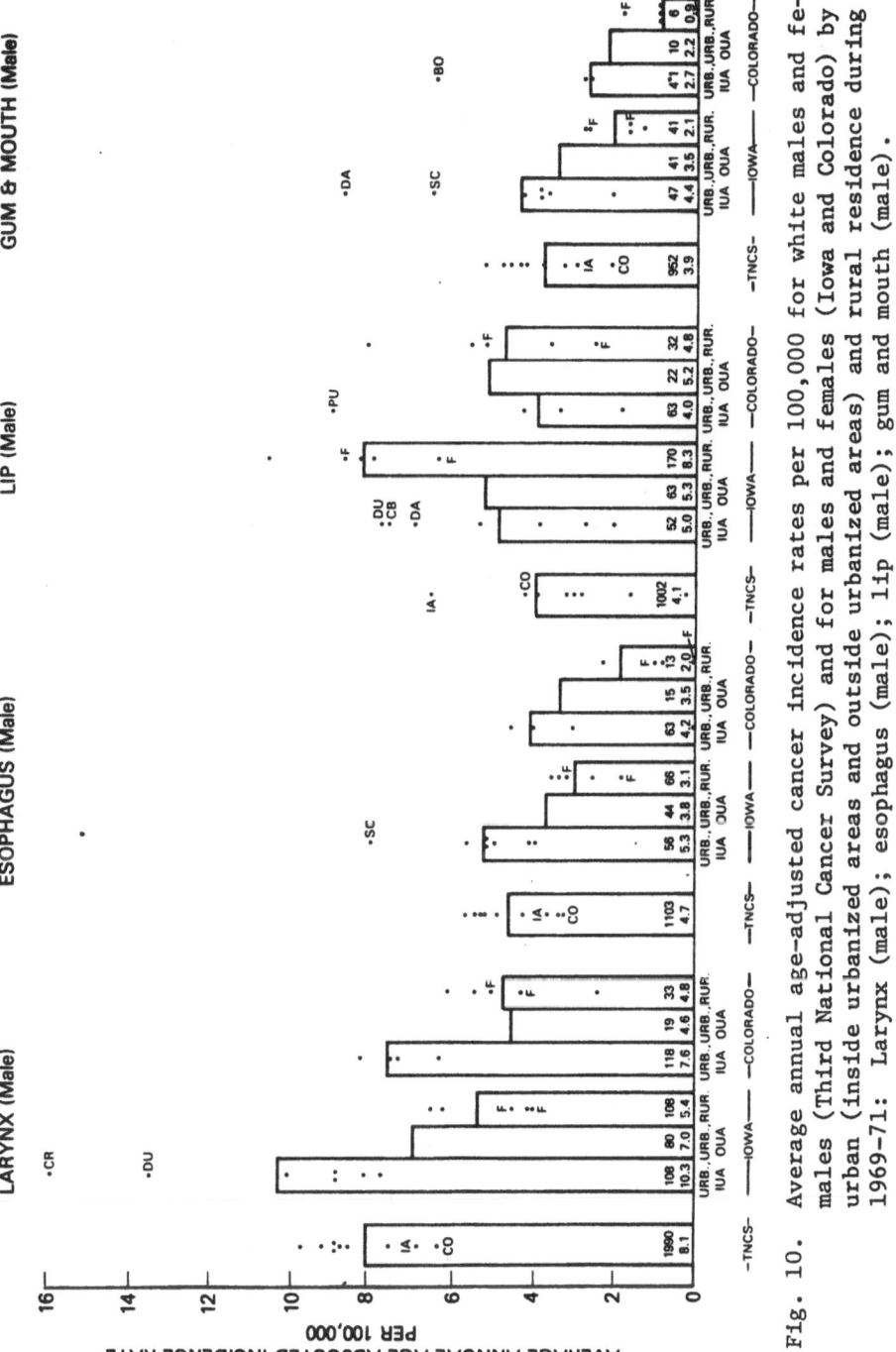

Fig. 10. Average annual age-adjusted cancer incidence rates per 100,000 for white males and females (Third National Cancer Survey) and for males and females (Iowa and Colorado) by
urban (inside urbanized areas and outside urbanized areas) and rural residence during
1969-71: Larynx (male); esophagus (male); lip (male); gum and mouth (male).

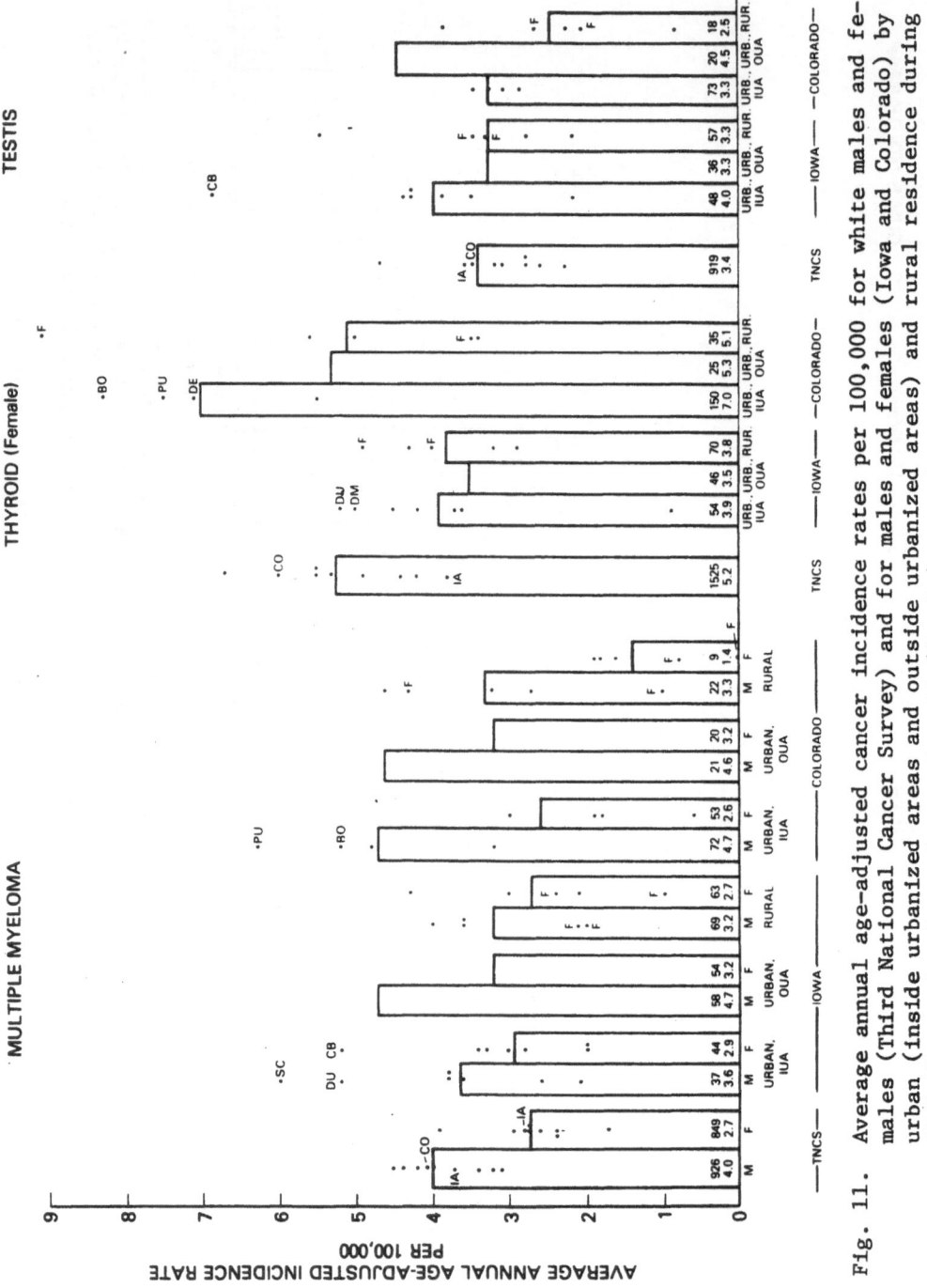

Fig. 11. Average annual age-adjusted cancer incidence rates per 100,000 for white males and females (Third National Cancer Survey) and for males and females (Iowa and Colorado) by urban (inside urbanized areas and outside urbanized areas) and rural residence during 1969-71: Multiple myeloma; thyroid (female); testis.

Lung, bronchus and trachea. Overall rates in Iowa and
Colorado were the lowest of all the participants in the TNCS (Fig.
3). In both states, rates among rural residents were significantly
less than among urban residents; rural residents of counties having
the highest concentration of farmers had the lowest rates of all.
The low rank of Colorado among the TNCS participants was also due
to the relatively low rates for this disease in both large and
small cities of that state.

Prostate. Colorado men had high rates for this disease and
would have ranked at the top of all TNCS participants if only urban
residents of that state were considered in the ranking (Fig. 3).
Urban-rural relative risks were significantly different in Colorado
but not in Iowa; in Iowa, the rate among residents of small cities
was low and no different from that among rural residents while in
Colorado, the rate among residents of small cities was more like
the high rate for residents of large cities.

Breast (female). A consistent rate gradient from high among
urban residents of large cities, to lower among urban residents of
smaller cities, to the lowest among rural residents was evident
among women of both Iowa and Colorado (Fig. 3). However, the
gradient was much stronger in Colorado than in Iowa. Breast cancer
incidence rates among all urban residents of the two states were
similar; the rural rate was significantly less than the urban rate
in Colorado but the urban-rural difference was not significant in
Iowa.

Colon excluding rectum. As for breast cancer, a consistent
rate gradient was observed for colon cancer; the gradient was
stronger in Colorado than in Iowa (Fig. 4). Incidence rates were
much lower in Colorado than in Iowa within each residence
category. Sex differences in colon cancer incidence rates were
smaller in these two states than to those for most other
participants of the TNCS, especially in Iowa. Rates among Iowa
women were the highest of any TNCS participant.

Rectum and rectosigmoid junction. Urban-rural differences in
risk were minimal; there was a tendency for urban residents of
small cities to have the highest rates (Fig. 4). Rates were low in
Colorado, especially among women, compared to other TNCS
participants, but this cannot be explained by urban-rural
differences.

Urinary system. The high rates among residents of small
cities in Colorado and the low rates among rural residents of both
Iowa and Colorado (especially in counties with high concentrations
of farmers) are prominent features of bladder cancer (Fig. 5).
Differences in urban-rural relative risks were statistically
significant for men in both states and for women in Iowa.   In

contrast to bladder cancer, urban-rural differences were minimal
for cancer of the kidney and renal pelvis.

Female genital system. Cervix cancer incidence rates were
high among residents of large cities in Iowa but not in Colorado
(Fig. 6). Urban-rural differences for corpus cancer were virtually
absent in Iowa while a moderate rate gradient was seen in
Colorado. The ovarian cancer incidence rate was relatively high
among urban residents of small cities in Iowa.

Stomach and Pancreas. No consistent patterns were seen for
these sites (Fig. 7). The low incidence rate for pancreatic cancer
among women in Iowa cannot be solely explained by urban-rural
differences.

Leukemia. No strong gradient in rates with type of residence
was observed for leukemia (Fig. 8). The high incidence rates among
men in Iowa and the low rates among men in Colorado cannot be
explained by urban-rural differences.

Lymphomas. Residents of small cities in both Iowa and
Colorado had somewhat higher rates for this disease than residents
of large cities or rural residents (Fig. 8). Overall urban-rural
differences were not remarkable and they cannot account for the low
lymphoma rates in Colorado.

Urban and rural incidence rates for several less common cancer
sites are shown in Figures 9 to 11; although the rates for most
Iowa and Colorado subgroups were based on very small numbers, some
patterns are worthy of comment. Urban-rural differences were not
large for melanomas of skin, especially in Iowa, and they cannot
account for the low rates of this disease in that state (Fig. 9).
In contrast, the low rates for laryngeal and esophageal cancer
among male residents of both Iowa and Colorado can be largely
attributed to the low rates among their rural residents (Fig.
10). Rural male residents of Iowa, but not Colorado, had a
significantly increased risk for lip cancer (Fig. 10). A
consistent gradient in rates -- highest among residents of large
cities to lowest among rural residents -- was observed for cancer
of the gum and mouth among men of both states (Fig. 10). Residents
of small cities tended to have high rates of multiple myeloma (Fig.
11). The low rate for thyroid cancer among women in Iowa cannot be
explained by urban-rural differences; rates were high in Colorado,
especially so among female residents of large cities (Fig. 11).

Change in Iowa Cancer Rates Between 1950 and 1969-71

Sex- and age-specific incidence rates and relative risks for
cancer (all sites excluding skin cancer) among urban and rural
residents of Iowa for 1950 and 1969-71 are shown in Table 4. Among

Table 4. Urban and Rural Incidence Rates and Relative Risks for Cancer (all sites combined excluding skin cancer) by Sex and Age; Iowa, 1950 and 1969-71

Sex, Type of Residence and Age	Number of Cases		Ave. Annual Incidence Rate per 100,000		Relative Risk[†]	
	1950[‡]	1969-71	1950[‡]	1969-71	1950[‡]	1969-71
Males:						
Urban:						
0-14	32 (25)	96	20.7 (16.2)	14.0	1.59 (0.98)	0.92
15-29	39 (32)	139	28.1 (23.0)	23.6	2.11** (1.26)	1.07
30-44	122 (107)	286	99.8 (87.5)	76.9	1.65** (1.22)	1.15
45-59	440 (440)	1506	429.8 (429.8)	431.7	1.53** (1.53)**	1.26**
60-74	806 (806)	3325	1193.8 (1193.8)	1471.2	1.40** (1.40)**	1.23**
75+	456 (445)	2326	2264.5 (2209.9)	2519.4	1.09 (1.04)	1.05
Total[±]	1895 (1855)	7678	276.5 (270.0)	301.1	1.35** (1.29)**	1.17**
Rural:						
0-14	27 (34)	84	13.1 (16.4)	15.2		
15-29	19 (26)	79	13.3 (18.2)	22.0		
30-44	82 (97)	189	60.5 (71.6)	66.9		
45-59	327 (327)	1062	281.1 (281.1)	343.1		
60-74	670 (670)	2626	852.9 (852.9)	1191.7		
75+	516 (527)	1990	2084.7 (2129.1)	2408.3		
Total[±]	1641 (1681)	6030	200.9 (206.5)	255.8		
Females:						
Urban:						
0-14	25 (19)	63	16.8 (12.7)	9.6	2.05 (1.13)	0.97
15-29	53 (53)	184	35.1 (35.1)	29.1	1.31 (1.31)	1.22
30-44	266 (245)	599	205.2 (189.0)	153.9	1.64** (1.33)**	1.06
45-59	680 (640)	1873	613.5 (577.4)	486.6	1.23** (1.08)	1.11**
60-74	807 (807)	2895	1039.3 (1039.3)	938.9	1.14* (1.14)*	1.12**
75+	491 (461)	2393	1811.0 (1700.4)	1443.7	1.28** (1.10)	0.99
Total[±]	2322 (2225)	8007	303.6 (290.3)	249.4	1.25** (1.14)**	1.07**
Rural:						
0-14	16 (22)	52	8.2 (11.3)	9.9		
15-29	36 (36)	85	26.8 (26.8)	24.0		
30-44	163 (184)	418	125.5 (141.7)	144.6		
45-59	540 (580)	1360	498.5 (535.5)	437.4		
60-74	664 (664)	1920	909.9 (909.9)	841.0		
75+	348 (378)	1574	1417.6 (1539.8)	1450.9		
Total[±]	1767 (1864)	5409	240.7 (254.2)	229.0		

[†] * (**) = significantly different from 1.00 at p < 0.05 (0.01).

[‡] ( ) = Adjusted for the over-reporting of urban residence in 1950 (see Appendix).

[±] Incidence rates are age-adjusted (1950 U.S. standard).

men, incidence rates increased over time for urban residents aged 60 and older and for rural residents aged 45 and older. Increases over time were greater for rural residents and the relative risks decreased between 1950 and 1970. Among women, incidence rates decreased at nearly all ages for both urban and rural residents. Decreases over time were greater for urban residents and the relative risks decreased between 1950 and 1970.

Urban-rural relative risks in 1950 were higher than in 1970 due in part to the more likely misclassification of some rural cases in the 1950 survey; it was not possible to systematically check the reported address of cancer cases against census tract maps or street maps to the extent this was done in the 1969-71 survey. A crude method for adjusting the 1950 data for this

probable bias is presented in the Appendix and the results of this
exercise are shown by the figures in parentheses in Table 4. The
adjustment reduced the difference between 1950 and 1970 relative
risks (particularly so at young ages) but the risks for urban
residents generally remain greater in 1950 than in 1970 even after
this adjustment.

Changes in cancer incidence between 1950 and 1970 are
presented for selected primary sites in Table 5. The increased
incidence for all cancer sites combined among men in Iowa was
primarily due to the large increase in lung cancer while the
decreased incidence among women was primarily due to decreases in
cancers of the cervix and stomach. These patterns were similar to
those seen in the large cancer surveys in the U.S. (8). For most
cancer sites, if the incidence was increasing, it increased more
among rural residents of Iowa and if it was decreasing, it
decreased less among rural residents. One unexpected finding was
the large increase for tumors of lymphatic tissue among rural men
and women.

Recent Changes in Iowa Cancer Rates

SEER data from Iowa were analyzed to see if the changes in
incidence between 1950 and 1970 for tumors of lymphatic tissue
persisted during more recent years. Changes in Iowa cancer rates
between 1969 and 1978 (1972 excluded) were examined for pseudo
urban-rural subgroups of the population (residents of highly rural
counties, highly urban counties, and the remaining suburban
counties). These findings are summarized in Tables 6 and 7.
Incidence rates during the years 1969-71, 1973-75 and 1976-78 are
presented for multiple myeloma, Hodgkin's disease, the remaining
lymphomas (non-Hodgkin's lymphomas), and (for comparison purposes)
leukemia.

No significant changes over recent years occurred in the
incidence of Hodgkin's disease among Iowa men in any of the
residence subgroups (Table 6). Among women less than 35 years of
age, Hodgkin's disease incidence increased (significantly for urban
women), while at older ages incidence decreased (significantly for
suburban women 65 years of age and older). For the non-Hodgkin's
lymphomas, significant increases in incidence at ages 65 and older
were observed among female residents of rural counties and male
residents of urban counties.

Incidence rates for multiple myeloma increased to a greater
extent among rural residents than among other residence subgroups
(Table 7). A significant trend was observed for males 35-64 years
of age residing in rural counties. Overall changes for leukemia
were not remarkable although a significant increase in disease
incidence occurred among young rural women.

Table 5. Age-adjusted (1950 U.S. Standard) Cancer Incidence Rates
for Selected Primary Sites by Sex; U.S. Surveys (1948/49
and 1969-71), Urban and Rural Iowa (1950 and 1969-71)

Primary Site and Area	Males Circa 1950	1969-71	% Change	Primary Site and Area	Females Circa 1950	1969-71	% Change
Lung, bronchus and trachea				Lung, bronchus and trachea			
U.S. Surveys	29.5	68.0	+ 131	U.S. Surveys	6.7	14.9	+ 122
Urban Iowa	(29.9)	65.4	+ 119	Urban Iowa	(8.1)	11.2	+ 38
Rural Iowa	(10.7)	46.8	+ 337	Rural Iowa	(6.3)	7.1	+ 13
Colon excluding rectum				Colon excluding rectum			
U.S. Surveys	23.8	29.0	+ 22	U.S. Surveys	26.0	24.8	- 5
Urban Iowa	25.4	29.6	+ 17	Urban Iowa	28.3	29.4	+ 4
Rural Iowa	17.4	26.8	+ 54	Rural Iowa	23.3	26.6	+ 14
Rectum and recto. junct.				Rectum and recto. junct.			
U.S. Surveys	20.7	16.0	- 23	U.S. Surveys	13.9	9.6	- 31
Urban Iowa	16.3	15.7	- 4	Urban Iowa	10.0	9.5	- 5
Rural Iowa	12.4	13.8	+ 11	Rural Iowa	11.0	9.2	- 16
Stomach				Stomach			
U.S. Surveys	32.4	12.1	- 63	U.S. Surveys	17.8	5.8	- 67
Urban Iowa	24.7	10.2	- 59	Urban Iowa	13.1	4.7	- 64
Rural Iowa	24.7	10.7	- 57	Rural Iowa	14.1	4.9	- 65
Pancreas				Pancreas			
U.S. Surveys	8.9	10.7	+ 20	U.S. Surveys	5.6	6.5	+ 16
Urban Iowa	9.0	10.3	+ 14	Urban Iowa	5.7	5.2	+ 9
Rural Iowa	5.1	8.7	+ 71	Rural Iowa	4.4	4.8	+ 9
Lymphomas incl. mult. myeloma				Lymphomas incl. mult. myeloma			
U.S. Surveys	(12.0)	(16.7)	+ 39	U.S. Surveys	(7.6)	(11.3)	+ 49
Urban Iowa	12.2	15.6	+ 28	Urban Iowa	7.2	10.7	+ 49
Rural Iowa	6.1	14.5	+ 138	Rural Iowa	5.5	11.1	+ 102
Leukemia				Leukemia			
U.S. Surveys	9.0	11.0	+ 22	U.S. Surveys	6.9	6.7	- 3
Urban Iowa	(14.4)	12.1	- 16	Urban Iowa	(10.9)	7.3	- 33
Rural Iowa	(11.4)	13.2	+ 16	Rural Iowa	(7.2)	7.1	- 1
Prostate				Breast			
U.S. Surveys	37.4	45.2	+ 21	U.S. Surveys	73.6	73.3	- 0
Urban Iowa	37.8	46.6	+ 23	Urban Iowa	78.0	70.6	- 9
Rural Iowa	34.2	42.8	+ 25	Rural Iowa	62.4	66.3	+ 6
Bladder				Cervix			
U.S. Surveys	17.2	21.3	+ 24	U.S. Surveys	38.3	15.1	- 61
Urban Iowa	20.2	20.6	+ 2	Urban Iowa	46.8	19.3	- 59
Rural Iowa	12.9	16.8	+ 30	Rural Iowa	26.4	15.6	- 41
Kidney and other urinary				Corpus and uterus NOS			
U.S. Surveys	5.6	8.4	+ 50	U.S. Surveys	22.9	23.2	+ 1
Urban Iowa	4.9	9.4	+ 92	Urban Iowa	21.2	20.8	- 2
Rural Iowa	3.6	7.6	+ 111	Rural Iowa	17.3	21.4	+ 24

Rates shown in parentheses are not entirely comparable to others for that site: Iowa rates for "lung, bronchus and trachea" in 1950 do not include cancers of the trachea; U.S. survey rates for "lymphomas including multiple myeloma" include lymphomas of specific organs other than lymphatic tissue; Iowa rates for "leukemia" in 1950 include all cancers of the spleen.

Relatively high rates for the various lymphomas among residents of suburban counties were observed during 1969-71 but this pattern was not sustained in subsequent years.

DISCUSSION

Urban-rural differences in risk for cancer of some primary sites were observed in analyses of data from Iowa and Colorado, 1969-71. Excess risks for urban residents over rural residents were the most common finding in this study as in others (2,9,10). Interpretation of differences in risk is made difficult due to the

Table 6. Time Trends in Hodgkin's and Non-Hodgkin's Lymphoma
Incidence Rates by Sex and Age for Residents of "Rural",
"Suburban", and "Urban" Counties in Iowa, 1969-78

Primary Site, Type of County, and Age	Males						Females					
	No. of Cases			Age-adjusted Rate[†]			No. of Cases			Age-adjusted Rate[†]		
	1969 -71	1973 -75	1976 -78	1969 -71	1973 -75	1976 -78	1969 -71	1973 -75	1976 -78	1969 -71	1973 -75	1976 -78
Hodgkin's Disease:												
'Rural':												
<35	12	14	16	2.7	2.7	2.9	8	10	14	1.8	2.0	2.7
35-64	14	11	12	4.2	3.4	4.0	6	6	1	1.8	1.9	0.3
65+	13	9	9	9.9	6.8	6.8	11	8	5	6.3	4.2	2.6
Total	39	34	37	3.9	3.4	3.6	25	24	20	2.2	2.2	1.9
'Suburb.':												
<35	36	35	28	3.6	3.3	2.4	23	19	29	2.3	1.8	2.7
35-64	29	14	18	5.5	2.6	3.5	16	13	15	2.9	2.3	2.9
65+	18	15	19	9.3	7.9	10.1	19	16	8	6.8	5.8	3.0*
Total	83	64	65	4.7	3.5	3.5	58	48	52	3.0	2.4	2.8
'Urban':												
<35	12	32	23	1.4	3.3	2.2	13	20	34	1.4	2.0	3.3**
35-64	27	36	17	6.3	8.1	3.8	15	12	7	3.2	2.5	1.5
65+	10	10	6	8.5	8.6	5.0	14	9	9	7.8	5.0	4.9
Total	49	78	46	3.7	5.4	3.0	42	41	50	2.6	2.5	2.9
Non-Hodgkin's Lymphoma:												
'Rural':												
<35	8	9	7	1.7	1.7	1.3	2	6	6	0.4	1.2	1.2
35-64	28	39	35	8.5	11.5	10.6	32	33	42	9.1	9.5	12.2
65+	56	49	57	42.2	37.2	43.8	49	46	95	28.4	26.2	51.2**
Total	92	97	99	7.9	8.4	8.5	83	85	143	6.0	6.3	9.6*
'Suburb.':												
<35	12	14	9	1.2	1.3	0.9	8	11	11	0.8	1.0	1.1
35-64	76	54	78	14.0	10.0	14.5	62	51	52	10.8	8.8	9.1
65+	75	85	80	38.8	44.4	42.3	82	73	103	29.7	26.4	35.4
Total	163	153	167	9.0	8.4	9.3	152	135	166	6.9	6.0	7.0
'Urban':												
<35	14	13	11	1.6	1.3	1.1	7	8	7	0.8	0.9	0.7
35-64	60	48	58	13.9	10.9	13.0	34	46	41	7.3	9.6	8.5
65+	37	46	63	31.7	38.6	52.8*	46	71	66	24.5	37.2	34.4
Total	111	107	132	8.5	8.1	10.0	87	125	114	5.2	7.2	6.5

[†] Age-adjusted rate (1970 U.S. standard); * (**) = trend significant at p < 0.05 (0.01).

likely influence of uncontrolled factors. The effects of biasing
factors such as better access to the medical care system for urban
residents, more complete ascertainment of cancer cases in urban
areas, errors in residency determination, in- and out-of-state
migration, and internal migration from rural to urban areas of
people in failing health are particularly difficult to evaluate
(2,9-11). However, differences between urban and rural residents
in cigarette smoking habits, alcohol consumption, and occupational
exposure to carcinogens are more likely to account for the excess
urban risks for mouth, pharynx, lung, larynx, esophagus, and
bladder cancer. Whether urban-rural differences in exposure to
these factors can explain all of the excess urban risk found for
these sites (in particular, lung cancer) has been argued pro (12)

Table 7. Time Trends in Multiple Myeloma and Leukemia Incidence
Rates by Sex and Age for Residents of "Rural", "Suburban",
and "Urban" Counties in Iowa, 1969-78

Primary Site, Type of County, and Age	Males						Females					
	No. of Cases			Age-adjusted Rate†			No. of Cases			Age-adjusted Rate†		
	1969 -71	1973 -75	1976 -78	1969 -71	1973 -75	1976 -78	1969 -71	1973 -75	1976 -78	1969 -71	1973 -75	1976 -78
Multiple Myeloma:												
'Rural':												
<35	0	0	1	0.0	0.0	0.2	0	0	0	0.0	0.0	0.0
35-64	10	12	22	2.8	3.6	6.4*	11	10	18	3.2	2.7	5.0
65+	30	49	36	22.6	37.0	27.3	29	40	38	17.8	22.8	20.6
Total	40	61	59	3.1	4.8	4.8*	40	50	56	2.8	3.1	3.6
'Suburb.':												
<35	0	0	1	0.0	0.0	0.1	0	0	1	0.0	0.0	0.1
35-64	16	30	26	2.9	5.5	4.7	25	21	23	4.3	3.7	3.9
65+	61	67	55	32.2	35.0	28.8	42	55	50	15.7	20.1	17.0
Total	77	97	82	4.1	5.2	4.4	67	76	74	2.9	3.2	3.0
'Urban':												
<35	0	0	0	0.0	0.0	0.0	0	0	0	0.0	0.0	0.0
35-64	17	16	27	4.0	3.6	6.1	8	20	18	1.7	4.2	3.7
65+	30	28	40	25.6	23.9	33.8	46	43	45	25.5	20.8	22.1
Total	47	44	67	3.8	3.5	5.3	54	63	63	3.1	3.4	3.4
Leukemia:												
'Rural':												
<35	30	23	21	5.7	4.4	4.0	6	11	15	1.2	2.2	3.1*
35-64	35	46	35	10.2	13.9	10.1	27	27	29	7.7	7.7	8.2
65+	121	140	112	89.9	105.4	83.8	84	106	100	47.0	56.6	49.4
Total	186	209	168	15.4	17.4	13.9	117	144	144	7.8	9.3	9.3
'Suburb.':												
<35	35	43	38	3.5	4.3	3.8	15	29	27	1.6	3.0	2.8
35-64	72	73	66	13.3	13.3	12.3	44	43	48	7.6	7.4	8.2
65+	158	177	177	81.4	90.8	91.4	124	119	136	44.5	39.9	43.6
Total	265	293	281	14.3	15.7	15.2	183	191	211	7.7	8.1	8.6
'Urban':												
<35	32	30	27	3.5	3.3	3.0	23	23	18	2.5	2.6	2.1
35-64	49	46	55	11.5	10.4	12.4	36	35	35	7.7	7.3	7.2
65+	93	101	115	79.5	86.1	96.5	96	96	87	51.2	48.6	42.5
Total	174	177	197	13.6	13.7	15.2	155	154	140	9.0	8.6	7.7

† Age-adjusted rate (1970 U.S. standard); * (**) = trend significant at p < 0.05 (0.01).

and con (13). The possibility that air pollution contributes
substantially to the excess lung cancer risk among urban residents
is still uncertain despite considerable research (12-14).

The association of cancer incidence with measures of
socioeconomic status has been investigated in Iowa and Colorado
based on the census tract of residence for cases residing in large
cities (15-17). For several sites where urban risks were greater
in Colorado than in Iowa (prostate, breast, colon, and corpus), a

significant direct association with income (increasing risk with
increasing affluence) was found for these sites in Colorado but not
in Iowa (16,17). The lack of an association with income among
residents of large cities in Iowa may reflect a homogeneity of the
population in cultural or nutritional risk factors for these
sites. If such homogeneity exists in large cities, it may extend
to smaller cities and even to rural areas of Iowa, thus explaining
the smaller urban-rural differences for these sites in Iowa
compared to Colorado. In Colorado, socioeconomic status may be an
important confounding factor in the urban-rural patterns observed
for these sites. Other studies have shown that the urbanization
effect for colon cancer (but not breast cancer) disappears when
social class differences are controlled (18).

For cervical cancer, where a significant excess urban risk was
found in Iowa but not in Colorado, strong indirect associations
with income and education were found in both states (16,17). Thus,
socioeconomic status is an unlikely confounding factor leading to
the high rates for women living in large cities in Iowa and the low
rates for women living in large Colorado cities.

Appreciable increases in Iowa cancer rates over time between
1950 and 1969-71 were observed for lung cancer among men,
especially rural men, and for tumors of lymphatic tissue among
rural men and women. Such changes for lung cancer can probably be
attributed to changes in cigarette smoking habits (12). There is
some evidence that exposure of agricultural workers to chemicals
may be a causative factor for lymphoma (19).

Examination of trends in lymphoma incidence rates over more
recent years in urban-rural subgroups of the Iowa population
revealed different temporal patterns by histologic subtype.
Multiple myeloma rates increased between 1969-71 and 1976-78
primarily among rural residents (both men and women) and urban male
residents. Rates for Hodgkin's disease decreased in most residence
subgroups. Only older rural women and older urban men experienced
significant increases for non-Hodgkin's lymphoma. Interpretation
of these temporal changes in rates is complicated by likely
improvements in the diagnosis and classification of lymphomas over
time (20-22). Also, the analyses presented here do not include the
extranodal diagnoses of non-Hodgkin's lymphoma. While strong
evidence of real changes in the occurrence of these diseases may be
lacking, that possibility remains and additional studies of
apparently high risk subgroups (e.g., rural residents for multiple
myeloma) seem warranted.

The significant excess risk for lip cancer among rural men in
Iowa undoubtedly reflects an increased risk for this disease among
farmers in the state (23). Male farmers (women were not studied)
were also at significantly increased risk of death during 1971-78

from stomach and prostate cancer and from leukemia, lymphoma, and multiple myeloma (23). Urban-rural relative risks among both men and women in Iowa during 1969-71 were less than one (but not significantly so) for several of these same diseases, namely stomach cancer, leukemia and lymphoma. This may reflect an increased risk for these diseases among farmers and farm workers regardless of sex although the urban-rural and farmer-nonfarmer differences for stomach cancer may be confounded by more important ethnic differences (18). The higher risk among young farmers compared to old farmers for a wide array of primary sites (23) suggested to Archer (24) that these cancers "might be related to fertilizers or pesticides that have been introduced in the last 20 or 30 years." A similar suggestion was made by Cantor (25) to account for the significantly elevated risk for reticulum-cell sarcoma among younger farmers in Wisconsin.

Knowledge of urban-rural differentials in cancer risk can be used in the study of suspected risk factors. Urban-rural relative risks for breast cancer in Iowa have been contrasted with corresponding urban and rural distributions of age-at-first-birth and population nutrition, variables putatively related to breast cancer incidence (26). Changes over time in relative risk correlated better with changing nutritional patterns than with changing age-at-first-birth patterns (26). Attempts to find correlates of urban-rural risks for other cancers of undetermined etiology with personal or environmental factors might also be rewarding.

APPENDIX

A crude method for adjusting the 1950 Iowa data for the likely misclassification of some rural cases is presented here. The sex- and age-specific incidence rates for urban Iowa residents in 1969-71 were compared to those from the TNCS and rates for urban Iowa residents in 1950 were compared to those from the Second National Cancer Survey (SNCS) which was conducted at about the same time (8). Only data from seven areas common to both the TNCS and the SNCS were utilized in this analysis in order to make comparisons over time more meaningful (8). The sex- and age-specific cancer incidence rates for the TNCS seven common areas (SCA) were very similar to those for urban Iowa, 1969-71 (none was significantly different), while rates for the SNCS-SCA were quite often substantially lower than rates for urban Iowa, 1950.

It was assumed that the ratios of rates (National Survey to Iowa) in the 1950 data would have been the same as those for the 1969-71 data if the urban residence bias had been eliminated from the 1950 Iowa data. Modified sex- and age-specific cancer incidence rates for urban Iowa, 1950, were obtained by applying the 1969-71 ratios to the SNCS-SCA rates (except that in those

instances where the ratios for the earlier data were larger than in
the more recent data, the observed rate for urban Iowa, 1950, was
not adjusted). The adjusted rates were multiplied by the sex- and
age-specific urban Iowa populations to obtain the estimated number
of urban Iowa cases in 1950 under this assumption. The difference
between the estimated number of urban cases and the observed number
was assumed to be the urban excess due to the bias in classifying
residence. The urban excess was subtracted from the observed
number of urban cases and added to the observed number of rural
cases, then estimated urban and rural incidence rates were
calculated along with urban-rural relative risks.

This procedure for modifying the 1950 Iowa data in an attempt
to reduce the bias in the data due to misclassification of urban
residence resulted in reclassifying 40 of the 1,855 urban males
(2.1%) and 97 of the 2,225 urban females (4.4%) as rural cases.
The adjusted figures are shown in parentheses in Table 4.

REFERENCES

1.   Cutler, S. J. and J. L. Young, Jr. (eds.), "Third National
     Cancer Survey: Incidence Data," National Cancer Institute
     Monograph 41, Washington, DC (1975).
2.   Haenszel, W., S. C. Marcus, and E. G. Zimmerer, "Cancer
     Morbidity in Urban and Rural Iowa," Public Health Monograph
     No. 37, Washington, DC (1956).
3.   Young, J. L., Jr., C. L. Percy and A. J. Asire (eds.),
     "Surveillance, Epidemiology, and End Results: Incidence and
     Mortality Data, 1973-77," National Cancer Institute Monograph
     57, Washington, DC (1981).
4.   Armitage, P., The chi-square test for heterogeneity of
     proportions, after adjustment for stratification, J.R. Statis.
     Soc. B 28:150 (1966).
5.   Hakulien, T., A Mantel-Haenszel statistic for testing the
     association between a polychotomous exposure and a rare
     outcome, Amer. J. Epid. 113:192 (1981).
6.   Rothman, K. J. and J. D. Boise, "Epidemiologic Analysis with a
     Programmable Calculator," NIH Publication No. 79-1649,
     Washington, DC (1979).
7.   Tarone, R. E., On summary estimators of relative risk, J.
     Chron. Dis. 34: 463 (1981).
8.   Devesa, S. S., and D. T. Silverman, Cancer incidence and
     mortality trends in the United States: 1935-74, JNCI 60:545
     (1978).
9.   Levin, M. L., W. Haenszel, B. E. Carroll, P. R. Gerhardt, V.
     H. Handy, and S. C. Ingraham, II, Cancer incidence in urban
     and rural areas of New York State, JNCI 24:1243 (1960).
10. Nasca, P. C., W. S. Burnett, P. Greenwald, K. Breannan, P.
     Wolfgang, and K. Carlton, Population density as an indicator
     of urban-rural differences in cancer incidence, upstate New
     York, 1968-1972, Am. J. Epid. 112:362 (1980).

11. Melton, L. J., III, D. D. Brian and R. L. Williams, Urban-rural differential in breast cancer incidence and mortality in Olmstead County, Minnesota, 1935-1974, Int. J. Epid. 9:155 (1980).

12. Doll, R., and R. Peto, The causes of cancer: Quantitative estimates of avoidable risks of cancer in the United States today, JNCI 66: 1192 (1981).

13. Karch, N. J. and M. A. Schneiderman, "Explaining the Urban Factor in Lung Cancer Mortality," A Report to the Natural Resources Defense Council, Clement Associates, Washington, DC (1981).

14. National Research Council, Subcommittee on Airborne Particles, Committee on Medical and Biologic Effects of Environmental Pollutants, "Airborn Particles," University Park Press, Baltimore (1979).

15. Berg, J. W. and R. R. Connelly, Economic status and cancer incidence in Colorado, in: "Cancer Centers: Interdisciplinary Cancer Care and Cancer Epidemiology," E. Grundmann and J. W. Cole, eds., Gustav Fischer Verlag, Stuttgart, 1979, pp. 203-213.

16. Devesa, S. S., A study of the association of cancer incidence with income and education among whites and blacks, Ph.D. dissertation, Johns Hopkins University, School of Hygiene and Public Health (1979).

17. Devesa, S. S. and E. L. Diamond, Association of breast cancer and cervical cancer incidence with income and education among whites and blacks, JNCI 65:515 (1980).

18. Hoover, R., T. J. Mason, F. W. McKay, and J. F. Fraumeni, Jr., Geographic patterns of cancer mortality in the United States, in: "Persons at High Risk of Cancer," J. F. Fraumeni, Jr., ed., Academic Press, New York, (1975).

19. Hardell, L., M. Eriksson, P. Lenner and E. Lundgren, Malignant lymphoma and exposure to chemicals, especially organic solvents, chlorophenols and phenoxy acids: A case-control study, Br. J. Cancer 43:169 (1981).

20. Blattner, W. A., A. Blair, and T. J. Mason, Multiple myeloma in the United States, 1950-1975, Cancer 48:2547 (1981).

21. Cantor, K. P. and J. F. Fraumeni, Jr., Distribution of non-Hodgkin's lymphoma in the United States between 1950 and 1975, Cancer Res. 40: 2645 (1980).

22. Linos, A., R. A. Kyle, W. M. O'Fallon, and L. T. Kurland, Incidence and secular trend of multiple myeloma in Olmstead County, Minnesota: 1965-77, JNCI 66:17 (1981).

23. Burmeister, L. F., Cancer mortality in Iowa farmers, 1971-1978, JNCI 66:461 (1981).

24. Archer, V. E. (Letter to the ed.), Cancer mortality in Iowa farmers, JNCI 67:743 (1981).

25. Cantor, K. P., Farming and mortality from non-Hodgkin's lymphoma: A case-control study, Int. J. Cancer (to be published, 1982).

26. Pawlega, J. and R. Wallace, Nutrition and age at first birth
     in breast-cancer risk, Br. J. Cancer 41:941 (1980).

                              DISCUSSION

Q. MANALE: Have you controlled for in-migrations into urban
    areas over the 20-30 years prior to your study? Also, did you
    include health data on migrant workers?

A. CONNELLY: In the routinely collected data being analyzed, we
    do not learn how long a cancer case has been a resident of the
    area where he was diagnosed with cancer. Such information is
    important, but is best gathered during special studies, e.g.
    case-control interview studies. Residence at the time of
    diagnosis for Iowa cancer patients is probably a fair
    indicator of their residence 20-30 years earlier (i.e. at the
    time of exposure) since the population of Iowa is less mobile
    than most.

    If I understand the second question to be, "Did you include
    cancer cases diagnosed among migrant workers in your incidence
    rates?", the answer is 'no' if such workers revealed they were
    non-residents of the study area at the time of diagnosis. All
    cases of cancer diagnosed among non-residents of the study
    area were excluded from the incidence rate calculations.

CANCER RISKS ASSOCIATED WITH AGRICULTURE:

EPIDEMIOLOGIC EVIDENCE

Aaron Blair

Environmental Epidemiology Branch
National Cancer Institute
Bethesda, Maryland 20205

INTRODUCTION

Farmers are rather self-sufficient and routinely perform tasks normally associated with other occupations such as machine repair, carpentry, welding, equipment operating, pesticide application, and livestock handling. They may come in contact with a wide spectrum of chemical, physical, and biologic agents in the performance of these tasks. Of particular concern are pesticides; zoonotic viruses, microbes, and fungi; solvents, fuels and oils; dusts; metal fumes; and mycotoxins. The subset of exposures experienced by individuals would vary, however, according to the specific type of farming operation.

General Mortality Experience of Farmers

Despite likely exposures to numerous known or suspect hazardous agents, the mortality from all causes among farmers is lower than that of the general population (1-3) (Table 1) with standardized mortality ratios (SMRs) ranging from 83 to 92. A SMR is the ratio of the observed number to expected number of deaths multiplied by 100. A SMR of less than 100 indicates fewer deaths occurred than were expected while a SMR greater than 100 indicates more deaths occurred than were expected. SMRs for the two major causes of death, cardiovascular disease and cancer, are low. In fact among major cause of death categories, only accidents, poisonings, and violence are high among farmers.

Two possible explanations (not necessarily mutually exclusive) for the low mortality rates among farmers include: 1) selective

Table 1.   Standardized mortality ratios (SMR) for major causes of
           death among farmers

Study (Reference #)	All Causes	Cardiovascular All Disease	Cancer	Accidents, Poisoning, Violence
England and Wales (1)	91	82[1]	92	135
United States (2)	83	75	77	115
U.S. Veterans (3)	92	91	90	141

[1]Includes all circulatory disease.

bias, and 2) lifestyle factors. Selective bias is known in
occupational epidemiology as the healthy worker effect. Farming is
a rigorous occupation. Individuals lacking the strength, stamina,
and general good health required to perform necessary tasks may not
enter farming or may choose to leave it early in their working
career. The effect of such selection would, of course, lower the
mortality rate among farmers and increase it among the general
population. On the other hand, the lifestyle of farm families may
include factors thought to enhance good health (e.g., exercise,
fresh food, and clean air) and discourage deleterious habits (i.e.,
tobacco and alcohol use). Surveys of tobacco use have consistently
shown a larger proportion of non-smokers among farmers than among
the general population (3,4,5) (Table 2).

      A survey of World War I veterans (3) indicated that 35 percent
of the farmers had never smoked tobacco compared with 22 percent
among all veterans. In a study of cardiovascular disease in Evans
County, Georgia, in 1960-1962 (4), 47 percent of the farmers were
non-smokers vs. only 25 percent of the non-farmers. Similarly,
smoking patterns by occupation from the 1970 Health Interview
Survey from the National Center for Health Statistics (5) showed
that 31 percent of the farmers had never smoked, while only 23
percent of all men interviewed had never smoked tobacco. Farmers
smoke even less than groups such as physicians or other
professionals that are known for their low tobacco use.

      Tobacco use is a major contributor to ill health in the U.S.
(6). The persistence of low tobacco use among farmers over several
decades may partially explain their favorable mortality patterns,
especially the low mortality for lung cancer.

Cancer Mortality Among Farmers

      Despite the generally low overall mortality experience among
farmers compared to the general population, broad mortality surveys

Table 2. Smoking characteristics among farmers and other
          occupational groups, white males

Study Group (Reference #)	Non-Smokers	Smokers[1]
I. World War I Veterans (3)		
All White Men	22%	38%
Farmers	35%	30%
Physicians	21%	32%
II. Evans County (4)		
All White Men	34%	63%
Farmers	47%	50%
Non-farmers	25%	72%
III. Health Interview Survey (5)		
All White Men	23%	69%
Farmers	31%	69%
Professionals	28%	79%

[1]Row percentages may not total 100% because of unknown smoking
status for some persons.

of occupational groups, as well as studies of specific cancers have
noted excesses for certain tumors among farmers, and raise concerns
about agriculture related exposures.

Broad Occupational Surveys of Mortality Among Farmers

Several broad occupational surveys of varying epidemiologic
designs compare the cancer mortality among farmers with that of the
general population or other occupational groups.

A survey of mortality and occupation in England and Wales (1)
noted high mortality from certain cancers among farmers aged 15-64
(Table 3). Mortality from cancer of the lymphatic and
hematopoietic system (SMR=131) and colon (SMR=120) were
significantly elevated. Sites with slightly elevated mortality,
that were not statistically significant, include lymphosarcoma
(SMR=112), and cancers of the esophagus (SMR=113) and prostate
(SMR=122). Mortality was low for cancer of the lung (SMR=84),
bladder (SMR=70), and other urinary organs (SMR=81). In a survey
of mortality and occupation among U.S. men (2), mortality from
leukemia was elevated (SMR=116) among farmers. On the other hand,
SMRs were depressed for cancers of the oral cavity (SMR=62),
stomach (SMR=89), colon and rectum (SMR=69), lung (SMR=55), and
bladder and other urinary organs (SMR=73). A mortality study of
World War I veterans (3) is particularly noteworthy because

AARON BLAIR

Table 3. Standardized mortality ratios (SMR) for selected cancers among farmers

I. From England and Wales, aged 15-64, 1970-1972 (1).

Site	SMR
Esophagus	113
Colon	120*
Prostate	122
Lymphatic and Hematopoietic System	131*
Lymphosarcoma	112

II. From the United States, aged 20-64, 1950 (2).

Site	SMR
Leukemia	116*

III. From the United States who were World War I veterans, aged 35-84, 1953 (3).[+]

Site	SMR
Pharynx	169
Lymphoma	110
Leukemia	113

*Statistically significant at p<0.05.
[+]SMRs adjusted for smoking.

information on individual use of tobacco was available allowing
adjustment for smoking differences among occupations. Among
farmers more deaths than expected occurred from lymphoma (SMR=110),
leukemia (SMR=113), and cancer of the pharynx (SMR=169), while
fewer deaths occured than expected from cancers of the esophagus
(SMR=61), colon and rectum (SMR=75), lung (SMR=83), and bladder
(SMR=50).

Other surveys of mortality and occupation utilized the
relative frequency of causes of death to estimate cancer risk.
Death certificates contain information on usual occupation or
industry as well as cause of death. These data can be used to
calculate the proportion of deaths from a specific cause among
decedents from a particular occupation which can be compared to an
expected proportion (often based on the experience of the general
population). These proportions, adjusted for age and year of
death, are used to calculate a proportionate mortality ratio
(PMR). The interpretation of the PMR is similar to the SMR, i.e.,
a value of less than 100 means fewer deaths occurred than expected,
while a value greater than 100 means more deaths occurred than

expected. The major limitation of the PMR is that the sum of
proportions for all causes of death must equal 100. A mortality
deficit for a particular cause must, therefore, be countered by an
excess among other causes.

Milham (7), using the PMR approach, noted increased
frequencies for several cancers among farmers from the state of
Washington (Table 4). Increased frequencies for cancer of the lip
were noted among general farmers (PMR=160) and specifically among
wheat and grain farmers (PMR=288). Mortality from stomach cancer
was high among general (PMR=177), dairy (PMR=143), and poultry
(PMR=133) farmers. PMRs for cancer of the prostate were greater
than 100 for all farmers, but were highest among ranchers
(PRM=133), dairy farmers (PMR=128), and poultry farmers
(PMR=124). The relative proportion of deaths from kidney cancer
was high among ranchers (PMR=211) and wheat and grains farmers
(PMR=186), while excess deaths from malignant melanoma of the skin
was noted only among wheat and grain farmers (PMR=148). Mortality
from cancer of the brain was high among ranchers (PMR=176),
dairymen (PMR=187), and poultry farmers (PMR=220). Mortality from
cancer of the connective tissues was elevated among general farmers
(PMR=166), but few deaths occurred among other farmer categories.
The frequency of deaths from leukemia was high among dairymen
(PMR=134), wheat and grain farmers (PMR=147), and poultry producers
(PMR=269). PMRs for lung cancer were low among all farmer
categories except orchardists (PMR=133) where past exposure to

Table 4. Proportionate mortality ratios for selected cancers among
farmers from Washington state, 1950-1971

Site	General Farmers	Orchardists	Ranchers	Dairy	Wheat and Grain	Poultry
Lip	160*	--	--	--	288	--[1]
Stomach	117*	67	90	143*	98	139
Prostate	104	108	133*	128	109	124
Kidney	87	109	211*	45	151	92
Melanoma	67	--	--	--	148	--
Skin (non-melanoma)	136*	--	162	--	186	--
Brain	106	88	176*	187*	97	220
Connective Tissue	166*	--	--	--	--*	--
Leukemia	108	84	106	134	147	269*
Colon	90*	106	69*	105	101*	104
Lung	81*	133*	75	56*	62	56

[1]-- = less than 4 deaths observed.
*Statistically significant at p<0.05.

arsenicals may be involved. The number of deaths due to colon
cancer was about as expected except among ranchers (PMR=69) and
general farmers (PMR=90) where there were deficits.

Peterson and Milham (8), using an approach similar to the
Washington state survey (7), reported the proportionate mortality
experience of California farmers dying from 1959 to 1961. The
relative frequency of deaths due to cancers of the skin (non-
melanotic) (PMR=155), lymphatic leukemia (PMR=136), and Hodgkin's
disease (PMR=134) were high, while the PMR for lung cancer (PMR=72)
was low.

Burmeister (9) using 1971-1978 mortality data from Iowa,
reported elevated PMRs and SMRs for several cancer sites among
farmers. The patterns for SMRs and PMRs were similar; however, the
SMRs were generally larger than the PMRs. Because the SMRs are
based on extrapolated denominators, only PMRs will be presented
here. Among Iowa farmers excess cancer deaths were reported for
leukemia (PMR=110), non-Hodgkin's lymphoma (PMR=114), multiple
myeloma (PMR=127), Hodgkin's disease (PMR=122), and cancers of the
lip (PMR=162), stomach (PMR=114), and prostate (PMR=110). As in
other studies, fewer deaths due to lung cancer occurred than were
expected (PMR=78).

Williams et al. (10) and Decoufle et al. (11) used data from
the Third National Cancer Survey and the Roswell Park Memorial
Institute, respectively, in case-control studies designed to
uncover associations between cancers and occupations. The Third
National Cancer Survey (10), after adjustments for age, race,
education, and tobacco and alcohol use, indicated that farmers had
a two-fold risk of cancer of the oral cavity [Odds Ratio (OR)=2.0],
and elevated risks of cancer of pancreas (OR=1.4), and prostate
(OR=1.5) compared to other occupational groups. Too few cases of
lymphatic and hematopoietic cancer occurred for meaningful
interpretation. Findings from a study of patients at Roswell Park
Memorial Institute (11) noted elevated risks among dairy farmers
for cancer of the prostate (OR=4.8) and bladder (OR=3.2), and an
elevated risk of melanoma (OR=3.1) among general crop and livestock
farmers.

In summary, broad mortality surveys raise the possibility that
certain cancers may be more common than would be expected among
farmers (Table 5). Although excesses for several sites have been
reported, the association between farming and cancer is most
consistent for cancers of the lymphatic and hematopoietic system
(particularly leukemia), prostate, skin, and stomach. Since these
studies have all made multiple comparisons between occupations and
cancers, some associations due entirely to chance would be
expected.

Table 5. Summary of reported associations between specific cancers and farming from mortality surveys of occupations

Data Source (Reference #)	Cancer Site							
	Stomach	Prostate	Skin	Brain	Connective Tissue	Leukemia	Lymphoma	Hodgkin's Disease
England and Wales (1)		✓					✓	
U.S. Men (2)						✓		
WWI Veterans (3)						✓	✓	
Washington (7)								
General Farmers	✓		✓		✓	✓		
Ranchers		✓	✓	✓				
Dairymen	✓							
Wheat and Grain			✓			✓		
Poultry	✓	✓	✓	✓		✓		
California (8)			✓			✓		✓
Iowa (9)	✓	✓				✓	✓	✓
TNCS (10)		✓						
Roswell Park (11)		✓	✓					

Studies of Specific Cancers

Studies of specific cancers are also available to evaluate the association between farming and cancer. The research effort has been very uneven with lymphatic and hematopoietic cancers receiving by far the most attention. A few reports, however, that deal with the farming question are available for cancers of the brain, skin, prostate, and stomach.

Lymphatic and Hematopoietic Cancer. In studies investigating the association between farming and cancer of the lymphatic and hematopoietic system, most of the attention has been focused on leukemia. Death certificate studies from Nebraska, Iowa, and Wisconsin (12-14), indicated that farmers were at higher risk of leukemia than other occupations. The risk of leukemia was greatest among farmers born after 1900 and dying before age 65 suggesting that, if the association is causal, recent changes in agricultural techniques and practices may be involved. However, not all studies have shown this association. A study of leukemia incidence in Olmsted County, Minnesota, suggested farmers were at high risk (15), however, a later, more detailed, case-control study found no association (16). The specfic types of leukemia associated with farming are not clear. Acute lymphatic and unspecified lymphatic leukemia were the cell types most strongly associated with farming in the Nebraska (12) and Iowa (14) studies, however, among Wisconsin farmers chronic myeloid leukemia showed the stronger association (13).

Table 6. Studies of farming (or farm-related exposures) and cancer

Geographic Area (Reference #)	Study Design	Findings
I. Lymphatic and Hematopoietic Cancer		
California (17)	Mortality (SMR)	Leukemia excess among farm residents (men and women)
Minnesota (16)	Case-control	No excess risk for leukemia among farmers
Washington and Oregon (18)	Death certificate (Case-control)	Excess risk of leukemia and multiple myeloma, high risk among poultrymen
Southeastern U.S. (19)	Geographic correlation	Leukemia mortality rates were not high in poultry-producing counties
Poland (23)	Geographic correlation	A higher hospital admission rate for leukemia among persons from areas where bovine leukemia occurred
Sweden (24)	Geographic correlation	No relationship between geographic location of human and bovine leukemia
United States (26)	Geographic correlation	Association between corn production and acute myeloid and chronic lymphatic leukemia, no association with dairying
Iowa (27)	Geographic correlation	High rates for acute lymphatic leukemia in counties with bovine leukemia
Wisconsin (13)	Death certificate (Case-control)	Excess risk for leukemia among farmers from dairying counties, but similar risks for general farmers and dairy farmers
Nebraska (12)	Death certificate (Case-control)	Excess leukemia among farmers particularly those from heavy corn-producing counties
Iowa (14)	Death certificate (Case-control)	Excess of leukemia among farmers from dairying and corn-producing counties
Finland (28)	Case-control	Childhood leukemia associated with the parental occupation of farming
United States (30)	Geographic correlation	No association between multiple myeloma and farming
Texas (31)	Geographic correlation	Multiple myeloma higher in areas with more persons employed in agricultural industries

Table 6. Continued

Geographic Area (Reference #)	Study Design	Findings
Sweden (32-34)	Case-control	High risk of soft-tissue sarcoma, Hodgkin's disease and non-Hodgkin's lymphoma among persons having contact with herbicides
Wisconsin (38)	Death certificate (Case-control)	High risk from non-Hodgkin's lymphoma associated with wheat production
Israel (39)	Case-control	No association between Hodgkin's disease and farming as an occupation

II. Brain Cancer

Minnesota (41)	Mortality	The proportion of rural-farm residents was greater among brain cancer deaths than among the general population
Baltimore, MD (42)	Case-control	Children with brain cancer were more likely to have lived on farms than were controls

III. Skin Cancer

England (45)	Mortality	Skin cancer rates were higher among farmers

IV. Prostate Cancer

United States (46)	Geographic correlation	Association between mortality from prostate cancer and poultry production
California (47)	Death certificate (Case-control)	Prostate cancer more common among gardeners, grounds-keepers, and persons in horticultural services (includes farmers)
Minnesota (48)	Case-control	Fewer persons with prostate cancer were farmers than were controls

V. Stomach Cancer

Iceland (49)	Death certificate	Mortality from stomach cancer greatest among farmers
New York (50)	Case-control	Among persons with stomach cancer a greater proportion had been exposed to grain dusts than had controls

One of the earliest investigations of farming and lymphatic and hematopoietic cancer used mortality statistics and 1960 U.S. Census data from California to compare mortality rates of leukemia and of lymphoma among farm and non-farm residents (17). Although mortality from all cancer was significantly lower among farm than non-farm residents, the rates of leukemia among farmers was greater than expected among men and women (SMR=114 for each sex). In contrast to leukemia, mortality from Hodgkin's disease, non-Hodgkin's lymphoma, and multiple myeloma was not elevated among farm residents.

Milham (18), using death certificates from Washington and Oregon in a case-control approach reported a significantly elevated risk for leukemia and multiple myeloma among farmers. The risk of leukemia, although seen for several types of farmers, was greatest among poultrymen, suggesting that oncogenic viruses (fowl leukosis) may be involved. This association, however, between leukemia and poultry production was not seen in other studies (12-14, 19). Relationships between multiple myeloma and particular types of farming were not investigated.

Considerable attention has also been focused on the possible association between human leukemia and bovine leukosis. An infectious virus has clearly been established as the primary agent in bovine lymphoma and can cross species barriers (20). However, it has not been demonstrated that it can be transferred to humans (21). Possible human contact with the virus from infected cattle and unpasteurized milk (22) indicates concern over human exposure should not be dismissed lightly. Geographic correlations between cattle populations and human leukemia rates are inconsistent (23-26). The frequency of leukemia among cattle in certain geographic areas was correlated positively with hospital admissions for leukemia among humans in Poland (23). However, no such association was noted in studies from Sweden (24), Russia (25), or the United States (26). In a descriptive study of leukemia in Iowa, Donham et al. (27) found that rates of acute lymphatic leukemia (ALL) among men were higher in counties where dairying was an important agricultural activity. Furthermore, the rates for ALL were highest among persons from counties where dairy herds were known to be infected with the bovine leukemia virus. These findings suggest exposure to bovine leukemia viruses may play a role in the etiology of human leukemia. In a study of leukemia in Wisconsin (13), a state noted for its dairy trade, the risk of leukemia was slightly elevated among farmers from dairy counties. Information regarding herd infection with the bovine leukemia virus was not available. However, the risk of leukemia among those specifically identified as dairy farmers (whether from death certificate notation or county agent reports) was similar to farmers in general and, therefore, does not strongly support the contention that dairy farmers in particular are at unusual risk for leukemia. In a study of Nebraska farmers (12), the risk of lymphatic leukemia (mostly chronic) was greater among farmers from counties heavily engaged in cattle production, but not among farmers from heavy dairying areas. Burmeister et al. (14), using a design similar to the Nebraska study, noted higher risks for lymphatic leukemia among Iowa farmers from dairying counties.

Corn production has also been associated with the risk of leukemia among farmers from Nebraska (12) and Iowa (14), but not Wisconsin (13). The particular exposures associated with this risk of leukemia have not been identified, however, there was little evidence for a relationship between leukemia and use of insecticides or herbicides. In an interesting study from Finland (28), the risk of leukemia among children was associated with the parental occupation of farming on both the paternal and maternal sides.

Few investigations of the role of agricultural factors in the origin of lymphatic and hematopoietic cancer other than leukemia are available. Multiple myeloma was more common among farmers from Washington and Oregon than among non-farmers (18). Among Nebraska farmers, the risk of multiple myeloma was higher among decedents from corn and cattle producing counties (29), neither association, however, was statistically significant. In a geographic survey of multiple myeloma during 1950-1975 in the U.S., mortality rates were higher in urban areas and were not correlated with farm-related parameters (30). In a similar approach, however, mortality rates among state economic areas in Texas were positively related to the proportion of the population employed in agricultural industries (31).

The strongest epidemiologic evidence concerning agricultural factors in the origin of lymphomas comes from Sweden where in a case-control study the risk of malignant lymphoma (Hodgkin's disease and non-Hodgkin's lymphoma) following exposure to herbicides was increased five-fold (32). The risks for Hodgkin's disease and non-Hodgkin's lymphoma were similar. Cantor (33), using a death certificate case-control approach similar to that used in studies of leukemia in Nebraska (12), Wisconsin (13), and Iowa (14), found that Wisconsin farmers from heavy wheat producing and insecticide using counties had increased risks of non-Hodgkin's lymphoma, particularly reticulum cell sarcoma. As with leukemia, the association of non-Hodgkin's lymphoma and farming was stronger among decedents less than 65 years than among those dying at older ages. However, aside from the Swedish study of herbicide exposure (32), I am unaware of any additional reports tying Hodgkin's disease to farming (34) or agricultural exposures (35).

Soft-tissue Sarcomas. The likely use of herbicides by many farmers also makes the Swedish reports of an increased risk of

soft-tissue sarcoma among persons with herbicide exposure
particularly relevant (36,37). Although soft-tissue sarcomas have
been noted among industrial populations exposed to herbicides (38-
40), lymphomas have not been excessive, however, the populations-
at-risk were very small.

Brain Cancer. The higher mortality due to cancer of the brain
and central nervous system noted among farm residents than non-farm
residents in Minnesota (41) is consistent with the report of higher
mortality for this cancer among Washington ranchers and poultrymen
(7). In a recent study of children (42), those with brain cancer
were more likely to have lived on farms than normal children (i.e.,
those with no known malignancies). There was also a greater
tendency for the children with brain tumors to have had previous
reported contact with insecticides than normal children. These
differences, however, may be partially due to selective recall,
since children with brain cancer did not differ in regards to
exposure to insecticides from children with other tumors.

Skin Cancer. Reports of excess mortality from skin cancer
among farmers (7,8,11) are consistent with epidemiologic findings
implicating ultraviolet radiation as a major agent in the origin of
these tumors (43, 44). Furthermore, data from the Manchester
Regional Tumor Registry indicate that farmers had twice the number
of skin cancers expected (with expected numbers based on general
population rates) (45).

Prostatic Cancer. Cancer of the prostate was associated with
farming in several of the large mortality surveys (7,9-11). The
positive correlation between county mortality rates for prostatic
cancer and the number of chickens inventoried (46) is consistent
with the excess mrotality for this tumor noted among Washington
poultrymen (7). In a review of occupation and industry on death
certificates from Alameda and San Francisco Counties, California,
gardeners and groundskeepers and persons in horticultural services
(which included farmers) had elevated risks for prostate cancer
(47). However, an interview case-control study of prostate cancer
in Minnesota found no elevated risk among farmers (48).

Stomach Cancer. Elevated risks of mortality from stomach
cancer among farmers has also been reported in Washington state
(7), Iowa (9), and Iceland (49). A related and intriguing finding
from a study of stomach cancer at Roswell Memorial Park Institute
in New York showed an association with exposure to grain dusts
(primarily encountered while farming) (50). However, these reports
may be confounded by social class, since the risk of stomach cancer
is inversely related to socioeconomic status (51).

Studies of Related Occupations

The mortality experience of veterinarians is of interest because of certain exposures they have in common with farmers, particularly insecticides and zoonotic viruses (52-56). Veterinarians experience high mortality from cancer of the lymphatic and hematopoietic system, brain and central nervous system, and skin (55), as do farmers. This raises suspicion that exposures common to both groups may be involved in the etiology of these tumors. Analysis by type of veterinary practice sheds additional light on the role of specific exposures associated with veterinary activities. The increased relative frequency of skin cancer is confined to non-small animal practitioners in accord with their presumed greater exposure to sunlight. Mortality from cancer of the brain and lymphatic and hematopoietic system was excessive among all types of veterinarians (i.e., small animal, large animal, and non-practitioners such as regulators and meat inspectors). The excess is, therefore, unlikely to be due to animal-related exposures. In a larger study of deaths among veterinarians (56), the leukemia excess was most striking among veterinarians practicing during the 1950's and 1960's, a period when use of radiography was growing rapidly but safety procedures were lax, suggesting that exposure to diagnostic x-rays may be involved. The role of zoonotic animals viruses is possible, but unlikely, since we have no information to suggest that the level of contact by veterinarians with supposedly infectious animal agents has varied appreciably over the past several decades. In summary, although the mortality pattern among veterinarians resembles that among farmers, except for cancer of the skin, there is little evidence that common environmental agents are involved.

Swedish studies of soft-tissue sarcomas and malignant lymphomas (32-34) suggest that contact with herbicides may be involved in the origin of these tumors. The cancer risks associated with herbicides were very high, 5 or 6 times that among unexposed persons. Exposures in Sweden were mainly associated with forestry, but similar chemicals are sometimes used in agriculture in the U.S. and raise serious concern.

SUMMARY

Despite their generally favorable mortality experience, general occupational surveys of farmers suggest they have elevated risks of cancer of the lymphatic and hematopoietic systems, stomach, prostate, brain, and skin. Since farmers often serve in the role of mechanic, carpenter, welder, pesticide applicator, and veterinarian, they may be exposed to many potentially hazardous substances. The types and levels of exposures have been discussed by others earlier in the program.

The evidence is strongest for the association between farming and risk of leukemia. However, the specific leukemogenic agent or agents have yet to be identified. Leukemia excesses among poultrymen and dairy farmers suggest involvement of zoonotic viruses, while associations with crop production is more indicative of pesticide usage.

The associations regarding other cancers (i.e., Hodgkin's disease, non-Hodgkin's lymphoma, multiple myeloma, soft-tissue sarcoma, and cancers of the stomach, brain, and prostate) are even less clear. However, the Swedish reports of high risk of soft-tissue sarcomas and lymphomas among persons exposed to herbicides is particularly disconcerting and underscores the urgent need for similar epidemiologic studies in the U.S.

Several case-control interview studies are underway that should help clarify the role of agricultural factors in the origin of various cancers. NCI is sponsoring studies of leukemia and non-Hodgkin's lymphoma among men from Minnesota and Iowa. Detailed information on farm practices and pesticide usage is being gathered. A study of soft-tissue sarcoma, Hodgkin's disease, and non-hodgkin's lymphoma also has just been initiated. This investigation is located in Kansas, a major wheat producing area. A wheat producing area was selected because herbicides are more heavily used on this crop than insecticides. The major objective of this project is to evaluate the role of herbicides in the origin of these cancers. A case-control study of brain cancer has also recently been initiated. Although this study focuses on contact with petrochemicals, a complete work history will be obtained and would note any farm experience. These data may help clarify the reported association between brain cancer and farming.

REFERENCES

1. The Registrar General's Decennial Supplement, England and Wales, 1961: Occupational Mortality Tables. Her Majesty's Stationery Office, London (1971).
2. Guralnick, L. Mortality by occupation and cause of death. Vital Statistics Special Report 53(3), DHEW (PHS), Washington, DC (1963).
3. Walrath, J. (Personal communication.)
4. Cassel, J., S. Heyden, A. G. Bartel, B. H. Kaplan, H. A. Tyroler, J. C. Cornoni, C. G. Hames. Occupational and physical activity and coronary heart disease. Arch. Intern. Med. 128:920-928 (1971).
5. Sterling, T. D. and J. J. Weinkam. Smoking characteristics by type of employment. J. Occup. Med. 18:743-754 (1976).
6. Smoking and Health--A Report of the Surgeon General. DHEW Publ. No. (PHS) 79-50066, USGPO, Washington, DC (1979).

7. Milham, S., Jr. Occupational mortality in Washington state,
    1950-1971. DHEW Publ. No. (NIOSH, NIH) 76-175-A, Rockville,
    MD (1976).

8. Petersen, G. R., S. Milham, Jr. Occupational mortality in the
    state of California, 1959-1961. DHEW Publ. No. (NIOSH, NIH)
    80-104, Rockville, MD (1980).

9. Burmeister, L. F. Cancer mortality in Iowa farmers, 1971-
    1978. Journal of National Cancer Institute 66:461-464
    (1981).

10. Williams, R. R., N. L. Stegens, and J. R. Goldsmith.
    Associations of cancer site and type with occupation and
    industry from the Third National Cancer Survey Interview.
    Journal of National Cancer Institute 59:1147-1185 (1977).

11. Decoufle, P., K. Stanislawizyk, L. Houten, I. D. J. Bross and
    E. Viadana. A retrospective survey of cancer in relation to
    occupation. DHEW (NIOSH) Publ. No. 77-178, Cincinnati, OH
    (1977).

12. Blair, A. and T. L. Thomas. Leukemia among Nebraska
    farmers: A death certificate study. Am. J. Epidemiol.
    110:264-273 (1979).

13. Blair, A. and D. W. White. Death certificate study of
    leukemia among farmers from Wisconsin. Journal of National
    Cancer Institute 66:1027-1030 (1981).

14. Burmeister, L. F., S.F. Van Lier, and P. Isacson. Leukemia
    and farm practices in Iowa. Am. J. Epidemiol. 115:720-728
    (1982).

15. Linos, A., R. A. Kyle, L. R. Elveback, and L. T. Kurland.
    Leukemia in Olmstead County, Minnesota, 1965-1974. Mayo Clin.
    Proc. 53:714-718 (1978).

16. Linos, A., R. A. Kyle, W. M. O'Fallon, and L. J. Kurland. A
    case-control study of occupational exposures and leukemia.
    Intern. J. Epidemiol. 9:131-135 (1980).

17. Fasal, E., E. W. Jackson, and M. R. Klauber. Leukemia and
    lymphoma mortality and farm residence. Am. J. Epidemiol.
    87:267-274 (1968).

18. Milham, S. Leukemia and multiple myeloma in farmers. Am. J.
    Epidemiol. 94:307-310 (1971).

19. Priester, W. A. and T. J. Mason. Human cancer mortality in
    relation to poultry population by county in 10 Southeastern
    states. Journal of National Cancer Institute 53:45-49 (1979).

20. Heath, C. W., G. G. Caldwell, and P. C. Feorino. Viruses and
    other microbes, in: "Persons at high risk of cancer," J. F.
    Fraumeni, Jr., ed., Academic Press, New York (1975).

21. Donham, K. J., M. J. VanDerMooten, J. M. Miller, B. C. Kruse
    and M. J. Rubino, Sero-epidemiologic studies on the possible
    relationships of human and bovine leukemia: Brief
    communication. Journal of National Cancer Institute 59:851-
    853 (1977).

22. Ferrer, J. F., S. J. Kenyon, and P. Gupta. Milk of dairy cows
    frequently contains a leukemia virus. Science 213:1014-1016
    (1981).

23. Wolska, A. Human and bovine leukemias. The Lancet I;1155 (1968).

24. Kvarnfors, E., B. Henricson and G. A. Hugoson. A statistical study on farm and village level on the possible relations between human leukemia and bovine leukosis. Acta. Vet. Scand. 16:163-169 (1975).

25. Khokhlova, M. D. Epidemiological studies of leukemias and lymphomas in the USSR, in: "Cancer Epidemiology in the USA and USSR," D. L. Levin ed., NIH Publ. No. 80-2044, Bethesda, MD (1980).

26. Blair, A., J. F. Fraumeni, Jr. and T. J. Mason. Geographic patterns of leukemia in the United States. J. Chron. Dis. 33:251-260 (1980).

27. Donham, K. J., J. W. Berg and R. S. Sawin. Epidemiologic relationships of the bovine population and human leukemia in Iowa. Am. J. Epidemiol. 112:80-92 (1980).

28. Hemminki, K., I. Saloniemi, T. Salonen, T. Partanen and H. Vainio. Childhood cancer and parental occupation in Finland. J. Epidemiol. Comm. Hlth. 35:11-15 (1981).

29. Blair, A. (Unpublished data.)

30. Blattner, W. A., A. Blair, and T. J. Mason. Multiple myeloma in the United States, 1950-1975. Cancer 48: 2547-2554 (1981).

31. Agu, V. U., B. L. Christensen and P. A. Buffler. Geographic patterns of multiple myeloma: Racial and industrial correlates, state of Texas, 1969-71. Journal of National Cancer Institute 65:735-738 (1980).

32. Hardell, L., M. Eriksson, P. Lenner and E. Lundren. Malignant lymphoma and exposure to chemicals, especially organic solvents, chlorophenols, and phenoxy acids: A case-control study. Br. J. Cancer. 43:169-176 (1981).

33. Cantor, K. Farming and mortality from non-Hodgkin's lymphoma: A case-control study. Int. J. Cancer. 29:239-247 (1982).

34. Abramson, J. H., H. Pridan, M. I. Sacks, M. Avitzour and E. Peritz. A case-control study of Hodgkin's disease in Israel. Journal of National Cancer Institute 61:307-314 (1978).

35. Gutensohn, N. and P. Cole. Epidemiology of Hodgkin's disease. Seminars in Oncology 7:92-102 (1980).

36. Hardell, L. and A. Sandstrom. Case-control study: Soft-tissue sarcomas and exposure to phenoxyacetic acids and chlorophenols. Br. J. Cancer. 39:711-717 (1979).

37. Eriksson, M., L. Hardell, N. O. Berg, T. Moller and O. Axelson. Soft-tissue sarcomas and exposure to chemical substances: A case-referent study. Br. J. Industr. Med. 38:27-33 (1981).

38. Ott, M. G., B. B. Holder and R. D. Olson. A mortality analysis of employees engaged in the manufacture of 2,4,5-trichlorophenoxyacetic acid. J. Occup. Med. 22:47-50 (1980).

39. Zack, J. A. and R. R. Suskind. The mortality experience of
     workers exposed to tetrachlorodibenzodioxin in a
     trichlorphenol process accident. J. Occup. Med. 22:11-14
     (1980).
40. Cook, R. R. Dioxin, chloracne, and soft-tissue sarcoma. The
     Lancet I:618-619 (1981).
41. Choi, N. W., L. M. Schuman, and W. H. Gullen. Epidemiology of
     primary central nervous system neoplasms. I. Mortality from
     primary central nervous system neoplasms in Minnesota. Am. J.
     Epidemiol. 91:238-259 (1970).
42. Gold, E., L. Gordis, J. Tonascia and M. Szklo. Risk factors
     for brain tumors in children. Amer. J. Epidemiol. 109:309-319
     (1979).
43. Fears, T. R., J. Scotto and M. A. Schneiderman. Mathematical
     models of age and ultraviolet effects on the incidence of skin
     cancer among whites in the United States. Am. J. Epidemiol.
     105:420-427 (1977).
44. Enamett, E. A. Ultraviolet radiation as a cause of skin
     tumors. CRC Crit. Rev. Toxicol. 2:211-255 (1975).
45. Whitaker, C. J., W. R. Lee and J. E. Downes. Squamous cell
     skin cancer in the Northwest of England, 1967-69, and its
     relation to occupation. Br. J. Industr. Med. 36:43-51 (1979).
46. Blair, A. and J. F. Fraumeni, Jr. Geographic patterns of
     prostate cancer in the United States. Journal of National
     Cancer Institute 61:1379-1384 (1978).
47. Ernester, V. L., S. Selvin, S. M. Brown, S. T. Sacks, W.
     Winkelstein and D. F. Austin. Occupation and prostatic
     cancer. J. Occup. Med. 21:175-183 (1979).
48. Schuman, L. M., J. Mandel, C. Blackard, H. Bauer, J. Scarlett
     and R. McHugh. Epidemiologic study of prostatic cancer:
     Preliminary report. Cancer Treat. Rep. 61:181-186 (1977).
49. Siguyonsson, J. Occupational variations in mortality from
     gastric cancer in relation to dietary differences. Brit. J.
     Cancer 21:651-656 (1967).
50. Kraus, A. S., M. L. Levin and P. R. Gerhardt. A study of
     occupational associations with gastric cancer. Am. J. Public
     Hlth. 47:961-970 (1957).
51. Buell, P., J. E. Dunn and L. Breslow. The occupational-social
     class risks of cancer mortality in men. J. Chron. Dis.
     12:600-621 (1960).
52. Botts, R. P., S. Edlavitch and G. Payne. Mortality of
     Missouri veterinarians. J. Amer. Vet. Med. Assoc. 149:499-504
     (1966).
53. Fasal, E., E. W. Jackson and M. R. Klauber. Mortality among
     California veterinarians. J. Chron. Dis. 19:293-306 (1966).
54. Schnurrenberger, P. R., R. J. Martin and J. F. Walker.
     Mortality in Illinois veterinarians. J. Amer. Vet. Med.
     Assoc. 170:1071-1075 (1977).

55. Blair, A. and H. M. Hayes, Jr. Cancer and other causes of
    death among U.S. veterinarians, 1966–1977. Int. J. Cancer.
    25:181–185 (1980).
56. Blair, A. and H. M. Hayes, Jr. Mortality patterns among U.S.
    veterinarians, 1947–1979: an expanded study. Int. J.
    Epidemiol., in press (1982).

DISCUSSION

Q. GENTILE: Are future case control studies going to be
    conducted in Iowa and Colorado in an attempt to correlate
    those data with the SEER urban-rural patterns developed for
    those states?

A. BLAIR: A case-control study of leukemia and non-Hodgkin's
    lymphoma is underway in Iowa. The information collected will
    be much more detailed then in the TNCS or SEER projects. A
    residential history of each study is being obtained, however,
    and can be used to look for similarities in urban-rural risk
    patterns suggested by Dr. Connelly for these cancers.

Q. MANALE: Did you include health data on migrant workers in
    your studies?

A. BLAIR: Cancer cases for the case-control studies are
    identified from tumor registrees. Therefore, if a migrant
    worker was diagnosed in the area covered by the study, he or
    she would be included. Very few are likely to occur, however.

Q. PUTTER: Could some of the differences in cancer rates between
    urban and rural areas be explained by different capabilities
    for diagnosis in the two areas, i.e. better diagnoses in urban
    areas?

A. BLAIR: Variability in diagnostic capabilities undoubtedly
    occur. However, diagnosis is less sophisticated in rural
    areas and adjustments for this bias would accentuate the
    excesses seen among farmers.

Q. HAWORTH: What is the tonnage of agrichemicals used in this
    country post-WWII vs. pre-WWII? If the tonnage is greater
    post-WWII, then would you expect that current cancer data for
    farmers is or might be a great underestimate of induced
    cancers in farmers?

A. BLAIR: I don't know the specific tonnage. Clearly the use of
    herbicides was rare before WWII but has increased dramatically
    since then. Occupational studies have generally indicated
    that 25–30 years are necessary before we see an effect of an

occupational carcinogen. Herbicides have been in use for approximately that length of time. However, heavy use has probably occurred only during the last 10-15 years.

Q.   ZWEIG: What herbicides were used in the Swedish studies?

A.   BLAIR: Phenoxyacetic acids and chlorophenols.

EXTRAPOLATION OF MUTAGENICITY TESTING TO THE HUMAN

Mortimer L. Mendelsohn

Biomedical Sciences Division
Lawrence Livermore National Laboratory
Livermore, California 94550

Agricultural genetic toxicology is typical of the challenging problems now being encountered in the rapidly growing field of environmental mutagenesis. Both fields involve a rich diversity of important chemicals, some already known mutagens, a few known carcinogens; both have some hints of human toxicity, but by and large no concrete human data; and both are floundering in the scientific and legal definition of human risk, as well as in regulatory confusion over when and to what degree to control.

The stakes in agricultural genetic toxicology are enormous. We have an absolute requirement for food and a heavy dependence on agricultural chemicals. But we also have the deep-seated concern that food growing, food preparation, and food consumption may well hold the key to the dramatic patterns of cancer incidence found among the countries of the world. Will it be genes versus butter? Do we need food more than we need genetic integrity? Or is it possible to have both? Can we find ways to feed the world, to gain safe and effective methods of chemical control, and simultaneously to reduce one of the dominant causes of human mortality by understanding and alleviating a potentially large component of environmental carcinogenesis?

The answer at present is yes, we should eventually be able to have it all, but no, we do not yet know how. Yes, we have remarkable new tools to study mutagenicity, but no, they remain inadequate for the task. Yes, we could do much harm by over-reacting too soon, but no, so far this has not happened. Yes, we need intensified research in environmental mutagenesis and carcinogenesis, but no, this does not seem to be forthcoming.

In the last two decades there has been rapid progress in the
measurement of mutagenicity using well-designed tests in microorganisms, cells, and some plants and animals. These accomplish-
ments, exciting as they are, will not provide the answers to our
problems until we better understand three things: the complex
relationships among the various genetic tests; the relationship
between mutagenicity and carcinogenicity; and the relationship
between mutagenicity in laboratory models and mutagenicity in the
human.

The broad spectrum of laboratory genetic tests is both an
ingenious resource and a regulatory nightmare. We know how to test
for single base changes, frameshifts, deletions, exchanges, cross-
overs, and aneuploidies; we can define forward or back mutations;
we can use raw DNA and prokaryotic or eukaryotic chromosomes; we
can disarm repair and enhance metabolic activation; we can measure
mutagenic effects in specific organs; and we can compare somatic
and heritable effects.

In theory each of these endpoints could give different
responses to a mutagen; the painful reality is that in practice
each one does give different results and sometimes the differences
can be dramatic. Thus it is the rule rather than the exception for
tests to disagree with each other. The discordance is enhanced in
test batteries which deliberately combine tests that are least
correlated and most divergent.

Is it any wonder, then, that there is so much disagreement in
how to interpret test results? At one extreme there are those who
would insist on complete concordance, i.e. that every test be positive before labelling a substance mutagenic. At the other extreme
one positive test is enough to indict, as judged by protocols which
go from negative test to negative test, and exonerate a compound
only when it achieves a perfect score. The former approach will
recognize only a small fraction of reasonable mutagens; the latter
will litter the field with false positives. We must find a stable,
rational, intermediate position in which testing is sufficiently
broad to identify all types of relevant genetic damage, and sufficiently redundant to control false alarms. In the absence of this,
we are creating indigestibly large lists of inconclusively positive
chemicals, regulators are being overwhelmed, industry is being
discouraged, and the public is being frightened or dulled into
fatalistic apathy. Like inquisitors, we have learned to point the
finger of suspicion, but we have yet to know how to bring in a
final, equitable verdict.

How does mutagenesis relate to carcinogenesis? The answer
remains unclear in spite of the obvious empirical correlation
between mutagens and carcinogens, and the mechanistically attractive idea that initiation involves genetic damage. On the

mutagenesis side of the issue, we lack insight into which of the
many types of genetic lesions (or genetic tests) are relevant. Is
it intragenic damage or chromosome damage or both? Is organ
specificity as important in mutagenesis as it is in carcinogenesis,
and therefore, must we develop genetic tests in all major cancer-
forming organs before we can relate the two? And if organ specificity prevails, where does that leave bacterial mutagenicity
tests? On the carcinogenesis side, there remains a profound confusion about the definitions of complete or incomplete carcinogen,
initiator, and promoter. We do not know how to exclude promoters,
and thus to limit the data to the relationship between initiators
and mutagens. Without this we cannot test whether all initiators
are mutagenic or whether all mutagens are initiators. In the
absence of clear insight, we hesitate to let mutagenicity be the
operating distinction between initiation and promotion. We do not
know how much the non-concordance between mutagens and carcinogens
is the result of errors in mutagenicity testing and how much is due
to errors in the bioassay for carcinogenicity. Since mutagenicity
tests are inherently more sensitive than carcinogenicity tests, we
question on what basis and at what point we are justified in extrapolating from the former to the latter.

     Can we infer human somatic or heritable genetic damage from
laboratory tests? Here again, we know some of the questions, but
few of the answers. We do not have a single validated test for
human in vivo somatic gene mutation. We have tests for induced
human heritable mutation, but no demonstrated example of heritable
mutagenesis in man induced by a chemical or by any other
modality. A valiant attempt to show heritable damage in the children of A-bomb survivors in Japan has just come up empty-handed in
spite of the overwhelming scientific evidence that radiation is
universally mutagenic. The human is not magically resistant to
mutagenesis; rather we human scientists lack the technical skill to
measure induced heritable mutation at near-background rates in our
complex, randomly breeding population. We know there are large
variations in metabolic activation and DNA repair among animals and
people. We know that in animals few somatic mutagens are capable
of giving delayed heritable mutations, but we do not understand why
this is or whether it applies to the human. We presently have no
way to handle complex mixtures of mutagens, co-mutagens, antimuta-
gens, etc., such as probably exist in the human diet. Nor can we
address the challenging technical and social problem of the genetic
susceptibles, those who are repair defectives and pharmacologic
outliers and who face extraordinary risk of mutagenic damage. How
are we to identify such people? What are we to do with them once
we know who they are? Do we, for example, ban an important
agricultural insecticide because one person in a thousand or in a
hundred-thousand is known to be hypersensitive to it?

The rapid progress in mutation research has opened this bewildering array of questions, but also suggests general strategies for finding many of the answers. Obviously, one way to tackle discordance among genetic endpoints is to generate an improved understanding of genetic mechanism. Once we focus on the idea that mutagenicity is not monolithic, the substructure should become rapidly apparent. The same may conceivably be true for the relation to carcinogenesis. That is, mutagenesis substructure may provide improved correlations and sharpened insights into carcinogenesis. But here, and certainly in the area of laboratory versus human mutagenesis, I believe the key development will be good tests for human mutagenicity. By far the best cancer data base is the human record. The most relevant way to tap this data base is to have a somatic mutagenicity profile on each new cancer patient. It would soon become clear whether mutagenicity correlates with carcinogenicity, and which mutagenicity test is best for which cancer. Armed with this knowledge, we could then find the biological, environmental, and occupational correlates for the pertinent mutagenesis. With the right insights and the right tests, the problem of mutagenic and potentially carcinogenic vectors in agriculture or in any other setting should be addressable using the same strategies and expecting the same success as has been achieved in fighting infectious diseases. Again, with appropriate test development and application, the same opportunities should be available for heritable mutagenesis in the human. There is no reason why we should have to remain blind to this horrendously important deleterious potential of a modern chemical society. Technology raised the threat, and technology should provide the ultimate defense.

What form will these human mutagenicity tests take? Some will be extensions of present methods, such as cytogenetic analyses with improved sensitivity and throughput; some will involve new chemistry, such as multidimensional protein mapping to characterize hundreds of inherited gene products in serum or other samples; and some will involve new technologies such as the detection of rare somatic or germinal cells which produce mutated gene products. To return to the agricultural perspective, the seeds for these advances are already germinating.

GENOTOXIC AGENTS IN THE AGRO-ECOSYSTEM

CHAIRMAN'S COMMENTS

Dennis P. H. Hsieh

Department of Environmental Toxicology
University of California
Davis, California 95616

In our agro-ecosystem, there are at least four classes of genotoxic agents that have been detected and characterized:

1. Genotoxic metabolites produced by plants and fungi.
2. Genotoxic heavy metal salts found in the soil.
3. Genotoxic man-made chemicals used as pesticides and other agricultural chemicals.
4. Genotoxic substances generated during the heat processing of foods or the burning of agricultural wastes.

Due to the recent advancement in the use of short-term sensitive genotoxicity tests, the number of detected genotoxic agents in the agro-ecosystem is increasing rapidly. Based on our current understanding of genetic toxicology, these genotoxic agents are all potentially capable of initiating genetic damages that may eventually lead to the development of cancer and birth-defects. The first paper in this section surveys various classes of genotoxic agents in the agricultural environment of Egypt as an example of the agro-ecosystem.

Despite the large number of genotoxic agents in our agro-ecosystem, not all of these are of legitimate health concern to man, because some agents may only be active to a particular test system and others may not actually be present in sufficiently high concentrations to result in significant human exposure. Thus, for a genotoxic agent to warrant a legitimate safety concern, it must at least meet the following two criteria:

1. Toxic to a meaningful battery of short-term tests.
2. Present in the environment at high enough concentrations to constitute a significant exposure situation.

Based on this consideration, the most signifcant classes of mutagens in the agro-ecosystem are perhaps those occurring naturally in foodstuffs and those occurring during cooking processes. Understandably, these unintentionally encountered genotoxic agents in our food chain are most difficult to avoid. Examples of naturally occurring genotoxic agents in foodstuffs are fungal toxins such as aflatoxins produced by Aspergillus flavus or plant alkaloids such as pyrrolizidine alkaloids produced by Senecio jacobaea. Mutagenic nitrosamines and heterocyclic amine derivatives generated during the cooking processes of meat and fish have been well described in the recent literature.

Of the unintentionally encountered genotoxic agents found in food, aflatoxins stand out as a towering example of genotoxic agents in the agro-ecosystem of occupational safety and public health concern. Aflatoxin B_1, the major member of the family, is an extremely potent mutagen to most mutagenicity test systems and an extremely potent hepatocarcinogen in several test animals; it occurs widely in grains, oil seeds, and tree nuts; and epidemiological studies have shown an association between aflatoxin exposure and increased incidence of liver cancer in certain populations. Recent frequent detection of aflatoxin residues in cow milk and dairy products has brought the public concern over genotoxic agents in the agro-ecosystem to a climax.

The second and the third papers will use aflatoxin as an example to illustrate the occurrence, detection, toxic actions, and biological effects of a genotoxic agent. This is of particular interest because much information is now available on aflatoxin, making it a model genotoxic agent in the agro-ecosystem.

Research in this area has been proceeding at a great pace, and a large volume of information is now available in the literature. Following are samples of references on the subject of genotoxic agents in general:

1. Naturally Occurring Carcinogens-Mutagens and Modulators of Carcinogenesis. Ed. E. C. Miller, J. A. Miller, I. Hirono, T. Sugimura, and S. Takayama. Japan Scientific Societies Press, Tokyo (1979).
2. Mycotoxin Teratogenicity and Mutagenicity. A. W. Hayes. CRC Press (1981).
3. Mycotoxins and N-Nitroso Compounds: Environmental Risks. R. C. Shank. CRC Press (1981).
4. Carcinogens in Industry and the Environment, J. M. Sontag, ed. Marcel Dekker, New York (1981).
5. Chemical Mutagens, Vol. 1-4, A. Hollaender, ed., Plenum (1976).
6. Mutagenic Effects of Environmental Contaminants, H. E. Sutton and M. I. Harris, ed. Academic Press (1972).

MUTAGENIC AND CARCINOGENIC CHEMICALS IN THE EGYPTIAN AGRICULTURAL

ENVIRONMENT

A. H. El-Sebae and S. A. Soliman

University of Alexandria Research Center and Department
of Pesticide Chemistry, Faculty of Agriculture,
Alexandria University, Alexandria, Egypt

INTRODUCTION

Egypt is a semi-arid country where the roughly 2.5 million
acres of arable land lie in the Nile River delta and valley. On
this narrow strip, almost all of Egypt's 42 million people live
and work. The Nile water is used for irrigation as well as for
industrial and domestic purposes. The river is also used for the
disposal of agricultural waste water. Industrial wastes may also
be flowing into the river and its tributaries.

In this densely populated and limited area, more than 30,000
metric tons of formulated pesticides (mainly insecticides) are
imported and used annually. More than 70% of these imports are
used to protect Egypt's main cash crop, cotton, from attacking
insects such as leaf- and bollworms. Containment of pests is,
therefore, of major importance in maintaining the health of the
Egyptian economy.

To eliminate them expeditiously, aerial spraying is used to
apply more than 75% of the pesticides, a method which is particularly
hazardous to the inhabitants of the crowded villages lying within
the spray zone. This congestion makes it particularly difficult
to implement an evacuation and re-entry program. Moreover, herbicides, fungicides, fertilizers (mainly nitrates and trace elements),
mulluscicides, food additives, and synthetic dyes are other sources
of chemical pollution. Insecticides are also used in towns and
cities to control the spread of insects hazardous to man.

MUTAGENICITY AND CARCINOGENICITY OF PESTICIDES

It is inevitable that pesticides be used to limit loss to agricultural production to an acceptable level. The urgency of this need coupled with the increasing resistance of many pests to older and more well investigated pesticides has spurred interest in less well known agents. The main reason for the rapid shift from one group to another is the ability shown by the Egyptian cotton leafworm S. littoralis and other insects to develop resistance to applied insecticides. Table 1 lists the insecticides to which the Egyptian cotton leafworm developed resistance. This situation necessitated the introduction of new insecticides which were not yet toxicologically evaluated for chronic side effects and, in many cases, were not yet even approved for distribution in the country where they were produced.

Table 2 lists the major insecticides and the quantities in which they were imported from 1950 to 1980. Although the list comprises about 70% of total imported insecticides, herbicides, fungicides, other pesticides are also widely used. For example, roughly 5 metric tons of the herbicide atrazine, a member of the triazine family, are imported and applied on agricultural regions annually.

Chu et al. (1) found toxaphene to be a carcinogen which induces liver and hepatocellular tumors when fed to either male or female mice. Hooper et al. (2) also demonstrated mutagenicity in

Table 1.   Insecticides to which Egyptian Cotton Leafworm
           Developed Resistance*

Insecticide	Year of Announced Resistance
Toxaphene	1961
DDT	1968
Lindane	1971
Carbaryl	1965
Trichlorfon	1967
Methyl parathion	1965
Sumithion	1967
Monocrotophos	1972
Methamidophos	1976
Guthion	1976

*Data from Ministry of Agriculture and our laboratory
 records.

Table 2. Amounts of Major Insecticides Imported and Used in Egypt (1950-1980)*

Compound	Imported Quantity** (metric tons)	Years of Consumption
Toxaphene	54,000	1955 - 1961
Endrin	10,500	1961 - 1981
DDT	13,500	1952 - 1971
Lindane	11,300	1952 - 1978
Carbaryl	21,000	1961 - 1978
Trichlorfon	6,500	1961 - 1970
Monocrotophos	8,300	1967 - 1978
Leptophos	5,500	1968 - 1975
Chlorpyriphos	9,500	1969 - 1981
Phosfolan	4,500	1968 - 1981
Mephosfolan	6,000	1968 - 1981
Methamidophos/Azinphos-methyl	4,500	1970 - 1979
Triazophos	3,500	1977 - 1981
Profenofos	4,000	1977 - 1981
Methomyl	3,500	1976 - 1981
Fenvalerate	4,500	1976 - 1981
Cypermethrin	2,300	1976 - 1981
Decamethrin	1,400	1976 - 1981

*Data from Ministry of Agriculture records.
**Active ingredient in each insecticide.

this insecticide. Shirasu et al. (3, 4) performed reverse mutation tests which indicated that the insecticide trichlorfon or Dipterex was a direct mutagen using S. typhimurium and E. coli WP2 hcr. Waters et al. (5) reported further that trichlorfon shows positive mutagenicity using the Ames, E. coli, WP2, and S. cerevisiae, tests with or without metabolic activation. Waters et al. (5) and Shirasu et al. (4), using the same tests, found that the insecticide monocrotophos can induce direct mutations. The Waters group (5) also found that azinphos-methyl was mutagenic using the Ames and D3 tests, and Chu et al. (1) found evidence of carcinogenicity in male rats in the same compound. The Waters group (5) also found chlorpyrifos mutagenicity when tested in the E. coli polA and B. subtilis rec in vitro tests. Uchiyama et al. (6) reported that the insecticide carbaryl might be transformed into nitrosocarbaryl, a potent mutagen, in acidic media. And Shawky et al. (7) showed that the pyrethroid insecticide fenpropathrin was mutagenic when submitted to the Ames test.

Many other mutagenic and potentially carcinogenic insecticides have been used, but in lower quantities. More than 450 metric tons of the insecticide dimethoate are imported and used annually (Record of the Ministry of Agriculture, 1975-1978). Recent data compiled by Shirasu et al. (4) indicated that this insecticide induces mutations in S. typhimurium and E. coli WP2 hcr. The same group demonstrated that the insecticide pirimiphos-methyl is also mutagenic. Introduced to the Egyptian environment as Actelic, 56 metric tons have been imported in 1978 alone, according to the Record of the Ministry of Agriculture.

More than 300 metric tons of the insecticide chlordan were imported and used in 1976 alone. Chu et al. (1) found evidence for carcinogenicity when chlordan-fed male and female mice developed liver and hepatocellular tumors. The insecticides phosmet, chlorfenvinphos, thiometon, fenitrothion, salithion, and vamidothion have been introduced in the Egyptian environment as Imidan, SD-7859, Ekatin, Sumithion, Salithion, and Kilval, respectively. Shirasu et al. (4) recently demonstrated mutagenicity in all of these chemicals in microbial test systems.

Disulfoton and acephate, known as Disyphon and Orthene, respectively, have also been recommended and used. About 5 metric tons of Orthene were imported in 1977. Waters et al. (5) and Shirasu et al. (4) have reported mutagenic activity in both these insecticides. In addition, dichlorvos or DDVP, an insecticide used both outdoors and indoors, has shown carcinogenicity in male mice and mutagenicity when tested by reverse mutation, according to Chu et al. (1) and Shirasu et al. (3).

Aldrin and dieldrin, two classic chlorinated hydrocarbon insecticides, were used heavily in the fifties and early sixties. Using male mice, Chu et al. (1) reported carcinogenicity after administration of aldrin and evidence to suggest carcinogenicity when the animals were fed dieldrin.

Waters et al. (5) reported that carbofuran or Furadan was not mutagenic. Shirasu et al. (4) have, however, recently demonstrated the mutagenicity of carbofuran.

MUTAGENICITY AND CARCINOGENICITY OF OTHER TOXIC SUBSTANCES

Genotoxic herbicides and fungicides have also been used in Egyptian agriculture. Youssef et al. (8) reported that paraquat, a widely used herbicide, is mutagenic when submitted to the Drosophila sex-linked recessive lethal test. Triazine herbicides like atrazine and simazine among others are also used in significant levels. Waters et al. (5) reported mutagenicity in simazine using the same test as the Youssef researchers. In addition, Wolfe et al. (9) found nitrosamine formation products in drinking water contaminated with atrazine. Moreover, Preussmann et al. (10-12) demonstrated that triazines are potential carcinogens, the most affected structures being the kidney and central nervous system and, less frequently, the heart. Captan, Ferbam, Ziram, and Folpet are some of the fungicides of known mutagenicity, according to Waters et al. (5) and Shirasu et al. (4). Not all of these, however, are currently used in Egypt.

The molluscicide niclosamide, also known as Bayer 73 or Baylucide, is used to combat the Bilharzia snails which cluster in canals. This compound induces hepatic and kidney lymphosarcoma in B. regularis (toads) when administered daily at 10 ppm for 2-5 mo, according to El-Mofty et al. (13).

Food additives, fertilizers, synthetic dyes, and industrial wastes are other sources of potential mutagens and carcinogens. Synthetic dyes used in textiles, a major industry, are being imported in increasing quantities. Fishbein (14) demonstrated carcinogenicity and/or mutagenicity in many dyes as well as food additives. For example, the aziridines which are used for dyeing and printing are highly reactive alkylating agents (14, 15). The monomer of one of these compounds, polyethylenimine, was found to be carcinogenic in mice after oral administration, producing liver cell and pulmonary tumors according to IARC researchers (16). Van Duuren et al. (17) found other aziridines to be carcinogenic in mice, producing malignant tumors at the site of injection.

EFFECTS OF CHRONIC EXPOSURE TO ENVIRONMENTAL POLLUTANTS

Davies et al. (18) indicated that at the current rate of pesticide use, workers who formulate and apply these materials are risking both acute and chronic exposure. More than 2000 cases of cancer have been registered in one city alone, Alexandria. Table 3 presents the distribution of types of cancer among those patients. Although the incidence of cancer in the city's total population (~ 3 million) is less than that reported in the United States and other industrialized nations, it is, nevertheless, significant. In addition, accidental and occupational poisoning are a major concern in developing countries where safety assurance methods have not kept pace with advances in agricultural technology. The Davies researchers also mention that male sterility, neurological dysfunction, behavioral disorders, renal diseases, cancer, and other abnormalities may be related to contamination by pesticides and other environmental pollutants.

These chronic effects may result from either incidental or long-term exposure to sublethal doses of the toxicants which may act directly or be transformed metabolically into toxic forms.

Table 3.   Cancer Cases Registered in Alexanderia, Egypt*

| | % Distribution | |
| | Male
(1086 cases) | Female
(918 cases) |
Cancer Type		
Breast	1.7	18.9
Bladder	13.0	3.9
Brain Tumor	4.6	2.8
Lymphosarcoma	8.7	3.6
Stomach	2.7	0.4
Uterus	-	3.4
Other cases	69.3	67.0

*Cases were registered at the Medical Research Institute, Alexandria University (June - December, 1980).

The lipophilic nature of most of these agents (19, 20) allows accumulation and retention in lipoproteins and body fat.

SUMMARY AND CONCLUSIONS

The introduction and heavy use of pesticides, insecticides, and other toxic substances in the Egyptian environment is suspected to correlate with the growing incidence of cancer and other abnormalities in the nation. The spread of malnutrition, lack of proper immunization, and the existence of endemic diseases also contribute to the damaging effects of environmental pollutants. Precise determination of the effects of chronic exposure is, therefore, urgently needed.

REFERENCES

1. Chu, K.C., C. Cueto, Jr., and J.M. Ward, 1981, Factors in the evaluation of 200 National Cancer Institute carcinogen bioassays, J. Toxicol. Environ. Health, 8:251-280.
2. Hooper, N.K., B.N. Ames, M.A. Saleh, and J.E. Casida, 1979, Toxaphene, a complex mixture of polychloroterpenes and a major mutagenic insecticide, Science, 205:591-593.
3. Shirasu, Y., M. Moriya, K. Kato, A. Furuhashi, and T. Kada, 1976, Mutat. Res., 40:19-30.
4. Shirasu, Y., M. Moriya, H. Tezuka, and S. Teramoto, 1981, Mutagenicity screening studies on pesticides. Presented at the Third Int. Conf. on Environmental Mutagens, Tokyo, Japan.

5. Waters, M.D., V.F. Simmon, A.D. Mitchell, and T.A. Jorgenson, 1980, An overview of short-term tests for the mutagenic and carcinogenic potential of pesticides, J. Environ. Sci., Health, B15:867-906.

6. Uchiyama, M., M. Takida, T. Susuki, and K. Yoshikawa, 1975, Mutagenicity of nitroso derivatives of N-methylcarbamate insecticides in the microbiological method, Bull. Environ. Contamn. Toxicol., 14:389-394.

7. Shawky, A.S., S.M. Hamza, and A.M. Kadry, 1981, Mutagenicity of the pyrethroid insecticide fenpropathrion in S. typhimurium. Presented at the Proceedings of the Int. Congress of Soil Pollution, Zagazig Univ., Egypt.

8. Youssef, M.K., A.Y. Abou-Yousef, A.A. Omar, E. Badr, and A. El-Bendary, 1981, Mutagenicity effect of paraquat in D. melanogaster. Presented at the Proceedings of the Int. Congress of Soil Pollution, Zagazig Univ., Egypt.

9. Wolfe, N.L., R.G. Zepp, J.A. Gardon, and R.C. Fincher, 1976, N-nitrosamine formation from atrazine, Bull. Environ. Contamn. Toxicol., 15:342-346.

10. Preussmann, R., H. Druchrey, S. Ivankovic, and A. Von Hodenberg, 1969, Chemical structure and carcinogenicity of aliphatic hydrazo-, azo- and azoxy compounds and of triazines, potential in vivo aklylating agents, Ann. N.Y. Acad. Sci., 163:697-716.

11. Preussmann, R., A. Von Hodenberg, and H. Hengy, 1969, Mechanism of carcinogenesis with 1-aryl-3,3-dialkyltriazines, enzymatic dealkylation by rat liver microsomal fraction in vitro, Biochem. Pharmacol., 18:1-13.

12. Preussmann, R., S. Ivankovic, C. Landschutz, J. Gimmy, E. Flohr, and U. Griesbach, 1974, Carcinogene wirkung von 13 aryldialkyl triazenen an BD-ratten, Z. Krebsforsch., 81:285-310.

13. El-Mofty, M., M. Renber, A.H. El-Sebae, and I. Sabry, 1981, Induction of neoplastic lesions in toads (B. regularis) with Baylucide (niclosamide or Bayer 73). Presented at the Proceedings of Int. Symposium on Prevention of Occupational Cancer, Helsinki, Finland.

14. Fishbein, L., 1979, Potential Industrial Carcinogens and Mutagens, Elsevier Press, Amsterdam. pp. 93-120.

15. Fishbein, L., 1980, Potential carcinogenic and mutagenic industrial chemicals. I. Alkylating agents, J. Toxicol. Environ. Health, 6:1133-1177.

16. International Agency for Research on Cancer, 1975, in: "IARC Monographs on the Evaluation of the Carcinogenic Risk of Chemicals to Man," Vol. 9, pp. 37-46, 47-49, 61-65, IARC, Lyon, France.

17. Van Duuren, B.L., S. Melchionne, R. Blair, B.M. Goldschmidt, and C. Katz, 1971, Carcinogenicity of isoesters, epoxides and lactones: Aziridine ethanol, propane sultone and related compounds, J. Natl. Cancer Inst., 46:143-150.

18. Davies, J.E., V.H. Freed, H.F. Enos, A. Barquet, C. Morgade,
     and J.X. Danauskas, 1980, Minimizing occupational exposure to
     pesticides: Epidemiological review. in: "Residue Rev.,"
     F.A. Gunther and J.D. Gunther, eds., 75:7-20.
19. Brooks, G.T., 1974, Chlorinated Insecticides, Vol. 1, CRC
     Press, Cleveland, OH.
20. Eto, M., 1974, Organophosphorus Pesticides: Organic and
     Biological Chemistry, CRC Press, Cleveland, OH.

DISCUSSION

Q.   KADO: What is the Egyptian government's policy regarding
     importation of pesticides suspended or banned in the U.S.?
A.   EL-SEBAE: The Egyptian Ministry of Agriculture has the regula-
     tory authority to accept any compound registered in the produc-
     ing developed countries on the basis of the efficacy screening
     which lasts at least 3 years. However, it is the right of the
     Egyptian authorities to suspend any new or old compound when
     there is an adverse effect to humans or non-target organisms.
Q.   BYARD: Many of the carcinogenic chemicals which you have
     reported to be used in Egyptian agriculture are hepatocarcino-
     gens. Do you know the incidence of liver cancer in Egypt?
A.   We do not have a complete national registry for liver cancer
     in Egypt that can be correlated to pesticide exposure.

BIOLOGICAL CHARACTERISTICS OF THE AFLATOXIN-INDUCED HEPATIC TUMOR

Avril D. Woodhead

Biology Department
Brookhaven National Laboratory
Upton, NY 11973

INTRODUCTION

Human diseases resulting from the contamination of food by fungal products have been recorded since the Middle Ages. The terrifying convulsions, dancing mania and, finally, the gangrene of "St. Anthony's fire" a common epidemic disease of the tenth and eleventh centuries, came from eating rye infected with the ergot fungus, Claviceps purpurea. Under suitable conditions of high humidity, fungi can grow on almost any plant and plant product. It is not surprising, therefore, that epidemics of mycotoxicosis have been recorded from many parts of the world; early this century, "yellow rice disease" in Japan and alimentary toxic aleukia in Russia killed large numbers of people (18).

The connection between ergotism and fungal toxins was recognized in the 1850s, but for more than a century afterwards molds on foods were regarded as no more than a nuisance, and there was little interest in their toxicity. Referring to this period, Ciegler and Bennett (18) termed mycotoxicoses the "neglected diseases of human and animal medicine." The discovery of penicillin and its many benefits encouraged this complacency. These ideas were severely jolted in the early 1960s however, when it was found that some mold poisons could be highly dangerous to man and animals. Intensive research on the subject started when hundreds of thousands of turkeys and ducklings in the United Kingdom died with acute liver necrosis - the so-called Turkey X disease - as a result of eating a commercial diet containing Brazilian ground nuts (10,78). At the same time, the first report was published in the United States concerning a high incidence of hepatic carcinoma amongst hatchery-reared trout (100); this

127

epidemic coincided with a marked change in their food from a wet
mixture of animal offals to dried pellets, which included cottonseed meal (99). Outbreaks of hepatic toxicity in cattle, pigs and
sheep in Britain were also reported at that time which were related
to the presence in their fodder of nuts from Uganda, heavily
contaminated with fungus. The inclusion of Ugandan nuts in poultry
food was also associated with a widespread death of ducks in Kenya
(78). It was quickly established that the Brazilian groundnuts
from the suspect shipment fed to guinea-pigs caused their death
within three weeks (14). Rats given the same diet did not succumb,
but after 30 weeks they developed severe liver damage (14,52).
Very shortly afterwards, investigators on both sides of the
Atlantic isolated the agents responsible for the illness from the
nuts and cotton-seed meal, and named them "Aflatoxins" after the
mold that produced them, Aspergillus flavus. Two major components
and several smaller ones were distinguished, and named aflatoxin B
and G on the basis of their blue or green fluorescence (29,65).
The findings indicated strongly that the aflatoxins were not only
acutely toxic but probably also carcinogenic when ingested over a
long period. These early results have been well confirmed.

The fungus, Aspergillus flavus has a worldwide distribution in
agricultural products and in soil and a few strains (and also
strains of A. parasiticus) will produce aflatoxin under suitable
conditions of high humidity and temperature. Crops left standing
in the field in contact with damp soil or damaged by rain and snow
may become contaminated with molds. Fungal growth is encouraged
when crops are stored under damp warm conditions. As methods of
harvesting, storage, and preservation have improved, the prevalence
of fungal contamination of foodstuffs has decreased, and today
there is no great hazard from aflatoxin poisoning in the developed
countries. Liver cancer incidence is low, at about 2 cases per
year for 100,000 people (9,26,81). Aflatoxin contamination is
still a considerable problem in some underdeveloped nations of the
world, where liver cancer may account for the major part of all
recorded cancers (Figure 1).

Nevertheless, aflatoxin is present in low amounts in many of
our foods (88), especially in those eaten by children, such as
cereals and peanut butter, and consumption of low levels of what is
now known to be a powerful carcinogen and mutagen would seem undesirable (36).

EPIDEMIOLOGY

Epidemiological studies have shown a correlation between the
level of aflatoxin in the diet and liver cancer in humans, although
a cause and effect relationship has not been proven. In several

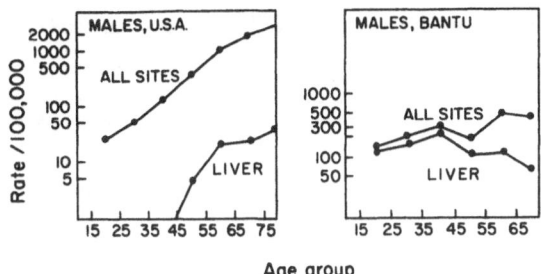

Fig. 1.   A comparison between the incidence of liver cancer in
males in the U.S.A. and Bantu males (adapted from
Higginson, 40).

areas of Africa, India, and Thailand, the correspondence is particularly striking between the frequency of mold contamination of
staple foods and the regional incidence of liver cancer, as shown
in Table 1, (2,44,71). The highest known intake in the world
occurs in Mozambique, with a mean daily ingestion of 15 µg; this
country has the highest known rate of liver cancer (91). In Kenya
it was shown that levels of fungal contamination in the homes of
cancer patients were higher than in the dwellings of unaffected
individuals (71,72). Similarly, Aleksandrowicz and Smyk (1) surveyed 380 houses in Poland, and found Aspergillus flavus and other
fungal flora present in the homes of people with liver cancer, but
absent from those of healthy people. Surprisingly, although agricultural practices and climate in parts of South America are
similar to those in Africa, there have been no reports of high
incidences of liver cancer (81).

The association between aflatoxin toxicity and human mortality
has been highlighted in several dramatic events. The best-known
incident occurred in Western India in 1974, when unseasonal rains
in a chronically drought-stricken area drenched the maize crops.
These became moldy, and subsequently 397 people from 200 villages
became ill, with vomiting and jaundice from eating the contaminated
maize, and 106 of these people died with massive gastrointestinal
hemorrhage. The contaminated maize was pale, shrivelled, and
covered with mold; the levels of aflatoxin ranged from six to 15
parts per million (49). Isolated cases of aflatoxin poisoning have
also been reported among people who handle the substance. Thus a
42-year old biochemist died, and his young assistant was gravely
ill after spending some months purifying aflatoxin from mold
cultures (24). Dvorachova (27) has reported the deaths from pulmonary cancer of two men who worked with contaminated peanut-meal
and had inhaled the dust.

Table 1.   Aflatoxin Intake and Hepatoma Incidence in Kenya

	Average daily intake aflatoxin B_1 (ng/kg bodyweight)		Hepatoma incidence cases/100,000/year	
	Male	Female	Male	Female
Low areas, 3,500 ft	14.81	10.03	12.92	5.44
Middle area, 6,000	7.84	5.86	10.80	3.28
High area, 12,000 ft	4.88	3.46	3.11	1/10,000/4yr

Adapted from Peers and Linsell (72).

The World Health Organization Report on Mycotoxins (102) con-
cludes that aflatoxin ingestion may increase the risk of liver
cancer, the extent of risk depending upon the amount eaten. The
U.S. Food and Drug Administration also hold that mycotoxins may be
some of the most significant pollutants known, and may be the cause
of many diseases of unknown etiology. Accordingly in 1965, the FDA
restricted the permissible level of aflatoxin in food to 30 ppb,
and further lowered the limit to 20 ppb in 1969. Aflatoxin is
present in many foods at low levels - especially in cereals, nuts,
dairy products, pulses, and dried fruits (63,88), but generally the
level is below the limit set by the FDA (32,35). However, Consumer
Reports in 1978 (23) tested two samples from 38 brands of peanut
butter, and found that only 9 of these had no detectable
aflatoxin. At least one sample from every brand tested contained
some aflatoxin, and three had levels exceeding the current limit.

The problem of keeping aflatoxin to a minimum in foodstuffs in
the developed countries is one of careful monitoring. Food that is
visibly moldy has an unacceptable taste, but low levels of
aflatoxin contamination may be masked by the substrate, for
example, in peanut butter. The problem is also a seasonal one, and
mycotoxins may be confined to the occasional nut; thus Fuller et
al. (34) found one contaminated walnut amongst 28 thousand, and
one moldy almond in 26 thousand. Careful hand sorting or
electronic sorting is usually efficacious. Visibly moldy nuts can
safely be made into peanut-oil, since the extraction processes
remove virtually all the aflatoxin. Chemical decontamination can
be used for animal feed, and this is cheaper than discarding large
batches of nuts.

AFLATOXIN AS A CO-CARCINOGEN

People with the highest risk for developing liver cancer are
those whose diet consists of rather few staple foods, which may

easily become contaminated with mold. Where the epidemiological
studies have been detailed enough, they usually show a simple dose-
response relationship between aflatoxin intake and liver cancer
(Figure 2) indicating that aflatoxin may be a complete carcinogen
(97). Other data suggest that additional factors may cooperate or
possibly be a prerequisite for cancer development, for example,
hepatitis-B infection, malnutrition, and protozoan or other parasitic infections. Malnutrition in children may cause liver damage,
and so predispose the organ to cancer from agents encountered later
in life. Oettle (68) suggested that liver cancer has a multifactorial origin and points out that viral hepatitis is common amongst
the poorly nourished peoples of the underdeveloped nations. Woodfield et al. (101) detected hepatitis-B antigen in the serum of 82%
of their liver cancer patients in Papua, New Guinea. A high incidence of liver cancer in Taiwan has been associated with low-level
contamination of many dried fruits; viral hepatitis is also common
in Taiwan, and Sung (85) found antigen in the blood of over 50% of
his liver cancer patients. Lin et al. (55) have studied the long-
term effects of aflatoxin B, and viral hepatitis in experiments
with marmosets. Viral hepatitis did not induce hepatic tumors, but
the double injury of hepatitis and aflatoxin caused much more
severe effects than when the chemical was given alone. Thus the
association between viral hepatitis and liver cancer is persuasive
(4,11,56,69), but requires further substantiation (81).

Being male significantly increases the risk of developing
liver cancer, both in animals and humans, as shown in Figure 2,
(13,15,52,66,82). This may be partly related to hormonal background, since the adminstration of diethylstilbestrol or the cas-

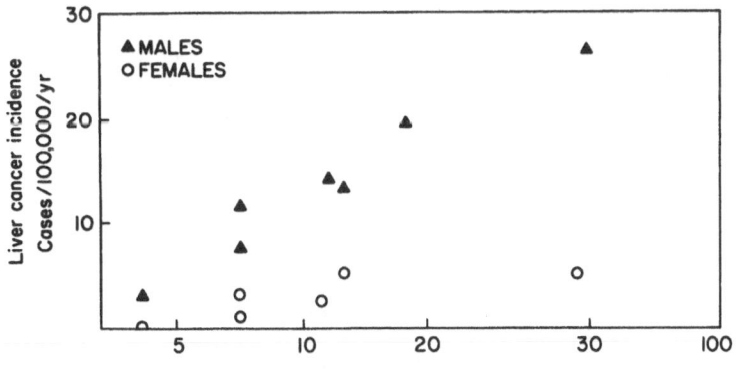

Fig. 2. The Relationship between Liver Cancer Incidence and Daily
         Aflatoxin Intake in the Diet. The data were obtained in
         surveys in Kenya, Mozambique and Thailand (adapted from
         Shank, 81).

tration of male rats inhibits aflatoxin carcinogenesis (15,66).
About twice as many men as women have been the victims of outbreaks
of aflatoxin poisoning (49), and this does not seem to be related
to differences in their diet, although the aflatoxin intake in
females is generally somewhat less. On the other hand, viral hepatitis is much commoner in males than in females (45,82,85). Coady
(19) believes that concurrent protozoan or schistosomal infections
may suppress the immune response to viral invasion. In some parts
of the world, parasitic diseases and hepatoma both occur at an
increased rate, for example, in Northern Thailand, but in other
areas, such as Mauritania and Senegal, liver cancer is common but
schistosomiasis is not (68). In experiments with chickens, Thaxton
et al. (86) showed that aflatoxin itself may be an
immunosuppressant, and so could account for the enhanced
susceptibility to infectious agents seen during aflatoxicosis.

COMPARATIVE ASPECTS OF AFLATOXICOSIS

     The acute toxicity of aflatoxin has been demonstrated in a
diversity of species. No species are known to be refractory, but
there is a wide range of sensitivity which bears no apparent relationship to their taxonomic standing. Closely related species may
show large differences in sensitivity, the best example being the
salmonid fishes. Halver et al. (38) found that coho salmon,
Oncorhynchus kisutch, were 10 to 30 times more resistant and showed
less extensive and less specific liver damage after exposure to
aflatoxin than the closely related rainbow trout, Salmo
gairdnerii. It is now recognized that differences in hepatic aflatoxin metabolism may underlie species and strain variability and
may also be a component of the sex differences in mortality. A
proviso might be added here: aflatoxins are insoluble in water but
are soluble in dimethylformamide and in dimethylsulfoxide. Dimethylformamide, which was used as a solvent in many early studies has
been shown to be unsuitable since it may by itself cause
significant pathological changes in the liver (59). Some earlier
comparative studies may require confirmation.

     The carcinogenic effects of aflatoxin also differ between
strains, sex and with age. Wogan (96) showed that a level of 150
ppm aflatoxin in the diet of random-bred mice given over their
lifespan did not induce liver tumors, but newborn mice of a hybrid
strain developed many tumors following injections of aflatoxin
during the prenatal period. Carcinogenicity may be also increased
by a poor diet, an important factor since malnutrition is widespread in countries where food is more likely to be contaminated
with molds (40). One of the most sensitive species to aflatoxin is
the rainbow trout, its response exceeding that of the duckling, the

animal commonly used in toxicology testing. The Mount Shasta strain is particularly sensitive, and the addition of 8 ppb of aflatoxin B_1 to their diet for 12 months caused hepatomas in 85 to 100 percent of the fish. Levels as low as 0.4 to 0.5 ppb gave rise to a significant increase in cancer incidence (83). Sensitivity also differs at different stages of the trout's life span, and in common with many other animals, the young are particularly vulnerable (83,89,94). Trout eyed-ova show a 40 percent increase in cancer incidence some ten months after exposure to 0.5 ppm aflatoxin B_1 for 1 hour and as short and exposure as 15 minutes produces a significant increase in tumor incidence. Coho salmon, which are resistant as adults, also show much greater sensitivity as embryos.

    The Amazon molly, Poecilia formosa, is very sensitive to afla- toxin and 7-day old fish, exposed to 3 ppb for 24 hours have a 100 percent incidence of liver tumors after nine months (Woodhead and Setlow, unpublished). Hepatomas have been induced in guppies, Lebistes reticulatus, by feeding a diet with 6 ppm aflatoxin for 9 to 11 months (60). Hepatic neoplasms have been seen in a surpris- ingly large number of feral fishes. The Registry of Tumors in Lower Animals from 1966 to 1979 lists 17 species with liver tumors, some having multiple records. By contrast, there is only one record for amphibia and three for reptiles. The total number of records for tumors of any kind in these two classes, however, is less than half those recorded for fishes and this probably reflects the frequency with which they are sampled, rather than any class difference in susceptibility to liver cancer. Experimental studies with the amphibian species, Bombina and Rana have shown that they exhibit developmental abnormalities after exposure to aflatoxin (73).

    Some birds are very sensitive to the toxic effects of aflatoxin, and the duckling is routinely used as a test animal. Doses of 30 ppb in the diet for 14 months induced tumors in over 80 percent of exposed turkeys (16). The chick embryo has also been widely used in toxicology assays (92). Other species of birds may be more resistant and Marks and Wyatt (57) have recently developed, by selective breeding, lines of Japanese quails resistant to afla- toxin, which may be useful as an animal model in investigating the physiological basis of resistance (Table 2).

    It would generally appear that the exposures required to cause tumors in mammals are 10 to 100 times higher than those effective in the duckling and rainbow trout. Wogan et al. (98) demonstrated that aflatoxin B_1, was carcinogenic in male Fischer rats at a dose of 1 ppb when given for 105 weeks; Tisdel et al. (87), working with the same strain of rats over the same period, found hepatomas after

Table 2. Mortality of Japanese Quail from Acute Aflatoxicosis

Generation		S1	S2	S3	S4	S5
Control	2.5 mg/kg	40	72.5	79.0	787.3	75.0
Selected		14.4	36.9	22.4	11.6	6.3
Control	3.0 mg/kg	71.6	88.5	97.0	78.3	82.9
Selected		39.7	42.0	35.6	12.4	10.0

Adapted from Marks and Wyatt (57).

exposure to 5 ppb. In general, humans and monkeys are classed in
an intermediate group for sensitivity, guinea-pigs are more
sensitive and mice less so (28,58,76). Often there is no
immediately obvious correlation between the toxic and the
carcinogenic dose, and it may be difficult to relate differences in
sensitivity to the pathways of metabolism (75). Within a normal
outbreeding species there is also a great deal of inherent
variability in response. Thus, groups each of five mink exposed to
a single dose of 300, 500 or 900 µg aflatoxin B_1 showed one, two
and four deaths respectively, but those animals which survived were
no different from the untreated controls, except that their livers
contained more fat (17). Reddy et al. (74) fed tree shrews with a
total of 24 to 66 mg aflatoxin over periods of 74 to 172 weeks and
found that while some animals showed severe postnecrotic scarring
of the liver, others had only mild portal fibrosis.

THE LIVER TUMOR

     Four sequential stages have been distinguished in the develop-
ment of liver carcinomas in rats. The first stage is marked by the
appearance of areas of pale, hyperplastic cells with irregular,
enlarged nuclei. Next to appear are foci or hyperplastic nodules
in which the cells have a large hyperchromatic nucleus and
granular, acidophilic cytoplasm. The following stage in development is the neoplastic nodule. The nucleus of the neoplastic cell
is larger and more hyperchromatic than in earlier lesions and
occupies a bigger area of the cell, while the cytoplasm is less
abundant, granular, and basophilic. Large hyperbasophilic malignant foci develop from these nodules.

Similar morphological changes have been described in afla-toxin-treated rainbow trout, although Sinnhuber et al. (83) point out that their sequential nature and their homology with the cellular stages in the rat have not been unequivolcally estab-lished. Areas of hyperplastic, pale cells in the livers of fish increase in extent with the dose of aflatoxin and the length of exposure. Sinnhuber and his associates (83) believe that these areas result from the toxic action of aflatoxin and are not an early stage in the development of a liver tumor. They suggest that as the hepatocytes undergo degeneration and necrosis, loci of regeneration appear and that a mutant cell among these may lead to the development of cancer. Some degree of degeneration and regeneration may be a prerequisite for malignant change (21,103), and could arise where the regenerative process "overshoots the mark."

The role of the eosinophilic nodule in hepatocarcinogenesis is currently under debate, particularly in fishes. Sinnhuber et al. (83) believe that eosinophilic cells have a minimal contribution to neoplasia, and they have not observed an eosinophilic to basophillic change in trout. In support of this view, they demon-strated that eosinophilic cells elicit a host immune response, which presumably destroys them. However, Wales (95) from similar observations in trout assumed that the transformation does take place. We have not seen mixed nodules in the Amazon molly and, in general, eosinophilic nodules were rare. Other investigators have described the occurrence of small numbers of basophilic cells (or small basophilic nodules) within eosinophilic nodules (5,79).

Basophilic nodules vary in size from small groups of cells to nodules which may occupy 30 to 40 percent of the liver. The nodules are usually unencapsulated, non-compressing and the cells are arranged in broad widely-spaced chords of three to four cells. Mitoses are often seen. Sinnhuber et al. (83) believe that for the most part neoplastic development in trout liver begins directly at this stage; basophilic nodules rarely elicited an immune reaction in trout.

There is disagreement upon whether the basophilic nodule is benign or an early developmental stage of the mature malignant neoplasm. Sinnhuber and his associates favor the latter hypothesis, and have used a variety of features to distinguish between benign nodules and liver carcinomas, including increased width of the liver chords and increased mitotic activity. Meta-stases, usually regarded as the hallmark of malignant neoplasia, are rarely seen in the trout, and I have not seen any in the Amazon molly. Trout liver tumors do not metastasize until late in life, after about three to six years, and often the rapidly enlarging primary tumor causes the death of the fish from massive hemorrhage at an earlier age (83). In mammals, also, longer periods of exposure to the carcinogen may be required before metastases appear (80).

We have investigated this problem further with the Amazon
molly as our experimental model. The Amazon molly exists in nature
as several all-female clones, reproducing gynogenetically, so that
the offspring of a single original female, all females, are genetically homogenous. Thus cells and tissues transplanted between
members of a clone are not rejected and survive as long as the
recipient. Interclone transplants are, however, eliminated. We
treated one-week old mollies from Clone 2 with aflatoxin B_1, and
nine months later killed the fish and removed their livers. Tumors
can readily be seen as white areas within the normal pinkish-brown
liver tissue (Figure 3 a, b). The tumors were carefully dissected
free under sterile conditions, homogenized to give a suspension of
single cells, the cells washed and resuspended in phosphate-
buffered saline at a concentration of 200,000 cells in 0.2 μl.

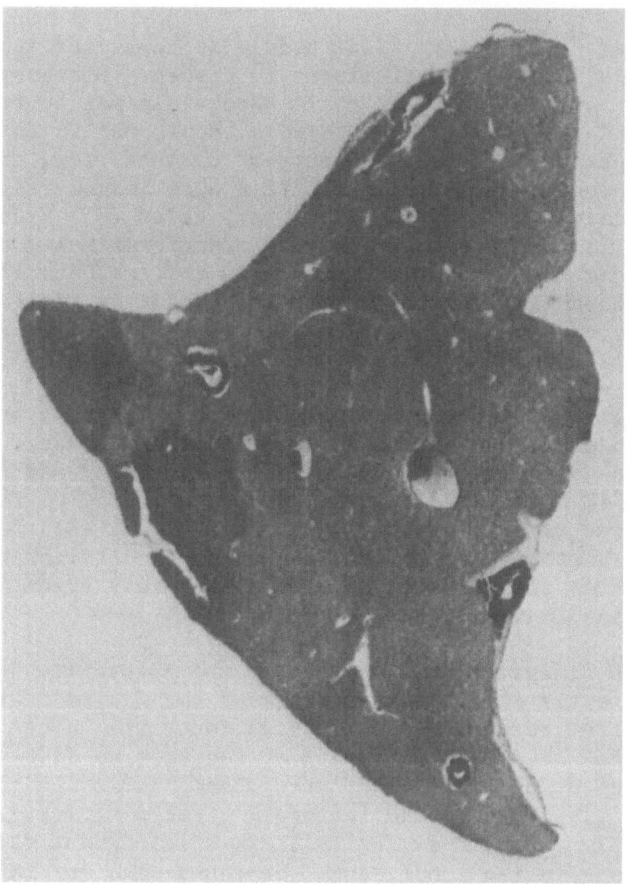

Fig. 3 (a) Section through the Liver of 9 Month Old Amazon Molly,
           Exposed to 3 ppb Aflatoxin for 24 Hours at 7 Days of Age.
           There are two well developed basophilic nodules. (Mag x35;
           reduced 23% for reproduction.)

This suspension was injected intraperitoneally into homologous
recipients (intraclone transfer) and also into mollies from Clone 4
(interclone tranfer). Nine months later the fish were examined
histologically. We found that 37 out of 40 fish from the
intraclone transfer had enlarged livers, with nodules replacing
more than half of the normal liver. Nodules were present in 14 out
of 30 interclone recipients but had replaced only ten percent of
normal liver tissue. In contrast to the rarity of eosinophilic
nodules found after exposure to aflatoxin, eosinophilic cells
occurred in 60 percent of the intraclone recipients, and 20 percent

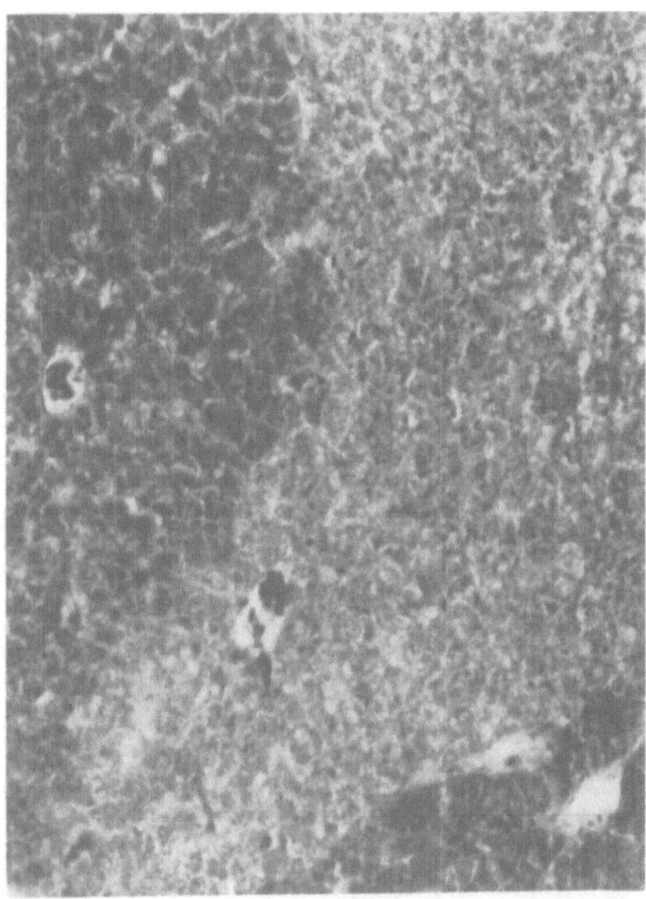

Fig. 3 (b) A High-Power Photograph of the Basophilic Nodules in
        3a, with Normal Liver Tissue in between. (Mag x250; re-
        duced 23% for reproduction.)

of the interclone recipients, often occurring in close proximity to
basophilic nodules. Tumors in which basophilic cells were
intermingled with eosinophilic cells (mixed nodules) were still
rather few in number; they were seen in seven of the 40 intraclone
transfer fish and in two of the interclone recipients. The fact
that the injected tumor cells gave rise to liver tumors in
interclone transfer argues that cellular transformation had
occurred and that the original basophilic nodules, from which the
cells were derived, were in fact early neoplasms. Our results have
not clarified the status of the eosinophilic nodule in liver carcinogenesis in fishes (Woodhead and Setlow, unpublished).

TUMORS AT OTHER SITES

     The pathological lesions resulting from aflatoxin administra-
tion are mainly found in the liver, but have also been recorded
from other sites. In some of the earliest assays in rodents aflatoxin was given subcutaneously and some twenty weeks later, sarcomas and fibrosarcomas developed at the site of injection (25).
Salmon and Newberne (77) noted that rats fed aflatoxin in their
diet developed kidney tubule adenomas, as well as hepatomas. Aflatoxin-induced lesions have now been seen in several other sites,
including the colon (24,97), the lung (27,43), and kidney (37).

     During the years 1970-1971 there was an outbreak of hepatomas
among hatchery-reared trout in Japan resulting from the presence of
aflatoxin in fish food. Kimura et al. (46) observed that many of
the trout had adenomatous polyps in their stomachs, and that the
frequency of polyps was much higher in fish reared in ponds with a
gravel bottom than in trout from ponds with beds of dead leaves.
The development of the polyps was believed to result from repeated
mechanical injury to the stomach when gravel was accidentally swal-
lowed, and aflatoxin accelerated the development of the lesion.
Stomach polyps were noted in yellowtails (Serola quinqueradiata)
and sea bream (Pagrus major) given commercial pellets.

     There is evidence that aflatoxin (or its metabolites) can pass
the placental barrier and induce malformations in the fetus. Munoz
(64) showed in experimental animals that aflatoxin may be embryo-
toxic early in the first half of pregnancy, and teratogenic if
given later in the first half of pregnancy. The compound acts as a
transplacental carcinogen only when given in the second half of
pregnancy. Vesselinovitch (93) suggested that the largest
nonhazardous level to the human female may be carcinogenic to the
fetus. The fetus may be placed at higher risk for liver cancer in
other ways. Blumberg et al. (12) found that 70 to 80 percent of
the mothers of their liver cancer patients were carriers of viral -
hepatitis antigen, and suggest that an infection acquired in utero
could readily develop later into chronic persistent hepatitis and
predisposition to cancer.

IN VITRO ASSAYS

Attempts have been made to associate morphological changes in cells treated in vitro with aflatoxin with their ability to induce tumors in syngenic hosts. Evans and DiPaola (30) treated cultures of fetal guinea-pig cells with aflatoxin and saw some loss of cell orientation after five days, but marked changes did not become apparent until 4 months or more and this did not coincide with the onset of the capacity of the cells to produce tumors in genetically compatible recipients. Tumorigenicity did not correlate with changes in plating efficiency, doubling time, or chromosomal alterations, but there was an apparent relationship with the ability of the cells to form colonies in soft agar. Noyes (67) exposed human liver parenchymal cells to 0.01 µg per ml aflatoxin and noted that subsequently some cells become enlarged, with pale eosinophilic cytoplasm and hyperchromatic nuclei - similar to the changes seen in vivo after exposure. Auletta and Suk (6) also found morphological transformation in rat embryo cells at 0.01 µg and 0.05 µg, together with a 50 percent reduction in plating efficiency; the transformed cells lacked contact inhibition and grew in semisolid agar. Beniumovich (8) showed that the damage caused by aflatoxin was greatest in hepatocytes undergoing mitosis, but under conditions of retarded propagation, the resistance of hepatocytes may be higher than that of other types of cells. Lines of rat liver cells resistant to aflatoxin have been established by Iype et al. (42). An exposure to 0.5 µg per ml aflatoxin for three weeks is needed to transform these cells to multinucleate ones, which will form colonies in soft agar.

ASSAYS FOR MUTAGENESIS

Assays for mutagenicity have been conducted with various prokaryotic and eukaryotic cells, in order to detect aflatoxin in foodstuffs (and its metabolites in biological material from exposed people) and to probe the nature of the molecular damage caused by the compound. Over the years, the level of detection has been progressively lowered and quantification increased. Recently, enzyme immunoassays using monoclonal antibodies have been developed which reliably detect aflatoxin B_1 - DNA adducts at levels of one residue per 250,000 nucleotides (39).

The naturally occurring aflatoxins are inactive in prokaryotic cells which do not have metabolic activation systems. Ames and his colleagues (3) devised a simple, rapid assay, the His[+] revertant assay, to measure the mutational ability of chemicals using different strains of Salmonella typhimurium in the presence of rodent liver microsomes (S-9 fraction) as the activating system.

This test has been widely used (3,22,41,50,62,90). By the use of specially constructed mutant strains of the bacterium, one of which detects base-pair substitutions and others which detect frameshift mutants, it has generally been shown that aflatoxin B_1 is a reactive frameshift mutant. However, Coles, Lindsay Smith and Garner (20) chemically synthesized a model of the metabolically active epoxide of aflatoxin, the compound 3a,8a - dihydrofuro [2,3-b] benzofuran, and tested its mutagenicity against Salmonella. They concluded that aflatoxin may cause base-pair substitution as well as frameshift mutations. Aflatoxin is also mutagenic in Neurospora crassa in the presence of an activation system (50,61,70).

Mutation tests with Drosophila melanogaster have in general confirmed the findings from prokaryotic assays. Exposure of male flies to doses of 0.02 mg per ml aflatoxin caused the appearance of recessive lethal mutations in their offspring. Surveys of successive broods fathered by the treated males indicated that the compound had affected the premeiotic spermatogonia, suggesting that nuclear division is important in aflatoxin-induced mutagenicity (51,54). Fahmy et al. (31) also used the Drosophila assay to compare the activity of aflatoxin B_1, and aflatoxin-chloride, a model of the oxidative metabolite of aflatoxin. Aflatoxin-chloride had a spermicidal efficiency a thousand times greater than the parent compound. The authors concluded that the biological effects of aflatoxin were due to structural alterations in the compound during metabolism, and that the main site of attack in the cell was the N-7 guanine of DNA.

The cytotoxicity and mutagenicity of aflatoxin B_1 and B_2 have been examined using Chinese Hamster V79 cells (48). Many cultured mammalian cell lines also lack mixed-function oxidase enzyme activity, so that an activation system is added. In the presence of the S-9 fraction from rat livers, the mutagenic activity of several aflatoxins in V79 cells paralleled their carcinogenic activity as found in other assays (Table 3). Several investigators have proposed using such eukaryotic cell assays as screening tests for presumptive carcinogens (53,84). The carcinogenic activity of aflatoxin has also been assessed by other methods including stimulation of unscheduled DNA synthesis in human intestinal mucosa cells (33) and sister chromatid exchanges and chromosomal aberrations in V79 cells (7,47).

CONCLUSIONS

There is a well-documented association between the intake of food contaminated with aflatoxin and the occurrence of liver cancer in underdeveloped nations and there may be real opportunities for drastically reducing its incidence. It is encouraging that

Table 3.   Relative Potency of Various Naturally—Occuring
           Aflatoxins and Their Metabolites

Type	Relative mutagenicity percent	Carcinogenicity
AFB_1	100	Most potent in rat, rainbow trout
AFL	22.8	50% activity of AFB_1 in trout
AFG_1	3.3	Less active than AFB_1 in rat and trout
AFM_1	3.2	One third of AFB_1 in trout: less active in rat
AFH_1	2.0	----------
AFQ_1	1.1	Not active in rat and trout
AFB_2	0.2	Weak activity (1/150th AFB_1) in rat and trout
AFP_1	0.1	----------
AFG_2	0.1	Inactive in trout
AFB_{2a}	0	----------
AFG_{2a}	0	----------

Adapted from Krahn and Heidelberger (48).

prevention of liver cancer has largely been accomplished in the developed nations by the efforts of food producers and manufacturers. There is now no great risk from aflatoxin contamination of food, and continued careful monitoring of foods can maintain protection of humans and livestock. The problem, however, is a great one in underdeveloped countries, and its solution calls for a vast improvement in crop handling and storage, together with the instigation of health and nutrition programs to prevent a background of chronic liver damage.

ACKNOWLEDGEMENT

This research was carried out at the Brookhaven National Laboratory under the auspices of the U. S. Department of Energy.

REFERENCES

1. Aleksandrowicz, J. and B. Smyk. 1973. The association of neoplastic diseases and mycotoxins in the environment. Tex. Rep. Biol. Med., 31, 715.

2.   Alpert, M.E., M.S.R. Hutt, G.N. Wogan and C.S. Davidson.
     1971. The association between aflatoxin content of food and
     hepatoma frequency in Uganda. Cancer, (Philadelphia) 28,
     253.
3.   Ames, B.N., W.E. Durston, E. Yamasaki and F.D. Lee. 1973.
     Carcinogens are mutagens: A simple system combining liver
     homogenates for activation and bacteria for detection. Proc.
     Natl. Acad. Sci. USA, 70, 2281.
4.   Anthony, P.P. 1976. Precursor lesions for liver cancer in
     humans. Cancer Res., 36, 2579.
5.   Ashley, L.M. and J.E. Halver. 1961. Hepatomagenesis in
     rainbow trout. Fed. Proc. Fed. Am. Soc. Exp. Biol., 20, 290.
6.   Auletta, A.E. and W.A. Suk. 1977. Transformation of the
     Fischer rat embryo cell system by two carcinogenic
     mutagens. Proc. Am. Assoc. Cancer Res., 18, 137.
7.   Batt, T.R., J. L. Hsueh, H. H. Chen, and C. C. Huang. 1980.
     Sister chromatid exchange and chromosome aberrations in V79
     cells induced by aflatoxin B1, B2, G1 and G2 with or without
     metabolic activation. Carcinogenesis, 1, 759.
8.   Beniumovich, M.S. 1973. Effect of aflatoxins on animal
     cells in tissue culture. Farmakol. Toksikol (Kiev), 36, 497.
9.   Berglund, F. 1975. Mycotoxicosis in Europe in the 20th
     century. Lakartidningen, 72, 5065.
10. Blount, W.P. 1961. Turkey "X" disease. Turkeys, 9, (2) 52.
11. Blumberg, B.S. 1977. Australia antigen and the biology of
     hepatitis B. Science, 197, 17.
12. Blumberg, B.S., B. Laurouze, W.T. London, B. Werner, J.E.
     Hesser, I. Millman, G. Saimot, and M. Payet. 1975. The
     relation of infection with the hepatitis B antigen to primary
     hepatic carcinoma. Am. J. Pathol., 81, 669.
13. Butler, W.H. 1971. The toxicology of aflatoxin, pp. 141–
     165. In Mycotoxins in Human Health. Purchase, J. F. H., ed.
     Macmillan Press, London.
14. Butler, W.H. and J.M. Barnes. 1964. Toxic effects of
     groundnut meal containing aflatoxin to rats and guinea-
     pigs. Br. J. Cancer, 17, 699.
15. Cardeilhac, P. T. and K. P. Nair. 1973. Inhibition by
     castration of aflatoxin-induced hepatoma in carbon
     tetrachloride-treated rats. Toxicol. Appl. Pharmacol., 26,
     393.
16. Carnaghan, R. B. A. 1965. Hepatic tumors in ducks fed a low
     level of toxic groundnut meal. Nature, (London), 208, 308.
17. Chou, C. C., E. H. Marth and R. M. Shackelford. 1976. Ex-
     perimental acute aflatoxicosis in mink (Mustela vison). Am.
     J. Vet. Res., 37 , 1227.
18. Ciegler, A. and J. W. Bennett. 1980. Mycotoxins and
     mycotoxicoses. BioScience, 30, 512.
19. Coady, A. 1976. Tropical cirrhosis and hepatoma. J. Roy.
     Coll. Physicians, London, 10, 133.

20. Coles, B. F., J. R. Lindsay Smith, R. C. Garner. 1977.
Mutagenicity of 3A, 8A-dihydrofuro [2,3-B] dibenzofuran, a
model of aflatoxin B for Salmonella typhimurium TA 100.
Biochem. Biophys. Res. Commun., 76, 888.

21. Columbano, A., S. Rajalatshni, and D. S. R. Sarma. 1981.
Requirement of cell proliferation for the initiation of liver
carcinogenesis as assayed by three different procedures.
Cancer Res., 41, 2079.

22. Commoner, B. 1976. Reliability of bacterial mutagenesis
techniques to distinguish carcinogenic and noncarcinogenic
chemicals. Environ. Prot. Agency (U.S.) Report No. EPA-
600/1-76-022. Washington, DC, 114 pp.

23. Consumer Reports. 1978. Peanut butter. Consumer Reports,
43, 435.

24. Deger, G. E. 1976. Aflatoxin in human colon
carcinogenesis. Anns. Intern. Med., 85, 204.

25. Dickens, F. and H. E. H. Jones 1964. The carcinogenic
action of aflatoxin after its subcutaneous injection in the
rat. Br. J. Cancer, 17, 691.

26. Doll, R. and T. Vodopiga (eds). 1973. International Agency
for Research on Cancer Sci. Publ. No. 7. Lyon, France.

27. Dvorachova, I. 1976. Aflatoxin inhalation and alveolar cell
carcinoma. Br. Med. J., 60, 691.

28. Edwards, G. S., T. D. Rintel, and C. M. Parker. 1975. Aflatoxicol as a possible predictor for species sensitivity to
aflatoxin B_1. Proc. Am. Soc. Cancer Res., 16, 133.

29. Engebrecht, R. H., J. L. Ayres and R. O. Sinnhuber 1965.
Isolation and determination of aflatoxin B_1 in cottonseed
meals. J. Assoc. Offic. Anal. Chemists, 4, 815.

30. Evans, C.H. and J.A. DiPaolo. 1975. Neoplastic transformation of guinea-pig fetal cells in culture induced by chemical
carcinogens. Cancer Res., 35, 1035.

31. Fahmy, M.J., O.G. Fahmy and D.H. Swenson. 1978. Aflatoxin
B_1-2,3-dichloride as a model of the active metabolite of
aflatoxin B_1 in mutagenesis and carcinogenesis. Cancer Res.,
38, 2608.

32. Fletcher, D.C. 1977. Is the aflatoxin level in peanut
butter hazardous to man? Letter, J. Am. Med. Assoc. 238,
518.

33. Freeman, H.J. and R.H.C. San. 1980. Use of unscheduled DNA
synthesis in freshly isolated human intestinal mucosal cells
for carcinogen detection. Cancer Res., 40, 3155.

34. Fuller, G., W.W. Spooncer, A.D. King, J. Schade and B.
Mackey. 1977. Aflatoxins in Californian tree nuts. J. Am.
Oil Chemists. Soc., 54, 231A.

35. Gilchrist, A. 1977. Is the aflatoxin level in peanut butter
hazardous to man? Letter, J. Am. Med. Assoc., 238, 518.

36. Gloag, D. 1981. Contamination of food: mycotoxins and
metals. Br. Med. J., 282, 879.

37. Gurtoo, H. and L. Motycka. 1976. Effect of sex differences
    on the in vitro and in vivo metabolism of aflatoxin B by the
    rat. Cancer Res., 36, 4663.
38. Halver, J.E., L.M. Ashley and R.R. Smith. 1969. Aflatoxins
    in coho salmon. Natl. Cancer Inst. Monogr., 31, 141.
39. Haugen, A., J.D. Groopman, I-C. Hsu, G.P. Goodrich, G.N.
    Wogan and C.C. Harris. 1981. Monoclonal antibody to afla-
    toxin B_1-modified DNA detected by enzyme immunoassay. Proc.
    Natl. Acad. Sci. USA, 78, 4124.
40. Higginson, J. 1963. The geographical pathology of primary
    liver cancer. Cancer Res., 23, 1624.
41. Ichinotsubo, D., H.F. Mower, J. Setliff and M. Mandel.
    1977. The use of rec bacteria for testing of carcinogenic
    substances. Mutation Res., 46, 53.
42. Iype, P.T., T.D. Allen and D.J. Pillinger. 1975. Certain
    aspects of chemical carcinogenesis in vitro using adult rat
    liver cells. pp. 425-440. In Gene Expression and Carcino-
    genesis in Cultured Liver. Schinson, L.E. and E.B. Thompson,
    eds. Academic Press, New York.
43. Kay, K. 1976. A brief overview of the toxicological and
    epidemiological background to the detection and prevention of
    cancer in agricultural workers. Cancer Detect. Prev., 1,
    107.
44. Keen, P. and P. Martin. 1971. Is aflatoxin carcinogenic in
    man? The evidence in Swaziland. Trop. Geogr., Med., 23, 44.
45. Kew, M.C., R. Marcus and E.W. Geddes. 1977. Some character-
    istics of Mozambican Shangaars with primary hepatocellular
    cancer. S. Afr. Med. J., 51, 306.
46. Kimura, I., T. Miyake, S. Kubota, A. Kamata, S. Morkawa and
    Y. Ito. 1976. Adenomatous polyps in the stomachs of
    hatchery-grown salmonids and other types of fishes. Prog.
    Exp. Tumor Res., 20, 181.
47. Korte, A. 1980. Comparative analysis of chromosomal abbera-
    tions and sister-chromatid exchanges in bone marrow cells of
    Chinese hamsters after treatment wth aflatoxin B_1, patulin
    and cyclophosphamide. Mutation Res., 74, 164.
48. Krahn, D.F. and C. Heidelberger. 1977. Liver homogenate-
    mediated mutagenesis in Chinese Hamster V79 cells by
    polycyclic aromatic hydrocarbons and aflatoxins. Mutation
    Res., 46, 27.
49. Krishnamachari, K.A.V.R., R.V. Bhat, V. Nagarajan and T.B.G.
    Tilak. 1975. Hepatitis due to aflatoxicosis. An outbreak
    in Western India. Lancet, May 10, 1975, 1061.
50. Kuczuk, M.H., P.M. Benson, H. Heath and H. Hayes. 1978.
    Evaluations of the mutagenic potential of mycotoxins using
    Salmonella typhimurium and Saccharomyces cerevisiae.
    Mutation Res., 53, 11.
51. Lamb, M.J. and L.J. Lilly. 1971. Induction of recessive
    lethals in Drosophila melanogaster by aflatoxin B_1. Mutation
    Res., 11, 430.

52. Lancaster, M.C., F.P. Jenkins and J. McL. Philip. 1961. Toxicity associated with certain samples of ground nuts (letter). Nature, (London,) 192, 1095.

53. Langenbach, R., H.J. Freed and E. Huberman. 1978. Liver cell-mediated mutagenesis of mammalian cells by liver carcinogens. Proc. Natl. Acad. Sci. USA., 75, 2864.

54. Lilly, L.J. and M.J. Lamb. 1972. Review of the genetic effects of aflatoxins and a report on the induction of recessive lethals in Drosophila melanogaster by aflatoxin B_1. EMS Newletter, 6, 26.

55. Lin, J.J., C. Liu and D.J. Svoboda. 1974. Long-term effects of aflatoxin B_1 and viral hepatitis on marmoset liver. A preliminary report. Lab. Invest., 30, 267.

56. Linsell, C.A. and F.G. Peers. 1977. Field studies on liver cancer, pp. 549-556. In Origins of Human Cancer. Book A. Incidence of Cancer in Humans. Hiatt, H.H., J.D. Watson and J.A. Winsten, eds. Cold Spring Harbor Conferences on Cell Proliferation.

57. Marks, L.H. and R.D. Wyatt. 1979. Genetic resistance to aflatoxin in Japanese Quail. Science, 206, 1329.

58. Masri, M.S., A.N. Booth and D.P. Hsieh. 1974. Comparative metabolic conversion of aflatoxin B_1 to M_1 and Q_1 by monkey, rat and chicken liver. Life Sci., 15, 203.

59. Mathew, T., R. Karunanithy, M. H. Yee, and P. N. Natarajan, 1980. Hepatotoxicity of dimethyl formamide and dimethyl sulfoxide at and above levels used in some aflatoxin studies. Lab. Invest., 42, 257.

60. Matsushima, T. and T. Sugimura, 1976. Experimental carcinogenesis in small aquarium fishes. Prog. Exp. Tumor Res., 20, 367.

61. Matzinger, P. K. and T-M. Ong. 1976. Mutation induction of rodent liver microsomal metabolites of aflatoxin B_1 and G_1 in Neurospora crassa. Mutation Res., 37, 27.

62. McCann J., N. E. Spingarn, J. Kobori, and B. N. Ames 1975. Detection of carcinogens as mutagens: bacterial tester strains with R factor plasmids. Proc. Natl. Acad. Sci. USA., 72, 979.

63. Ministry of Agriculture, Fisheries and Food. 1980. Steering group on food surveillance, Working party on mycotoxins. Survey of Mycotoxins in the United Kingdom. H. M. S. O., London.

64. Munoz, N. 1976. Prenatal exposure and carcinogenesis. Tumori, 62, 157.

65. Nesbitt, B. F., K. O'Kelly, K. Sargeant, and A. Sheridan. 1962. Toxic metabolites of Aspergillus flavus. Nature, (London), 195, 1062.

66. Newberne, P. and G. Williams. 1969. Inhibition of aflatoxin carcinogenesis by diethylstilbestrol in male rats. Arch. Environ. Health, 19, 489.

67. Noyes, W. F. 1975. Aflatoxin-induced changes in human hepatocytes in organ culture. Proc. Am. Assoc. Cancer Res., 16, 26.

68. Oettle, A. G. 1964. Cancer in Africa, especially in regions south of the Sahara. J. Natl. Cancer Inst., 33, 383.

69. Ohta, Y. 1976. Viral hepatitis and hepatocellular carcinoma, pp. 73-81. In Hepatocellular Carcinoma. Obuda, K. and R. L. Peters, eds. John Wiley and Sons, New York.

70. Ong, T-M. 1970. Mutagenicity of aflatoxins in Neurospora crassa. Mutation Res. 9, 615.

71. Peers, F. G., G. A. Gilman, and C. A. Linsell. 1976. Dietary aflatoxin and human liver cancer. A study in Swaziland. Int. J. Cancer, 17, 167.

72. Peers, F. G. and C. A. Linsell. 1973. Dietary aflatoxins and liver cancer: A population-based study in Kenya. Br. J. Cancer, 27, 473.

73. Puscariu, F., V. V. Papillian, M. Gabor and C. Deac. 1973. Toxicity and morphopathologic effect of aflatoxin in frog tadpoles. Arch. Roum. Pathol. Exp. Microbiol., 32, 255.

74. Reddy, J. K., D. J. Svoboda, and M. S. Rao. 1976. Induction of liver tumors by aflatoxin B_1 in the tree shrew (Tupaia glis), a non-human primate. Cancer Res., 36, 151.

75. Roebuck, B. D. and G. N. Wogan 1977. Species comparison of in vitro metabolism of aflatoxin B_1. Cancer Res. 37, 1649.

76. Salhab, A. S. and G. S. Edwards 1977. Comparative in vitro metabolism of aflatoxicol by liver preparations from animals and humans. Cancer Res., 37, 1016.

77. Salmon, W. D. and P. M. Newberne. 1963. Occurrence of hepatomas in rats fed diets containing peanut meal as a major source of protein. Cancer Res., 23, 571.

78. Sargeant, K., A. Sheridan, J. O'Kelly, and R. B. A. Carnaghan. 1961. Toxicity associated with certain samples of groudnuts (letter). Nature, (London), 192, 1096.

79. Scarpelli, D. G., M. H. Greider and W. J. Frajola. 1963. Observations on hepatic cell hyperplasia, adenoma and hepatoma of rainbow trout (Salmo gairdnerii). Cancer Res., 23, 848.

80. Shalkop, W. T., and B. H. Armbrecht. 1974. Carcinogenic response of brood sows fed aflatoxin for 28 to 30 months. Am. J. Vet. Res., 35, 623.

81. Shank, R. C. 1977. Epidemiology of aflatoxin carcinogenesis, pp. 291-318. In Advances in Modern Toxicology. Kraybill, H. F. and M. A. Mehlman, eds. John Wiley and Sons, New York.

82. Sherlock, S. 1976. Predicting progression of acute type-B hepatitis to chronicity. Lancet, 2, 1976, 354.

83. Sinnhuber, R. O., J. D. Hendricks, J. H. Wales and G. B. Putnam, 1977. Neoplasms in rainbow trout, a sensitive animal model for environmental carcinogenesis. pp. 389-408. In Aquatic Pollutants and Biological Effects with Emphasis on Neoplasia. Kraybill, H. F., C. J. Dawe, J. C.

Harshbarger, and R. G. Tardiff, eds. New York Academy of
Science, New York.

84. Stich, H. F. and B. A. Laishes, 1975. The response of xeroderma pigmentosum cells and controls to the activated mycotoxins, aflatoxins and stregmatocystin. Int. J. Cancer, 16,
266.

85. Sung, J. L. 1973. Hepatitis and hepatoma in Taiwan. Jpn. J.
Gastroenterol. , 70, 977.

86. Thaxton, J. P., H. T. Tung, and P. B. Hamilton. 1974. Immunosuppression in chickens by aflatoxin. Poult. Sci., 53,
721.

87. Tisdel, M. O., P. O. Nees, D. L. Harris and G. E. Mann.
1977. Aflatoxicosis in rats fed low levels of aflatoxin
either chemically pure or as a natural contaminant. Toxicol.
Appl. Pharmacol., 41, 166.

88. Torrey, G. S. and E. H. Marth. 1977. Isolation and toxicity
of molds from foods stored in homes. J. Food Protection, 40,
187.

89. Toth, B. 1968. A critical review of experiments in chemical
carcinogenesis using newborn animals. Cancer Res., 28, 727.

90. Ueno, Y., K. Kubota, T. Ito and Y. Nakamura. 1978. Mutagenicity of carcinogenic mycotoxins in Salmonella
typhimurium. Cancer Res. 38, 536.

91. Van Rensburg, S. J., J. J. Van der Watt, I. F. H. Purchase,
I. Pereira Coutinho, and R. Markham. 1974. Primary liver
cancer rate and aflatoxin intake in a high cancer area. S.
Afr. Med. J., 48, 2508.

92. Verrett, J. M., J. P. Marliac, and J. McLaughlin, Jr.
1974. Use of chick embryo in the assay of aflatoxin
toxicity. J. Assoc. Agr. Chemists, 47, 1003.

93. Vesselinovitch, S. D. 1974. Transplacental and neonatal
carcinogenesis: experimental approach. Proc. Fifth Int.
Symp. Biol. Characterization of Human Tumors, pp. 135-150.
Bologna, April, 1973.

94. Vesselinovitch, S. D., N. Mihailovich, G. N. Wogan, L. S.
Lombard and K. V. N. Rao. 1972. Aflatoxin B_1, a hepatocarcinogen in the infant mouse. Cancer Res., 32, 2289.

95. Wales, J. H. 1970. Hepatoma in rainbow trout, pp. 351-
365. In A Symposium on Diseases of Fishes and Shellfishes.
Vol. 5. Snieszko, S. F. ed. American Fisheries Society,
Washington, D.C.

96. Wogan, G. N. 1977. Mycotoxins and other naturally occurring
carcinogens, pp. 263-290. In Advances in Modern
Toxicology. Kraybill, H. F. and M. A. Mehlman, eds. John
Wiley and Sons, New York.

97. Wogan, G. N. and P. M. Newberne. 1967. Dose-response characteristics of aflatoxin B_1 carcinogenesis. Cancer Res., 27,
2370.

98.   Wogan, G. N., S. Paglialunga and P. M. Newberne. 1974.
      Carcinogenic effects of low dietary levels of aflatoxin B_1 in
      rats. Food Cosmet. Toxicol., 12, 681.
99.   Wolf, H. and E. W. Jackson. 1963. Hepatomas in rainbow
      trout: descriptive and experimental epidemiology. Science,
      142, 676.
100. Wood, E. M. and C. P. Larson. 1961. Hepatic carcinoma in
      rainbow trout. Arch. Pathol., 71, 471.
101. Woodfield, D. G., Y. Endo, and T. Matsuhashi. 1974. Primary
      liver cancer, alpha 1 feto-protein and hepatitis-B antigen in
      Papua, New Guinea. Aust. N. Z. J. Med., 4, 3.
102. World Health Organization. 1979. Environmental Health
      Criteria. 11. Mycotoxins. World Health Organization, Geneva.
103. Ying, T. S., D. S. R. Sarma and E. Faber. 1981. Role of
      acute hepatic necrosis in the induction of early steps in
      liver carcinogenesis by diethylnitrosomine. Cancer Res., 41,
      2096.

MECHANISMS OF DIETARY MODIFICATION OF AFLATOXIN

B$_1$ CARCINOGENESIS[1,2]

George Bailey[3,4], Matthew Taylor, Daniel Selivonchick[5], Thomas Eisele, Jerry Hendricks, Joseph Nixon, Norman Pawlowski, and Russell Sinnhuber

Department of Food Science and Technology
Oregon State University
Corvallis, Oregon 97331

ABSTRACT

Trout were fed a range of dietary components which altered their carcinogenic response to aflatoxin B$_1$ (AFB$_1$). Dietary protein at levels substantially exceeding nutritional requirements were synergistic with AFB$_1$. Cyclopropene fatty acids (CPFA) were carcinogenic when fed alone at 20 or 55 ppm, and synergistic when fed with AFB$_1$. In contrast, several flavonoid and indole compounds, especially β—naphthoflavone (β—NF) and indole-3-carbinol, inhibited the carcinogenic response when fed prior to and along with AFB$_1$.

The mechanisms by which some of these dietary factors modulate AFB$_1$ carcinogenesis were investigated. Dietary β—naphthoflavone was shown to substantially induce the levels of mixed function oxidase (MFO) activities assayed <u>in vitro</u>. These changes were accompanied by alterations in AFB$_1$ metabolism and binding in freshly isolated hepatocytes. AFB$_1$ incubated in hepatocytes freshly isolated from

---

[1]Technical Paper No. 6020, Oregon Agricultural Experiment Station, Oregon State University.
[2]This work was supported in part by NIH grants CA-20990, CA-25766, N01-CP-85660, ES-00550, ES-00541, ES-01926, and CA-30087.
[3]To whom all correspondence should be addressed.
[4]Recipient of Mid—Career Development Award ES-00092-01 from NIH.
[5]Recipient of Young Environmental Scientist Health Research Grant ES-01702 from NIH.

fish fed β-NF diet was metabolized more rapidly, showed enhanced rates of detoxication reactions, and decreased accumulation of AFB_1-DNA adducts compared to control hepatocytes. These results suggest that β-NF inhibits AFB_1 carcinogenesis at least in part by altering MFO activities such that detoxication is enhanced and initial DNA damage by AFB_1 is reduced.

In contrast, high dietary protein is a synergist for AFB_1 carcinogenesis, and this appears to occur primarily by enhancing the transformation probability for AFB_1-initiated genome damage. Fish treated with AFB_1 as embryos and then reared on high protein diets had substantially higher incidences of hepatocellular carcinoma (86%) than similarly treated fish fed normal protein diet (44%) or high protein controls without AFB_1 exposure (0-2%).

The synergistic behavior of dietary CPFAs also appears to partially involve enhanced transformation following DNA damage by AFB_1. Fish exposed as embryos to AFB_1 and then fed CPFA-containing diets are known to show promotion effects similar to the high protein results (Hendricks, J. D., Proc. 11th Int. Symp. of the Princess Takamatsu Cancer Research Fund, in press.)

However, factors other than promotion are involved in the synergism between CPFA and AFB_1. Preliminary studies indicate that dietary CPFAs repress MFO activities and depress DNA damage by AFB_1 in vitro. If this occurs in vivo, then the net synergistic effect of dietary CPFAs would involve depression of initial AFB_1-induced DNA damage, but highly efficient promotion of transformation from the remaining lesions.

INTRODUCTION

Mycotoxins, including aflatoxin B_1 (AFB_1), are among the most potent agriculturally related genotoxic substances known. AFB_1 is highly carcinogenic in a range of experimental animals (1, 2) and has been implicated in human liver cancer in some areas of the world (3). AFB_1 is also generally similar in metabolism and mutagenic behavior to the polycyclic aromatic hydrocarbons, which are another broad and ubiquitous class of compounds of environmental concern. As such, studies on the mechanisms of AFB_1 carcinogenesis, and especially on the means for reducing or preventing the carcinogenic response to such compounds, may ultimately contribute to improved human health.

Mechanisms of carcinogenesis by AFB_1 have been investigated in several animal and fish models. AFB_1 is metabolized by mixed function oxidase systems to a highly reactive 2,3-oxide intermediate capable of binding covalently to cellular macromolecules (4). The principal DNA adduct formed in rats, trout, and mice (5, 6) is the N-7-guanine adduct of AFB_1 (2,3-dihydro-2-(N-7-guanyl)-3 hydroxy)

aflatoxin B_1). This adduct is converted spontaneously to afla-
toxin-formamidopyrimidine derivatives by opening of the guanyl
imidazole ring (7). These products, once formed, are apparently
repaired only slowly in vivo and may thus be especially important
in tumor initiation (8).

Several enzymatic reactions have been described which are in
competition with AFB_1 adduct formation (9-12). These include:
formation of glutathione conjugate by the oxide, reduction of AFB_1
to aflatoxicol; hydroxylation of AFB_1 at various positions to produce aflatoxin M_1, P_1, or Q_1; transferase reactions to form sulfate
and glucuronide conjugates; and hydrolysis of the oxide intermediate. Mechanism studies in mice and coho salmon have revealed
unusually low rates of formation of the oxide intermediate relative
to detoxication reactions (12, 13), accompanied by reduced DNA
damage from AFB_1 in vivo (12). Both species are unusually
resistant to AFB_1 carcinogenesis (12, 14). These mechanism studies
suggest that AFB_1 carcinogenesis is initiated by DNA damage in
target cells, and that genetic factors which alter AFB_1 metabolism
and DNA damage rates may be responsible at least in part for
species differences in carcinogenic susceptibility to AFB_1.
Species differences in DNA repair to AFB_1 adducts have not, to our
knowledge, been described.

In addition to genetic variation, a number of chemical factors
or dietary components have been identified which may influence the
response to certain carcinogens. Compounds which elevate tumor
response by alterations in post-initiation processes are called
promoters. A classic example of promotion is the striking enhancement of polycyclic hydrocarbon-induced skin cancer caused by
delayed application of phorbol ester compounds (15). By contrast,
some compounds administered before or during carcinogen exposure
can reduce or inhibit the carcinogenic response. Examples of such
compounds, called inhibitors, include antioxidants, flavonoids,
selenium, and certain vitamins (16-18). To complicate our understanding, certain compounds such as phenobarbital have been shown
to inhibit if administered prior to or along with carcinogen
exposure (19) but promote if applied after (20).

Inhibitors of chemical carcinogenesis have come under
increasing study, not only because they provide information on
basic mechanisms of carcinogenesis, but also for their obvious
appeal as candidates for reduction of cancer in man. Those compounds which can be shown to have consistent protective effects
across animal systems, without significant noxious behavior under
any protocol, might then receive priority for possible human
study. It is essential that the mechanisms by which any dietary
compound inhibits carcinogenesis be thoroughly understood; consistency in mechanisms among animal species might strongly suggest
that a similar mechanism would operate in humans. At present,

information on dietary modulation of mycotoxin carcinogenesis is
very limited. This report describes some of our studies on the
mechanisms of modulation of AFB_1 carcinogenesis in rainbow trout
(Salmo gairdneri) by three classes of dietary factors - excessive
dietary protein, toxic lipids (cyclopropene fatty acids), and
several flavonoid and indole compounds.

Materials and Methods

Chemicals. AFB_1 (Cal Biochem) and $^3H-AFB_1$ (Moravek) were
checked for purity by thin layer chromatography (benzene-acetone-
ethyl acetate 55:15:30 or chloroform-acetone-isopropanol
82.5:15:2.5). The dietary inhibitors β-naphthoflavone (Sigma),
quercetin, flavone, indole-3-carbinol, and β-ionone (Aldrich), were
used without further purification. A mixture of tangeretin and
nobilitin was a generous gift of Dr. James Tatum (Citrus and Sub-
tropical Products Laboratory, Winter Haven, Florida). Cyclopropenoid fatty acids were obtained from Sterculia foetida oil as
previously reported (21). The preparation and use of fish protein
concentrate for trout diets has been described (22).

Animals. Rainbow trout were reared from brood stock at the
Oregon State University Food Toxicology and Nutrition Laboratory
and have been developed over 18 years as a derivative of the Shasta
strain. Protocols for carcinogenesis studies, including diet
preparation, carcinogen feeding or embryo exposure, and histology
procedures have been described (22-25).

Hepatocyte Studies. Isolated hepatocytes were prepared by
modifications (26) of the two-step perfusion procedures of Hazel
and Prosser (27). Viabilities were routinely measured at various
times in each experiment by Trypan Blue exclusion (28), lactate
dehydrogenase leakage (29, 30) and glutathione content (31). Cells
were suspended to a final concentration of $2-6 \times 10^6$/ml in 4 ml
incubation buffer (2.5 mM $CaCl_2$, 110 mM NaCl, 20 mM KCl, 1 mM
$MgSO_4$, 8 mN $NaHCO_3$, 10 mM glucose 40 mM Hepes pH 7.4, 2% Sigma
fraction V bovine serum albumin) supplemented with amino acids
(32). $^3H-AFB_1$ dissolved in ethanol was added to 40 volumes incubation buffer less albumin, rotary evaporated to remove all but
traces of ethanol (26), and restored to initial weight with H_2O.
Incubations were started by adding 1 ml of this solution (4 µCi,
3.3. µg AFB_1) to 4 ml cells. Each flask was continuously gassed
with 95 O_2:5 CO_2 on a metabolic shaker at 20°. After 1 h, cells
were rapidly sedimented, washed with 4 ml incubation buffer less
albumin, and frozen at -80°. The medium and wash from each flask
were combined, acidified with 20 µl acetic acid to retard further
tritium exchange and stored at -80°. DNA was purified from each
cell pellet and its specific activity determined as described elsewhere (26).

Analysis of Unbound AFB$_1$ Metabolites. Supernatants from each incubation were made 10% in methanol and twice passed slowly through a SepPak C18 minicolumn (Waters Associates). (Prior to use each column was washed with 20 ml methanol and 10 ml of a 50 mM potassium acetate pH 5.0 buffer containing 10% methanol.) The column was then washed with 10 ml 10% methanol buffer to remove exchanged tritium and incubation buffer components. AFB$_1$ and its metobolites (AFL, AFM$_1$, and polar conjugates) were eluted slowly with 10 ml 60% buffered methanol and evaporated to dryness. Isotope recovery was routinely 80–100%. Samples were reduced in volume to 250 µl and an aliquot injected onto a microbondpak C18 column (3.9 x 300 mm, 10 micron, Waters Associates). The column was pumped at 1 ml/min with 28% acetonitrile in 20 mM potassium acetate pH 5.0 and 32 drop fractions were collected. Detection was by UV (345 nm) and liquid scintillation counting.

Analysis of Mixed Function Oxidase Activities. Three to fifteen pools of 5 livers each were extracted, fractionated, and assayed as previously described for cytochrome P450 (33), benzo(α) pyrene mono-oxygenase (34), epoxide hydrase (35), ethoxycoumarin-O-deethylase (36), glutathione tranferase (37) and p-nitroanisole-O-demethylase (38).

Results

Dietary Modulators of Aflatoxin B$_1$ Carcinogenesis. The carcinogenic response of rainbow trout to AFB$_1$ can be altered by a number of natural and synthetic dietary components. Table 1 shows that the level of protein in the diet influences final tumor

Table 1. The influence of dietary protein on AFB$_1$-induced hepatocellular carcinoma incidence in rainbow trout

Diet	Carcinoma incidence[a]	
	Total	Percent
40% protein[b]	0/2	0
" + AFB$_1$[c]	33/99	33
50% protein	0/100	0
" + AFB$_1$	48/100	48
60% protein	0/100	0
" + AFB$_1$	67/98	68
70% protein	5/96	5
" + AFB$_1$	90/101	90

[a]Histologically confirmed.
[b]Fish protein concentrate.
[c]AFB$_1$ was fed at 20 ppb for 4 weeks.

Table 2. The influence of dietary cyclopropenoid fatty acids on
AFB$_1$-induced hepatocellular carcinoma incidence in
rainbow trout

Diet	Hepatocellular carcinoma incidence					
	6 month	(%)	9 month	(%)	12 month	(%)
Control	0/60	(0)	0/60	(0)	0/74	(0)
0.5 ppb AFB$_1$[a]	0/60	(0)	0/60	(0)	15/76	(20)
2 ppb AFB$_1$	3/60	(5)	10/60	(15)	46/77	(61)
20 ppm CPFA	0/60	(0)	1/60	(2)	11/76	(15)
50 ppm CPFA	2/60	(3)	6/60	(10)	32/77	(42)
0.5 ppb AFB$_1$ + 20 ppm CPFA	2/60	(3)	19/30	(63)	119/122	(98)
0.5 ppb AFB$_1$ + 50 ppm CPFA	3/60	(5)	47/60	(78)	126/129	(98)
2 ppb AFB$_1$ + 20 ppm CPFA	23/60	(39)	54/60	(90)	129/131	(99)
2 ppb AFB$_1$ + 50 ppm CPFA	29/60	(49)	115/120	(96)	--	

[a]All diets were fed continuously for the entire study.

incidence. Populations fed the normal 40% fish protein concentrate
(FPC) diet before and during AFB$_1$ exposure showed 33% incidence of
hepatocellular carcinoma 9 months after AFB$_1$ exposure. By comparison those fed 70% FPC had an 89% incidence. Casein as a
dietary protein source shows similar effects (data not shown). The
highest level tested here, 70% protein, not only enhanced AFB$_1$
response but induced a significant incidence of "spontaneous" carcinoma (5%). Whether this represents de novo carcinogenesis or
promotion-like enhancement of a low level of spontaneous events is
at present unclear.

Lipids are known to influence the response to chemical carcinogens in a number of animal models (39-40). Cyclopropenoid fatty
acids (CPFA), structurally unique common constitutents of human
foods derived from cottonseed and kapok oil, are carcinogens as
well as potent synergists for AFB$_1$ hepatocellular carcinoma in
trout (Table 2; 41). For example the incidence of carcinoma after
9 months continuous feeding of 0.5 parts per billion (ppb) AFB$_1$ was
0, for 20 parts per million (ppm) CPFA was 2%, but for the combination 0.5 pb AFB$_1$ plus 20 ppm CPFA was 63%. The behavior of
CPFA as a carcinogen and as a synergistic co-carcinogen were both
dose-responsive.

A number of natural and synthetic dietary components have been
examined for their ability to inhibit AFB$_1$ carcinogenesis in the
trout model. The results in Table 3 show that several substances
including β-naphthoflavone, indole-3-carbinol, and possibly
quercetin and tangeretin-nobilitin, reduce the carcinogenic
response of trout populations when fed prior to and during AFB$_1$
exposure. These compounds have also proved effective to varying
degrees as inhibitors of carcinogenesis for other animals and

Table 3. Effects of flavonoid and indole compounds on hepatocellular carcinoma incidence after exposure to 20 ppb AFB_1 for 10 days

Diet	Hepatocellular carcinoma incidence	
	Total	Percent
Negative control	0/118	0
AFB_1 only	53/118	45
β-Napthoflavone, 50 ppm	23/117	20
β-Napthoflavone, 500 ppm	9/120	8
Flavone, 1000 ppm	54/120	45
Tangeretin-nobilitin, 1000 ppm	37/118	31
Quercetin, 2000 ppm	40/115	35
β-Ionone, 1000 ppm	50/118	42
Indole-3-carbinol, 1000 ppm	6/118	5

carcinogens (42-44). In contrast, dietary cruciferous vegetables (cauliflower, broccoli, brussels sprouts) and associated isothiocyanate compounds were not effective against AFB_1 carcinogenesis in trout (45) even though inhibitory in other systems (46). The basic mechanisms by which dietary protein, CPFA, and flavonoids enhance or reduce the response to AFB_1 are examined below.

Promotion of AFB_1 Carcinogenesis. Embryos 21 days old were immersed for up to 1 h in solutions of AFB_1 (.05 to .5 ppm), rinsed, and returned to hatchery trays. At feeding onset fingerlings were placed on control diet or diet containing varying amounts of FPC or casein. The tumor incidences were determined at 9 and 12 months and are shown in Table 4. The results were similar to those in Table 1 - higher dietary protein caused a higher carcinogenic response to AFB_1. Since the enhancement by dietary protein occurred well after completion of AFB_1 metabolism and DNA binding in the exposed embryos (6), high dietary protein behaves as a promoter of AFB_1 carcinogenesis in trout.

We have previously shown that dietary CPFAs also promote carcinogenesis following embryo exposure to AFB_1 (47). Hence the co-carcinogenic behavior of CPFAs resides in part in their ability to enhance the probability of transformation from lesions initiated by AFB_1.

Alterations of Mixed Function Oxidase (MFO) Enzymes by Dietary Effectors of AFB_1 Carinogenesis. One possible mechanism by which dietary components elevate or reduce response to a chemical

Table 4. Effect of dietary protein on hepatocellular carcinoma
incidence after embryo exposure to AFB_1

Embryo Treatment	Diet	Gross incidence of hepatocellular carcinoma			
		9 month	(%)	12 month	(%)
--	40% protein[b]	0/74	(0)	0/118	(0)
AFB_1[a]	"	8/64	(12)	50/115	(44)
--	50% protein	0/67	(0)	0/120	(0)
AFB_1	"	18/74	(25)	55/114	(48)
--	60% protein	0/69	(0)	0/116	(0)
AFB_1	"	28/70	(40)	93/117	(80)
--	70% protein	1/69	(2)	0/119	(0)
AFB_1	"	49/72	(68)	99/115	(86)

[a]Embryos were immersed for 0.5 h. in a 0.5 ppm solution of AFB_1.
[b]Fish protein concentrate.

carcinogen is to alter the relative levels of enzyme activities
which compete for carcinogen activation and detoxication
reactions. The influence of dietary β-naphthoflavone and of CPFAs
on various xenobiotic metabolism activities is shown in Table 5.
β-naphthoflavone was a strong inducer of several activities assayed
in vitro including benzo(α)pyrene monooxygenase (aryl hydrocarbon
hydroxylase), deethylase and demethylase activities, and glutathione transferase. Assays using AFB_1 substrate also indicated a
substantial increase in the rate of formation of the detoxication
products aflatoxicol-M_1 and aflatoxin M_1 (AFM_1) (data not shown).
By contrast CPFA repressed the specific activities of most of these
enzyme systems. Cruciferous vegetables and their associated
isothiocyanates were found to have no effect on MFO enzyme levels
(data not shown).

It is difficult to relate such activity changes measured in
vitro to AFB_1 metabolism and DNA binding in vivo - some of the
assays cannot be carried out with AFB_1 as substrate, rate-limiting
reactions are unknown, and other in vivo cosubstrates and effectors
may be lost. To the extent that these assays reflect AFB_1 metabolism in vivo, dietary β-NF may be expected to enhance the overall
rate of AFB_1 metabolism and detoxication to AFM_1. In contrast
CPFAs appear to generally repress mixed function oxidase activity
and may be expected to depress cellular rates of AFB_1 metabolism.
However, the magnitude and direction of any changes in DNA binding
which may result are difficult to predict.

AFB_1 Metabolism and DNA Adduct Formation in Isolated
Hepatocytes. Many of the limitations of metabolism studies with

Table 5. The effects of dietary β—naphthoflavone (β-NF) and
cyclopropene fatty acids (CPFA) on the rainbow trout
mixed function oxidase system

Function Assayed	Control Diet[a]	β-NF 500 ppm[a]	CPFA 450 ppm[b]
Cytochrome P-450 (nmole/mg)	0.428±0.034	0.715±0.153[c,d]	0.124±0.006[c]
Benzo(α)pyrene monooxygenase (nmole/mg/min)	0.056±0.025	0.762±0.230[c]	0.022±0.019[c]
Epoxide Hydrase (nmole/mg/min)	2.70±0.67	2.17±0.45[c]	1.75±0.49[c]
Ethoxycoumarin-O-deethylase (nmole/mg/min)	0.052±0.015	0.281±0.057[c]	0.004±0.001[c]
Glutathione Transferase[e] (nmole/mg/min)	7.46±1.17	11.24±1.55[c]	6.93±2.47
p-nitroanisole-O-demethylase (nmole/mg/min)	0.27±0.30	2.43±0.29[c]	0

[a]Fifteen groups of five trout; mean ± S.D. β-NF fed for six weeks.

[b]Three groups of five trout; mean ± S.D. CPFA fed for six weeks.

[c]Statistically significant from controls (P<0.05) by Student's "t" test.

[d]Maximum absorbance at 448 nm, expressed using cyt. P-450 extinction coefficient.

[e]Measured on 105,000 XG supernatant. Enzyme activities expressed on mg protein basis.

broken cell extracts may in principle be avoided using freshly
isolated hepatocytes. The metabolism and binding of AFB₁ in
isolated group hepatocytes have been extensively characterized and
appear to reflect in vivo cellular metabolic properties (26).
Hepatocytes were freshly isolated from each of 14 fish (7 on
control diet, 7 on β-NF diet) and incubated 1 h with ³H-AFB₁ under
defined conditions (26) using 3 to 6 replicate flasks per fish.
The pattern of unbound AFB₁ metabolites released into the medium
and cell cytosol of each flask was examined by HPLC. DNA was also
purified from each flask and the specific activity for adduct
formation determined.

A typical HPLC profile of unbound AFB₁ metabolites is shown in
Figure 1. The major peaks represent conjugates and any other
highly polar metabolites (I), AFM₁ (II), unreacted AFB₁ (III), and
AFL (IV). Other minor peaks remain as yet unidentified. The AFB₁-
DNA adducts formed in this system are described elsewhere (26) and
consist primarily of the N-7-guanyl adduct of AFB₁ and its guanyl
ring-opened derivitives. The results of 7 paired experiments
(control vs. β-NF) are given in Table 6 and Figure 2, where dietary
pretreatment with β-NF is seen to significantly alter AFB₁ metabolism and DNA bindng. The most striking alteration is the 10 to

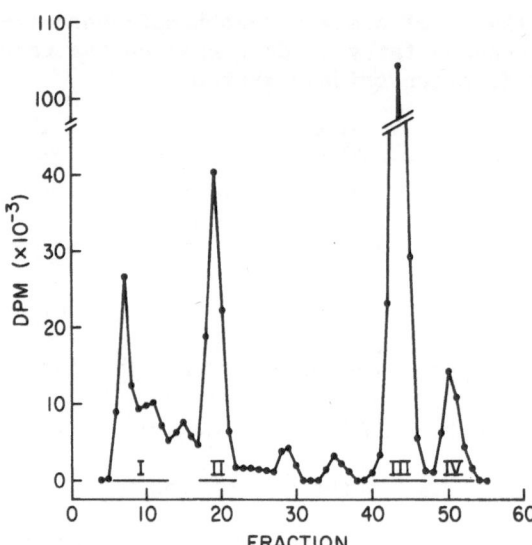

Fig. 1.   HPLC profile of AFB_1 and its soluble metabolites after
incubation in hepatocytes from fish fed β-naphthoflavone
diet.   Hepatocytes were suspended at 3×10^6 cells/ml and
incubated 1 h at 20° with ^3H-AFB_1 (4 μCi, 3.5 μg).
Initial viability by LDH retention was 93% and was 85%
after 1 h.   Cells were centrifuged, rinsed and the
combined supernatants passed through Sep-Pak as described
in Methods. 5.21×10^5 DPM were applied to the column,
with 99% recovered.

20-fold enhancement of AFM_1 formation in hepatocytes from β-NF fish
(Figure 2). AFM_1, which is known to be far less carcinogenic than
AFB_1 (48), changes from a minor to a major unbound metabolite of
AFB_1.   Conversely the level of AFL, a metabolite equally carcinogenic with AFB_1 whose production appears to correlate with
species carcinogenic response (49), is reduced 3-fold.   Polar metabolites were always equal or greater in β-NF hepatocytes compared
to controls (individual data not shown).   Overall recovery of unreacted AFB_1 is reduced in β-NF fish, indicating greater rates of
total AFB_1 metabolism in these cells.

     The statistical significance of these changes depends on how
the experiments are grouped for comparison.   In Figure 2, the 7 β-
NF or control values are averaged as independent experiments and
the error bars represent standard deviations on this average.   In
this case there is no significance in the change in conjugates
(P<.1) while other changes are highly significant (P<.005).
However, the experiments were actually performed as 7 paired
independent tests and when analyzed this way (Student's T test for

Table 6. AFB$_1$-DNA adduct formation in hepatocytes isolated from trout fed control and β-naphthoflavone diets

| | DNA specific activity (DPM/μg) | | | | | | |
| | Experiment | | | | | | |
	1	2	3	4	5	6	7
Control	1295(218)[a]	1319(112)	1679(116)	1163(60)	1235(171)	1429(186)	1401(227)
β-NF	539 (16)	470 (17)	1469(161)	626(13)	697 (42)	1236 (59)	916 (33)
Significance	P<.025	P<.005	NS	P<.005	P<.025	NS	P<.05
Cumulative[b] significance						P<.001	

[a]Mean (±S.D.), n = 3. Each experiment used a separate control and β-NF fish, with 3-6 flasks incubated from each for DNA analyses.

[b]Paired difference T test for 7 experiments.

independent samples, n = 7) all differences are accumulatively significant (P<.001; individual experiments not shown).

The enhanced detoxication reactions in hepatocytes isolated from fish fed β-NF are accompanied by a decreased rate of accumulation of AFB$_1$-DNA adducts in our 1 h assay period (Table 6). The contribution, if any, of differential DNA repair rates in these short-term _in vitro_ incubations has yet to be evaluated. Comparable experiments on CPFA-fed fish are in progress.

DISCUSSION

Among the parameters which may influence response to a chemical procarcinogen are: initial pharmacokinetic distribution and target cell uptake, relative rates of activation and detoxication, initial rate of DNA damage, rate of damage repair and other post-initiation factors which might influence final transformation probability. We have investigated some of these processes in an attempt to understand the mechanisms by which selected dietary factors alter the carcinogenic response to AFB$_1$.

The synthetic flavonoid β-naphthoflavone was shown in the present study to be highly effective as a dietary inhibitor of AFB$_1$ carcinogenesis in rainbow trout. Analysis of cell extracts revealed major induction of several mixed function oxidase activities, and alterations in extract-mediated AFB$_1$ metabolism after dietary β-NF treatment. A more thorough and integrated assessment of AFB$_1$ metabolism changes was provided using hepatocytes isolated from β-NF and control fish. These studies revealed an overall enhancement of AFB$_1$ metabolism rate, enhanced

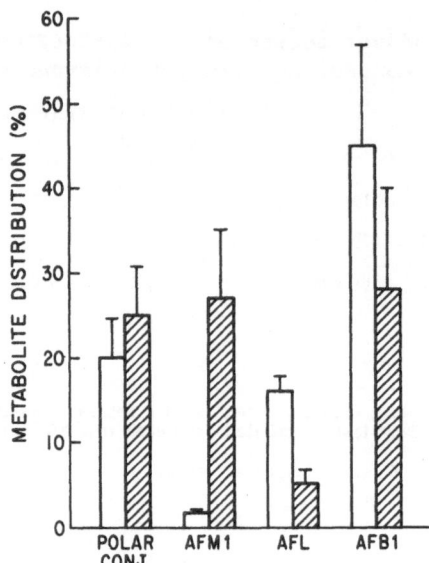

Fig. 2.   The influence of dietary β-naphthoflavone on formation of
          unbound metabolites of AFB_1 in isolated hepatocytes. Each
          bar represents the mean (± S.D.) of seven experiments from
          Table 6, treated here as independent (unpaired)
          experiments. Hatched bars are values determined using
          hepatocytes from β-NF-treated fish, and plain bars are
          controls.

detoxication reactions, and reduced DNA adduct formation in hepatocytes from β-NF compared to controls. The results suggest that the
inhibitor β-NF operates at least in part by modulation of enzyme
activities such that AFB_1 detoxication is enhanced and initial DNA
damage for a given AFB_1 exposure is reduced.

     Further mechanism studies are necessary, however, before the
in vivo effects of dietary β-NF are clear. We have not compared
the pharmacokinetic distribution, target binding, and dosage
effects of injected versus dietary AFB_1, nor the effect of dietary
β-NF on these parameters. It is also essential to examine the
possible influence of β-NF on DNA repair and other post-initiation
factors. Since the extent of DNA binding reduction seen in vitro
(30-40%) is less than the observed extent of tumor protection, one
or more of these additional factors may contribute to β-NF inhibition of AFB_1 carcinogenesis.

     High levels of dietary protein are co-carcinogenic in rainbow
trout when fed simultaneously with AFB_1. Although 50% or more
protein was required to see this effect, these results should be
considered in light of the animal's protein requirement. Trout

require about twice the dietary protein of laboratory rats for adequate nutrition, and even 60% dietary protein does not repress growth. Yet this level substantially promotes AFB_1-induced carcinogenesis and 70% elevates the incidence of "spontaneous" carcinoma. It is conceivable that levels of dietary protein which substantially exceed nutritional requirements of mammals including man, could have similar effects.

Feeding experiments with fish previously exposed to AFB_1 as embryos demonstrated that high dietary protein behaves as a promoter of AFB_1 carcinogenesis. Since the potencies of high protein as co-carcinogen-like and promoter-like activities are approximately equal, it is likely that the co-carcinogenic effect in trout is primarily one of post-initiation promotion of AFB_1 lesions. We have not, however, carried out studies which rule out some contribution of high dietary protein as a modulator of AFB_1 metabolism and binding.

The importance of such studies is illustrated by the results for dietary CPFAs, which appear to have several modes of action. This class of compounds was shown to behave as an efficient promoter of AFB_1 carcinogenesis by embryo studies, to be carcinogenic by feeding studies, and to be a potent synergist when fed simultaneously with AFB_1. Hepatocyte experiments similar to those for β-NF are currently being carried out to test whether CPFAs are synergistic by virtue of induced alteration in AFB_1 metabolism leading to increased DNA damage by AFB_1 metabolites. Preliminary results indicate that this is not so --dietary CPFAs appear to substantially repress AFB_1 binding to DNA in hepatocytes. These results are in agreement with the repression of MFO activities reported here. Dietary CPFAs may, therefore, actually repress initial DNA damage from AFB_1, but greatly enhance the probability of effective transformation of the remaining lesions, leading to a net synergistic effect. Again, the effects of CPFAs on repair, other post-initiation processes, and direct DNA damage by CPFAs themselves, are presently unknown. These dietary compounds are known to substantially perturb normal hepatocyte membrane architecture (50) and this may in some way greatly increase the probability of transformation for cells with spontaneous or chemically-induced genome damage.

ACKNOWLEDGEMENT

We wish to thank Pat Loveland, Janet Wilcox, Ted Will, and John Casteel for their technical assistance.

REFERENCES

1. Cooper, P. Aflatoxins and the liver, Food Cosmet. Toxicol. 17:408 (1979).

2. Newberne, P. M. and W. H. Butler, Acute and chronic effects of
    aflatoxin on the liver of domestic and laboratory animals: A
    review, Cancer Res. 29:236 (1969).
3. Peers, F. G. and C. A. Linsell, Dietary aflatoxins and liver
    cancer – a population based study in Kenya, Br. J. Cancer
    27:473 (1973).
4. Swenson, D. H., E. C. Miller, and J. A. Miller, Aflatoxin B_1-
    2,3-oxide as a probable intermediate in the covalent binding
    of aflatoxins B_1 and B_2 to rat liver DNA and ribosomal RNA in
    vivo, Cancer Res. 37:172 (1977).
5. Croy, R. G. and G. N. Wogan, Quantitative comparison of
    covalent aflatoxin-DNA adducts formed in rat and mouse livers
    and kidneys, J. Natl. Cancer Inst. 66:761 (1981).
6. Croy, R. G., J. E. Nixon, R. O. Sinnhuber, and G. N. Wogan,
    Investigation of covalent aflatoxin B_1-DNA adducts formed in
    vivo in rainbow trout (Salmo gairdneri) embryos and liver,
    Carcinogenesis 1:903 (1980).
7. Lin, J., J. A. Miller, and E. C. Miller, 2,3-Dihydro-2-(guan-
    7-yl)-3-hydroxy-aflatoxin B_1, a major acid hydrolysis product
    of aflatoxin B_1-DNA or ribosomal RNA adducts formed in hepatic
    microsome-mediated reactions and rat liver in vivo. Cancer
    Res. 37:4430 (1977).
8. Wang, T. V. and P. A. Cerutti, Formation and removal of afla-
    toxin B_1 induced DNA lesions in epithelilioid human lung
    cells, Cancer Res. 39:5165 (1979).
9. Decad, G. M., K. K. Dougherty, D. P. H. Hsieh, and J. L.
    Byard, Metabolism of aflatoxin B_1 in cultured mouse hepato-
    cytes: Comparison with rat and effects of cyclohexene oxide
    and diethyl maleate, Toxicol. Appl. Pharmacol. 50:429 (1979).
10. Campbell, T. C. and J. R. Hayes, The role of aflatoxin meta-
    bolism in its toxic lesion, Toxicol. Appl. Pharmacol. 35:199
    (1976).
11. Degen, C. H. and H. G. Neumann, The major metabolite of afla-
    toxin B_1 in the rat is a glutathione conjugate, Chem.-Biol.
    Interact. 22:239 (1978).
12. Degen, G. H. and H. G. Neumann, Differences in aflatoxin B_1-
    susceptibility of rat and mouse are correlated with the
    capacity in vitro to inactive aflatoxin B_1-epoxide, Carci-
    nogenesis 2:299 (1981).
13. Whitham, M., J. E. Nixon, and R. O. Sinnhuber, In vivo binding
    of aflatoxin B_1 to liver DNA as a measure of hepatocarcinoma
    initiation in rainbow trout, J. Natl. Cancer Inst., in press
    (1982).
14. Wales, J. H. and R. O. Sinnhuber, Hepatomas induced by
    aflatoxin in the sockeye salmon (Oncorhynchus nerka), J. Natl.
    Cancer Inst. 48:1529 (1972).
15. Baird, W. M. and R. K. Boutwell, Tumor-promoting activity of
    phorbol and four diesters of phorbol in mouse skin. Cancer
    Res. 31:1074 (1971).

16. Wattenberg, L. W., Naturally occurring inhibitors of chemical carcinogenesis, Proc. 9th Internatl. Symp. of Princess Takamatsu Cancer Res. Rund, 315 (1979).

17. Wattenberg, L. W. and V. L. Sparnins, Inhibitory effects of butylated hydroxyanisole on methylazoxymethanol acetate-induced neoplasia of the large intestine and on NAD-dependent alcohol dehydrogenase activity in mice, J. Natl. Cancer Inst. 63:219 (1979).

18. Griffin, C., Role of selenium in the chemoprevention of cancer, Adv. Cancer Res. 29:419 (1979).

19. Peraino, C., R. J. M. Fry and E. Staffeldt, Reduction and enhancement by phenobarbital of hepatocarcinogenesis induced in the rat by 2-acetylaminofluorene. Cancer Res. 31:1506 (1971).

20. Kitagawa, T., H. C. Pitot, and J. A. Miller, Promotion by dietary phenobarbital of hepatocarcinogenesis by 2-methyl-N,N-dimethyl-4-aminoazobenzene in the rat. Cancer Res. 39:112 (1979).

21. Nixon, J. E., T. A. Eisele, J. D. Hendricks, and R. O. Sinnhuber, Reproduction and lipid composition in rats fed cyclopropene fatty acids, J. Nutrition 107:574 (1977).

22. Lee, D. J., R. O. Sinnhuber, J. H. Wales, and G. B. Putnam, Effect of dietary protein on the response of rainbow trout (Salmo gairdneri) to aflatoxin B₁. J. Natl. Cancer Inst. 60:317 (1978).

23. Sinnhuber. R. O., J. D. Hendricks, J. H. Wales, and G. B. Putnam, Neoplasms in rainbow trout, a sensitive animal model for environmental carcinogenesis, Ann. N. Y. Acad. Sci. 298:389 (1977).

24. Wales, J. H., R. O. Sinnhuber, J. D. Hendricks, J. E. Nixon, and T. A. Eisele, Aflatoxin B₁ induction of hepatocellular carcinoma in the embryos of rainbow trout (Salmo gairdenri), J. Natl. Cancer Inst. 60:1133 (1978)

25. Hendricks, J. D., R. O. Sinnhuber, P. M. Loveland, N. E. Pawlowski, and J. E. Nixon, Hepatocarcinogenicity of glandless cottonseeds and cottonseed oil to rainbow trout (Salmo gairdneri), Science 208:309 (1980).

26. Bailey, G. S., M. J. Taylor, and D. P. Selivonchick, Metabolism and DNA binding of aflatoxin B₁ in isolated hepatocytes from rainbow trout (Salmo gairdneri), Carcinogenesis, in press (1982).

27. Hazel, J. R. and C. L. Prosser, Incorporation of 1-¹⁴C-acetate into fatty acids and sterols by isolated hepatocytes of thermally acclimated rainbow trout (Salmo gairdneri), J. Comp. Physiol. 134:321 (1979).

28. Moldeus, P., J. Hogberg, and S. Orrenius, Isolation and use of liver cells, Meth. Enzymol. 52:60 (1978).

29. Kornberg, A., Lactic dehydrogenase of muscle, Meth. Enzymol. 1:441 (1955).

30. Walton, M. J. and C. B. Cowey, Gluconeogenesis by isolated
     hepatocytes from rainbow trout (Salmo gairdneri). Comp.
     Biochem. Physiol. 62:75 (1979).
31. Hissin, P. J. and R. Hilf, A fluorometric method for
     determination of oxidized and reduced glutathione in tissues,
     Anal. Biochem. 74:214 (1976).
32. Hogberg, J. and A. Kristoferson, A correlation between
     glutathione levels and cellular damage in isolated
     hepatocytes, Europ. J. Biochem. 74:77 (1977).
33. Omura, T. and R. Sato, The carbon monoxide-binding pigment of
     liver microsomes, I. Evidence for its hemoprotein nature. J.
     Biol. Chem. 239:2379 (1964).
34. de Pierre, J. W., M. S. Moron, K. A. M. Johannesen, and L.
     Ernster, A reliable, sensitive, and convenient radioactive
     assay for benzpyrene monooxygenase, Anal. Biochem. 63:470
     (1975).
35. Oesch, F., D. M. Jerina, and J. Daly, Radiometric assay for
     hepatic epoxide hydrase activity with [7-^{3}H]styrene oxide,
     Biochem. Biophys. Acta. 227:685 (1971).
36. Ullrich, V. and P. Weber, The O-dealkylation of 7-
     ethoxycoumarin by liver microsomes, Hoppe-Seyler's Z. Physiol.
     Chem. 353:1171 (1972).
37. James, M. O., J. R. Fouts, and J. R. Bend, Hepatic and
     extrahepatic metabolism in vitro of an epoxide (8-^{14}C-styrene
     oxide) in the rabbit. Bioche. Pharm. 25:187 (1976).
38. LaDu, B. N., H. G. Mandel, and E. L. Way, Fundamentals of Drug
     Metabolism and Drug Disposition. Williams and Wilkins,
     Baltimore, 1971, pp. 566-577.
39. Carroll, K. K., Neutral fats and cancer. Cancer Res. 41:3695
     (1981).
40. Brown, R. R., Effects of dietary fats on incidence of
     spontaneous and induced cancer in mice, Cancer Res. 41:3741
     (1981).
41. Lee, D. J., J. H. Wales, and R. O. Sinnhuber, Promotion of
     aflatoxin-induced hepatoma growth in trout by methyl malvate
     and sterculate, Cancer Res. 31:960 (1971).
42. Wattenberg, L. W., Inhibition of chemical carcinogenesis, J.
     Natl. Cancer Inst. 60:11 (1978).
43. Loub, W. D., L. W. Wattenberg, and D. W. Davis, Aryl
     hydrocarbon hydroxylase induction in rat tissues by naturally
     occurring indoles of cruciferous plants, J. Natl. Cancer Inst.
     54:985 (1975).
44. Wattenberg, L. W., Inhibition of carcinogenic effects of
     polycyclic hydrocarbons by benzyl isothiocyanate and related
     compounds, J. Natl. Cancer Inst. 58:395 (1977).
45. Haight, L. E., J. E. Nixon, J. D. Hendricks, and R. O.
     Sinnhuber, Null effect of cruciferous vegetables on aflatoxin
     B$_1$ induced carcinogenesis in rainbow trout, Fed. Proc. 40:948
     (1981).

46. Stoewsend, G. S., J. B. Babish, and H. C. Wimberly, Inhibition of hepatic toxicities from polybrominated biphenyls and aflatoxin B_1 in rats fed cauliflower, J. Environ. Pathol. and Toxicol. 2:399 (1977).
47. Hendricks, J. D., The use of rainbow trout (Salmo gairdneri) in carcinogen bioassay, with special emphasis on embryonic exposure, in Phyletic Approaches to Cancer, C. J. Dawe et al. (eds.), Japan Sci. Soc. Press, Tokyo, In Press (1981).
48. Sinnhuber, R. O., D. J. Lee, J. H. Wales, M. K. Landers, and A. C. Keyl, Hepatic carcinogenesis of aflatoxin M_1 in rainbow trout (Salmo gairdneri) and its enhancement by cyclopropene fatty acids, J. Natl. Cancer Inst. 53:1285 (1974).
49. Salhab, A. S. and G. S. Edwards, Compartive in vitro metabolism of aflatoxicol by liver preparations from animals and humans. Cancer Res. 37:1016 (1977).
50. Selivonchick, D. P., J. L. Williams, and H. W. Schaup, Alteration of liver microsomal proteins from rainbow trout (Salmo gairdneri) fed cyclopropenoid fatty acids, Lipids 16:211 (1981).

TOXIC AGENTS IN THE AGRO-ECOSYSTEM

CHAIRMAN'S COMMENTS

Gordon W. Newell

National Academy of Sciences
Washington, DC 20418

As we begin the session concerned with Toxic Agents in the Agro-Ecosystem, it seems proper to consider additional ways in which a chemical may interact with its target. While the first portion of this session dealt principally with the direct effects of mycotoxins acting on receptor systems, the following papers will offer possibilities wherein exposures to combinations of chemicals can complicate an assessment of associated health hazards. How, then, does the risk to health from exposure to a combination of chemicals compare to an estimated risk from exposure to a single chemical by itself? This question recently was considered by a National Research Council panel concerned with maritime personnel exposed to multiple cargo vapors. The following comments reflect certain observations and conclusions of this panel.

First, the literature may be searched for laboratory, clinical or epidemiological data that specifically deal with exposures to combinations of chemicals of interest.

Second, laboratory and/or epidemiological studies may be initiated to specifically test for interactive effects of certain combinations of chemicals, when and if concern for a specific combined exposure arises.

And third, if there is knowledge of toxicokinetic and toxicodynamic characteristics of individual chemicals, such knowledge may be used to judge the potential for altered health risk arising from exposure to specific combinations of such chemicals.

A prerequisite for the development of an approach to understand what is meant by "toxicological interactions" requires a

167

definition which is generally accepted by many investigators. A
definition of this type might be as follows: "A toxicological
interaction is a circumstance in which exposure to two or more
chemicals results in a qualitatively or quantitatively altered
biological response relative to that predicted from the actions of
a single chemical. Multiple-chemical exposures may be simultaneous
or sequential in time, while the altered response may be greater or
smaller in magnitude."

Injury produced by a chemical in a living organism is proportional to the quantity of the biologically active form of the chemical that is available for reaction with critical responsive sites;
that is, the targets. Thus, toxicological interations can be perceived in general as occuring in two forms: (1) the quantity of an
active form of one or more chemicals available for target-site
interactions is altered by the presence of one or more other chemicals, or (2) the reactivity of the target macromolecule with the
active form(s) of one or more chemicals is altered by the presence
of one or more other chemicals that may or may not be capable of
eliciting a response. The first form involves primarily sites of
inactivation or loss (i.e., sites of detoxification, excretion,
storage, or neutralization) or sites of activation of a chemical.
The second involves interaction at sites of action; affinity for or
intrinsic activity at the site of action may be altered.

At least three general mechanisms of reaction among chemicals
may be involved in toxicological interactions:
     (A) Chemical-Chemical Reactions. As a result of a combined
exposure, one chemical may react with another in such a way that
the potentially injurious chemical never reaches the target site in
an active form. Examples that might be cited include: neutralization reactions among acids and bases, chelation reactions such
as those with heavy metals, and direct reactions between organophosphates and aldoximes. An example of the chemical-chemical
reaction is the formation of nitrosamines from secondary amines and
nitrites in the stomach. Because many nitrosamines are carcinogenic, this particular chemical-chemical interaction could be
classed as one yielding enhanced risk of injury.
     (B) Chemical Competition at Macromolecules. This general
mechanism of toxicological interation is probably the most frequently encountered and the most thoroughly studied. It involves
the relative affinities of exogenous chemicals for a limited number
of reaction sites on cellular macromolecules, which may be the
molecular sites of absorption, activation, detoxification, injurious action, or excretion. Competition for binding or reaction at
various sites may result in either enhanced or reduced toxicity.
     (C) Altered Cellular Responsiveness or Reactivity. A third
general mechanism for toxicological interactions is one in which a
cell or tissue is altered by one chemical, in such a way that the
cell's or tissue's response to a second chemical is altered, even

if the first chemical is no longer present. This type of interaction is more likely to result when the chemical events are separated in time. Promotion by one compound of chemical carcinogenesis that is initiated by another chemical would be included in
this classification.

In many other situations, toxicological interactions develop
only when exposures occur in a certain order. When attempting to
predict interactions between combinations of chemicals solely on
the basis of kinetic data on individual chemicals, one should keep
in mind that the nature, mechanism, and duration of the cellular
injury are critical factors.

The frequency of exposure can also determine whether or not a
toxicological interaction will occur. Obviously, the more often
there is exposure to a chemical, the greater the statistical probability that it will occur in the presence of, or close in time to,
the exposure to another possibly interacting chemical.

These theoretical considerations of chemical interactions are
brought to your attention as a prelude to several of the subjects
to be presented in this volume.

VIRUSES AS ENVIRONMENTAL CARCINOGENS: AN AGRICULTURAL PERSPECTIVE

Murray B. Gardner

Department of Pathology
School of Medicine
University of California
Davis, California 95616

ABSTRACT

Under natural circumstances tumor viruses can be considered as risk factors which in themselves are neither necessary nor sufficient to produce cancer; they may do so, however, if provided with suitable genetic and environmental conditions. It follows that a reduction in amount of virus or other environmental cofactors may prevent the associated tumors. In this paper we will consider four major families of viruses associated with cancer in animals and man, and will highlight the exogenous cofactors and related preventive measures. We will mention those agricultural practices that have resulted in significant economic loss from virus induced cancer in farm and domestic animals and will summarize some of the occupational hazards from environmental agents other than tumor viruses.

VIRUSES ASSOCIATED WITH CANCER IN ANIMALS AND MAN

There are four major families of viruses associated with cancer in animals; 1) retroviruses, 2) herpesviruses, 3) papovaviruses, and 4) hepatitis B virus (Table 1). Retroviruses have not yet been incriminated in human cancer despite extensive research (21).

Retroviruses (RNA Tumor Viruses)

These agents are mostly nonpathogenic and noncytolytic, but they do cause important disease in many, but not all, avian and mammalian species (64). Included are avian leukosis of chickens, reticuloendotheliosis of turkeys, leukemia and breast cancer in

Table 1. Viruses Associated with Cancer in Animals and Man

Virus	Animals	Diseases	Transmission	Genetic Control	Environmental Factors	Prevention
Retroviruses	Chickens, Turkeys, Ducks, Mice, Cats, Cows, Horses, Sheep, Goats, Primates	None Leukemia Sarcoma Breast Ca. Anemia Adenomatosis CNS	Genetic and Horizontal	Cellular and Immune Levels	Chemicals Radiation Other viruses Living conditions Vaccines	Selective breeding Vaccine
Herpesviruses	Frog, Rabbit, Chicken, Primates, Man	None Infect. Mono. Lymphoma Cervical Ca. CNS	Horizontal	Cellular and Immune Levels	Temperature Living conditions Malaria Bacterial or plant products Sexual contact	Selective breeding Vaccine
Papova	Mice, Hamster, Rabbit, Dog, Cattle, Horse, Sheep, Deer, Primate, Man	None Warts Fibroma CNS	Horizontal	Cellular and Immune Levels	Chemicals Radiation Living conditions	
Hepatitis B	Woodchuck, Squirrel, Man	None Hepatitis Liver Ca. Arteritis	Horizontal	Cellular and Immune Levels	Living conditions Chemicals	Vaccine

mice, and lymphoma in cows, domestic cats, and gibbon apes. Sarcomas are less commonly produced in chickens, mice, cats, and primates. Other non-neoplastic, naturally occurring diseases caused
by retroviruses are anemia in chickens, mice, cats, and horses;
encephalitis and arthritis in goats; pulmonary adenomatosis
(jagziekte), and demyelination (visna) in sheep; and neuromotor
paralysis in wild mice. Avian and bovine leukosis are of major
economic importance and feline leukemia is a major concern to pet
owners and veterinarians (11). Although retroviruses have the
capacity to be transmitted by both genetic (32) (DNA provirus) and
horizontal (RNA tumor virus) means they cause disease only when
spread horizontally between cells of an individual animal and between animals of the same species. In lymphoma-prone inbred mice,
such as the AKR strain, the leukemia virus is transmitted genetically, whereas the leukemia viruses of chickens, wild mice (15),
and gibbon apes are transmitted mainly by maternal, nongenetic
means. The mammary tumor virus of mice is transmitted both genetically and by milk. The bovine and feline leukemia viruses are
transmitted primarily by contact after birth, although maternal
congenital transmission can also occur. Retrovirus contamination
of infectious disease vaccines used in chickens and cows has also
been a source for virus spread. We found that vaccination of
newborn chickens against Marek's disease herpesvirus may have been
a source of leukosis virus spread and resultant solid tumors
(27). A common denominator in the pathogenesis of many of these
retrovirus-associated diseases is lifelong, persistent and productive infection and relative immunologic tolerance to the virus.
However, in bovine leukosis, feline leukemia, and visna the host
immune response apparently plays an important role in regulating
viral latency. Feline leukemia virus may itself be immunosuppres-
sive, thus predisposing infected cats to other infections. Chemical
carcinogens, X-irradiation, and DNA tumor viruses, such as polyoma
and herpesvirus, may activate latent retroviruses in vitro, but
there is no convincing evidence that these environmental agents
behave as retrovirus cocarcinogens under natural circumstances. In
particular, we know of no evidence suggesting that agricultural
chemicals induce cancer in farm or domestic animals, including wild
mice, or activate latent RNA or DNA tumor viruses in vivo. Far and
away the most important factors determining retrovirus virulence in
domestic and farm animals are the degree of genetic suceptibility
and closeness of contact with other animals of the same species.
Prolonged and intimate exposure from crowded housing conditions is
the principal environmental circumstance predisposing to infection
and disease with the avian and mammalian retroviruses outside of
the laboratory, as manifested by outbreaks of leukosis in captive
chickens, turkeys, ducks, cats, cows, rhesus monkeys, and gibbon
apes (60). Virtually all commercial chickens are heavily infected
with leukosis virus. Since the tumors induced are not grossly
apparent until about 20 weeks of age, this virus is not economically as important as is the Marek's disease herpesvirus which

induces tumors by 6-8 weeks of age. Bovine leukemia virus is widespread in commercial dairy herds; more than 20% of dairy cows and
60% of herds surveyed in the U.S.A. are infected (9). Although
present in milk and viable milk cells, the virus is probably spread
mainly by insects. Since only a few cows develop leukosis late in
life this virus is not of major economic significance. However,
if transstate shipment of cattle or sperm were ever restricted to
viral antibody-free animals this would become an important consideration. Spread of feline leukemia virus and related disease among
domestic cats in multicat households has been well documented (14)
and we have recently observed the spread of feline leukemia virus
from domestic to exotic cat within a household (56). Of course,
these crowded conditions for farm and domestic animals are man-made
and, thus, not truly natural. Without human intervention the naturally-occurring animal retroviruses would indeed be largely nonpathogenic.

     Prevention of retrovirus disease in mice and chickens through
introduction of virus resistance genes by selective breeding is
potentially effective (18). Retrovirus resistance genes have been
best defined in inbred mice where they operate at both the intra-
cellular and immune levels (43). By contrast, the genetic control
of retrovirus infection in chickens is exerted at the cell membrane
level. Elimination or isolation of infected animals has also
helped to control exogenous spread of bovine and feline leukemia
viruses. Active immunization has worked well against cell to cell
spread of endogenous leukemia virus in certain laboratory strains
of mice (31). Passive immunization has been effective in preventing retroviral disease in inbred (16) and feral mice (36) and
active immunization has blocked chronic infection with leukemia
virus under experimental conditions in domestic cats
(24,35,42,50). Vaccination trials against bovine leukosis are now
underway at the University of California at Davis (G. Theilen,
pers. comm.).

     The animal retroviruses apparently present only the remotest
public health risk. Despite constant concern and ample testing of
various high risk groups (e.g. lab workers, veterinarians, dairy
workers, FeLV household contacts), there has been no proven human
infection with or immunologic evidence of exposure to any of the
animal retroviruses. Numerous earlier reports of such virus antibodies in human sera were erroneously based upon nonspecific reactions (2). That humans do have the capacity to respond immunologically to these agents has been shown by experimental inoculation
of cancer patients with murine leukemia virus. But under other
exposure conditions these agents do not infect humans because they
cannot pass external barriers or are rapidly lysed by human complement (65). Millions of years ago certain retroviruses may have
spread horizontally and infected the germ cells of unrelated
species (63), but there is no proof of cross species spread in
contemporary times.

Previous reports of exogenous retroviruses isolated from human cells in vitro were laboratory contaminants because they closely resembled or were identical with the already known monkey leukemia viruses. However, a new candidate retrovirus (29,51) associated with some, but not all, adult T-cell leukemias in the U.S.A. and Japan deserves serious attention. Seroepidemiologic studies suggest that this virus, which is unrelated to any of the extant animal retroviruses, may be spread horizontally among humans, although it does not necessarily cause any disease. If confirmed, it will be the first human retrovirus to be discovered.

An extensive search for an endogenous inherited human retrovirus has so far been negative. Nor are there any confirmed retrovirus isolates in higher apes or in certain household pets, such as dogs or parakeets, where they have been sought (10,22). There is no solid evidence that endogenous retroviruses play any useful or necessary role in evolution, in embryonic growth and differentiation or in tumor immunosurveillence, except the latter possibly in the cat (8). On the other hand, retroviruses have provided a magnificent tool for molecular biologists to probe the structure and function of the cellular genes (3). Their ability to behave like a bacterial transposon (37) and potential to activate and recombine with cellular oncogenes are of great heuristic value regardless of how important or frequent these events are in the real world. Except in a special rat cell virus system (57), it has not been possible to recreate in the laboratory the conditions required to reproducibly rescue endogenous oncogenes with helper retroviruses. Presumably, this recombination is also a very low probability event in vivo, but nevertheless, it has already provided a total of 15 different oncogenes that have been characterized in chickens, mice, cats, and woolly monkeys (7). Each of these oncogenes encodes a protein with tyrosene phosphokinase activity that probably performs a normal function in cell growth. When incorporated into a replicating helper retrovirus these cellular oncogenes produce several hundred fold excess of their product whose presence is essential to the initiation and maintenance of cell transformation in vitro and rapid induction of tumors in vivo. Most of these animal oncogenes are highly conserved in evolution and, in contrast to virogenes, are also represented by closely homologous genes and proteins in humans (66). Recently, transformation-specific genes have been identified in human cancer cells by their ability to transform mouse cell cultures by DNA transfection techniques (39,46). It will be interesting to determine if these molecularly cloned "cancer genes" resemble known retroviral or cellular oncogenes in their structure and function and whether or not they segregate in accord with mendelian inheritance in pedigrees of genetically determined human cancer. It might prove possible to link this transfection property with other assays of cancer susceptibility in these families, such as susceptibility of fibroblasts to

transformation by rodent sarcoma virus (55), thus adding credence
to the possible cancer-causative significance of these
transfectable nucleotide sequences. Importantly, activation of
transformation-specific oncogenes might well serve as the basis for
a badly needed short-term bioassay for potential environmental
carcinogens using human cells.

    Turning animal retroviruses to a useful purpose may also prove
feasible. In cell cultures retroviruses can serve as a vector for
transporting unrelated genes into the host cell genome. Such hybrid viruses can now be synthesized by recombinant DNA techniques,
and thus might eventually be used to purposely convey desirable
genes for genetic engineering. Introduction of nonpathogenic retroviruses as foreign immunogens into heterologous species may open
a new approach toward cancer immunotherapy.

Herpesviruses

    Viruses of this group are associated with naturally-occurring
kidney cancer in the frog and lymphoma in rabbits, chickens, and
New and Old World monkeys. In humans, the Epstein Barr virus (EBV)
is associated with Burkitt's lymphoma and nasopharyngeal carcinoma
(NPC), and the herpes simplex virus (HSV) with cervical carcinoma.
Cytomegalovirus is associated with Kaposi's sarcoma. As with retroviruses, the herpesviruses are also ubiquitous, usually latent
and nonpathogenic. They are spread by solely horizontal means and
usually held in check by the host's immune response and genetic
resistance at the cellular level. EBV is a normal parasite of B-
cells in the nasopharynx and genital HSV normally hides out in the
autonomic ganglion cells of the sacral paraspinal plexus. When
activated in lymphoid or epithelial target cells the herpesviruses
generally replicate, cause cell lysis and acute inflammation, and
only rarely do the infected cells become nonproductive and oncogenic. The herpesvirus transformed cells contain integrated viral
genes which are regulated by the host cell. EBV transformed cells
usually retain an entire viral genome whose expression is strongly
restricted whereas cells transformed by HSV contain only a fraction
of the viral genome which is usually more actively expressed (58).

    Herpesvirus of chickens does cause a T-cell lymphoma of major
economic importance, namely Marek's disease. This cancer can kill
10 to 20% of chickens before 8 weeks of age. The causative virus
is shed from feather follicles and spreads through the dander, but
the virus-transformed lymphocytes are, of course, nonproductive.
The obvious environmental cofactor in this disease is man-made,
intense, environmental crowding of chickens customary in commercial
frier operations. Over 100,000 chickens are housed in each shed.
Prevention could probably follow the selective breeding of virus-
resistant chickens (23), but a vaccine, made from a viable but
nonpathogenic related herpesvirus of turkeys, has proved more prac-

tical and efficacious (53). To date this is perhaps the best
example of vaccine prevention of a virus-induced cancer. Interestingly, the Marek's disease herpesvirus can also cause paralysis
in chickens by damaging myelin in the peripheral nerves and setting
forth a cellular autoimmune reaction (52).

In captive primates indigenous herpesvirus is rarely associated with spontaneous T-cell lymphomas in New World monkeys and
B-cell lymphomas in Old World monkeys. Close crowding of baboons
in a laboratory colony in Russia led, however, to activation and
spread of their latent herpes virus and occurrence of many lymphomas (40). The experimental induction of lymphomas in marmosets
by New World primate herpesviruses was prevented by vaccination
(41). The major environmental factors associated with Burkitt's
lymphoma in man are an early age of infection and coincident
malaria. Nitrosamines, herbal drugs, and noxious fumes have been
suggested, but not confirmed as cocarcinogens for EBV-related nasopharyngeal carcinoma. Genital herpes is clearly a venereal disease
in its epidemiologic characteristics. CMV associated Kaposi's
sarcoma may also be venereally transmitted in homosexual males
(33). From the environmental standpoint then, each of these
herpesvirus-related cancers is related primarily to sociologic and
hygienic features, rather than to well-defined chemical or physical
agents. Of course, genetic susceptibility is also a critical determinant as evidenced by the relatively high NPC risk of Chinese
and the susceptibility of males with an x-linked immunodeficiency
to overwhelming EBV infection and resultant severe mononucleosis,
agammaglobulinemia, or lymphoma (54). It appears that reduction in
malaria incidence has also reduced the incidence of Burkitts's
lymphoma, thus negating the need for and avoiding possible risks of
an EBV vaccine. No sound rationale exists for using an EBV vaccine
against NPC because the natural history of this disease remains so
obscure (28). Antiherpes drugs, interferon, and improved hygiene
appear the most promising approaches towards control of herpesvirus
infection in man. None of the animal herpesviruses are infectious
for humans.

Papovaviruses

This family consists of the papilloma viruses and the polyoma
viruses. Members of the papilloma virus genus are ubiquitous in
many mammalian species (cattle, horses, sheep, goats, dogs, monkeys, rabbits, hamsters) including man in which they induce benign
epithelial or connective tissue tumors that regress and are highly
host and tissue-specific. Papillomaviruses are transmitted by
close contact including venereal transmission and are usually maintained in a latent state by T-cell immune mechanisms. However,
papillomaviruses in rabbits, cattle, and man can be associated with
squamous cell carcinoma. Lack of a cell culture system for replication of papillomaviruses had impeded an understanding of their

molecular biology. However, human and bovine papillomaviruses have
been molecularly cloned and shown to share common transforming
sequences (30). Similar to other oncogenic DNA viruses the formation of a tumor (papilloma or fibroma) results from the abortive
infection of germinal cells. Virus production is induced by the
keratinizing process and may result in an abnormal DNA synthesis in
terminally differentiating cells that would normally be restricted
for DNA synthesis. This masking of virus in Shope papillomas of
the wild cottontail rabbit was the first model for studying viral
oncogenesis in mammals (12). The importance of genetic constitution and environmental cofactors in viral oncogenesis was also
first shown in this model by enhancing effect of chemical carcinogens on experimental virus-induced papillomas in the domestic rabbit. It is not known, however, whether extrinsic factors are involved in the malignant conversion of Shope papillomas under
natural conditions.

The bovine fibropapilloma viruses (BPV) consist of at least 3
types that cause skin, teat, genital, and alimenteric warts in
cattle. The skin and genital growths do not become malignant but
regress and have little economic significance. Based upon the
detection of BPV-specific DNA by molecular hybridization it was
suggested that subcutaneous fibromas (sarcoids) in the horse may be
caused by horizontal spread of BPV (38). Most remarkable, however,
is the evidence of a strong cocarcinogenic interaction of dietary
bracken fern and BPV in cattle with urinary bladder tumors suffering chronic enzootic hematuria (47), and in malignant transformation of alimentary tract papillomas that occur in high incidence (2.5%) in cattle raised in the Scottish highlands (34). The
alimentary, cutaneous, and genital viruses are each a distinct type
of BPV. Only the alimentaric BPV DNA is found in the GI tract
papillomas or carcinomas to which they give rise (6). These are
squamous cell carcinomas in the tongue, orophayrnx, esophagus and
rumen, and adenocarcinomas in the intestine. None of the animal
papillomaviruses are infectious for man.

At least six different species of papillomavirus cause skin,
anogenital (condyloma), and laryngeal warts in humans (48).
Malignant transformation to squamous cell carcinoma occurs in
families with a rare, recessively inherited disorder called epider-
modysplasia verruciformis. A defect in cellular immunity predi-
sposes these patients to life-long persistence of the virus and
sunlight promotes malignant transformation of the warts. The possibility has been raised that the venereally transmitted condyloma
virus might be associated with cervical and vulvar dysplasia and
carcinoma, although initial attempts to detect viral DNA sequences
in cervical carcinomas were negative. Preliminary studies to detect bovine or human papilloma virus DNA in colon polyps or carcinomas were also negative (67). Papillomas in man or animal are
often responsive to treatment with autogenous vaccines or inter-

feron. The latter has been especially useful in treating recurrent laryngeal papillomas in children.

The small DNA viruses, polyoma, SV40, and adenovirus are oncogenic only after experimental inoculation into heterologous cells or newborn animals. Under natural conditions indigenous polyoma virus is nononcogenic in aging laboratory and wild mice (17). Humans are infected with two distinct types of polyoma virus, designated JC and BK viruses. These agents are ubiquitous, worldwide in distribution, and most adults have antibodies to both viruses by young adulthood. Both viruses persist throughout life and become activated in immunologically compromised individuals where they are usually shed in the urine. Activation of the JC virus in brain oligodendroglia is associated with a demyelinating disease called progressive multifocal leukodystrophy. A similar disease with papovavirus particles was described in immunocompromised rhesus monkeys (26). BKV and JCV are oncogenic for newborn hamsters and JCV can induce brain tumors in owl monkeys. Transformed cells and tumors induced in animals by BKV and JCV contain the intranuclear T-antigen. However, a search for the antigen or other evidence of papovavirus in human cancer has so far been negative (62). Similarly, a thorough search for adenovirus in relation to human cancer has also been negative (25).

Hepatitis B Virus

Life-long persistent infection with hepatitis B virus (HBV) is a major risk factor for development of chronic active hepatitis, cirrhosis, and primary hepatocellular carcinoma (PHC) (4). This tumor is relatively rare in the U.S.A. and Europe, but it is the most common cancer of males in parts of China, Taiwan, southeast Asia, and most of Africa. It is indeed one of the most common and fatal cancers in the world causing between 500,000 and 1,000,000 deaths annually. Infection occurs by directly horizontal transmission. Chronic carriers, which make up 5 to 20% of these high risk populations, usually arise as a result of neonatal infection acquired from their mothers or siblings who are also chronic carriers. Like other DNA tumor viruses, the virus DNA appears to be integrated into the genome of the tumor cells, and it is also present and expressed in the nonmalignant hepatocytes (59). In the chronic carrier state both free and integrated HBV DNA have been found in the liver, but only the former is associated with virus production (5). An immune response to the persistent HBV infection results in continuing damage to infected hepatocytes. Continuous liver-cell regeneration results which likely sets the stage for cocarcinogenic interaction with other environmental carcinogens. Aflatoxin B, a mycotoxin that commonly contaminates peanuts, grains, and human foodstuffs; alkaloids in medicinal plants; and nitrosamines are the most probable candidates. Aflotoxin has caused epidemics of liver cancer in lower animals and has been

detected in the environment in those areas that have a high incidence of PHC. Genetic suceptibility to persistent HBV infection
and a marked male predominance also occur. Different subtypes of
surface antigen (HBsAg) show specific geographic localizations. The
virus will not infect cell cultures, but a tissue culture cell line
isolated in 1975 from an African patient with PHC has been shown to
continually produce small amounts of viral HBsAg (1). No evidence
of HBV DNA or other viral markers was found in many American and
African patients that lacked HBsAg in their blood suggesting that
in those populations with low incidence of HBV infection PHC must
be caused by factors other than HBV (44).

     Prevention might be aimed at eliminating aflatoxin from the
areas involved, but this would require major changes in the economics and agricultural practices. A vaccine program against HBV has
been carried out since 1978 in Senegal, an area of endemic HBV
infection (86% of the population has a marker of past or present
infection) and high PHC prevalence (75 to 150 per 100,000). The
immunogen is purified from HBsAg positive sera from healthy blood
donors and inactivated with formaldehyde. Pregnant women (64%) and
3 to 6 month old infants (92%) responded to the vaccine by developing anti-HBsAg antibodies and the incidence of HBsAg chronic
carriers was reduced from 15% to 2% (45). Thus, it should eventually be possible to completely eradicate HBV infection and associated PHC in this high risk population.

     A naturally-occurring model of chronic hepatitis, cirrhosis,
and hepatocellular carcinoma associated with an indigenous hepatitis virus has recently been found in woodchucks in the eastern
U.S.A.(61) and squirrels in California. These animal hepatitis
viruses are related to, but distinct from, HBV and appear to be
highly analogous in their ability to produce excess surface
antigen, and lead to hepatitis in about 75% and primary liver
tumors in about 25% of the captive animals. As with HBV in humans,
hepatocellular injury probably results from an immunologic
interation with viral antigens on liver cells. Carcinogenesis most
likely results from a similar mechanism as that which occurs in
man, although no environmental cofactors have been defined in this
animal model. A search for similar viruses in other wild rodents,
including feral mice from southern California, is underway.

CONCLUSIONS

     The studies summarized in the previous paragraphs lead to the
following conclusions: 1) Retroviruses are widely prevalent in
animals, but are seldom pathogenic. In the proper genetic and
environmental setting they may be spread horizontally and result in
both neoplastic and nonneoplastic diseases. Their natural history
is not effected, however, by environmental or agricultural chemicals. The DNA tumor viruses are also ubiquitous and widely preva-

lent in animals and man. Under natural conditions they, too, are
generally latent and harmless, but after activation they may be
associated with cell killing via the host's immune response. Only
very infrequently do they integrate into the chromosomes as nonproductive infections and cause cancer, sometimes in conjunction
with recognized environmental cofactors (e.g. bracken fern and
aflatoxin). 2) The most important extrinsic factors enhancing the
incidence of virus tumors in both animals and man are related to
living conditions. Close crowding and poor hygiene enhance the
opportunities for horizontal spread of the viruses early in life
and allow for them to "get a jump" on the immune system and establish the chronic carrier state. Conditions of immunosuppression
can lead to an increased level of infection and occasionally an
increased tumor incidence. From the agricultural standpont, closed
or semiclosed containment of animals (such as chickens or cows or
cats) is a major culprit fostering spread of herpes, papova, and
retroviruses. A similar conclusion applies to the spread of herpes, papova, and hepatitis viruses in man. 3) Selective breeding
of farm animals for economically favorable attributes, such as
rapid weight gain, may also increase their genetic susceptibility
to these agents. The intensive inbreeding of mice has created an
obvious artifactual biology by selection for the inheritance of
certain properties, such as infectious virogenes, recombination
among endogenous virogenes, and genetic permissiveness to
endogenous virus replication. This does not occur in outbred feral
mice (19). 4) Vaccine induced protection against the naturally-
occurring virus-associated tumors is of proven value with lymphoma
and breast cancer in mice, lymphoma in cats, Marek's disease in
chickens and hepatitis in man. Reduced exposure to important
cofactors, such as malaria and bracken fern, improved hygiene, and
more "breathing room" may be equally effective in prevention of the
associated tumors. 5) The animal tumor viruses are highly species-
specific and are not infectious for humans. Even in high exposure
situations no convincing evidence exists for even a single human
infection, past or present, with any of the animal tumor viruses.
This applies also to humans inadvertently inoculated years ago with
vaccines contaminated with avian leukosis virus or SV40 and laboratory workers accidentally inoculated with animal retroviruses
(13). There is, thus, no reason to consider the animal tumor viruses as public health risks.

Occupational Hazards

By contrast, occupational hazards for farm workers from environmental agents other than tumor viruses pose a more realistic
threat. Farm workers, veterinarians, and lab technicians face
possible injury from accidents, bites, or scratches, in addition to
infections from animals or their ectoparasites. Infections caused
by farm animals include tuberculosis, anthrax, brucellosis, lepto-
spirosis, salmonella, streptococcus, staphlococcus, Q fever, and

viral or fungal infections. Recent outbreaks of ornithosis in
veterinarians from exposure to ducks in poultry processing plants
are a pertinent example (49). Animal-related allergies or
allergies indirectly related to animals - such as farmer's lung
from mouldy hay - also present a potential health risk. The presence of fecal bacteria and germ negative endotoxins in dust of
intensive poultry and swine units may contribute to organic dust
disease, such as byssinosis. Acute toxicity from pesticides with
consequent accidental injury or death is a definite risk to farm
laborers working in close contact with agricultural chemicals. The
potential genetic risk to farm worker of chronic exposure to agricultural chemicals is discussed in other papers in this volume.

The current revolution in biotechnology and introduction to
agribusiness of advanced techniques of genetic engineering raise
exciting prospects, but also some cautionary notes. As more and
more commercial livestock and cat breeding operations take place in
crowded, closed, or semiclosed units we can anticipate further
outbreaks of leukemia, papillomatosis, and other infectious diseases among animals and increased exposure of farm workers to the
other occupational hazards mentioned above. Another concern, expressed also by plant breeders, is that intensive inbreeding and
selection for certain properties in livestock and domestic animals
may narrow the genetic reserves necessary to maintain the health of
present species. Such losses to the gene pool may not be replaced
by genetic engineering. A vivid example of the beneficial effect
of genetic diversity was observed by this author in his study of
retroviruses in feral mice. A strong retrovirus restriction gene
not present in laboratory mice was discovered to be polymorphic in
wild mice (20). Upon crossing wild mice bearing this gene with
leukemia prone inbred (AKR) mice the spread of infectious leukemia
virus was blocked and the associated tumors prevented. The Fl mice
were large, long-lived, and healthy, a remarkable illustration of
hybrid vigor! According to this model and other similar examples
in animal and plant breeding, it seems wise to make efforts towards
preserving the gene pool of our crops and livestock. Introducing
new traits by breeding domestic plants and animals with wild or
foreign species may contribute much towards a better farm
product. Genetic engineering has indeed opened a dramatic, new
approach towards improved animal and crop management, but it cannot
yet serve as substitute for the natural wealth of genetic diversity.

REFERENCES

1.   Alexander, J., G. Macrab, R. Saunders. Studies on In Vitro
     Production of Hepatitis B Surface Antigen by a Human Cell
     Line. Perspect. Virol. 10:103, 1978.

2. Barbacid, M., D. Bolognesi, S. A. Aaronson. Humans Have Anti-
    bodies Capable of Recognizing Oncoviral Glycoproteins: Demon-
    stration That These Antibodies are Found in Response to Cellu-
    lar Demonstration of Glycoproteins Rather than as Consequences
    of Exposure to Virus. PNAS 77:1617, 1980.

3. Bishop, J. M. The Molecular Biology of RNA Tumor Viruses: A
    Physician's Guide. NEJM 303:675, 1980.

4. Blumberg, B. S., B. Larouze, W. T. London, B. Werner, J. E.
    Hesser, I. Millman, G. Saimot, M. Paget. The Relation of
    Infection with the Hepatitis B Agent to Primary Hepatic Carci-
    noma. Am. J. Path. 81:669, 1975.

5. Brechot, C., M. Hadchonel, J. Scotto, F. Degos, P. Charnoy, C.
    Trepo, P. Tilollos, Detection of Hepatitis B Virus DNA in
    Liver and Serum: A Direct Appraisal of the Chronic Carrier
    State. The Lancet II, 765, 1981.

6. Campo, M. S., M. W. Moar, W. F. H. Jarrett, H. M. Laird. A
    New Papillomavirus Associated with Alimentary Cancer in
    Cattle. Nature 286:180, 1980.

7. Coffin, J. M., H. E. Varmus, J. M. Bishop, et al. A Proposal
    for Naming Host Cell-Derived Inserts in Retrovirus Genomes. J.
    Virol. 40:953, 1981

8. Essex, J., A. Sliski, S. M. Cotter, R. M. Jakowski, W. D.
    Hardy. Immunosurveillance of Naturally-Occurring Feline Leu-
    kemia. Science 190:790, 1975.

9. Ferrer, J. F., S. F. Kenyon, P. Gupta. Milk of Dairy Cows
    Frequently Contains a Leukemogenic Virus. Science 213:1014,
    1981.

10. Gardner, M. B. Current Information on Feline and Canine Can-
    cers and Relationship or Lack of Relationship to Human Cancer.
    JNCI 46:281, 1971.

11. Gardner, M. B. Feline Oncogenic Viruses: A Brief Overview.
    Mod. Vet. Prac. Feb. 1980, 127.

12. Gardner, M. B. Historical Background (Chapter 1) In: Mole-
    cular Biology of RNA Tumor Viruses J. R. Stephenson (ed).
    Acad. Press, N.Y., P. 1, 1980.

13. Gardner, M. B. Avian and Murine RNA Tumor Viruses: Modes of
    Transmission. In: Biohazards in Biological Research Eds. A.
    Hellman, M. N. Oxman, R. Pollack. Cold Spring Harbor Labora-
    tory, p. 143, 1973.

14. Gardner, M. B., J. C. Brown, H. P. Charman, et al. FeLV Epi-
    demiology in Los Angeles Cats: Appraisal of Detection
    Methods. Int. J. Cancer 19:581, 1977.

15. Gardner, M. B., A. Chiri, M. F. Dougherty, J. Casagrande, J.
    D. Estes. Congenital Transmission of Murine Leukemia Virus
    from Wild Mice Prone to Development of Lymphoma and
    Paralysis. JNCI 62:63, 1979.

16. Gardner, M. B., J. D. Estes, J. Casagrande, S. Rasheed. Pre-
    vention of Paralysis and Supression of Lymphoma in Wild Mice
    by Passive Immunization to Congenitally Transmitted Murine
    Leukemia Virus. JNCI 64:359, 1980.

17. Gardner, M. B., B. E. Henderson, H. Menck, J. Parker, J. D.
    Estes, R. J. Huebner. Spontaneous Tumor Occurrence and C-Type
    Virus Expression in Polyoma Infected Aging Wild Mice. JNCI
    52:979, 1974.
18. Gardner, M. B., V. Klement, B. E. Henderson, H. Meier, J D.
    Estes, R. J. Huebner Genetic Control of Type C Virus of Wild
    Mice. Nature 259:143, 1976.
19. Gardner, M. B., S. Rasheed. Retroviruses in Feral Mice.
    Inter. Rev. Exp. Pathol., 23:209-267, 1982.
20. Gardner, M. B., S. Rasheed, B. K. Pal, J. D. Estes, S. T.
    O'Brien, Alvr-1, A Dominant Murine Leukemia Virus Restriction
    Gene, is Polymorphic in Leukemia-Prone Wild Mice. PNAS
    77:531, 1980.
21. Gardner, M. B., S. Rasheed, S. Shimizu, R. W. Rongey, B. E.
    Henderson, R. M. McAllister, V. Klement, H. P. Charman, R. V.
    Gilden, R. L. Heberling, R. J. Huebner. Search for RNA Tumor
    Virus in Humans. In: Origins of Human Cancer. Eds. H. H.
    Hiatt, J. D. Watson, J. A. Winster. Cold Spring Harbor Labo-
    ratory p. 1235, 1977.
22. Gardner, M. B., R. W. Rongey, P. Sarma, P. Arnstein. Electron
    Microscopic Search for Retrovirus Particles in Spontaneous
    Tumors of the Parakeet. Vet. Pathol. 18:700, 1981.
23. Gavora, J. S., J. L. Spencer. Marek's Disease in Chickens:
    Genetic Resistance to a Viral Neoplastic Disease. A Review.
    In: Genetic Control of Natural Resistance to Infection and
    Malignancy Eds: E. Skamene, P. A. L. Kongshavn, M. Landy.
    Acad. Press, p. 361, 1980.
24. Grant, C. V., G. deNoronha, E. Tusch, M. T. Michalek, M. F.
    McLane. Protection of Cats Against Progressive Fibrosarcomas
    and Persistent Leukemia Virus Infection by Vaccination with
    Feline Leukemia Virus. JNCI 65:1285, 1980.
25. Green, M., W. S. M. Wold, J. K. Mackey, P. Rigden. Analysis
    of Human Tonsil and Cancer DNAs and RNAs for DNA Sequence of
    Group C (Serotypes 1.2.5.6.) Human Adenoviruses. PNAS
    76:6606, 1979.
26. Gribble, D. H., C. C. Haden, L. W. Schwartz, R. V.
    Henrickson. Spontaneous Progressive Multifocal Leukoen-
    cephalopathy (PML) in Macaques. Nature 254:602, 1975.
27. Henderson, B. E., M. B. Gardner, H. P. Charman, E. Y. Johnson,
    T. Rucio, P. Sarma, B. Alena, R. J. Huebner. Investigation of
    an Increase of Solid Tumors in Chickens Vaccinated Against
    Marek's Disease. Avian Diseases 18:58, 1974.
28. Henderson, B. E, E. Louie, J. Jing, P. Buell, M. B. Gardner.
    Risk Factors Associated with Nasopharyngeal Carcinoma. NEJM
    295:1101, 1976.
29. Hinuma, Y., K. Nagata, M. Hanoka, M. Nakai, T. Matsumoto, K.
    Kinoshita, S. Shirakawa, I. Miyoshi. Antigen in an Adult T-
    Cell Leukemia Cell Line and Detection of Antibodies to the
    Antigen in Human Sera. PNAS 78:6476, 1981.

30. Howley, P. M., M. F. Low, C. Hellman, L. Engel, M. C. Alonso, M. A. Israel, D. R. Lowy. Molecular Characterization of Papilloma Virus Genomes. In: Viruses in Naturally-Occurring Cancer. Eds: M. Essex, G. J. Todaro, H. Zur Hausen. Cold Spring Harbor Laboratory, p. 233, 1980.

31. Huebner, R. J., R. V. Gilden, R. Toni, R. W. Hill, R. W. Trimmer, D. C. Fish, B. Sass. Prevention of Spontaneous Leukemia in AKR Mice by Type-Specific Immunosuppression of Endogenous Ecotropic Virogenes. PNAS 73:4633, 1976.

32. Huebner, R. J., G. J. Todaro. Oncogenes of RNA Tumor Viruses as Determinants of Cancer. PNAS 64:1087, 1969.

33. Hymes, H. B., J. B. Greene, A. Marcus, D. C. William, T. Cheung, N. S. Prose, H. Ballard, L. F. Laubenstein. Kaposi's Sarcoma in Homosexual Men - A Report of Eight Cases. Lancet II 598, 1981.

34. Jarrett, W. F. H., P. E. McNeil, W. T. R. Grimshaw, I. E. Selman, W. I. M. McIntyre. High Incidence Area of Cattle Cancer with a Possible Interaction Between an Environmental Carcinogen and a Papilloma Virus. Nature 274:215, 1978.

35. Jarrett, W. O., J. Jarrett, H. Mackey, H. Laird, C. Hood, D. Hay. Vaccination Against Feline Leukemia Virus Using a Cell Membrane Antigen System. Int. J. Cancer 16:134, 1975.

36. Kelloff, G. J., R. L. Peters, R. M. Donahoe, I. Ghazzouli, B. Sass, R. M. Nims, R. J. Huebner. An Approach to C-Type Virus Immunoprevention of Spontaneously Occurring Tumors in Laboratory Mice. Cancer Res. 36:622, 1976.

37. Kleckner, N. Translocatable Elements in Procaryotes. Cell 11:11, 1977.

38. Lancaster, W. D., G. H. Theilen, C. Olson. Hybridization of Bovine Papilloma Virus Type 1 and Type 2 DNA to DNA from Virus-Induced Hamster Tumors and Naturally-Occurring Equine Tumors. Intervirology 11:227, 1979.

39. Lane, M. A., A. Sainten, G. M. Cooper. Activation of Related Transforming Genes in Mouse and Human Mammary Carcinomas. PNAS 78:5185, 1981.

40. Lapin, B. A., V. A. Agrba, A. F. Voevodin, A. G. Dyachenko, L. A. Yakovleva, L. V. Kokosha, G. N. Chuvirov, H. Rabin, F. Deinhardt, L. Folk. Characterization of the Baboon Herpesvirus (HVP) Associated with Malignant Lymphoma in the Sukhumi Hamadryas Baboon Colony. Adv. in Comparative Cancer Research, Eds: D. S. Yohn, B. A. Lapin, J. R. Blakeslee. Elsevier/North-Holland 1979, p. 413.

41. Laufs, R., H. Steinke. Vaccination of Non-Human Primates Against Malignant Lymphoma. Nature 253:71, 1975.

42. Lewis, M. G., L. E. Mathes, R. G. Olsen. Protection Against Feline Leukemia by Vaccination with a Subunit Vaccine. In Press.

43. Lilly, F., T. Pincus. Genetic Control of Viral Leukemogenesis. Adv. Cancer Res. 17:231, 1973.

44. Marion, P. L., W. S. Robinson. Hepatitis B Virus and Hepato-
    cellular Carcinoma. In: Viruses in Naturally-Occurring Can-
    cers Eds: M. Essex, G. J. Todara, H. Zur Hausen. Cold
    Spring Harbor Laboratory p.423, 1980.

45. Maupas, P. A. Goudeau, P. Coursaget, J. Drucker, P. Bagros.
    Hepatitis B Vaccine: Efficacy in High Risk Settings, A Two-
    Year Study. Intervirology 10:196, 1978.

46. Murray, M. J., B-Z Shilo, C. Shih, D. Cowing, H. W. Hsu, R. A.
    Weinberg. Three Different Human Tumor Cell Lines Contain
    Different Oncogenes. Cell 25:355, 1981.

47. Olson, C., D. E. Gordon, M. G. Robl, K. P. Lee. Oncogenicity
    of Bovine Papilloma Virus. Arch. Environ. Health 19:827,
    1969.

48. Orth, G. S., S. Jablonska, F. Breitburd, M. Favre, O. Crois-
    sant. The Human Papillomaviruses. Bull. Cancer 65:151, 1978.

49. Palmer, S. R. A Common-Source Outbreak of Ornithosis in Vete-
    rinary Surgeons. The Lancet II p.798, 1981.

50. Pedersen, N. C., G. H. Theilen, L. L. Warner. Safety and
    Efficacy Studies of Live and Killed Feline Leukemia Virus
    Vaccines. Amer. J. Vet. Res. 40:1120, 1978.

51. Poisez, B. J., F. W. Ruscetti, A. F. Gazdar, P. A. Bunn, J. D.
    Minna, R. C. Gallo. Detection and Isolation of Type C Retro-
    virus Particles from Fresh and Cultured Lymphocytes of a
    Patient with Cutaneous T-Cell Lymphoma. PNAS 77:7415, 1980.

52. Prineas, J. W., R. G. Wright. The Fine Structure of Peri-
    pheral Nerve Lesions in a Virus-Induced Demyelination Disease
    in Fowl (Marek's Disease). Lab. Invest. 26:548, 1972.

53. Purchase, H. G., Prevention of Marek's Disease: A Review.
    Cancer Research 36:396, 1976.

54. Purtilo, D. T., L. Paguin, T. Gindhart. Genetics of Neoplasia
    - Impact of Ecogenetics on Oncogenesis. Amer. J. Path.
    91:609, 1978.

55. Rasheed, S., M. B. Gardner. Growth Properties and Suscep-
    tibility to Viral Transformation of Skin Fibroblasts from
    Individuals at High Genetic Risk to Colorectal Cancer. JNCI
    66:43, 1981.

56. Rasheed, S., M. B. Gardner. Isolation of Feline Leukemia
    Virus from a Leopard Cat. Cell Line and Search for Retrovirus
    in Wild Felidae. JNCI 67:929, 1981.

57. Rasheed, S., M. B. Gardner. In Vitro Isolation of Stable Rat
    Sarcoma Viruses PNAS 75:2972, 1978.

58. Roizman, B., N. Frenkel, E. D. Kieff, P. G. Spear. The Struc-
    ture and Expression of Human Herpesvirus DNA in Productive
    Infection and in Transformed Cells. In: Origins of Human
    Cancer Cold Spring Harbor Laboratory p. 1069, 1977.

59. Skafritz, D. A., D. Skouval, H. J. Sherman, S. J. Hadziyarmis,
    M. C. Kew. Integration of Hepatitis B Virus DNA into the
    Genome of Liver Cells in Chronic Liver Disease and Hepatocel-
    lular Carcinoma. NEJM 305:1067, 1981.

60. Stowell, R. E., E. K. Smith, C. Espana, V. G. Nelson. Out-
     break of Malignant Lymphoma in Rhesus Monkeys. Lab. Invest
     25:476, 1971.

61. Summers, J., J. M. Smolec, R. L. Synder. A Virus Similar to
     Human Hepatitis B Virus Associated with Hepatitis and Hepatoma
     in Woodchucks. PNAS 75:4533, 1978.

62. K. K. Takemoto. Human Polyoma Viruses: Evaluation of Their
     Possible Involvement in Human Cancer. In: Viruses in Natu-
     rally-Occurring Cancers. Eds: M. Essex, G. J. Todaro, H.
     Hausen. Cold Spring Laboratory p. 311, 1980.

63. Todaro, G. T. Evolution and Modes of Transmission of RNA
     Tumor Viruses. Park-Davis Award Lecture. Am. J. Pathol.
     81:590: 1975.

64. Veterinary Cancer Medicine. Eds: G. H. Theilen, B. R. Made-
     well. Lea & Fieberger, p. 204, 1979.

65. Welsh, R. M., F. C. Jensen, N. R. Cooper, M. B. A. Oldstone.
     Inactivation and Lysis of Oncornaviruses by Human Serum.
     Virology 74:432, 1976.

66. Wong-Staal, F., R. Dalla-Favera, G. Franchini, E. P. Gelman,
     R. C. Gallo. Three Distinct Genes in Human DNA Related to the
     Transforming Genes of Mammalian Sarcoma Retroviruses. Science
     213:226, 1981.

67. Zur Hausen, H., W. Scheiber, G. W. Bornkama. Attempts to
     Detect Virus Specific DNA in Human Tumors: I: Nucleic Acid
     Hybridization with Complimentary RNA of Human Wart Virus.
     Int. J. Cancer 13:650, 1974.

DISCUSSION

Q.   SUGIMURA: An antibody reacting with the established T-
     lymphoma cell line was observed in more than 25% of healthy
     subjects on Kyushu Island. Could you explain more about
     encephalitis by retrovirus? Also, could you give more
     comments on arteritis by HB virus? In addition, is CMV the
     cause of Kaposi's sarcoma and pavova virus a cause of skin
     carcinoma? Are these acting as tumor promotors like
     phorbolester?

A.   GARDNER: Antibody reacting with the established T-lymphoma
     cell line was detected in more than 25% of healthy subjects
     living in areas of Kyushu Island where the occurence of adult
     T-cell lymphomas was endemic. Almost all sera from patients
     having T-cell lylmphoma in these areas also gave a positive
     result.

     Encephalitis, arthritis, and interstitial pneumonia are
     features of a widespread disease syndrome of goats which
     appears to be caused by a retrovirus related to the maedi-
     visna virus of sheep.

It has been estimated that hepatitis B antigen may be the inciting agent in 25-40% of patients with necrotizing vaculitis. Hepatitis B antigenemia and related circulating immune complexes have been found in high incidence in the sera of patients with polyarteritis nodosa. Furthermore, hepatitis B antigen, immunoglobulins and complement occur in the vascular lesions.

CMV appears to be causatively associated with some cases of Kaposi's sarcoma and may be venerally transmitted in homosexual males.

Papilloma virus is causatively associated with squamous cell carcinoma in the rare genetically recessive condition called epidermo-dysplasia verruciformis. Multiple warts occur in this condition and sunlight is a co-carcinogen in their transition to carcinoma.

One way that viruses may function as promoters is via the stimulation of cellular DNA replication. In addition, retroviruses may activate transcription of nearby cellular onc genes by virtue of the promoter sequences present at each end (long terminal repeat) of the proviral DNA.

Q.   KRISHINA: What is your opinion about the durability of interferon?

A.   GARDNER: The antiviral action of interferon has a very brief duration of activity lasting only, perhaps, a few days. Therefore, for clinical effectiveness, it must be given repeatedly at daily or more frequent intervals.

TRACE ELEMENTS AND TERATOLOGY: AN INTERACTIONAL PERSPECTIVE

Lucille S. Hurley, Carl L. Keen, and Bo Lönnerdal

Department of Nutrition
University of California
Davis, CA 95616

INTRODUCTION

Congenital malformations and developmental defects are at the present time the leading cause of infant mortality in the United States and Europe. Only about 30% of the causes of developmental defects are known, including those of genetic transmission. The biochemical mechanisms responsible for the remaining 65-70% of the developmental defects in humans are unknown (38). Several papers in this volume provide evidence of how congenital malformations may arise as a consequence of mutagenic agents in the environment.

It is our thesis that nutritional factors may also be involved in the development of these malformations. In this paper we will describe how the nutritional environment of the embryo and the fetus may dictate the occurrence of some congenital malformations. This idea will be discussed with regard to (a) simple dietary nutrient insufficiency (primary deficiency), (b) drug-induced nutrient deficiency, (c) genetic lesions which mimic nutrient deficient states, and (d) the interaction of the above factors. Although the list of nutrients that are essential to the processes of mammalian life is extensive (over 30 essential nutrients are recognized) we will focus this paper on the effects of deficiencies of the trace elements zinc, copper, and manganese on early development.

Trace Element Deficiency and Teratology

Zinc. The first report that congenital malformations could result from zinc deficiency during pregnancy was published by Hurley and Swenerton in 1966 (18). In this study, it was shown

that when a zinc deficient diet is fed to normal pregnant rats
during gestation only, about half of their embryos die before birth
and the other half are small and usually malformed. These
malformations include cleft lip and palate (42%), brain
malformations (47%), eye malformations (47%), skeletal deformations
(70%), malformations of the lung (50%) and numerous abnormalities
of the heart and urogenital system. The brain malformations
observed are especially striking with hydrocephaly, exencephaly,
and anencephaly predominating. The basic defect responsible for
the malformations observed in zinc deficiency appear to be the
result of abnormal nucleic acid synthesis. DNA synthesis is
depressed and the activities of DNA polymerase and thymidine kinase
are significantly lower in zinc deficient embryos than in control
embryos early in gestation (3-5,34). Chromosomal aberrations
including gaps, fragments, and terminal deletions are also found in
both maternal and fetal tissues in zinc deficient animals.
Maturational abnormalities in development of the lung, esophageal
tract, and pancreas are also found in cases of zinc deficiency
(12).

The devastating effects reported for zinc deficiency during
pregnancy are particularly alarming when considering the rapidity
with which zinc deficiency can occur. We have shown that in rats
plasma zinc concentration falls by 50% less than 16 hrs. after the
introduction of a zinc deficient diet (14). This rapid effect of
dietary zinc deficiency on plasma zinc has also been shown to occur
in humans, although the time period is somewhat longer, several
days rather than several hours (9). Thus, dietary zinc deficiency
is reflected in the plasma very rapidly and as maternal plasma is
the only source of zinc for the developing embryos, a zinc deficient diet can have an immediate effect on the developing
organism. Indeed, in the rat only a few days of zinc deficiency
during pregnancy is sufficient to produce congential malformations
(15). With this observation in mind, it is not surprising that
reports have appeared suggesting that inadequate maternal zinc
status may have a negative effect on the outcome of pregnancy in
humans (21).

Copper. The effects of copper deficiency during pregnancy are
quite different from those of zinc deficiency. The importance of
copper for normal prenatal development was first indicated by reports on the disease "enzootic ataxia" in sheep. This condition
occurs in the newborn and young lambs born to ewes grazing on copper deficient pastures. Afflicted lambs are ataxic and show
abnormal development of their brains marked in particular by amye-
lination and/or demyelination. This disease, once a major problem,
can be prevented by supplementation of the ewe with copper during
pregnancy (16). The teratogenicity of copper deficiency has also
been demonstrated in experimental animals. The offspring of guinea
pigs and rats fed copper deficient diets during pregnancy have

abnormalities of the central nervous system and are often born
dead. Surviving pups usually die of aneurysms. Deficient pups
have low levels of tissue copper (16). We have recently shown that
the mouse is especially sensitive to deficiency of this element
during gestation; fetuses show gross malformations, even when their
mothers have consumed a copper deficient diet for only a short
period of time (17). Copper deficiency in human infants has been
described under a variety of conditions (36), but teratogenic effects of copper deficiency during prenatal life in humans are not
documented.

The principal biochemical defects in copper deficiency which
lead to the observed abnormalities have not been agreed upon.
Three enzymes that have been implicated are: lysyl oxidase (the
enzyme responsible for cross-linking in connective tissue), copper-
zinc superoxide dismutase (the enzyme necessary for scavenging of
free radicals) and cytochrome oxidase. Reduced activities of these
enzymes are found in tissues of copper deficient animals (28).

Manganese. The essentiality of manganese in the diet of mammals was shown in 1931 by Orent and McCollum in rats (31) and by
Kemmerer et al. in mice (24). Orent and McCollum reported that
there was a high incidence of neonatal mortality in the offspring
of manganese-deficient rats; this high mortality was subsequently
shown to be due to congenital debility of the offspring (1). The
most striking effect of prenatal manganese deficiency is irreversible congenital ataxia in the offspring which is characterized by
lack of equilibrium, incoordination, and retraction of the head.
Research in our laboratory (12) has shown that these signs of manganese deficiency are caused principally by abnormal development of
the otoliths of the inner ear, the calcified structures essential
for normal vestibular function.

The principal biochemical lesion responsible for this anomaly
is probably depressed activity of the manganese-activated enzyme
glycosyl transferase. This enzyme catalyzes the addition of
hexoses to glycoproteins and mucopolysaccharides, which form the
primary matrix in which the crystalline otoconia comprising the
otoliths are embedded. In manganese-deficient animals the muco-
polysaccharide matrix is abnormal, supporting the hypothesis that
abnormal glycosylation is the biochemical lesion leading to the
ataxic condition. A similar explanation, that is, low activity of
glycosyl transferase, may be given for the observation that skeletal malformations are another important effect of manganese deficiency. Manganese deficiency during either prenatal life or the
postnatal growth period show various skeletal abnormalities characteristic of chondrodysplastic growth, suggesting that the lesion is
in the bone matrix rather than in calcification of the skeleton.
These abnormalities include disproportionate growth, with relative
shortening of the limbs in proportion to body length, curvature of

Table 1. Common Signs of Prenatal Trace Element Deficiencies

	Zinc	Copper	Manganese
Fetal death	+	+	-
Early neonatal death	+	+	+
Neurological abnormalities			
Spastic paralysis	-	+	-
Incoordination	-	+	+
Convulsive seizures	-	+	-
Abnormal brain morphology	+	+	-
Paucity of normal myelin	-	+	-
Inner ear abnormalities	?	?	+
Cardiovascular lesions			
Abnormal cardiac morphology	+	+	-
Aneurysms	-	+	-
Impaired cross-linking of elastin	?	+	-
Abnormal lung development	+	+	-
Skin and hair abnormalities	+	+	-
Multiple congenital malformations	+	-	-
Skeletal abnormalities	+	+	+
Anemia	-	+	-
Abnormal pancreatic function	+	-	+
Impaired membrane integrity	?	?	+
Chromosomal abnormalities	+	?	?
Abnormal immune function	+	+	+

the spine and of some of the long bones, and disproportionate shape of the skull (12).

The metalloenzyme manganese-superoxide dismutase (Mn-SOD), found primarily in mitochondria, also requires manganese. This enzyme catalyzes the dismutation of superoxide free radicals to hydrogen peroxide, a reaction considered critical for cell integrity. Without SOD, superoxide anions can form hydroxyl radicals, which can increase cellular peroxidation. In manganese deficient animals Mn-SOD activity is lower than normal in certain tissues (2,32). It has also been found that manganese deficiency may lead to abnormal mitochondrial membranes (19). We are investigating the hypothesis that this abnormality in membranes is due to an increased rate of membrane lipid peroxidation as a consequence of decreased Mn-SOD activity. The possible relationship between SOD activity, membrane defects, and lipid peroxidation is being studied with particular reference to its potential role in teratogenesis.

In summary, simple dietary deficiency of zinc, copper, or manganese can have severe consequences on the development of the fetus. The teratogenic expression of the deficiencies of these elements is quite different because of the different biochemical mechanisms affected by the respective deficiencies. Below, we discuss how a deficiency for the fetus can occur even when the maternal animal is taking in adequate amounts of the nutrient.

Trace Element-Gene Interactions

The importance of zinc, copper, and manganese during development can be demonstrated by genetic mutants that have errors of trace element metabolism. In general, the interaction of trace elements and genetic factors can be classified into two types. The first type involves mutant genes whose phenotypic expression is similar to the signs of deficiency or toxicity of an element, the second type involves strain differences within a species.

   Single Gene Interactions. A striking example of a genetic mutant related to trace element metabolism is acrodermatitis enteropathica, a disorder in which the phenotypic expression of the gene mimics zinc deficiency. This autosomal recessive disorder in humans is characterized by severe dermatitis, alopecia, and diarrhea. If the disease is not treated, infants with this condition usually die at an early age. All the signs of the disorder can be cured and prevented by zinc supplementation (29). Although the actual genetic defect in this disease is not known, it has been shown that there is an abnormality of zinc absorption from the intestine (20). An apparently analogous disorder has been recognized in the cow. The Adema disease of Friesian calves resembles very closely that of infants with acrodermatitis enteropathica and, similarly, all of the known effects of the mutant gene can be alleviated by feeding these animals high amounts of dietary zinc (8). It is believed that the underlying metabolic lesion in the Adema calf is malabsorption of zinc. It remains to be shown if the mechanism leading to the malabsorption is the same as in acrodermatitis enteropathica patients (25).

   A genetic disorder of copper metabolism is Menkes' disease in humans. The phenotypic expression of this disease is similar to the signs of copper deficiency. Infants with this X-linked disorder have severe neurological disturbances, abnormal hair similar to the steely wool of copper-deficient sheep, and other abnormalities that lead to death in the first years of life. Unfortunately, in contrast to acrodermatitis enteropathica, supplementation of the Menkes' patient with dietary copper has not been found to alleviate the phenotypic expression of the gene (28). It is important to note, however, that only postnatal supplementation has been investigated thus far. It is possible that copper supplementation during the prenatal period may be useful, but this remains to be determined.

An animal which may be useful to study Menkes' disease is the mottled mouse, which also has an X-linked disorder of copper metabolism. Studies in the mottled mouse have shown that part of the abnormality involves abnormal transport and/or sequestering of copper in some tissues leading to a copper deficiency in others. Like Menkes' patients, mottled mice die if untreated; however, in contrast to the Menkes' patient, injections of copper have been found to be beneficial for prolonging life (26). Two other mutations occurring in mice which are characterized in part by producing abnormal copper status are the autosomal recessive genes crinkled (cr) and quaking (qk). However, it should be noted that the strain in which these mutant genes are found can influence the degree to which copper metabolism is affected (17,33). (The effects of strain differences on trace element metabolism will be discussed below).

Finally, genes have been identified which affect manganese metabolism. The pallid mouse shows ataxia, head retraction, and abnormal development of the otoliths indistinguishable from those observed in the offspring of manganese deficient animals. If pregnant mice heterozygous for the gene pallid are given a diet containing large amounts of manganese, about 50 times normal, their mutant offspring show normal development of the otoliths and do not have ataxia (6). A gene analogous to pallid (screwneck) has been identified in mink, with abnormal or missing otoliths in the inner ear and severe ataxia. As with pallid, the effects of screwneck in mink can be prevented by giving manganese at high levels in the maternal diet during pregnancy (7).

In summary, pallid and screwneck are excellent examples of genetic lesions which mimic the effects of a nutrient deficiency, and whose phenotypic expression can be totally prevented by dietary intervention during critical phases of development. This observation, coupled with the finding that the previously lethal disorder acrodermatitis enteropathica in humans can be treated by zinc (although the treatment has to be continued throughout life) provides hope that some genetic disorders in man and animals may be controllable by dietary intervention.

Strain Variations. The second type of interaction between trace elements and genetic factors concerns strain differences. An important example of such an interaction is demonstrated by the work of Wiener and associates (37), who have investigated the relationship of the breed of sheep to their incidence of enzootic ataxia. These investigators found that the frequency of enzootic ataxia is quite different among breeds even when they are consuming the same forage, and the difference is due to differences in their absorption of copper. Thus, there is a strong influence of breed (genetic strain) on liver copper and plasma copper levels. Convincing evidence that differences in occurrence of enzootic ataxia are due to differences in maternal copper absorption and resulting copper status have come from embryo transfer studies. Wiener and his associates have shown that the maternal genotype and not the fetal genotype dictates the fetal tissue copper levels of the fetus.

A second example of strain influence on trace element requirements or metabolism is from our work on manganese deficiency. When pregnant mice of several different strains were fed diets containing either a normal (45 ppm) or a low amount of manganese (3 ppm), the effects on otolith development of their fetuses were quite different depending on their genetic background. All of the strains showed normal otolith development when fed the normal level of manganese. However, with the low manganese diet, some of the strains showed 30% of normal otolith development in their fetuses, while the others showed only 5% of normal otolith development (13). Thus, the two examples above show that the response to a deficiency of an element may be dependent on the strain background of the animal. It must be emphasized that none of these strains are regarded as "mutants" under normal circumstances. Similar examples could be cited for susceptibility to toxicity of various elements.

Trace Element-Drug Interactions

We have previously considered how the genetic background of an animal may affect its response to its trace element environment. Another factor which may influence an animal's trace element requirement is the presence of drugs or other chemicals which can interact with an element either as a primary or secondary consequence of the drug's action. For example, we have studied the interaction of zinc with the diuretic acetazolamide. The major pharmacological action of acetazolamide is the inhibition of carbonic anhydrase. This action is thought to be due to the sulfonamide moiety of the drug binding to the zinc ion at the active site of the enzyme (30). Acetazolamide is a potent teratogen with the principal abnormality being postaxial forelimb ectrodactyly. In addition, ocular defects, exencephaly, and bone defects are found (35). Because of the similarity of acetazolamide and zinc deficiency teratogenicity, we investigated the effects of zinc nutrition on acetazolamide teratogenicity. The level of zinc in the maternal diet was shown to have a pronounced effect on the frequency of ectrodactyly in rat fetuses from mothers fed acetazolamide. With no zinc (<0.5 µg/g) in the maternal diet during pregnancy, 100% of the fetuses alive at term showed this malformation. Increasing dietary zinc up to 100 µg/g reduced the incidence of the acetazolamide syndrome in a dose-response manner (10). The mechanisms of this effect are under investigation.

The above example shows the interaction of a drug with dietary zinc. Examples of drugs interacting with other trace elements are also known. We have been studying the teratogenicity of D-penicillamine (DP) in rats with regard to its effect on copper metabolism. D-penicillamine is a drug used in the treatment of several disorders including Wilson's disease, cystinuria, and rheumatoid arthritis. This drug is an effective chelating agent of copper and is known for its property of increasing the excretion of copper from the body. When D-penicillamine was given to rats during pregnancy in three different amounts, the frequency of resorption (embryonic and fetal death) was slightly but significantly higher than in control rats without the drug. More striking, the frequency of malformations was greatly increased in the rats receiving this drug. Thus, at the two higher levels of drug, 30% and 65% of the fetuses alive at term showed malformations. D-penicillamine also produced low concentrations of copper in the maternal plasma and liver and similar effects in the fetal tissues. Thus the teratogenicity of penicillamine may be related to the copper deficiency produced by the drug (23,27).

In summary, while under normal circumstances the trace element content of a maternal diet may be adequate, the presence of drugs such as acetazolamide and D-penicillamine may result in an increased requirement of the elements such that conditioned deficiency with resulting teratogenicity can occur.

Interactional Effects

Finally, trace elements can interact with drugs and with genetic factors in a multifactorial way. An example of this kind of multifactorial interaction is a study in which we used two strains of rats, Sprague-Dawley and Wistar, and investigated the teratogenic effects of salicylate in relation to the level of dietary zinc. This drug was investigated because its teratogenic expression is similar to that of zinc deficiency and its structure suggests a capacity to bind this element. Four different levels of salicylate were used and three different levels of dietary zinc were fed. Using a multivariant statistical analysis, we were able to show that the frequency of malformations was influenced by the level of dietary zinc, by the amount of salicylate given, by the interaction of the genetic strain and the zinc dietary level, and the interaction of the dietary zinc concentration and salicylate given (11).

Thus, the outcome of fetal development depends not only on the genetic background, dietary environment, and drugs given, but also on the interactions between diet and drugs, the interactions between genetic factors and drugs, and the interactions between the genetic factors and diet, as well as multifactorial interactions involving all of these different factors.

CONCLUDING REMARKS

Questions relating to the effects of potentially toxic substances on various populations, including man, may be approached from several directions. These substances are usually tested by toxicity studies and risk assessment in homogenous populations which are otherwise adequate to optimal in health status. We have addressed the issue of deleterious effects of toxic substances from a different viewpoint. Specifically, we emphasize the point that the effects of toxic materials depend not only on the characteristics of the materials themselves but also on the characteristics of the exposed subjects, including their nutritional status. Thus, deleterious toxic effects may result from an interaction between toxic chemicals, nutritional factors, and genetic factors. The interaction of these factors may be particularly important during pregnancy if the product of the interaction is severe enough to interfere with normal reproduction and development. It may be that interactions of such types, with resulting impairment of development, may be a significant risk factor in determining the number and severity of congenital abnormalities occurring in man and animals.

REFERENCES

1. Daniels, A.L., and G. J. Everson. The relation of manganese to congenital debility. J. Nutr. 9: 191-203.
2. deRosa, G., C.L. Keen, R.M. Leach, and L.S. Hurley. Regulation of superoxide dismutase activity by dietary manganese. J. Nutr. 110: 795-804, 1980.
3. Dreosti, I.E., P.E. Grey, and P.J. Wilkins. Deoxyribonucleic acid synthesis, protein synthesis and teratogenesis in zinc-deficient rats. S. Afr. Med. J. 46: 1585-1588, 1972.
4. Duncan, J.R., and L.S. Hurley. Thymidine kinase and DNA polymerase activity in normal and zinc deficient developing rat embryos. Proc. Soc. Exp. Biol. Med. 159: 39-43, 1978.
5. Eckhert, C.D., and L.S. Hurley. Reduced DNA synthesis in zinc deficiency: regional differences in embryonic rats. J. Nutr. 107: 855-861, 1977.
6. Erway, L., L.S. Hurley, and A. Fraser. Neurological defect: manganese in phenocopy and prevention of a genetic abnormality of inner ear. Science 152: 1766-1768, 1966.
7. Erway, L.C., and S.E. Mitchell. Prevention of otolith defect in pastel mink by manganese supplementation. J. Hered. 64: 111-119, 1973.
8. Flagstad, T. Intestinal absorption of ^{65}Zn in A46 (Adema disease) after treatment with oxychinolines. Nord. Vet. Med. 29: 96-104, 1977.
9. Gordon, P.R., C.W. Woodruff, H.L. Anderson, and B.L. O'Dell. Acute zinc deficiency in man impairs platelet aggregation. Fed. Proc. 40: 839, 1981.

10. Hackman, R.M., and L.S. Hurley. The effect of dietary zinc
     and genetic interaction on acetazolamide teratogenesis in
     mice. Teratology 23: 39–40A, 1981.
11. Hackman, R.M., and L.S. Hurley. The influence of dietary zinc
     and genetic strain on salicylate teratogenesis in rats. Tera-
     tology 23: 40A, 1981.
12. Hurley, L.S. Teratogenic aspects of manganese, zinc and
     copper nutrition. Physiol. Rev. 61: 249–295, 1981.
13. Hurley, L.S., and L.T. Bell. Genetic influence on response to
     dietary manganese deficiency. J. Nutr. 104: 133–137, 1974.
14. Hurley, L.S., P. Gordon, C.L. Keen, and L. Merkhofer. Cir-
     cadian variation in rat plasma zinc and rapid effect of
     dietary zinc deficiency. Fed. Proc. 39: 431, 1980.
15. Hurley, L.S., J. Gowan, and H. Swenerton. Teratogenic effects
     of short-term and transitory zinc deficiency in rats. Tera-
     tology 4: 199–204, 1971.
16. Hurley, L.S., and C.L. Keen. Teratogenic effects of copper.
     In: Copper in the Environment, Part II. Health Effects,
     edited by J. Nriagu. New York: Wiley, p. 33–36, 1979.
17. Hurley, L.S., C.L. Keen, and B Lönnerdal. Copper in foetal
     and neonatal development. In: Ciba Found. Symp. The
     Biological Roles of Copper. London: Excerpta Med. Found., p.
     227–245. 1980.
18. Hurley, L.S., and H. Swenerton. Congenital malformations
     resulting from zinc deficiency in rats. Proc. Soc. Exp. Biol.
     Med. 123: 692–697, 1966.
19. Hurley, L.S., L. Theriault, and I.E. Dreosti. Liver mito-
     chondria from manganese-deficient and pallid mice: function
     and ultrastructure. Science 170: 1316–1318, 1970.
20. Jackson, M.J. Zinc and di-iodohydroxyquinoline therapy in
     acrodermatitis enteropathica. J. Clin. Pathol. 30: 284–287,
     1977.
21. Jameson, S. Effects of zinc deficiency in human
     reproduction. Acta Med. Scand. Suppl. 593, 1976.
22. Keen, C.L., B. Lönnerdal, and L.S. Hurley. Abnormal copper
     status resulting from D-penicillamine administered during
     pregnancy. Teratology 23: 44A, 1981.
23. Keen, C. L., P. Mark-Savage, B. Lönnerdal, and L. S. Hurley.
     Abnormal copper status resulting from D-penicillamine admi-
     nistered during pregnancy. Teratology 23: 44A, 1981.
24. Kemmerer, A. R., C. A. Elvehjem, and E. B. Hart. Studies on
     the relation of manganese to the nutrition of the mouse. J.
     Biol. Chem. 92: 623–630, 1931.
25. Lönnerdal, B., C. L. Keen, and L. S. Hurley. Zinc binding
     ligands and complexes in zinc metabolism. In: Advances in
     Nutrition Research, edited by H. Draper. Vol. 5, Plenum
     Press. In press.
26. Mann, J. R., J. Camakaris, D. M. Danks, and E. M. Walliczek.
     Copper metabolism in mottled mouse mutants. Copper therapy of
     brindled (Mo^{br}) mice. Biochem. J. 180: 605–612, 1979.

27. Mark-Savage, P., C. L. Keen, B. Lönnerdal, and L. S. Hurley.
     Teratogenicity of D-penicillamine in rats. Teratology 23:
     50A, 1981.
28. Mason, K. E., A conspectus of research on copper metabolism
     and requirements of man. J. Nutr. 109: 1979-2066, 1979.
29. Moynahan, E. J., Acrodermatitis enteropathica: a lethal
     inherited human zinc-deficiency disorder. Lancet 2: 399-400,
     1974.
30. Mudge, G. H., Diuretics and other agents employed in the mobi-
     lization of edema. In: The Pharmacological Basis of
     Therapeutics, Sixth Ed., edited by A. G. Goodman, L. S.
     Goodman and A. Gilman. New York: Macmillan, pp. 892-915.
31. Orent, E. R. and E. V. McCollum. Effects of deprivation of
     manganese in the rat. J. Biol. Chem. 92: 651, 1931.
32. Paynter, D. J., Changes in activity of the manganese
     superoxide dismutase enzyme in tissues of the rat with changes
     in dietary manganese. J. Nutr. 110: 437-447, 1980.
33. Prohaska, J. R., Normal copper metabolism in quaking mice.
     Life. Sci. 26: 731-735, 1980.
34. Swenerton, H., R. Shrader, and L. S. Hurley. Zinc-deficient
     embryos: reduced thymidine incorporation. Science 166: 1014-
     1015, 1969.
35. Tellone, C. I., J. K. Baldwin and R. O. Sofia. Teratogenic
     activity in the mouse after oral administration of acetazol-
     amide. Drug Chem. Toxicol. 3: 83-98, 1980.
36. Walravens, P. A., Nutritional importance of copper and zinc in
     neonates and infants. Clin. Chem. 26: 185-189, 1980.
37. Wiener, G., Review of genetic aspects of mineral metabolism
     with particular reference to copper in sheep. Livestock Pro-
     duction Science 6: 223-232, 1979.
38. Wilson, J. G., Environmental effects on developmental terato-
     logy. In: Pathophysiology of Gestation, edited by N. S.
     Assali. Vol. 2, New York; Academic Press, pp. 269-320.

DISCUSSION

SHARMA: I don't have a question, but would like to add a
comment. We are further developing and standardizing an assay
to detect sister chromatid exchanges in mouse fetuses for
studying transplacental genetic damages and examining its
feasibility for routine testing of teratogens. Since this
assay is more sensitive than the chromosomal aberrations test,
it may provide a model system to study the teratogenic effects
of some of the factors discussed in this presentation.

PESTICIDES AS ENVIRONMENTAL MUTAGENS

Donald G. Crosby

Department of Environmental Toxicology
University of California
Davis, California 95616

CALIFORNIA PESTICIDES

The terms "pesticide" and "mutagen" seem continually to be
linked in the public mind. According to news accounts, almost
every pest-control chemical is a "potential mutagen" or "potential
carcinogen." In this chapter, I would like to explore the validity
of this assumption and present an environmental view which modifies
but does not entirely overcome it.

Pesticides are chemical substances used to control any type of
unwanted organisms (Table 1). Consequently, the term includes a
wide variety of chemicals applied in agriculture, public health and
safety, industry, recreation, homes, and many other places. In
California, about 1,000 different substances are classed and used
as pesticides; I will present only the 26 principal organic pesticides as examples (Table 2), with a somewhat longer list provided
for reference at the end (Table 10). Table 2 does not include the
many inorganic substances and petroleum products which also receive
major pesticide use.

The Table provides a reflection of some major pest-control
needs in California and perhaps some surprises. For example, nematodes and mites obviously present unusually severe problems, and
three of the twelve top-volume chemicals (DD-Telone, methyl
bromide, and EDB) are soil fumigants. Such unexpected names as
nitrofen, propargite and molinate are high on the list, and few of
the top 20, I suspect, are familiar to most scientists. The
principal uses likewise may be unexpected by many: DD and Telone
are applied most extensively in the production of sugar beets, to-
matoes, grapes; maneb receives its principal use on head lettuce;

Table 1. Major Pest Control Applications

Insects	Insecticide
Weeds	Herbicide
Fungi	Fungicide
Nematodes	Nematicide
Mites	Acaricide
Leaves	Defoliant
Bacteria	Bactericide
Rodents	Rodenticide
Snails	Molluscicide
Algae	Algicide
Plant growth	Plant Growth Regulator

nitrofen is applied primarily to broccoli and several other vegetable crops; and molinate goes almost entirely onto flooded rice
fields (1). The total use of pesticides in California agriculture
in 1980--even excluding most industrial and home uses--amounted to
over 120 million pounds (1).

Table 2. Organic Pesticides Used in California, 1980 (1)

Rank	Names	Use	Volume (1,000 lbs)
1*	Dichloropropene (DD/Telone)	Nemat	14,195
2*	Methyl bromide	Nemat,Ins	6,065
3*	Maneb	Fung	2,189
4*	Nitrofen	Herb	2,102
5	Propargite (Omite)	Acar	1,798
6	Methomyl (Lannate)	Ins,Acar	1,669
7	Molinate (Ordram)	Herb	1,637
8*	Chloropicrin	Nemat,Fung	1,444
9*	CDEC (Sulfallate)	Herb	1,346
10	DCPA (Dacthal)	Herb	1,304
11	Methamidophos (Monitor)	Ins	1,009
12*	Ethylene dibromide (EDB)	Nemat,Ins.	886
13*	Carbaryl (Sevin)	Ins	830
14	Chlorthalonil (Daconil)	Fung	813
15*	Parathion	Ins	806
16*	Captan	Fung	790
17	DEF	Defol	745
18*	Dinoseb (DNBP)	Herb	705
19*	Dimethoate (Cygon)	Ins	666
20	Dichloran (Botran)	Fung	663
21*	Acephate (Orthene)	Ins	610
22	MCPA dimethylamine salt	Herb	600
23	Oxydemeton methyl (Metasystox)	Ins	563
24	2,4-D dimethylamine salt	Herb	532
25	Dicofol (Kelthane)	Acar	522
*	PCP (Pentachlorophenol)	Herb,Fung,Ins	>500[a]

*Mutagenic in at least one assay.

[a]Estimated. Total use not covered by Ref. 1.

MUTAGENIC PESTICIDES

All of the pesticides listed in Table 2, and many others, have been tested for mutagenicity in at least one type of organism, and the results are reported in the literature. All together, a wide variety of tests have been used, often with conflicting results in the same test by different investigators. Tests include biochemical reversion in bacterial mutants (S. typhimurium or E. coli), sensitivity (toxicity) in bacteria (B. subtilis or E. coli), S. cerevisiae mitotic recombination, and unscheduled DNA repair systhesis (UDS) in human fibroblasts. Typical results for a broad cross-section of pesticide types--including most of the examples of Table 2--are presented in References 2-9. However, concentrations greater than 1,000 mg/l (1,000 ppm) often have been required to give clearly positive results.

For example, Simmons showed that 18 out of 39 common pesticides gave a positive response in at least one of a battery of 6 tests (2,3), and Shirasu's group found 9 out of 166 pesticides to produce bacterial revertants (4,5). (Recently, the figure reached 50 out of 228 (6).) Waters' chapter in this volume presents an up-to-date summary (7). If we include as mutagenic any pesticide which has provided a postive response in at least one standard test and is published in an authoritative report, 14 of the 26 compounds listed in Table 2 must be considered mutagenic (indicated by an asterisk). Only captan (number 16) gave almost uniformly postive results, most of the others being positive in only a single test. It should be noted that a number of the "pesticides" frequently cited as mutagenic (10,11)--hemel, hempa, and apholate, for example--actually have never been registered nor used in practice because of their genotoxicity.

Chemical reactivity offers a rationale for this high incidence of mutagenicity. Electrophilic (electron-seeking) reactivity has emerged as an important chemical characteristic common to many mutagens (12,13), including those with such functional groups as epoxide, hydroxylamine, phosphate, sulfate, reactive halide, and diazo (Table 3). Six of the pesticides listed in Table II contain such a group (Table 4). Alternatively, 6 of them also contain functional groups which can be toxicologically activated (by liver homogenates, for example) to provide mutagenic structures--they are promutagens (Table 5). It is predictable that many pesticides will be mutagenic in laboratory tests; interestingly, others elicit no response at all.

A large proportion of the organophosphorus insecticides, halo-alkane nematicides, and fungicides tested produced postive responses. Many of these can alkylate NH, SH, and OH groups, and several of the type have been shown to react with the 7-hydroxyl group of guanine. Penetration and reaction are simple when cells

Table 3. Some Genotoxic (Electrophilic) Groups

Group	Electrophile	Example
Cl-C=C	Cl-C$\overset{O}{\diagup}$C	Vinyl Chloride
ArNO$_2$	ArN-OH	4-Nitrobiphenyl
R'OCONHR	CON-OH	Ethyl Carbamate
(RO)$_3$PO	OPO-R	Trimethyl phosphate
(RO)$_2$SO$_2$	OSO-R	Dimethyl sulfate
R-Cl	X-R	Nitrogen Mustard
R$_2$NNO	N$_2$-R	Dimethylnitrosamine

are immersed in a medium containing relatively high concentrations
-- up to seven percent -- of the candidate chemical.

PESTICIDES IN THE ENVIRONMENT

The application of pesticides in the field involves conditions
greatly different from those pertaining in the laboratory tests.
For one thing, pesticides seldom are applied neat (except for
ultralow-volume use) but rather are formulated with presumably
inert diluents, wetting agents, adhesives, and other adjuvants.
These concentrates are again diluted by suspension in water, and
the dispersion is sprayed (or distributed on granules) by aircraft
or ground rig; fumigants are injected directly into the soil.
Typical application rates for many pesticides lie in the 1-2 kg/ha
range, although fumigants usually are applied in much larger
amounts because of their rapid dissipation and dilution.

The organophosphorus insecticide parathion (I) is weakly active in unscheduled DNA repair synthesis in cell cultures at 0.3
ppm in the medium; let us consider what happens in the practical
application of this compound to a peach orchard. An aerial spray
of one pound active ingredient per acre (1.12 kg/ha) in the form of
an emulsion in 400 gal (1600 l) of water corresponds to deposition
of about 15 µg/cm^2 on a flat surface (Fig. 1, A)(14). However, the

Table 4. Mutagenic Pesticide Structures

Rank	Pesticide	Electrophile
1*	Dichloropropene	Cl-CH$_2$C=C
2*	Methyl bromide	Br-R
4*	Nitrofen	ArO-R
12*	Ethylene dibromide	Br-R
21*	Acephate	OPO-R

Table 5. Promutagen Pesticide Structures

Rank	Pesticide	Type	Mutagen
1*	Dichloropropene	Cl–C=C	Cl–C$\overset{O}{-}$C
4*	Nitrofen	$ArNO_2$	ArNHOH
9*	CDEC	Cl–C=C	Cl–C$\overset{O}{-}$C
13*	Carbaryl	CO–NH	CO–N–OH
		C=C	C$\overset{O}{-}$C
15*	Parathion	SPO–R	OPO–R
16*	Captan	$SCCl_3$	$CSCl_2$

peach leaves actually received only a small portion of this amount, about 0.15 µg/cm^2 (18 ppm) immediately after spraying. At this time, the fruit was quite small, with a surface area of only a few cm^2. During the week following treatment, the parathion residue declined to below 0.01 µg/cm^2 (1.0 ppm), or less than 1/1000 of the calculated application rate (Fig. 1); the law prohibits workers from entering the orchard or picking fruit within at least 14 days, and by that time, the parathion residue was down to less than 0.5 ppm. Small wonder that 250 composites of grocery food taken throughout the United States by the Food and Drug Administration (FDA) (15) typically showed only 6 which contained measurable para- thion and those in a range of only 2-13 parts per billion (ng/g) (Table 6).

Where did the rest go? It did not "disappear". It was sub- jected to dissipative forces including bulk movement as spray drift, volatilization from surfaces, adsorption onto soil, and dissolution in water. Indeed, air sampling during and immediately

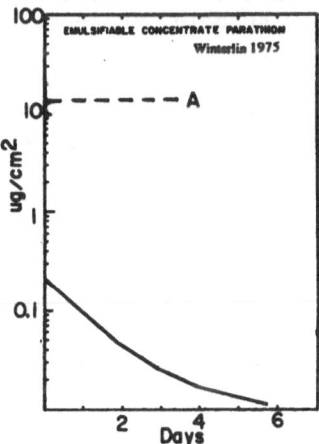

Fig. 1. Dissipation of Parathion from Peach Leaves. Application rate (A) was 1.12 kg/ha.

Table 6. Food Residues of Major Pesticides[a]

Rank	Pesticide	Positive[b]	Residue ppm
3*	Maneb	0	>0.01
10	DCPA	1	0.003
13*	Carbaryl	2	0.07
15*	Parathion	6	0.002-0.013
20	Dichloran	5	0.001-0.016
22	MCPA	0	>0.01

[a]Ref. 15.
[b]Out of 240 Composite Samples.

after application showed the presence of parathion as particles and vapor in the atmosphere within and adjacent to the treated orchard (16, 17) and in the top few millimeters of soil (18). However, as on the leaves, the parathion fell away rapidly (17, 18) except where it was difficult for the dissipative forces to be effective -- in well-water, for example.

Pesticide residues are subjected from the beginning to chemical reactions with environmental reagents. The principal reactions in the environment include oxidation, reduction, and nucleophilic displacements (Table 7) by natural NH, SH or OH groups and often can be shown to generate mutagenic intermediates. The initial reactions are nonbiological (19) and are followed by similar biochemical metabolism in plants, micro-organisms, and animals. (An especially interesting observation is the formation of N-nitroso compounds from amines and amides in the presence of dissolved nitrite or atmospheric nitrogen oxides (20)). The parathion of our example was rapidly oxidized in the atmosphere or on soil or leaf surfaces to give the corresponding phosphate ester, paraoxon (II) (17,18). It also was reduced in soil to aminoparathion (III), isomerized to S-ethylparathion (IV), and hydrolyzed via paraoxon to p-nitrophenol (V) (21). Although all of these products possess mutagenic or promutagenic structures, they actually proved to be only transient intermediates in the eventual conversion of parathion to environmentally unreactive (largely inorganic) end-products (22).

The situation is similar with DD-Telone (1,3-dichloropropene isomers VI), a soil-dispersed fumigant nematicide (Fig. 3). In treated soil, both cis- and trans-dichloropropene, as reactive allylic halides, were rapidly hydrolyzed to chloroallyl alcohol (VII) and then oxidized to chloroacrylic acid (VIII) and, eventually, to carbon dioxide and chloride ion (23, 24). Any which escaped to the atmosphere would be oxidized to the unstable epoxide (IX) which rearranges to chloropropionyl chloride (X) and goes on

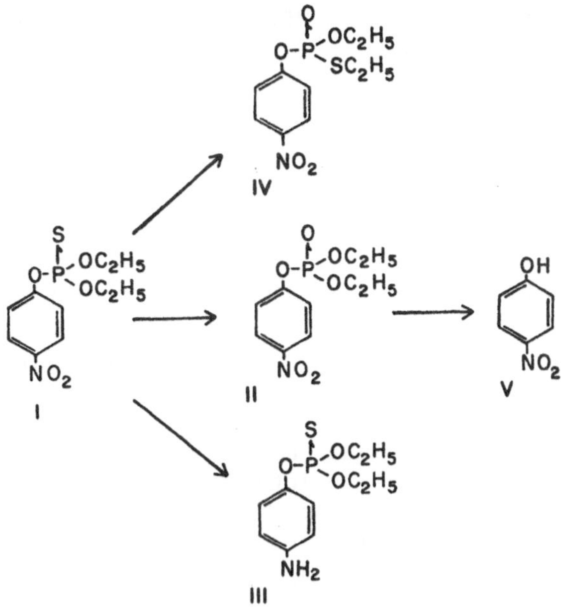

Fig. 2. Environmental Degradation Reactions of Parathion.

to the corresponding acid (XI) and then to the inorganic state
(25). Again, the intermediates have mutagen or promutagen
structures but are both short-lived and highly dilute.

Pentachlorophenol (PCP, XII) is an example of a true biocide,
a substance toxic to all forms of life. It is used primarily in
treatment of wood and other products against fungi and insects.
Although it can be dispersed widely in the environment (26), its
uses and properties make it especially likely to occur in water.
However, it, too, was rapidly degraded by both sunlight and soil
micro-organisms (Fig. 4) through a complex series of transient

Table 7. Environmental Generation of Mutagens

Reaction	Example (Rank)	Mutagen
Oxidation	Dichloropropene (1*)	$Cl-C\overset{O}{\frown}C$
	Propargite (5)	R_2SO_4
	Carbaryl (13*)	CON-OH
	Parathion (15*)	OPO-R
Reduction	Nitrofen (4*)	ArN-OH
Nucleo-philic	Captan (16*)	$CSCl_2$
	Carbaryl (13*)	$CON(NO)CH_3$

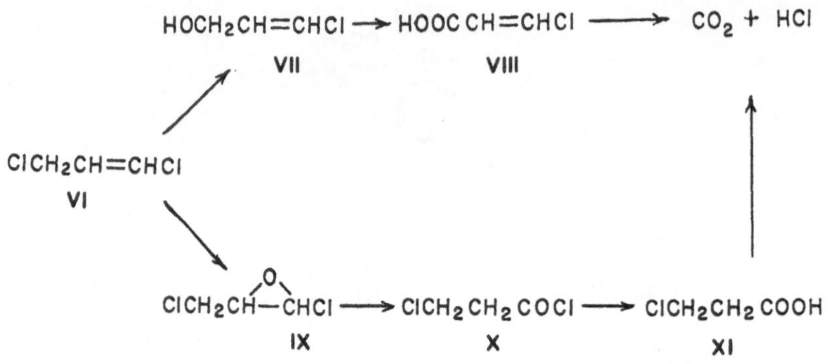

$$HOCH_2CH=CHCl \rightarrow HOOC\,CH=CHCl \longrightarrow CO_2 + HCl$$

VII   VIII

$$ClCH_2CH=CHCl$$

VI

$$ClCH_2\overset{O}{\overset{|}{CH}}-CHCl \longrightarrow ClCH_2CH_2COCl \longrightarrow ClCH_2CH_2COOH$$

IX   X   XI

Fig. 3. Environmental Degradation Reactions of Dichloropropenes.

intermediates to carbon dioxide and chloride (27). At no time would the level of any of these intermediates seem to present a meaningful exposure to humans; on the other hand, the absence of light and microbes led to detection of PCP, itself, in well-water (27).

If PCP is so unstable in the environment, why should it be of genotoxic concern? The mutagenic effect in microbial tests may be attributed to the presence of more stable dibenzo-p-dioxins, diben-zofurans, and hexachlorobenzene (HCB) as manufacturing by-products

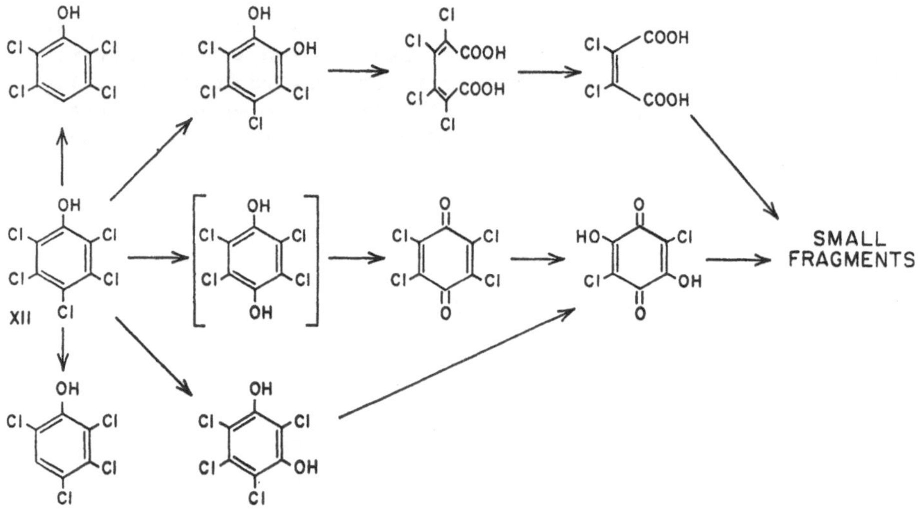

Fig. 4. Environmental Degradation Reactions of Pentachlorophenol (PCP).

in the technical pesticide (26). Mutagenic impurities now are
recognized to occur at significant levels in several pesticides
(Table 8) — up to several percent in the case of carbon tetrachloride in dichloropropenes and HCB in DCPA and PCP. Dialkylni-
trosamines have been found at levels of many ppm in certain pesticides; for example, dimethylnitrosamine (DMN) accompanies the amine
in dimethylamine salts of MCPA and 2,4-D, and dipropylnitrosamine
occurs in trifluralin formulations. Ethylenethiourea (2-imidazoli-
dinethione, ETU) is found in many dithiocarbamate fungicides and
also can be generated under food processing conditions (28).

Fortunately, most of these impurities also are subject to
facile environmental degradation. For example, the highly volatile
dipropylnitrosamine escapes to the atmosphere where it is oxidized
to dipropylnitramine and then on to other products (Fig. 5)(29),
while ETU tends to move into water where it is degraded quickly to
nontoxic ethyleneurea and glycine (30). The lower chlorodioxins,
such as the toxic 2,3,7,8-tetrachlorodibenzo-p-dioxin (TCDD), are
degraded to harmless products by light (31), but the more highly
chlorinated homologs are more stable. HCB is remarkably stable in
the environment (32).

EXPOSURE

While such exceptions exist, and the dissipation process does
take place over time, the general picture which emerges most often
is one of continual dispersion, degradation, and dilution. The
central question then seems to be not so much whether a pesticide
is mutagenic in a given test, but whether a particular organism of
interest — such as man — receives sufficient exposure to allow
the substance to survive environmental dissipation, absorption,
transport, and detoxication and reach the target cell. In recent
years, rather extensive field research has been conducted on farm-
worker exposure; parathion, for example, is toxicologically "safe"
for re-entry contact within 14 days of application according to
analysis and the fairly sensitive blood cholinesterase assay
(33). That does not mean that there will be zero exposure, and if

Table 8.   Genotoxic Impurities in Pesticides

Rank	Pesiticide	Impurity[a]
1	Dichloropropene	CCl_4
3	Maneb	ETU
10	DCPA	HCB
22	MCPA, 2,4-D	DMN
	PCP	Dioxins, HCB

[a]See text for explanation of abbreviations.

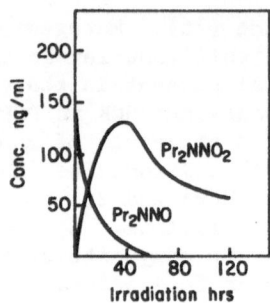

Fig. 5.   Degradation of Dipropylnitrosamine (Pr$_2$NNO) and Its
          Photoproduct Dipropylnitramine (Pr$_2$NNO$_2$) under Simulated
          Atmospheric Conditions (29).

one subscribes to the "one-hit" theory, which relates mutation to
reaction by a single mutagen molecule, only total cessation of
pesticide application would assure safety.

        In relation to that theory, however, let me refer to the her-
bicide, 2,4-D.   2,4-D is weakly positive at high levels in the E.
coli and B. subtilis mutagen toxicity tests and several others
(3,34) but not in reversion, UDS, or mouse dominant-lethal
assays.   Despite its lack of mutagenicity or teratogenicity in
intact mammals (34,35) and the very low probability of human exposure (34), human miscarriages and birth defects have been popularly
attributed to 2,4-D.   We now believe that we have linked the defect
instead to maternal consumption of milk containing alkaloids from
toxic range plants (36).   Considering that such powerful genotoxic
substances are present naturally in our everyday diet and environment (37,38), emphasis on a possible trace of a marginally
mutagenic pesticide seems rather incongruous.

CONCLUSION

        Even this brief consideration of pesticides as environmental
mutagens leads to several important conclusions:

    1.   Pesticides represent a very large (and still growing)
         input of chemicals into our environment, especially when
         their formulation ingredients and impurities are included.
    2.   Pesticides are reactive--primarily electrophilic--and
         they often form even more reactive electrophiles as
         intermediate products during environmental or metabolic
         degradation.

3. As electrophiles, many pesticides are predictable mutagens
    or promutagens in laboratory tests; in fact, a case could
    be made for expected mutagenicity or promutagenicity in
    <u>all</u> the technical-grade pesticides listed in Table 2, and
    the fact that half of them produce negative laboratory
    results is suprising.
4. Also due to their electrophilic properties, these pesti-
    cides generally do not persist in the environment, and
    their degradation products most often are short-lived and
    transient.
5. Exposure of the general public to agricultural pesticides
    via food, air, or water is very low or non-existent, and
    even then the processes of absorption, transport, and
    detoxication counteract genotoxicity.

This is not to say that present regulations cannot be improved
or that genotoxic potential should be considered insignificant in
evaluation of the environmental impact of pesticides. Rather, the
preceding discussion should underscore a number of the following
major research needs.

It may prove difficult to make a case for significant genotoxic exposure of the general public to agricultural pesticides.
In fact, even farmers often turn large-scale pesticide applications
over to a smaller group of licensed pest-control applicators;
where they do not, they themselves are required by law to undergo
training and licensing. However, workers who mix and load aircraft
and sprayers may not be adequately protected, and many employees of
formulation plants and disposal facilities surely have above-normal
exposure. In particular, the easy availability of pesticides to
home gardeners through nurseries, hardware stores, and even grocery
stores (Table 9) presents a source of largely uncontrolled
pesticide exposure — as much as 20% of total pesticide use in
California is through the home market. Surely, these populations
provide a preferred object of epidemiological investigation —
effects in such high-risk cohorts could provide leads for wider
evaluation, while negative genotoxic results would suggest safety
for the general public.

Perhaps not surprisingly, there seems as yet to be no verified
connection between pesticides applied in agriculture and incidents
of human or animal genotoxicity in practical, everyday life, despite extensive investigation by the EPA and other agencies for
over a decade. Several regulatory agencies already require or plan
to require data from a battery of genotoxicity tests before registration of new pesticide products, and the EPA's RPAR (Rebuttable
Presumption Against Registration) process includes genotoxicity (in
laboratory tests) as a trigger for re-evaluation of existing pesticides. Risks due to pesticide exposure must continually be placed
in a context of competing risks including accident, disease, and

Table 9.   Pesticides for Home Use[a]

Rank	Names[b]	% AI[c]	Use
3*	Maneb	80	Fung
10	DCPA (Dacthal)	5,5	Herb
13*	Carbaryl (Sevin)	27,10,10,	Ins
	"	50,4	Moll
14	Chlorthalonil (Daconil)	30,9	Fung
16*	Captan	25,14,5	Fung
19*	Dimethoate (Cygon)	23	Ins
21*	Acephate (Orthene)	16	Ins
22	MCPA, DMA salt	12,11	Herb
23	Oxydemeton methyl (Metasystox)	7,5[d]	Ins, Acar
24	2,4-D, DMA salt	12,10,3	Herb
25	Dicofol (Kelthane)	2,1,0.05[d]	Acar
*	PCP (Pentachlorophenol)	4.4[d]	Ins, Fung
	"	2.25,0.7	Herb

[a]Survey of a single store in Davis, Calif., November, 1981.

[b]Other mutagenic (*) home pesticides found in the survey:
allethrin, benomyl, binapacryl, bromacil, cacodylic acid,
dicamba, dichlorvos, folpet, simazine, thiram, zineb.

[c]AI=active ingredient.   Different brands listed separately.

[d]For indoor use.

the natural genotoxic background presented especially by food,
water, and the atmosphere.   However, the genotoxic effect of pesticides in combination with other natural and man-made substances
with which they are associated in food and the environment remains
largely unexplored.

Despite the large application volumes of some of the major
pesticides, there is as yet no instance of a complete accounting of
the environmental distribution and fate for any of them.   Although
the exposure to residues of the originally-applied pesticides
usually become demonstrably low within a short time, the genotoxic
significance of actual "weathered" (terminal) residues has not been
reported.   This especially includes environmentally more stable
impurities such as HCB and the higher chlorinated dioxins.

There is obvious need by regulatory agencies, the pesticide
industry, and agriculture for an agreed-upon battery of reliable
genotoxicity screening tests as an early-warning indicator for
further research and evaluation (certainly not as a regulatory tool
itself).   These tests must be sure to consider the physical and
chemical properties of each candidate pesticide, especially volati-
lity and hydrolysis which may cause loss of test compound during
the assay and (low) solubility which may present a very unrealistic
reservoir of excess test compound.   At present, apparently only 7
of California's top 25 pesticides have undergone such a coordinated

Table 10.   Top 100 Pesticides by Total Lbs. Applied in 1980 in the
State of California (1)

Rank	Total Lbs.	Acres	
1	26,823,616	1,268,621	Sulfur
2	13,396,261	116,092	D-D Mixture
3	11,656,680	295,890	Petroleum Oil, Unclassified
4	6,064,626	49,687	Methyl Bromide
5	4,005,037	432,226	Petroleum Hydrocarbons
6	3,749,553	1,043,518	Sodium Chlorate
7	3,162,852	110,050	Petroleum Distillates
8	2,301,551	743,111	Aromatic Petroleum Solvents
9	2,189,356	236,007	Maneb
10	2,185,834	1,019,416	Xylene
11	2,102,043	78,357	Nitrofen
12	1,880,710	53,869	Mineral Oil
13	1,797,892	983,828	Propargite
14	1,669,290	1,413,513	Methomyl
15	1,637,447	435,300	Molinate
16	1,443,820	45,547	Chloropicrin
17	1,346,090	51,679	CDEC
18	1,304,231	93,188	DCPA
19	1,008,522	425,709	Methamidophos
20	886,095	43,858	Ethylene Dibromide
21	876,471	1,608,635	Alkylaryl Polyoxyethylene Glycol
22	830,212	346,878	Carbaryl
23	815,220	106,460	Cryolite
24	812,904	190,291	Chlorothalonil
25	806,259	680,266	Parathion
26	798,920	6,743	1,3 Dichloropropene (See No. 2)
27	790,343	289,077	Captan
28	745,082	434,134	DEF
29	705,143	408,910	Dinoseb
30	665,678	482,577	Dimethoate
31	662,847	59,915	Dichloran
32	641,561	a	Vikane-R
33	610,048	332,656	Acephate
34	600,067	568,744	MCPA, Dimethylamine Salt
35	562,518	236,746	Oxydemeton Methyl
36	546,843	89,803	Copper Sulfate (Basic)
37	531,682	489,569	2,4-D Dimethylamine Salt
38	521,713	428,493	Dicofol
39	488,415	360,396	Diazinon
40	460,297	499,377	Petroleum Distillate, Aromatic
41	450,593	101,066	Toxaphene
42	449,139	99,969	Diuron
43	448,326	337,342	Azinphosmethyl
44	445,525	36,848	Copper Sulfate
45	439,794	19,919	Calcium Hydroxide
46	430,312	1,756,260	Paraquat Dichloride
47	409,196	33,960	Atrazine
48	407,261	85,207	Copper Hydroxide
49	371,104	87,570	Pronamide
50	368,795	63,470	Ziram
51	339,362	488,872	Xylene Range Aromatic Solvent
52	328,508	377,876	Disulfoton

Table 10.   Continued

53	326,890	137,711	Malathion
54	320,674	673,678	Free Fatty Acids and/or Amine Salts
55	306,453	525,561	Mevinphos
56	305,427	277,098	Methidathion
57	294,941	279,904	Endosulfan
58	290,415	495,869	Methyl Parathion
59	272,415	11,185	Chlordane
60	253,596	291,158	Phorate
61	251,447	219,850	Aldicarb
62	249,197	374,266	Benomyl
63	246,869	116,434	Maneb with Zinc Ion
64	243,140	445,048	Poly-1-Para-Menthene
65	238,185	51,838	Simazine
66	230,963	28,884	Glyphosate, Isopropylamine Salt
67	230,059	137,531	Imidan
68	217,671	29,383	Folpet
69	214,196	153,534	2,4-D, Alkanolamine Salts (See No. 37)
70	203,584	524,525	Mevinphos, Other Related (See No. 55)
71	189,990	230,322	Trifluralin
72	181,543	251,888	Monocrotophos
73	174,186	33,223	Copper Oxychloride Sulfate
74	167,131	76,850	Captafol
75	155,912	38,882	Alachlor
76	153,431	199,029	Chlorpyrifos
77	153,165	75,326	Difenzoquat
78	145,961	233,624	Sodium Cacodylate
79	145,036	3,036	Amitrole
80	141,864	138,821	Pendimethalin
81	126,516	182,995	Bromoxynil Octanoate
82	125,312	104,744	Naled
83	120,193	12,764	Sodium Arsenite
84	118,669	49,177	DNBP, Amine Salts (See No. 29)
85	114,806	66,334	Prometryn
86	112,845	19,596	EPTC
87	109,447	30,891	Copper
88	108,847	27,734	Propham
89	107,782	11,724	Copper-Zinc Sulfate Complex
90	102,282	101,249	Methoxychlor
91	100,564	52,572	Napropamide
92	100,341	a	Disodium Octaborate Tetrahydrate
93	98,960	1,396,624	Isopropyl Alcohol
94	95,380	1,432,894	Phosphoric Acid
95	92,700	170,323	Carbofuran
96	92,450	25,590	Propanil
97	90,314	73,812	Dichlorvos
98	88,571	348,445	Endothall, Mono (N,N-Diethylalkylamine) Salt
99	87,356	98,726	Cyhexatin
100	84,199	a	Carbon Tetrachloride
Total	117,353,564	30,308,197	

aNot applied to fields

group of assays (7); in this case, dichloran, methomyl, and parathion were totally inactive, while acephate, captan, CDEC and PCP
gave a positive result in at least one test. At the very least,
all of the major-use pesticides should be thoroughly tested.

However, it is increasingly incumbent upon genotoxicologists
as well as regulators to recognize the present superficiality of
such tests and the awesome power that accompanies their interpretation and the release of genotoxicity data to the public. A single
statement to the press that malathion was mutagenic (although not
supported by assay results) caused a near-panic this year in the
San Francisco Bay Area and delayed a crucial pest-control schedule
against the Mediterranian fruit fly; a statement by a State agency
concerning EDB mutagenicity and carcinogenicity presently has cargo
handlers refusing to load boxes of California fruit which contains
only nanogram levels of the nematicide; and the fear of 2,4-D mutagenicity and teratogenicity spread largely by "public interest"
groups has caused pregnant women to vacate their homes when distant
forests were to be sprayed.

To us, mutagenicity may only mean revertant bacterial colonies
on agar plates. To the general public, it conjures up monsters and
"The Creature from the Black Lagoon" and can lead to great expense,
hardship, and terror. We scientists cannot condone this
interpretation of our results if we are to retain our credibility
and meet our responsibilities to society.

ACKNOWLEDGEMENTS

I am grateful to John Knezovich and Ming-Yu Li for assistance
in gathering information for this report.

REFERENCES

1. California Department of Food and Agriculture, "Pesticide Use
    Report: Annual 1980", CDFA, Sacramento, 1981.
2. Simmons, V.F, A. D. Mitchell, and T. A. Jorgenson, "Evaluation
    of Selected Pesticides as Chemical Mutagens", EPA-600/1-77-
    028, US EPA, Research Triangle Park, NC, 1977.
3. Simmons, V. F., "In Vitro Microbiological Mutagenicity and
    Unscheduled DNA Synthesis Studies of 18 Pesticides", EPA-
    600/1-79-041, US EPA, Research Triangle Park, NC, 1979.
4. Kada, T., M. Moriya and Y. Shirasu, Screening of pesticides
    for DNA interactions by "rec-assay" and mutagenesis testing,
    and frameshift mutagens detected, Mutation Res. 26:243 (1974).
5. Shirasu, Y., M. Moriya, K. Kato, A. Furuhashi, and T. Kada,
    Mutagenicity screening of pesticides in the microbial system,
    Mutation Res. 40:19 (1976).

6. Shirasu, Y., M. Moriya, H. Tezuka, S. Teramoto, T. Ohta, and
    T. Inoue, Mutagenicity screening studies on pesticides,
    submitted for publication, 1981
7. Waters, M. D., Study of pesticide genotoxicity, This Volume.
8. Seiler, J. P., Evaluation of some pesticides for mutagenicity,
    Proc. Europ. Soc. Toxicol. 17:398 (1976).
9. Fishbein, L., Overview of potential mutagenic problems posed
    by some pesticides and their trace impurities, Environ. Health
    Perspect. 27:125 (1978).
10. Fishbein, L., W. G. Flamm, and H. G. Falk, "Chemical
    Mutagens", Academic Press, NY (1970).
11. Epstein, S. S., and M. S. Legator, "The Mutagenicity of Pesti-
    cides", MIT Press, Cambridge, 1971.
12. Miller, J. and E. Miller, in "Environmental Carcinogenesis"
    (P. Emmelot and E. Kriek, eds.), Elsevier, Amsterdam, 1979,
    p.25.
13. Weisburger, E. K., Mechanisms of chemical carcinogenesis, Ann.
    Rev. Pharmacol. Toxicol. 18:395 (1978).
14. Winterlin, W., J. B. Bailey, L. Langbehn, and C. Mourer, De-
    gradation of parathion applied to peach leaves, Pestic. Monit.
    J. 8:263 (1975).
15. Johnson, R. D. and D. D. Manske, Pesticide residues in total
    diet samples, Pestic. Monit. J. 11:117 (1977).
16. Stanley, C. W., J. E. Barney, M. R. Helton, and A. R. Yobs,
    Measurement of atmospheric levels of pesticides, Environ. Sci.
    Technol. $\underline{5}$, 430 (1971).
17. Woodrow, J. E., J. N. Seiber, D. G. Crosby, K. W. Moilanen, C.
    J. Soderquist, and C. Mourer, Airborne and surface residues of
    parathion and its conversion products in a treated plum
    orchard environment, Arch. Environ. Contam. Toxicol. 6:175
    (1977).
18. Spencer, W. F., T. D. Shoup, and R. C. Spear, Conversion of
    parathion to paraoxon on soil dusts as related to atmospheric
    oxidants at three California locations, J. Agr. Food Chem.
    28:1295 (1980).
19. Crosby, D. G., The fate of pesticides in the environment, Ann.
    Rev. Plant Physiol 24:467 (1973).
20. Kearney, P. C., Nitrosamines and pesticides, Pure Appl. Chem.
    52:499 (1980).
21. Archer, T. E., Dissipation of parathion and related compounds
    from field-sprayed spinach, J. Agr. Food Chem. 22:974 (1974).
22. Sethunathan, N., Degradation of parathion in flooded acid
    soils, J. Agr. Food Chem. 21:602 (1973).
23. Belser, N. O. and C. E. Castro, Biodehalogenation — the meta-
    bolism of nematocides cis- and trans-3-chloroallyl alcohol by
    a bacterium isolated from soil, J. Agr. Food Chem. 19:23
    (1971).
24. Roberts, T. R. and G. Stoyclin, The degradation of (Z)-and
    (E)-1,3-dichloropropenes and 1,2-dichloropropane in soil,
    Pestic. Sci. 7:325 (1976).

25. Crosby, D. G. and K. W. Moilanen, unpublished.
26. Crosby, D. G., The environmental chemistry of pentachloro-
    phenol, Pure Appl. Chem. 53:1051(1981).
27. Wong, A. S. and D. G. Crosby, Photodecomposition of penta-
    chlorophenol in water, J. Agr. Food Chem. 29:125 (1981).
28. Engst, R., Ethylenethiourea, Pure Appl. Chem. 29:675 (1977).
29. Crosby, D. G., J. R. Humphrey and K. W. Moilanen, The photo-
    decomposition of dipropylnitrosamine vapor, Chemosphere
    9:51(1980).
30. Ross, R. D. and D. G. Crosby, Photolysis of ethylenethiourea,
    J. Agr. Food Chem. 21:335 (1973).
31. Crosby, D. G. and A. S. Wong, Environmental degradation of
    2,3,7,8-tetrachlorodibenzo-p-dioxin (TCDD), Science 195:1337
    (1977).
32. Dime, R. A., "The Environmental Fate of Hexachlorobenzene",
    Ph.D. Thesis, Univ. of Calif., Davis, 1981.
33. Kilgore, W. W., and N. B. Akesson, Minimizing occupational
    exposure to pesticides: populations at risk, Residue Rev.
    75:21 (1980).
34. National Research Council of Canada, Phenoxy Herbicides--Their
    Effects on Environmental Quality, NRCC 16075, NRCC, Ottawa,
    Ontario, 1978.
35. Unger, T. M., J. Kliethermes, D. Van Goethem, and R. D. Short,
    Teratology and postnatal studies in rats of the propylene
    glycol butyl ether and isooctyl esters of 2,4-dichlorophen-
    oxyacetic acid, EPA-600/S1-81-035, US EPA, Research Triangle
    Park, NC, 1981.
36. Kilgore, W. W., D. G. Crosby, A. L. Craigmill, and N. K.
    Poppen, Toxic plants as possible human teratogens, Calif.
    Agric. 35(11):6 (1981).
37. Sugimura, T., Mutagens in cooked food, This Volume.
38. Ames, B. N., Mutagens, carcinogens, and anti-carcinogens, This
    Volume.

DISCUSSION

Q.   PLEWA: I agree that scientists should not speculate upon
      their data and scare people concerning the genotoxic
      properties of pesticides. However, we do not live in the most
      perfect of worlds. Certain agricultural agents are strong
      mutagens in short-term tests. Agents such as Captan should be
      handled with caution, and agricultural workers must be
      informed about the potential risk.

A.   CROSBY: Who could disagree? There should be (and is) a
      continuing effort to educate and train those who must work
      with pesticides to understand both the risks and necessary
      precautions. However, requiring the label to state "This
      product causes reversion of the histidine requirement in $\underline{S}$.

typhimurium TA-100" would not be very informative for most
people unless there were a much clearer connection with actual
damage in man or other nontarget species.

Q.   SUGIMURA: Could you comment on the pesticides which are
      applied after harvesting fruits and vegetables? One example
      is o-phenylphenol (OPP), a fungicide for oranges and lemons.
      OPP is important to avoid fungus growth and mycotoxin
      production. But there is suggestive data on its
      carcinogenicity in the urinary bladder.

A.   CROSBY: Other than use in home gardens, this may provide the
      most important opportunity for public exposure to
      'pesticides. The "California Pesticide Use Report" shows that
      3,700 pounds of o-phenylphenol was used here in 1980, mostly
      for washing oranges; however, a large amount of dichloran
      (Botran) was used similarly on other commodities. Clearly, a
      satisfactory exposure tolerance must be applied in such
      instances and accompanied by analytical monitoring at the very
      least; if possible, use of a safer wash would seem prudent.

ANALYSIS OF TOXICANTS IN AGRICULTURAL ENVIRONMENTS

James N. Seiber

Department of Environmental Toxicology
University of California
Davis, CA 95616

INTRODUCTION

It is axiomatic that the magnitude of biological effects is related to the dose of chemical to which an organism or group of organisms is exposed. Tremendous advances in analytical methodology during the past several years have furnished, in many instances, precise information on exposure. This ability to identify and quantify chemicals, even at very low concentration levels, is reflected in the assignment of finite chemical standards--tolerances, action levels, threshold limit values (TLV's), water and air quality standards, etc.--which belie the uncertainty in ascribing biological effects, particularly for diverse populations. This uncertainty is manifested in the relatively large safety factors used in assigning standards, rather than in the numerical standards themselves.

In a broad context, analysis plays two important roles in environmental toxicology (Fig. 1). Working in concert with laboratory testing and field observation of effects, analysis helps to define actual or potential problems with chemicals which may require some societal or regulatory action. For example, the epidemic outbreak of neurological disease in humans and animals in Minimata, Japan, dating from roughly 1953 to 1960, indicated the presence of a toxic agent(s) in that environment; chemical analysis of fish and shellfish samples showed abnormally high levels of methylmercury; and analysis further showed that the source was effluent from a local factory producing vinyl chloride. Controlled tests with animals showed clearly that the observed effects could be ascribed to methylmercury at the levels found in the Minimata samples. The action in this case was to prevent industrial

219

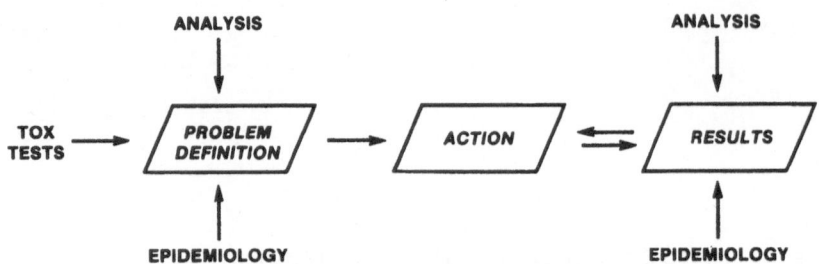

Figure 1. The role of analysis in defining and resolving problems
          associated with chemicals in the environment.

discharges containing mercury--an action which was embarrassingly
slow in its implementation (24). Once the cause-effect relationship had been established and steps were taken to correct the
situation, analysis then appeared in its second role, that of
monitoring the effectiveness of the action.

     This scenario has been acted out, to a greater or lesser ex-
tent, in many situations. The action followed as a result, at
least in part, of analytical findings may include banning the use
of a chemical, as in the case of DDT; closing a well or other
source of drinking water, as with DBCP; restricting the intake of
certain foods, as with endrin-contaminated ducks in a very recent
example (47), or the exposure to polluted air in the form of smog-
alerts in some areas; and in the general case of establishing
standards for permissable levels in foods, water, and industrial
atmospheres--standards which may need redefining as new toxicology
data or analytical findings come to light, or as use patterns
change.

     If the needs of the day have provided the driving force for
developments in analysis, the skills of the analyst augmented by
breakthroughs in technology have proved equal to the challenge.
Methods of ever increasing sensitivity and specificity have been
developed. The analytical process itself has, however, not changed
materially in the sense that all analyses conform to basic steps or
unit processes which vary little regardless of the application.
These steps include:

     Sampling: Obtaining a valid and representative sample of the
     environment or population of interest.

     Sample Preparation: A series of operations which includes
     extraction, to remove the analyte from the matrix bulk; cleanup
     of the extract, to remove potentially interfering
     coextractives; modification or derivatization, to chemically
     change the analyte to a more readily determinable form; and
     resolution, to separate the analyte or its derivative from
     other chemicals remaining in the prepared sample. Sample pre-

paration includes elements of concentration, in that a few micrograms or so of analyte are transferred from several grams or kilograms of sample to a small volume of solvent. It also includes elements of purification, in that one aims to isolate just one or a few chemicals from the thousands present in the raw sample.

Determination: One or more operations which include detection, that is, obtaining a response related to the structure and/or amount of analyte present, and measurement of the resulting response usually by reference to a standard of the chemical of interest or a close relative.

The strategy underlying these steps is to take advantage of physical and chemical properties unique to the analyte to concentrate, purify, and detect small amounts in whatever matrix is provided. This time-honored approach holds for analyses in the environmental, economic, and forensic fields of toxicology.

Much of the effort in analysis in recent years has been focused on the development of advanced techniques for resolution and detection (Fig. 2). In the 1940's and early 1950's, gravimetric and bioassay techniques were the mainstays in "trace" analysis, extending analyses to the then-frontier detection limits of about 1 ppm. Colorimetric and spectrophotometric methods held sway through the 1950's and early 1960's, providing improvements in both detection limits and specificity. The inroads of chromatography began roughly in the 1950's with paper and thin-layer chromatography, and achieved domination since that time culminating in the present widespread use of gas-liquid (GLC) and high performance liquid chromatography (HPLC). The now common use of GLC coupled with mass spectrometry (31) provides detection limits to 1 ppb routinely, with a few recent examples extending to ppt levels (9). These achievement in sensitivity and specificity have been costly such that equipping a modern laboratory for a broad spectrum of trace analyses can be undertaken only by the financially well-endowed. There appears to be some justification for the large capital investment in terms of cost per analysis. Finnegan et al. (15) and Schnute and Smith (41) have pointed out that analysis for 114 priority organic pollutants in a single water sample is actually less by GLC-MS than by GLC alone when one takes into account the number of gas chromatographs and operator time required if GLC were used. Recent advances in coupled HPLC-MS promise further applications of this pomising technique in much the same way as for GLC-MS (2).

One may question whether advances in analytical methodology have been responsible for the increased regulation of chemicals, or whether the promulgation of more stringent standards have been responsible for advances in analysis. Examples exist in support of both points of view. In the first instance may be cited the development of the electron-capture GLC detector and its use in

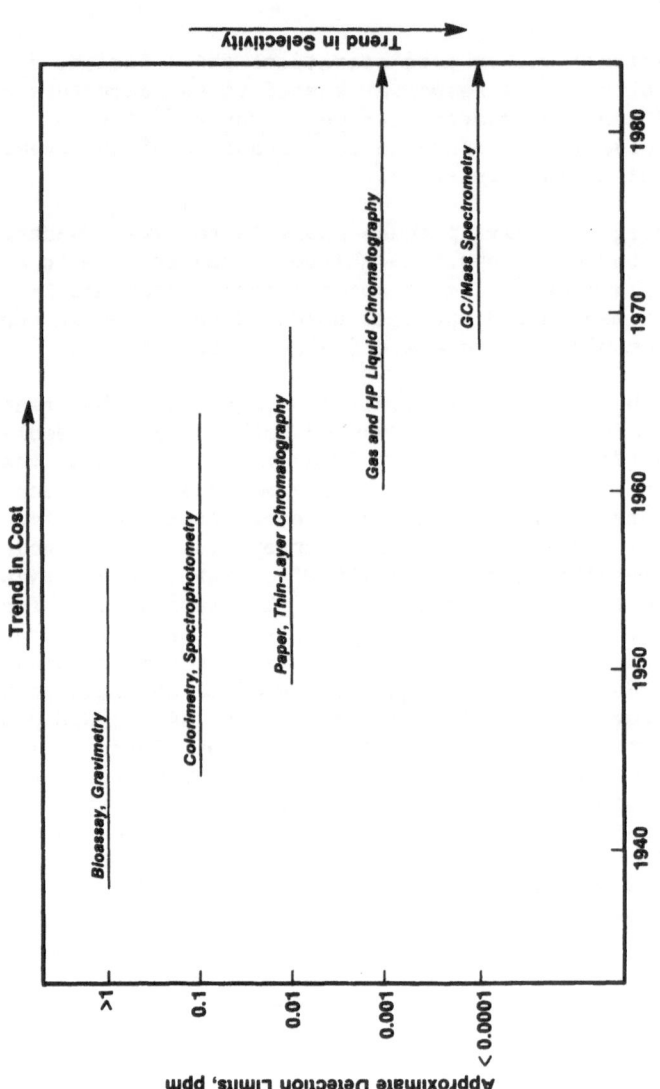

Fig. 2.   The evolution of analytical methodology for organic toxicants in environmental samples.

ascertaining the environmental stability and distributrion of organochlorine pesticides (50); the thermal energy analyzer applied similarly to nitrosamines in foods, and environmental samples (13, 14); and GLC-MS applied to priority organic pollutants (15). The second category includes the promulgation of the Clean Air Act (1970) and its 1977 amendments with the subsequent development of sophisticated automated instruments for routine monitoring of primary air pollutants (48) and advanced techniques for identification of trace hazardous substances in ambient air (5). It also includes the effect on analysis of the substantial lowering of the TLV for vinyl chloride in workplace air in 1974 (30), a situation for which the proposed lowering of TLV for ethylene dibromide may provide a current parallel (American Conference of Governmental Industrial Hygienists, 1980). At any rate, it is clear that trace analysis constitutes an integral part of hazard assessment and the regulation of those chemicals deemed hazardous.

In the remainder of this paper a few examples will be presented to show some of the current techniques available for trace analyses, their application to problems in agricultural environments, and some difficulties associated with these analyses. Excellent recent reviews of the spectrum of techniques for trace analysis may be found for pesticides (19), polynuclear aromatic hydrocarbons (7), air pollutants (5), water pollutants (25), and other categories of toxic substances (42).

Toxaphene

Toxaphene is a commercial insecticide used widely on a variety of food, feed, and fiber crops since its introduction in 1947. Recent concern over the continued use of this material in the U.S. has focused on its residual nature, leading to apparently widespread contamination of environments far removed from sites of application (6), its carcinogenic activity in rodents (36), and its mutagenic activity in the Ames Salmonella assay (22).

TOXICANT B   TOXICANT A-1   TOXICANT A-2

1   2   3

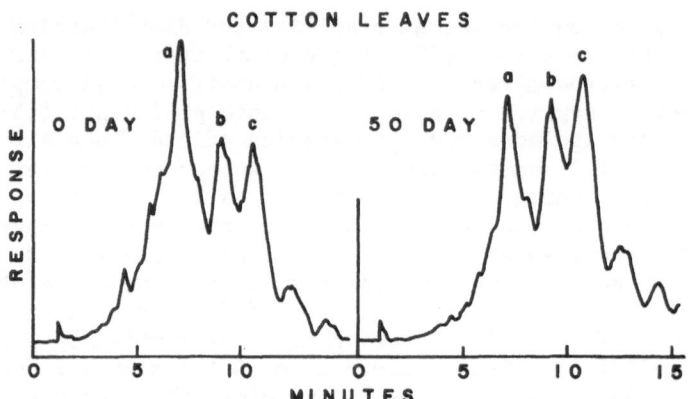

Figure 3.   Packed column gas chromatograms of toxaphene residue in
            0- and 14-day cotton leaf extracts.   From Seiber et al.
            (43).

An understanding of the evironmental behavior of toxaphene has
been slow in coming, in part because of the multicomponent nature
of the commercial product.   Holmstead et al.(21) showed technical
toxaphene to consist of at least 177 compounds.   Three compounds,
toxicant B (1) (37), and isomers A-1 and A-2 (2 and 3) (33, 46),
account for a significant proportion of the toxicity of technical
toxaphene to mice and houseflies (25a).

Tracking toxaphene in the environment thus involves two types
of problems; (1) the conventional, but very difficult problem in
the case of this complex mixture of isolating and determining residues free of interference by other organochlorine pesticides and
PCB's; and (2) the problem of analyzing individually for the more
hazardous components in the applied mixture.

Both problems are apparent in conventional, packed column gas
chromatograms of toxaphene residue from agroenvironmental samples
(Fig. 3).   The chromatograms are relatively diffuse compared with
the single peaks routinely obtained for DDT, DDE, dieldrin, and
most other organochlorine pesticides, resulting in higher limits of
detectability and less specificity in analyses for toxaphene.   And,
while some "weathering" of toxaphene is apparent from changes in
chromatographic profile with time for residues taken immediately or
several weeks after application, it would be impossible to analyze
for individual components by this conventional methodology.

To remove some interferences, a chemical cleanup technique may
be used in which chloroaromatic compounds, such as DDT, are
nitrated and thus removed from the sample, while stable chloroaliphatics, such as toxaphene, are left unchanged (26).   This

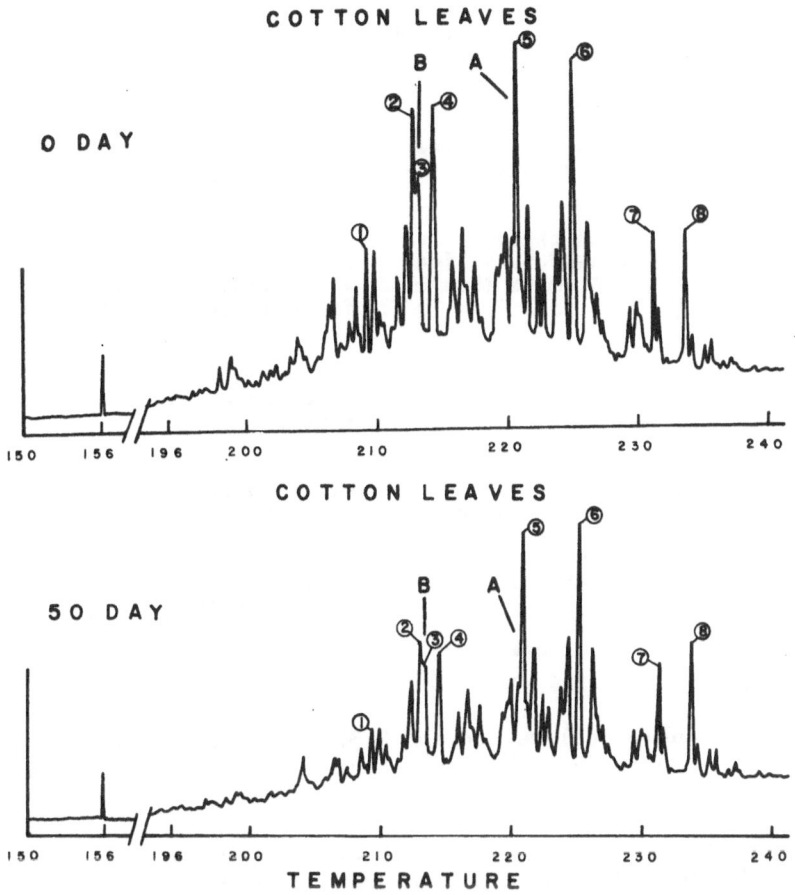

Figure 4.   Capillary gas chromatograms of toxaphene residue in 0-
            and 50-day cotton leaf extracts.   From Seiber et al.
            (43).

technique, when combined with the usual Florisil column
chromatography cleanup employed with many pesticide residues (39)
provides a reasonably clean sample for toxaphene analysis (43).

     For component resolution, gas chromatographic analyses may be
conducted with open-tubular (capillary) columns (20). Applied to
cotton leaf samples, this technique showed that toxicant B, and
others of the more volatile toxaphene components, were less residual than toxicant A isomer mixture and other less volatile components (Fig. 4). Analysis of air samples collected just adjacent to
the cotton field showed that the more volatile constituents of
toxaphene were enriched in the air, indicating that volatilization
was the major dissipation pathway for toxaphene from treated

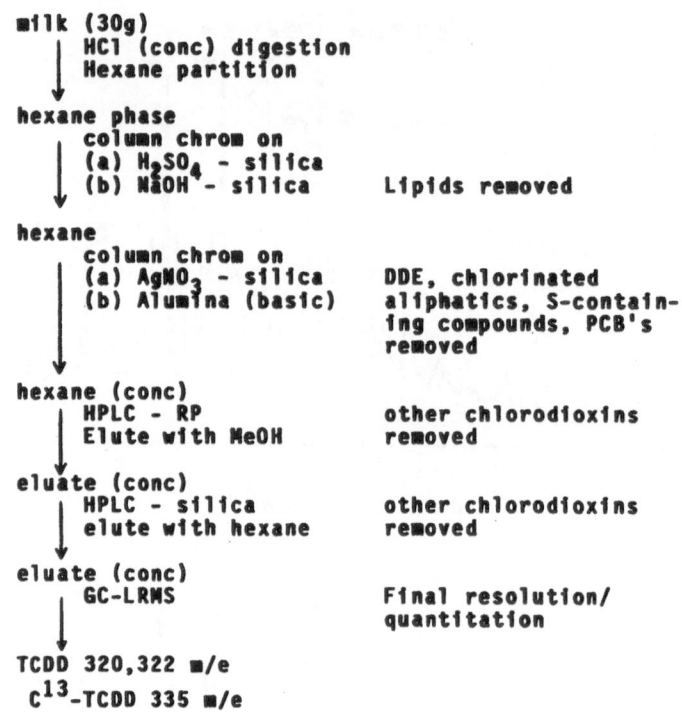

milk (30g)
  HCl (conc) digestion
  Hexane partition

hexane phase
  column chrom on
  (a) H₂SO₄ - silica
  (b) NaOH - silica   Lipids removed

hexane
  column chrom on
  (a) AgNO₃ - silica   DDE, chlorinated
  (b) Alumina (basic)   aliphatics, S-contain-
                               ing compounds, PCB's
                               removed

hexane (conc)
  HPLC - RP   other chlorodioxins
  Elute with MeOH   removed

eluate (conc)
  HPLC - silica   other chlorodioxins
  elute with hexane   removed

eluate (conc)
  GC-LRMS   Final resolution/
                               quantitation

TCDD 320,322 m/e
C^{13}-TCDD 335 m/e

Figure 5.   Analytical method for 2,3,7,8-tetrachlorodibenzo-p-
            dioxin in milk. From Langhorst and Shadoff (29).

foliage (43) and, coupled with its stability in the air, may
explain the distribution of toxaphene to remote environments (44).

A similar analysis of soil and sediment showed that microbial
degradation represents a major dissipation route for toxaphene in
anaerobic environments. Degradation yields products with fewer
chlorines than in the original mixture, resulting in chromatograms
with a larger proportion of early eluting GLC peaks and at least
partial destruction of Toxicants A and B (Fig. 5). This degradation can be rapid under conditions favoring high microbial
populations (34, 38), suggesting an approach to decontamination of
toxaphene at waste sites and other areas with high toxaphene
concentrations.

The use of a high performance gas chromatographic techniques
thus substantially increased the amount of information obtained
from toxaphene analyses. Application of this technique to wildlife, fish, and food animals may provide crucial information in the
poorly-understood area of food-chain accumulation and transfer of
toxaphene and the fate of the more hazardous constituents of toxaphene.

Dioxin

The limit of detectability achievable by state-of-the-art methodology when focused on single toxicants is best demonstrated by the polychlorinated dibenzo-p-dioxins, and the most toxic member of this chemical group, 2,3,7,8-tetrachlorodibenzo-p-dioxin ("dioxin"). Of particular concern are food chain transfer of dioxin to the human diet, passage of dietary dioxin to human milk, and human exposure to dioxin in air particulate matter (11, 28).

The extreme toxicity of dioxin to a range of organisms (3) mandates detection limits in the order of parts-per-trillion (ppt) in biological samples. This analytical problem has been placed in perspective by Lamparski and Nestrick (28) who point out that an analysis at 10 ppt in a matrix purified to 99.9% may still encounter interferences from as many as 10^5 compounds at concentrations up to 1000 times higher than the chemical of interest. Obviously, analyses at this level require unusual efficiencies in cleanup and resolution, and heroic selectivity and sensitivity in detection and measurement.

The historical trend in dioxin analysis is apparent in a sampling of methods forthcoming since 1973 (Table 1). The method of Woolson et al.(49) utilized conventional cleanup by chemical treatment, column chromatography, and electron-capture GLC to achieve a detection limit of 50 ppb in avian tissue. Baughman and Meselson (3) provided a dramatic lowering of detectability of over 1000-fold using a preparative GLC cleanup and, particularly, high resolution mass spectrometric detection. Lamparski et al.(27) described a method using a vigorous cleanup sequence involving chemical treatment, multiple column chromatography, and preparative HPLC prior to GLC/MS determination, achieving a detection limit of 10 ppt in trout. Langhorst and Shadoff (29) added a second preparative HPLC cleanup to achieve the current "frontier" limit for dioxin of 1 ppt in milk. Their method, outlined in Fig. 5, involved chemical treatment with hydrochloric acid during sample digestion, and subsequently with sulfuric acid and sodium hydroxide held on a chromatographic support to remove lipids; column adsorption chromatography on silver nitrate-impregnated silica gel and on basic alumina to separate DDE, chloroaliphatics, PCB's, and sulfur-containing coextractives; both reversed phase and adsorption HPLC to separate 2,3,7,8-dioxin from other chlorodioxins; and GLC-low resolution MS for selective detection of TCDD, referenced against an internal standard of C^{13}-TCDD. Brumley et al.(9) conducted an interlaboratory comparison of several TCDD methods, including that of the Dow group cited previously; the dual column HPLC method used 2 analysts working a total of 32 hours to conduct the extraction and cleanup of a 4 sample set. This is equivalent to 8 hours per sample (ie., roughly $125 per sample for skilled labor only).

Table 1.   Some Methods for the Trace Analysis of 2,3,7,8-
            Tetrachlorodibenzo-p-dioxin in Biological Samples

Samples	Approximate Detection Limit	Techniques	Reference
Bird	50 ppb	Chemical treatment Column Chromatogr EC-GLC	Woolsen et al. 1973 (49)
Beef (liver) Fish Crustaceans	20 ppt	Chemical treatment Prep GLC HR Mass Spec	Baughman and Meselsohn 1973 (3)
Trout	10 ppt	Chemical treatment Column Chromatogr (Multiple) HPLC GC/MS	Lamparski et al. 1979 (27)
Milk	1 ppt	Chemical treatment Column Chromatogr (Multiple) HPLC (2) GC/MS	Langhorst and Shadoff 1980 (29)

The dioxin analysis indicates that detection limits can be
extended using presently available techniques, providing that unusual care and time can be devoted in the process. For many
chemicals, a detection limit of 1 ppt may prove inaccessible, while
for most it would be unnecessary. It is, however, comforting to
know that, when health considerations require it, analysts can work
successfully at these levels.

Toxic Chemicals in Undefined Mixtures

In the toxaphene and dioxin examples, the analytical methods
were tailored to fit the chemicals of interest with no regard for
other substances present in the sample so long as they were removed
during sample preparation or were simply not detected in the final
determination. When the analyst is confronted with a biologically
active sample in which the components(s) responsible for the
activity are unknown, the analytical method must provide for all of
the components present which have even a remote chance of contributing to the activity.

An agricultural example lies with the observation of mutagenic
activity in the particulate matter of smoke from the burning of
crop residues (23). Sampling of smoke from controlled burns of
rice straw was carried out by filtration through glass fiber fil-
ters. Extraction of particulate matter, by sonication with a mixture of benzene and methanol, gave a complex mixture of organic

substances with mutagenic activity in the Ames <u>Salmonella</u> assay.
This result was not surprising given that combustion products of
other vegetative matter--cigarettes (7), leaf burning (16), and
wood burning (17)--including certain polynuclear aromatic and hete-
roaromatic compounds with mutagenic activity. For example, Hall
and DeAngelis (17) identified 33 specific and generic PAH's and
heterocyclics from wood-fired residential equipment, including
benzopyrenes, benzofluoranthenes, dibenzopyrenes, methylcholan-
threne, methylchrysene, and dibenzocarbazoles--all of which are
animal carcinogens. Fractionation of rice straw smoke extractives
was done with the goal of identifying organic compounds of several
classes (not restricted just to PAH's) present in fractions which
exhibited activity in the Ames assay. One fractionation scheme
employed normal phase HPLC using a cyano column eluted with a
hexane/acetone solvent gradient. Capillary column GLC of a single
HPLC fraction (Fig. 6) showed a complex mixture of chromato-
graphable components, any one of which could potentially contribute, at least in part, to biological activity. Six fractions
were collected in this manner, and all were, as expected, gross
mixtures. Over 30 individual chemicals have now been identified
primarily by GLC/MS, including several candidate PAH and
heterocyclic mutagens (32, 36a). However, it is not yet possible
to ascribe biological activity to any one compound or group of compounds in the whole smoke sample.

A multi-class fractionation sequence may also be required in
some analyses for pesticides when the sample is of unknown origin
or when it may contain residues of many chemicals. The common
multiclass residue procedures for pesticide use combinations of
liquid-liquid partition, column adsorption chromatographic fractionation, and GLC with several element-selective detectors for
determination. Examples include the Mills FDA procedure, primarily
for adipose tissue (Pesticide Analytical Manual, 39), and a silica
gel fractionation scheme (45) primarily for air, water, and soil
samples.

Analyzing for chemicals in complex mixtures and, particularly,
assigning biological activity to specific chemicals in such mixtures, is difficult, labor-intensive work which generally requires
a combination of analytical techniques, including GLC/MS. A close-
at-hand bioassay which can respond rapidly at low toxicant concentrations is critical for pin-pointing the source of activity.

SUMMARY AND CONCLUSIONS

Analytical chemists have made major progress during the past
20-30 years in increasing selectivity and decreasing limits of
detectability. Methodology as it now exists may be used in combination to achieve detection limits as low as 1 ppt in biological
matrices, although to do so can be extremely costly in terms of

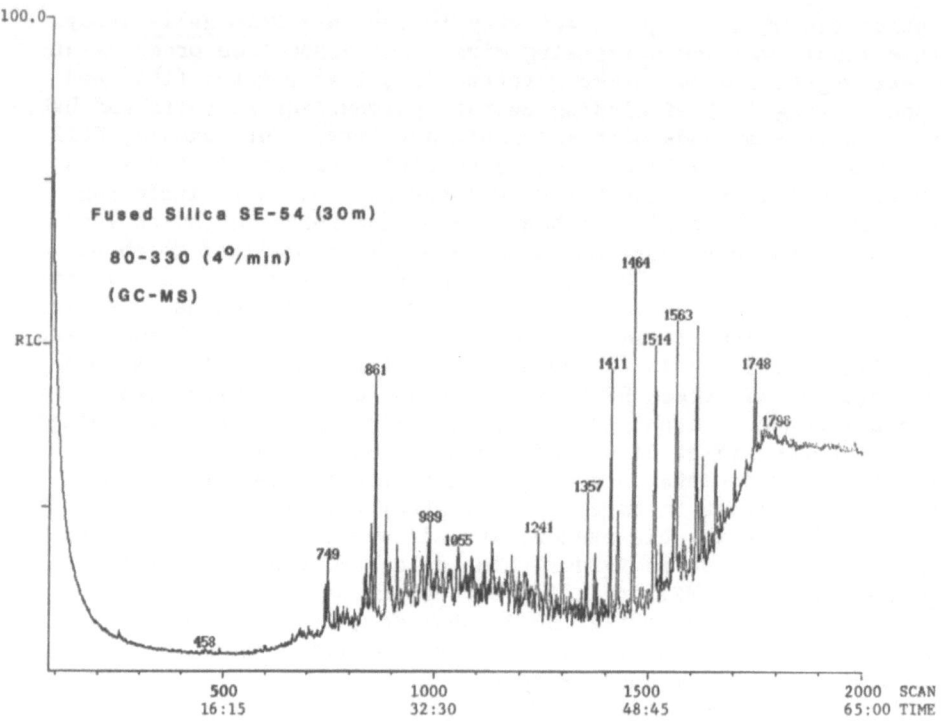

Figure 6. Capillary gas chromatogram of HPLC Fraction II from the fractionation of rice straw smoke extract.

labor and capital. Because labor is such a major contributor to analytical costs, much effort is now underway to automate some operations, including the evaporation of solvents, phase transfers, derivatization, chromatographic separations, and data processing (10). While total automation is several years down the road, the inroads of automation are beginning to be seen in some specific analyses, and for some parts of the general analytical sequence.

Time is a major roadblock in current trace-level analyses, particularly when the generator of the sample needs to know its contents quickly so that on-the-spot decisions can be made. The advent of the mobile laboratory may help, although for answers required in some instances, such as for reentry to pesticide-treated fields and exposure of applicators to pesticides, field tests may suffice to decide whether residues are above or below a set standard. A field test kit for organophosphorus pesticide residues was reported recently (4); immunoassay-based tests may offer room for further advances in this area (18, 40), as may re-discovery of the merits of bioassay (8).

Finally, a word of caution is in order regarding the quality of analytical results. A number of individuals and firms began to offer trace analytical services as a result of increasing demand in recent years, but lacking the needed expertise and experience. There are few licensing requirements and no mandatory quality assurance programs for such individuals. Given that wrong analytical results can be much more damaging than none at all, and every analysis can yield some number (right or wrong), it behooves knowledgeable environmental scientists in all parts of the country to expose the incompetent, and, where possible, provide remedial help to improve competency. These comments apply equally to contract analytical firms, University laboratories, and those of state and federal agencies.

Overall, however, the needs for trace analysis stimulated major improvements in instrumentation and the application of new instrumentation to real-world problems with generally high proficiency and competency. In this respect analysis has played an integral role in placing problems with chemicals in a quantitative perspective, and thereby contributing to the improvement in environmental quality overall.

REFERENCES

1. American Conference of Governmental Industrial Hygienist, Inc. 1980. Documentation of the Threshold Limit Values. Fourth Edition. Cincinnati, Ohio.
2. Arpino, P. J. and G. Guiochon. 1979. LC/MS coupling. Anal. Chem. 51: 682A-701A.
3. Baughman, R., and M. Meselson. 1973. An analytical method for detecting TCDD (dioxin): Levels of TCDD in samples from Vietnam. Environ. Health Perspectives 1973:27-35 (September).
4. Berch, B., Y. Iwata, and F.A. Gunther. 1981. Worker environment research: Rapid field method for estimation of organophosphorus insecticide residues on citrus foliage and in grove soil. J. Agric. Food Chem. 29:209-216.
5. Bertsch, W. 1981. Analysis of air and air pollutants. In: Applications of Glass Capillary Gas Chromatography, Jennings, W. G. (Ed). Marcel Dekker, New York. Chapter 4.
6. Bidleman, T. F. and C. E. Olney. 1975. Long-range transport of toxaphene insecticide in the western North Atlantic atmosphere. Nature 257:475-477.
7. Bjorseth, A., and A. J. Dennis (Eds). 1980. Polynuclear aromatic hydrocarbons; Chemistry and Biological Effects. Batelle Press, Columbus, Ohio.
8. Bowman, M.C., W.L. Oller, and T. Cairns. 1981. Stressed bioassay systems for rapid screening of pesticide residues. Part I. Evaluation of bioassay systems. Arch. Environ. Contamin. Toxicol. 10:9-24.

9. Brumley, W. C., J. A. G. Roach, J. A. Sphon, P. A. Dreifuss, D. Andrzejewski, R. A. Niemann, and D. Firestone. Low-resolution multiple ion detection gas chromatographic-mass spectrometeric comparison of six extraction-cleanup methods for determining 2,3,7,8-tetrachlorodibenzo-p-dioxin in fish. J. Agric. Food Chem. 29:1040-1046.

10. Burns, D. A. 1981. Automated sample preparation. Anal. Chem. 53:1404A-1418A.

11. Cairns, T., L. Fishbein, and R. K. Mitchum. 1980. Review of the dioxin problem. Mass spectrometric analyses of tetrachlorodioxins in environmental samples. Biomed. Mass Spec. 7:484-492.

12. Cooper, J. A. 1980. Environmental impact of residential wood combustion emissions and its implications. J. Air Pollut. Contr. Assn. 30:855-861.

13. Fine, D. H., R. Ross, D. P. Rounbuhler, A. Silvergleid, and L. Song. Analysis of nonionic nonvolatile N-nitroso compounds in foodstuffs. J. Agric. Food Chem. 25, 1416-1418 (1977).

14. Fine, D. H., D. P. Rounbuhler, N. M. Belcher, and S. S. Epstein. N-nitroso compounds in air and water. In: N-Nitroso Compounds, Analysis and Formation. International Agency for Research on Cancer, Publication No. 14, pp. 401-408.

15. Finnegan, R.E., D.W. Hoyt and D.E. Smith. 1979. Priority pollutants II - cost-effective analysis. Environ. Sci. Technol. 13, 534-541.

16. Friedman, L. and E. J. Calabrese. 1977. The health implications of open leaf burning. Revs. Environm. Health 2:257-258.

17. Hall, R. E., and D. G. DeAngelis. 1980. EPA's research program for controlling residential wood combustion emmissions. J. Air Pollut. Contr. Assn. 30:855-861.

18. Hammock, B. D. and R. O. Mumma. 1980. Potential of immunochemical technology for pesticide analysis. In: Pesticide Analytical Methodology, Harvey, Jr., J. and G. Zweig (Eds.), ACS Symposium Series 136, American Chemical Society, Washington, D. C. pp. 321-352.

19. Harvey, Jr., J., and G. Zweig (Eds.) 1980. Pesticide Analytical Methodology. ACS Symposium Series 136, American Chemical Society, Washington, D. C. 406 pp.

20. Hermann, B. W. and J. N. Seiber. 1981. Glass capillary gas chromatography of pesticides. In: Applications of Glass Capillary Gas Chromatography, Jennings, W. (Ed.), Marcel Dekker, New York. Chapter 6.

21. Holmstead, R. L., S. Khalifa, and J. E. Casida. 1974. Toxaphene composition analyzed by combined gas chromatography-chemical ionization mass spectrometry. J. Agric. Food Chem. 22:939-944.

22. Hooper, N. K., B. N. Ames, M. A. Saleh, and J. E. Casida. 1979. Toxaphene, a complex mixture of polychloroterpenes and a major insecticide, is mutagenic. Science 205:591-593.

23. Hsieh, D. P. H., J. N. Seiber, G. L. Fisher, T. J. Mast, E. H. Olsen, J. Woodrow, and J. F. Yee. 1981. Potential health hazards associated with particulate matter released from rice straw burning. Final Report: Project A8-093-31, California Air Resources Board, Sacramento, CA, 231 pp.

24. Katz, A. 1972. Mercury pollution: The making of an environmental crisis. CRC Crit. Rev. Environ. Contr. 1972:517.

25. Keith, L. W. (Ed.) 1976. Identification and Analysis of Organic Pollutants in Water. Ann Arbor Science, Ann Arbor, Mich.

25a. Khalifa, S., T. R. Mon, J. L. Engel, and J. E. Casida. 1974. Isolation of 2,2,5-endo,6-exo,8,9,10-heptachlorobornane and an octachloro toxicant from technical toxaphene. J. Agric. Food Chem. 22:653-657.

26. Klein, A. K., and J. D. Link. 1970. Elimination of interferences in the determination of toxaphene residues. J. Assoc. Off. Anal. Chem. 53:524-529.

27. Lamparski, L. L. and T. J. Nestrick. 1980. Determination of tetra-, hexa-, hepta-, and octachlorodibenzo-p-dioxin isomers in particulate samples at parts per trillion levels. Anal. Chem. 52:2045-2054.

28. Lamparski, L. L., T. J. Nestrick, and R. H. Stehl. 1979. Determination of part-per-trillion concentration of 2,3,7,8-tetrachlorodibenzo-p-dioxin in fish. Anal. Chem. 51:1453-1458.

29. Langhorst, M. L. and L. A. Shadoff. 1980. Determination of parts-per-trillion concentrations of tetra-, hexa-, and octachlorodibenzo-p-dioxins in human milk samples. Anal. Chem. 52:2037-2044.

30. Laramy, R. E. 1977. Analytical Chemistry of vinyl chloride--A survey. Amer. Lab. 1977:17-27 (December).

31. Ligon, Jr., W. V. 1979. Molecular analysis by mass spectrometry. Science 205:151-159.

32. Mast, T. J., J. E. Woodrow, and J. N. Seiber. 1981. Analysis of organic particulate matter from rice straw smoke. Paper No. 55 presented to the Division of Environmental Chemistry, 182nd National Meeting of the American Chemical Society, New York, NY, Aug. 23-28.

33. Matsumura, F., R. W. Howard, and J. O. Nelson. 1975. Structure of the toxic fraction A of toxaphene. Chemosphere 5:271-276.

34. Mirsatari, S. G. 1978. Some characteristics of toxaphene residues on foliage and in soil and sediment. Ph. D. Thesis, University of California, Davis, CA 95616. 112 pp.

35. Moye, H. A. (Ed.). 1980. Analysis of Pesticide Residues. Wiley, New York, 467 pp.

36. National Cancer Institute. 1979. Carcinogenesis Technical Report Series 37, Department of Health, Education, and Welfare Publication. NIH 79-837, Washington, DC.

36a. Olsen, H., J. Yee, T. Mast, J. Woodrow, G. Fisher, J. Seiber, D. Hsieh. "An Evaluation of PAH Content, Mutagenicity and Cytotoxicity of Rice Straw Smoke." Presented at 6th Interna-

tional Symposium on Polynuclear Aromatic HC's, Battelle, Columbus, Oct. 26–29, 1981.

37. Palmer, K. J., R. Y. Wong, R. E. Lundin, S. Khalifa, and J. E.
Casida. 1975. Crystal and molecular structure of 2,2,5-<u>endo</u>
6-<u>exo</u>, 8,9,10-heptachlorobornane, $C_{10} H_{11} Cl_7$, a toxic component of toxaphene insecticide. <u>J. Am. Chem.</u> Soc. 97:408–
413.

38. Parr, J. F. and S. Smith. 1976. Degradation of toxaphene in
selected anaerobic soil environments. <u>Soil Sci.</u> 121:52

39. <u>Pesticide Analytical Manual</u>, 1971. U. S. Department of
Healthy, Education, and Welfare, Food and Drug Adminstration,
Rockville, MD., Vol. I.

40. Rinder, D.F., and J.R. Flecker. 1981. A radioimmunoassay to
screen for 2,4-dichlorophenoxyacetic acid and 2,4,5-trichloro-
phenoxyacetic acid in surface waters. <u>Bull. Environ.</u>
<u>Contamin. Toxicol.</u> 26:325–330.

41. Schnute, W. C. and D. E. Smith. 1980. The application of
GC/MS in environmental analysis. <u>Amer. Lab.</u> <u>1980</u>:87–95
(July).

42. Schuetzle, D. (Ed.) 1979. <u>Monitoring Toxic Substances.</u> ACS
Symposium Series 94, American Chemical Society, Washington, DC
289 pp.

43. Seiber, J. N., S. C. Madden, M. M. McChesney, and W. L.
Winterlin. 1979. Toxaphene dissipation from treated cotton
field environments: Component residual behavior on leaves and
in air, soil, and sediments determined by capillary gas chromatography. <u>J. Agric. Food Chem.</u> 27:284–291.

44. Seiber, J. N., G. A. Ferriera, B. Hermann, and J. E.
Woodrow. 1980. Analysis of pesticidal residues in the air
near agricultural treatment sites. In: <u>Pesticide Analytical</u>
<u>Methodolgy</u>, Harvey, Jr., J. and G. Zweig (Eds.). ACS Sympo-
sium Series 136, American Chemical Society, Washington, DC,
Chapter 10.

45. Sherma, J. and T. M. Shafik. 1975. A m##lticlass, multi-
residue analytical method for determining pesticide residues
in air. <u>Arch. Environ. Contamin. Toxicol.</u> 3:55.

46. Turner, W. V., S. Khalifa, and J. E. Casida. 1975. Toxaphene
toxicant A. Mixture of 2,2,5-<u>endo</u>, 6-<u>exo</u>, 8,9,9,10-octa-
chlorobornane. <u>J. Agric. Food Chem.</u> 23:991–994.

47. Wallis, C. 1981. Bad news for the birds. <u>Time</u> 1981:52
(October 5).

48. Wilson, M. L. 1980. A review of monitoring methodology for
gaseous criteria pollutants. <u>Amer. Lab</u> <u>1980</u>:37–53 (February).

49. Woolsen, E. A., P. D. J. Ensor, W. L. Reichel, and A. L.
Young. 1973. Dioxin residues in Lakeland sand' and bald eagle
samples. In: <u>Chlorodioxins--Origin and Fate.</u> Blair, E. H.
(Ed.). ACS Symposium Series 120, American Chemical Society,
Washington, DC. Chapter 12.

50. Zweig, G. 1970. The vanishing zero: The evolution of pesticide analyses. In: <u>Essays in Toxicology</u>, Vol. 2, Academic
Press, New York. Chapter 3.

EXPOSURE ASSESSMENT FOR AGRICULTURAL CHEMICALS

David J. Severn

Hazard Evaluation Division
Office of Pesticides and Toxic Substances
Environmental Protection Agency
Washington, DC 20460

INTRODUCTION

Pesticides are toxic chemicals that are deliberately introduced into the environment to achieve control of pests. For agriculture, these pests include insects, mites, and nematodes which damage growing crops, weeds which compete for nutrients and decrease the value of the harvest, and fungi which cause plant diseases. The Federal Insecticide, Fungicide, and Rodenticide Act specifies that pesticides may be registered for use if that use will not cause unreasonable adverse effects on man or the environment. The potential for adverse effects on man is, of course, determined by both the inherent toxic properties of the pesticide and the extent of exposure to the pesticide. Thus an assessment of exposure is fully as important as the toxicological evaluation of a pesticide in making judgements about the overall risk of pesticide use.

The purpose of this paper is to review the status of our knowledge of the routes and extent of exposure to man from the application of pesticides to growing crops. Exposure in this context means contact with pesticide residues during all phases of caring for the crop, from preplant soil treatments with herbicides to harvesting, storage, and transportation of the crop. Although dietary exposure from consumption of food containing pesticide residues is of concern to the agency and is covered by established tolerances, that topic will not be considered in this review.

Agricultural Use of Pesticides

Human activities connected with the application of pesticides include the actual application process itself, and the associated activities of mixing and loading, cleanup, and maintenance of application equipment. Application practices vary widely in their potential for human exposure: orchard applicators operate air blast equipment which produces a very fine spray or mist of dilute pesticide directed upward into the trees, while other types of ground application result in coarse sprays which are directed downward and away from the applicator. Handheld spray equipment places the applicator in close proximity to the spray, while pilots are physically separated from the spray by the airplane cabin. On the other hand, spray pilots apply many types of pesticides throughout the year, so that they may be exposed over longer periods of time and to a wider variety of pesticides. Mixing and loading for all these types of application has the potential for considerable exposure, since mixers and loaders must handle concentrated pesticides. Equipment malfunction during operation, such as clogging of spray nozzles, can also result in exposure.

A different kind of exposure can result from entry into treated crops for purposes of harvesting, scouting for insect damage, or other types of fieldwork. Exposure in these situations is not to a pesticide concentrate or spray, but rather to a "weathered" or environmentally modified and dissipated residue, usually absorbed on foliar surfaces, surface dust, or soil.

Measurement of Exposure

For all of these widely varying human activities, measurements or estimates of actual exposure are needed in order to convert the toxicological characteristics of a pesticide into an assessment of risk. Two basic types of procedures are available to measure exposure: measurement of the amount of chemical that comes in contact with the body, and measurement of residues in the body or excreted in the urine.

The former procedure, generally termed "direct measurement", involves monitoring of dermal and inhalation exposure during typical field operations. Methods for these measurements have been developed and field tested over the last twenty years (2,4,17). For dermal exposure, pads constructed of layers of gauze or absorbent paper are taped to the skin or outside the clothing of the workers. Spray droplets or particulate matter containing the pesticide residues are retained by the pads; analysis of the pads gives a surface concentration of the pesticide for the part of the body being measured. Inhalation exposure is measured by small portable air samplers which collect air on filter casettes from the breathing zone of the workers, or by filter respirators worn by

the workers which trap vapor and particulates. In some cases high
volume air samples set up at the work site are used to collect
larger air samples for more sensitive analyses.

A special problem in field exposure monitoring is measurement
of exposure to the hands. The hands often have the highest
exposure, but the pads are not convenient since they interfere with
normal activity. Periodic washing of the hands with alcohol in
plastic bags has been used to measure surface residues, as have
absorbent cotton gloves. Each method has drawbacks: the hand
washing may underestimate exposure, since it can only be carried
out sporadically; also, repeated washing with solvent irritates the
skin. The absorbant gloves may overestimate exposure since they
may retain residues more efficiently than the skin.

When these direct methods of exposure monitoring are used, a
measure of the efficiency of absorption is needed in order to
convert the observed external exposure levels to an actual internal
dose. The absorption of chemicals through the skin is a complex
process, and data on extent of penetration of pesticides are
generally not available. Feldmann and Maibach (8) reported
absorption data for twelve pesticide chemicals applied in acetone
solution to the forearm of human subjects. The percent absorption,
calculated by measuring urinary excretion of radiolabelled material
and correcting for incomplete excretion, ranged from less than one
percent of the applied dose for diquat to 73.9% for carbaryl. The
extent of absorption varies with anatomic region (8); the presence
or absence of abrasions and the extent of perspiration also
influence the extent of absorption.

Measurement of actual residues in the body or in urine,
generally termed "indirect methods", circumvent these
difficulties. Clearly, detection of pesticide residues in human
tissue, blood or urine is prima facie evidence of exposure.
However, it is often difficult to back-calculate from an observed
residue level to the actual internal dose received, since data on
pharmacodynamics of pesticides in humans are usually not
available. For pesticides that are well studied and whose
metabolites are efficiently excreted in urine, such as phosphate
esters or phenoxy herbicides, exposure has been calculated by
analysis of urine for several days following a single instance of
either oral or dermal exposure (12, 15).

Another difficulty with these indirect methods is that the
observed residue levels in body tissues or fluids often cannot be
connected to a specific route or instance of exposure. This
consideration is very important when considering regulatory actions
designed to decrease exposure and risk. For example,
pentachlorophenol was found in 85 percent of human urine samples
collected in a nationwide survey, at a mean level of 6 ppb, while

occupationally exposed groups had much higher levels (7).
Pentachlorophenol is used as a wood preservative, a herbicide, a
slimicide, and as a preserving agent for adhesives, rubber,
textiles, oils, and other materials; it is also a degradation
product of other chlorinated organic compounds. It is difficult to
determine the source of the observed urinary levels in the general
population; in the absence of more specific information, EPA
concluded that the wood preservative use, which accounts for about
80% of the total use, was the most likely source (7).

Exposure Monitoring Results

A great many field monitoring studies of pesticide applicator
exposure have been carried out, using either the direct methods or
a combination of both types of methods. Generally, skin patches
are placed on several parts of the body, such as forehead, chest,
back, upper arms, and thighs. Dermal exposure is calculated by
multiplying the surface concentration as measured by each pad by
the area of the part of the body represented by the pad and summing
the results. Inhalation exposure is calculated either by
multiplying the observed air concentration by a standard breathing
rate or by simply using the amount found on the respirator
filter. The total exposure is the sum of the exposure by each
route, and is usually presented as milligrams per kilogram body
weight per hour of exposure.

One conclusion that may be drawn from all of these studies is
that the dermal route of exposure quite generally predominates
during pesticide application. Except in cases where the pesticide
in question is highly volatile, such as in the case of fumigants,
the amount of pesticide coming in contact with the skin appears to
be roughly two orders of magnitude greater than that available for
inhalation. Thus, even if dermal absorption is much less efficient
than absorption through the lung, the dermal route appears to make
the major contribution to the total exposure.

A second conclusion from these studies is that exposure of the
hands makes the largest contribution to the dermal exposure. Better
methods of measurement of hand exposure are thus important, not
only to quantify this exposure but also to evaluate the
effectiveness of the various types of glove material and design.

In principle, exposure monitoring studies could be carried out
for every pesticide, and for each application technique by which
the pesticide is applied. However, this would be a massive
undertaking, since an enormous number of pesticide products are
registered, and a large variety of application techniques are in
common use. Comparison of many studies carried out with different
pesticides but using the same application technique leads to the
conclusion that a dominant factor in many cases is the physical

process of application. In other words, the characteristics of the spray cloud, such as the type of carrier solvent, the number of spray droplets, their size, surface tensions, and trajectories, are often more important in determining deposition on skin than the identity of the pesticide dissolved in the spray solution. As an example, for high volume spraying of dilute aqueous suspensions of pesticides by speed sprayer equipment, exposure measurements from many field monitoring studies indicate that applicator exposure is generally in the range of about 10 - 100 milligrams per hour, or about 1 - 10 milligrams per kilogram per day for a 70 kilogram applicator working eight hours per day (1,10,18-21). These exposures were calculated from the field monitoring data on the basis that wor:ers were wearing minimal protective clothing, so the face, neck, forearms and hands would be exposed; also, these calculations make no assumption about the efficiency of absorption, but merely present the amount of pesticide deposited on the skin.

It appears from this type of data that reasonable assessments of applicator exposure may be made for other pesticides when they are applied by the same technique. Parameters unique to the exposure situation under consideration may easily by included, such as specific information about dermal absorption of a particular pesticide or the use of protective clothing. Exposure assessments based on this approach have been used by EPA as part of the risk assessment process (5).

There is less information available about exposure arising from other pesticide application techniques, although many studies are now being carried out by pesticide registrants, by the United States Department of Agriculture, by various State agencies, and by the Environmental Protection Agency. We hope in the near future to have compiled sufficient exposure data for many common pesticide application techniques to allow reasonable assessments of potential exposure to be made without the necessity of carrying out field studies.

Reentry Exposure

People who enter pesticide-treated fields incur exposure by different physical mechanisms, as noted earlier. The extreme variability of superficial pesticide residue levels in treated sites has made exposure assessment a much more uncertain endeavor. In recent years a few exposure monitoring studies similar to those described above for applicators have been carried out (3, 13, 16). One purpose of these studies has been to search for a correlation between the residues at the site and the resulting exposure. Such a correlation is heavily dependent on the crop and on the type of activity: picking citrus fruits involves much more foliar contact than thinning low-growing row crops, for example. The many difficulties involved in assessing persistence

of pesticide dislodgeable residues on crops and estimating the
levels of exposure to fieldworkers have been extensively reviewed
in recent publications (9,11). Availability of these correlations
would allow estimates of exposure to be made by measuring residues
at the site, using relatively simple techniques. The overall goal
of this research effort is to minimize exposure and risk, by
establishing periods of time after application before which workers
may not enter treated fields (called "reentry invervals"), by
specifying protective clothing, or perhaps other methods. Much
research needs to be completed in the general area of reentry
exposure assessment in order to obtain reliable estimates of this
type of exposure.

Research Needs

Reliable exposure assessment procedures require a vast array
of information about all facets of the exposure process. Our
general knowledge of human exposure to pesticides is much better
than it was a few years ago, but many gaps remain. More
information on efficiency of absorption of pesticides through the
skin is particularly needed, since the dermal route of exposure is
so important. The effectivenes of protective clothing needs
further study, since the potential for controlling and minimizing
exposure is very important. The use of mixing and loading devices
which permit transfer of concentrated pesticides by a competely
closed transfer system is a relatively recent development which
also may greatly diminish exposure; the potential of these devices
needs to be investigated (6). Finally, the different mechanisms of
exposure during entry into pesticide-treated work sites require
study in order to understand and limit this path of exposure.

CONCLUSIONS

In the past, the concern for human exposure was largely due to
the potential for acute toxic effects of pesticides. The chronic
toxicology properties of pesticides require more detailed
information regarding extent and duration of exposure. Risk
assessments for chronic effects generally involve some kind of
extrapolation from dose-response data generated in laboratory
animals, and reliable estimates of exposure are needed as input to
these extrapolations. Methods for field exposure monitoring have
been developed, and much data have been collected and evaluated.
Further research is needed on methods of controlling exposure.

REFERENCES
  1. Comer, S. W., D. C. Staiff, J. F. Armstrong, and H. R. Wolfe,
     1975. Exposure of Workers to Carbaryl. Bull. Environ.
     Contam. Tox. 13, 385-391.
  2. Davis, J. A., 1980. Minimizing Occupational Exposure to
     Pesticides: Personnel Monitoring. Res. Rev. 75, 33-50.

3. Davis, J. E., D. C. Staiff, L. C. Butler, and E. R. Stevens, 1981. Potential Exposure to Dislodgeable Residues after Application of Two Formulations of Methyl Parathion to Apple Trees. Bull. Environ. Contam. Tox., 27, 95-100.
4. Durham, W. F., and H. R. Wolfe, 1962. Measurements of the Exposure of Workers to Pesticides. Bull. WHO 26, 75-91.
5. EPA, 1978. Notice of Determination Concluding the Rebuttable Presumption Against Registration and Continued Registration of Pesticide Products Containing Chlorobenzilate; Availability of Position Document. Fed. Reg. 43, 29824-29828.
6. EPA, 1979. Closed System Packaging - Advance Notice of Proposed Rulemaking. Fed. Reg. 44, 54508.
7. EPA, 1981. Position Document No. 2/3: Creosote, Inorganic Arsenicals, Pentachlorophenol. January, 1981.
8. Feldmann, R. J., and H. I. Maibach, 1974. Percutaneous Penetration of Some Pesticides and Herbicides in Man. Tox. Appl. Pharm. 28, 126-132.
9. Gunther, F. A., Y. Iwata, G. E. Carman, and C.A. Smith, 1977. The Citrus Reentry Problem; Research on its Causes and Effects, and Approaches to its Minimization. Res. Rev. 67, 1-139.
10. Hickey, K. D. 1981. Dermal and Respiratory Exposure of Orchard Airblast Sprayer Operators to Benomyl, Mancozeb and Ethylene During Loading and Spraying. Final Report under Research Agreement No. 801-15-73, U. S. Dept of Agriculture/National Association of Pesticide Impact Assessment Program.
11. Knaak, J. B., 1980. Minimizing Occupational Exposure to Pesticides: Techniques for Establishing Safe Levels of Foliar Residues. Res. Rev. 75, 81-96.
12. Lavy, T. L., J. S. Sheppard, and J. D. Mattice, 1980. Exposure Measurements of Applicators Spraying (2,4,5-Trichlorophenoxy)-Acetic Acid in the Forest. J. Ag. Food Chem. 28, 626-630.
13. Maddy, K. T., W. Cusick, S. Edmiston, and C. Cooper, 1980. A Study of Dermal Exposure of Field Workers Picking Lemons to Residues of Chlorobenzilate in Ventura County, California. California Dept. of Food and Agriculture Report No. HS-781, November 28, 1980.
14. Maibach, H. I., and R. Feldmann, 1974. Systemic Absorption of Pesticides Through the Skin of Man. In Occupation Exposure to Pesticides (report to the Federal Working Group on Pest Management from the Task Group on Occupational Exposure to Pesticides, January 1974).
15. Morgan, D. P., H. L. Hetzler, E. F. Slach, and L. I. Lin, 1977. Urinary Excretion of Paranitrophenol and Alkyl Phosphates Following Ingestion of Methyl or Ethyl Parathion by Human Subjects. Arch. Environ. Contam. Tox. 6, 159-173.
16. Popendorf. W., 1980. Exploring Citrus Harvesters' Exposure to Pesticide Contaminated Foliar Dust. Am. Ind. Hyg. Assoc. J. 41, 652-659.

17. Siewierski, M., 1981 (ed.). Determination and Assessment of
     Pesticide Exposure. Proceedings of a Symposium, Hershey, PA,
     October 1980. In press.
18. Wojeck, G. A., H. N. Nigg, J. H. Stamper. and D. E. Bradway,
     1981. Worker Exposure to Ethion in Florida Citrus. Arch.
     Environ. Contam. Tox. In Press.
19. Wojeck, G. A., H. N. Nigg, R. S. Braman, J. H. Stamper, and R.
     L. Rouseff, 1981. Worker Exposure to Arsenic on Grapefruit in
     Florida. Arch. Environ. Contam. Tox., In press.
20. Wolfe, H. R., W. F. Durham, and J. F. Armstrong, 1967.
     Exposure of Workers to Pesticides. Arch. Environ. Health 14,
     622-633.
21. Wolfe, H. R., J. F. Armstrong, D.C. Staiff, and S. W. Comer,
     1972. Exposure of Spraymen to Pesticides. Arch. Environ.
     Health 25, 29-31.

MUTAGENS IN COOKED FOOD

Takashi Sugimura

National Cancer Center Research Institute
Tokyo, Japan

INTRODUCTION

The incidences of cancers in various organs of the body differ in different countries (14,100). For instance, in Japan stomach cancer is the predominant cancer of the digestive tract, but in most Western countries intestinal cancer is predominant. Japanese immigrants to the United States show a decrease in the incidence of stomach cancer with an increase in that of intestinal cancer, presumably because of change in their life style (34).

By the age of 50, humans have ingested an average of 10 tons dry weight of food (74) and 40 tons of water as components of food and drinks. Thus hazardous components of these foods and drinks may have had an appreciable impact. This may be especially true of mutagens and carcinogens, including tumor initiators and tumor promoters.

Components of food have been studied mainly from the standpoint of nutrient components in relation to the incidences of various cancers in different countries. Variations in the amounts of the main components of food, proteins, fats, carbohydrates and fiber, have various effects on the incidences of spontaneous and experimental cancer in animals, as already demonstrated in the early 1940s (86). Epidemiological data also clearly support the idea that food components greatly influence the incidences of cancer in various organs. For instance, fat intake shows an almost linear dose-relation with the incidence of breast cancer in various countries (4,10).

However, the detection of carcinogens or mutagens in foods was not studied extensively until the development of Ames' method for the detection of mutagens (3), because other methods were tedious

and unpractical, and only known carcinogens, such as aromatic
hydrocarbons, could be detected easily by chemical analyses.

However many compounds known to be probable human carcinogens,
such as aflatoxin B_1 (38), and nitrosamines (96), were found as
contaminants of foods and animal feeds. Most foods are agricultural products, and consequently the main source of mutagens and
carcinogens in food is related to agriculture.

Comprehensive information on these environmental mutagens is
integrated into various papers in this volume. Therefore this
paper is concerned mainly with mutagens and carcinogens recently
identified in the author's laboratories as constituents of foods.

MUTAGENS FORMED DURING COOKING

Pioneering studies were made on aromatic hydrocarbon analysis
of broiled foods by Lijinski and Shubik (44). Based on the observation of overlap of the mutagenic and carcinogenic potentials of
over several hundred compounds (49,67,81), an intensive search for
new carcinogens in cooked food was initiated by the microbial
mutation test. As shown in Figure 1, broiling of fish resulted in
the appearance of mutagenicity (57,75,78,79). Since pyrolysis of
protein was shown to cause the formation of mutagens (56),
pyrolysates of single amino acids were examined (78). As a result,
Trp-P-1 (3-amino-1,4-dimethyl-5H-pyrido[4,3-b]indole) and Trp-P-2
(3-amino-1-methyl-5H-pyrido[4,3-b]indole) were isolated as new
compounds from a tryptophan pyrolysate (77), Glu-P-1 (2-amino-6-

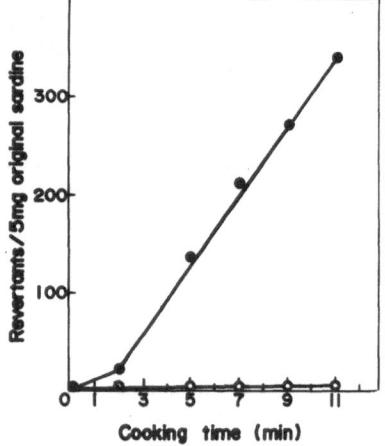

Fig. 1. Mutagenicity of sun-dried sardines broiled at various
         times. S. typhimurium TA98 with (●) and without (o) S9
         mix was used for the assay.

methyldipyrido[1,2-a:3',2'-d]imidazole) and Glu-P-2 (2-amino-dipyrido[1,2-a:3',2'-d]imidazole) were obtained from a pyrolysate of glutamic acid (104), Lys-P-1 (3,4-cyclopentenopyrido[3,2-a]carbazole) was obtained from a pyrolysate of lysine (95), Orn-P-1 (4-amino-6-methyl-1H-2,5,10,10b-tetraazafluoranthene) was obtained from a pyrolysate of ornithine (108) and Phe-P-1 (2-amino-5-phenylpyridine) was obtained from a pyrolysate of phenylalanine (77). AαC (2-amino-9H-pyrido[2,3-b]indole) and MeAαC (2-amino-3-methyl-9H-pyrido[2,3-b]indole) were isolated from a pyrolysate of soy bean globulin by Yoshida et al. (109). Trp-P-1, Trp-P-2, Glu-P-2, AαC and MeAαC were detected in broiled, fried, and grilled food stuffs, especially fish and meat (47,101-103).

New mutagens were also recently isolated from broiled sun-dried sardines; namely, IQ (2-amino-3-methylimidazo[4,5-f]quinoline) (40) and MeIQ (2-amino-3,4-dimethylimidazo[4,5-f]quinoline) (42). A new mutagen MeIQx (2-amino-3,8-dimethyl-imidazo[4,5-f]quinoxaline) was also isolated from fried beef (41). Most of these compounds are heterocyclic amines, and their abbreviated and chemical names and structures are given in Table 1. Table 2 shows the sources from which these compounds were first isolated and the substances in which they have since been found. Some of them have very strong mutagenicity toward Salmonella typhimurium, especially TA98, as shown in Table 3. Data on other typical carcinogens are also included in this table. It is clear that some newly isolated compounds are stronger mutagens than aflatoxin B_1.

The metabolisms of Trp-P-2 and Glu-P-1 have been studied most extensively. Cytochrome P-448, induced by 3-methylcholanthrene, is responsible for the conversion of the amino groups of these hetero-cyclic amines to hydroxylamino groups (39,106). These hydroxyl-amino groups are then acylated to yield ultimate forms that react readily with DNA bases (30). The structures of the adducts of Trp-P-2 and Glu-P-1 with guanine bases in DNA were found to be as shown in Figure 2 (28,29). One of the acylation reactions involves ATP, amino acids such as serine and amino acid activating enzymes. The ultimate form is probably seryl-hydroxylamino-derivative (107). Similar results were reported earlier for activation of 4-hydroxyaminoquinoline 1-oxide (83).

In vivo carcinogenicity experiments on Trp-P-1, Trp-P-2, Glu-P-1, Glu-P-2, AαC and MeAαC are complete, or will soon be complete. Results on Trp-P-1 and Trp-P-2 (46) are given in Table 4. It is noteworthy that female mice are more susceptible than males to these compounds. The additions of Glu-P-1 and Glu-P-2 at 0.05% to the diet and of AαC and MeAαC at 0.08% for 15 months produced many hepatomas, and as with Trp-P-1 and Trp-P-2, these heterocyclic amines induced more hepatomas in female mice than in males. A further interesting feature is that Glu-P-1, Glu-P-2,

Table 1.   Abbreviations, chemical names and structures of
             pyrolysate mutagens

Abbreviation	Chemical name	Structure
Trp-P-1	3-Amino-1,4,-dimethyl-5H-pyrido[4,3-b]indole	
Trp-P-2	3-Amino-1-methyl-5H-pyrido[4,3-b]indole	
Glu-P-1	2-Amino-6-methyldipyrido-[1,2-a:3',2'-d]imidazole	
Glu-P-2	2-Aminodipyrido[1,2-a:3',2'-d]-imidazole	
Lys-P-1	3,4-Cyclopentenopyrido-[3,2-a]carbazole	
Orn-P-1	4-Amino-6-methyl-1H-2,5,10,10b-tetraazafluoranthene	
Phe-P-1	2-Amino-5-phenylpyridine	
AαC	2-Amino-9H-pyrido[2,3-b]indole	
MeAαC	2-Amino-3-methyl-9H-pyrido-[2,3-b]indole	

Table 1. Continued

Abbreviation	Chemical name	Structure
IQ	2-Amino-3-methylimidazo-[4,5-f]quinoline	
MeIQ	2-Amino-3,4-dimethyl-imidazo[4,5-f]quinoline	
MeIQx	2-Amino-3,8-dimethyl-imidazo[4,5-f]quinoxaline	

AαC, and MeAαC induced hemoangioendothelial sarcomas in subcutaneous tissue between the scapulae in almost all mice even though the carcinogens were given orally, and there was no sex difference in the incidence of these sarcomas. The carcinogenicities of other heterocyclic amines, including IQ, are being examined. Although some heterocyclic amines are mutagenic, their carcinogenic potentials are not very high. In Figure 3, TD_{50} values, the doses inducing tumors in 50% of the animals, are shown on the ordinate and mutagenic potentials, expressed as numbers of revertants of Salmonella typhimurium either TA98 or TA100 per μg are shown on the abscissa. It is clear that plots for these new mutagens deviated greatly from those obtained for some typical carcinogens. Nevertheless these newly isolated mutagens may have a significant carcinogenic effect. AαC and MeAαC are 10^2 orders less mutagenic than Trp-P-1, Trp-P-2, Glu-P-1 and Glu-P-2, but their carcinogenicities are in the same order as those of other heterocyclic amines. The concentrations of AαC and MeAαC in protein pyrolysates are probably 10^2-fold greater and therefore these chemicals with lower specific mutagenic activity may be important as carcinogens.

We are now measuring the amounts of these heterocyclic amines in cooked foods by partial purification and gas chromatography/mass spectrometry with multiple ion detection (80). No standard method for their quantitative analysis suitable for routine assay has yet been established, but available data suggest that these hetero-cyclic amines are not present at sufficiently high concentrations in cooked foods to be strongly hazardous to humans. However, they may have synergistic actions with other environmental mutagens and multipotentiating actions with environmental tumor promoters, which

Table 2. Sources of isolation of pyrolysate mutagens and their
          presence in various materials

Compound	Source	Present in
Trp-P-1	Tryptophan pyrolysate	Broiled sardine Broiled beef
Trp-P-2	"	Broiled sardine
Glu-P-1	Glutamic acid pyrolysate	
Glu-P-2	"	Broiled sun-dried cuttlefish
Lys-P-1	Lysine pyrolysate	
Orn-P-1	Ornithine pyrolysate	
Phe-P-1	Phenylalanine pyrolysate	
AαC	Soybean globulin pyrolysate	Cigarette smoke condensate Grilled beef Grilled chicken Grilled Chinese mushroom
MeAαC	"	"
IQ	Broiled sardine	Heated beef extract
MeIQ	"	
MeIQx	Fried beef	

would greatly enhance their hazard to humans. Formation of these
mutagens during cooking could be reduced by avoiding over-cooking
of fish and meat, especially by not exposing these foods to a naked
flame.

It should be mentioned here that all these heterocyclic amines
are rapidly inactivated by dilute hypochlorite ion solution, such
as 1.5 ppm, which is almost equivalent to the concentration in city
tap water (90). All heterocyclic amines except IQ, MeIQ and MeIQx
were rapidly converted to hydroxy derivatives by deamination in the
presence of low concentration of nitrite ion at low pH (88,89).

Table 3. Specific mutagenic activities of pyrolysate mutagens and
          typical carcinogens toward S. typhimurium TA 98 and
          TA 100

	Revertants of TA98/μg		Revertants of TA100/μg
MeIQ[b]	661,000	AF-2[a]	42,000
IQ[b]	433,000	MeIQ[b]	30,000
MeIQx[b]	145,000	Aflatoxin B₁[b]	28,000
Trp-P-2[b]	104,000	MeIQx[b]	14,000
Orn-P-1[d]	57,000	4NQO[a]	9,900
Glu-P-1[c]	49,000	IQ[b]	7,000
Trp-P-1[b]	39,000	Glu-P-1[c]	3,200
AF-2[a]	6,500	Trp-P-2[b]	1,800
Aflatoxin B₁[b]	6,000	Trp-P-1[b]	1,700
Glu-P-2[c]	1,900	Glu-P-2[c]	1,200
4NQO[a]	970	MNNG[a]	870
B[a]P[b]	320	B[a]P[b]	660
AαC[d]	300	MeAαC[d]	120
MeAαC[d]	200	Lys-P-1[d]	99
Lys-P-1[d]	86	Phe-P-1[d]	23
Phe-P-1[d]	41	AαC[d]	20
DEN[d]	0.02	DMN[d]	0.23
DMN[d]	0.00	DEN[d]	0.15
MNNG[a]	0.00		

Amount of S9 per plate: a, without S9; b, 10 μl, c, 30 μl; d, 150 μl

AF-2, 2-(2-furyl)-3-(5-nitro-2-furyl)acrylamide, DEN, N,N-diethylnitrosamine;

DMN, N,N-dimethylnitrosamine; 4NQO, 4-nitroquinoline 1-oxide; MNNG,

N-methyl-N'-nitro-N-nitrosoguanidine.

This differential inactivation has been used for identification of
the percentage contributions of IQ-type mutagens (IQ, MeIQ and
MeIQx) and non-IQ type mutagens to the total mutagenic activity of
broiled food and examples are shown in Table 5.

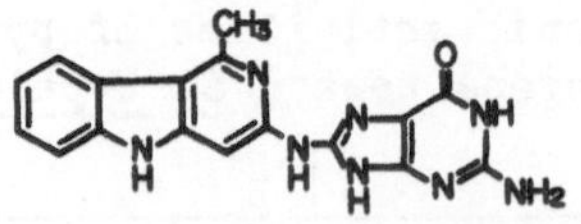

3-(C⁸-guanyl)amino-1-methyl-5H-pyrido[4,3-b]indole

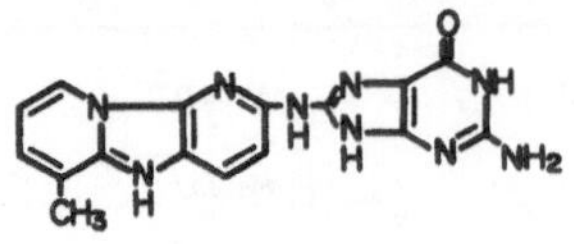

2-(C⁸-guanyl)amino-6-methyldipyrido[1,2-a:3',2'-d]imidazole

Fig. 2. Structures of the adducts of Trp-P-2 and Glu-P-1 with
         guanine base in DNA.

MUTAGENS IN BEVERAGES AND VEGETABLES

    Mutagens were found by Ames' test in coffee (1,60), tea
(60,85,92), alcoholic spirits (59), wines (85), and spices
(23,70). These mutagens could be divided into two classes. One
type, which is active without metabolic activation, is more active
on TA100 than TA98. This type of mutagen is found in coffee (1,60)
and evaporated residues of whisky and brandy (59), and its mutagenicity is almost completely abolished by incubation with S9

Table 4. Incidence of hepatic tumors in CDF_1 mice induced by
          Trp-P-1 and Trp-P-2

Treatment	Sex	Effective number	Hepatocellular tumor		Hemangioma	Total (%)
			Adenoma	Carcinoma		
Trp-P-1[a]	Male	24	1	4	0	5 (21)
	Female	26	2	14	0	16 (62)
Trp-P-2[a]	Male	25	1	3	0	4 (16)
	Female	24	0	22	0	22 (92)
None	Male	25	0	0	1	1 (4)
	Female	24	0	0	0	0 (0)

[a]0.02% of Trp-P-1 and Trp-P-2 in the diet was given.

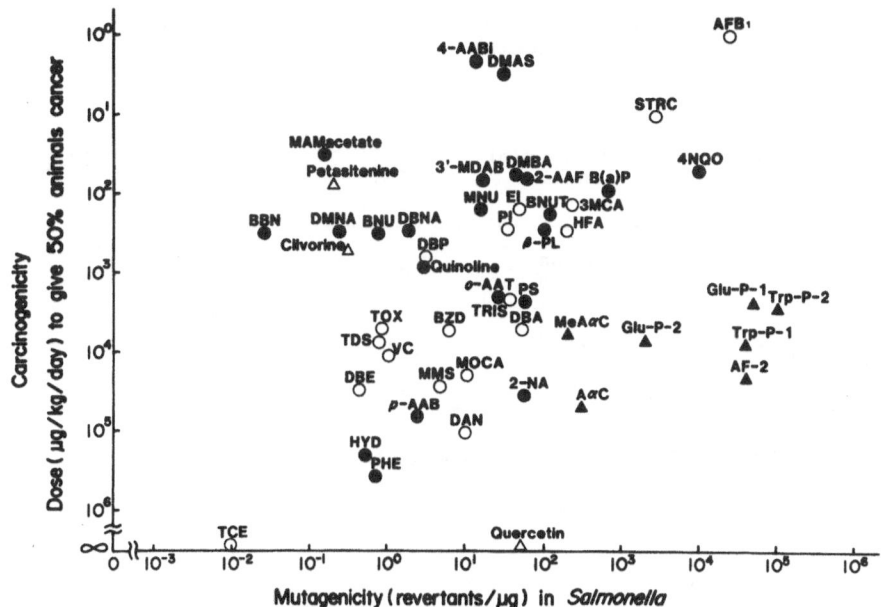

Fig. 3. Relationship between mutagenicity in S. typhimurium and
carcinogenicity. Abbreviations used: p-AAB, p-
aminoazobenzene; 4-AABi, 4-acetylaminobiphenyl; 2-AAF, 2-
acetylaminofluorene; o-AAT, o-aminoazotoluene; AFB₁,
aflatoxin B₁; BBN, N-butyl-N-butanolnitrosamine; BNU, N-n-
butyl-N-nitrosourea; BNUT, N-n-butyl-N-nitrosourethane;
B(a)P, benzo[a]pyrene; BZD, benzidine, DAN, 2,4-
diaminoanisole; DBA, dibenz[a,h]anthracene; DBE, 1,2-
dibromoethane; DBNA, N,N-di-n-butylnitrosamine; DBP, 1,2-
diboromochloropropane; DMAS, 4-dimethylaminostilbene;
DMBA, 7,12-dimethylbenz[a]anthracene; DMNA, N,N-
dimethylnitrosamine; EI, ethyleneimine; HFA, N-hydroxy-2-
acetylaminofluorene; HYD, hydralazine; MAM acetate,
methylazoxymethanol acetate; 3MCA, 3-methylcholanthrene;
3'-MDAB, 3'-methyl-4-dimethylaminoazobenzene; MMS, methyl
methanesulfonate; MOCA, 4,4'-methylene-bis(2-
chloroaniline); 2NA, 2-naphthylamine; PHE, phenacetin; PI,
propyleneimine; β-PL, β-propiolactone; PS, propane
sultone; STRC, sterigmatocystin; TCE, trichloroethylene;
TDS, toluenediamino sulfate; TOX, toxaphene; TRIS,
tris(2,3-dibromopropylphosphate); VC, vinylchloride.

mix. The other type, which is more active with metabolic
activation by S9 mix, is more effective on TA98 than TA100.
Mutagens in tea (60,92) and spices such as sumac (70) and dill
weed (23) and in certain vegetable pickles (84) and vegetable and
fruit juices (48) belong to this type.

Table 5. Mutagenicity of broiled sardines and fried beef after
          treatment with nitrite and hypochlorite

Basic fraction	$\dfrac{\text{Revertants/ml}}{\text{mg/ml}}$	Relative mutagenicity (%)		
		None	Nitrite (20mM)	Hypochlorite (2.5mM)
Sardines	$\dfrac{3,200}{0.20}$	100	37	12
Fried beef	$\dfrac{2,990}{1.70}$	100	53	2

Mutagenicity was assayed by S. typhimurium TA98 with S9 mix.

Reaction with nitrite was performed in 0.1N HCl for 30 min at 37°C.

The first class of mutagens are mainly produced by pyrolysis
of carbohydrate and found in substances such as caramel (43,73) and
their actual chemical structures have not yet been clarified.
Table 6 shows their mutagenic activities calculated per cup or
glass of coffee, whisky, and brandy. The mutagenic activity in
coffee was recently found to be inactivated by dilute sulfite
ion (82), as demonstrated in Figure 4. Brewed coffee, ordinary
instant coffee, and caffeine-free instant coffee showed similar
levels of mutagenic activity and this was abolished by sulfite.
There are epidemiological reports on the relation between coffee
drinking and the incidence of pancreatic cancer (45,64), so the
importance of mutagens in coffee should not be underestimated.
However, the presence of mutagens in coffee does not necessarily
mean the presence of carcinogens in coffee. It has been shown that
raw green coffee beans do not show any mutagenic activity so the
mutagens are probably produced during roasting of the beans. 1,2-
Dicarbonyls such as diacetyl and maltol have been found in
coffee (24). These compounds are mutagenic to Salmonella
typhimurium TA100 without metabolic activation (6) and the mutagenicity of diacetyl is abolished by adding sulfite (82). However,
it is not sure whether 1,2-dicarbonyls account for all the mutagenicity of coffee.

Addition of coffee powder to the diet did not induce cancer in
animals (99), but further studies are required in the isolation and
identification of mutagenic substances in coffee, and then in vivo

Table 6. Mutagenic activities induced by one cup of coffee or one glass of whisky and brandy

	Number of revertants[a]
Coffee[b]	135,000
Whisky[c]	3,600
Brandy[c]	8,000

[a]S. typhimurium TA100 without S9 mix was used.

[b]One cup contained 150 ml coffee

[c]One glass contained 30 ml whisky or brandy

long-term experiments on the carcinogenic effects of these mutagens in coffee should be carried out.

Whiskies, brandies, and apple brandy have mutagenic potentials (59). Evaporated residues from these alcoholic beverages were dissolved in DMSO and tested for mutagenicity. The mutagenic activities of different brands varied very much. Newly distilled whisky did not show mutagenic activity, but the mutagenicity seemed to appear during storage in a wooden barrel. In this connection it is interesting to note that the inside of some barrels is burned before the barrels are used for storage of whiskies and brandies. The mutagenicity of whisky was demonstrated without S9 mix and was stronger on Salmonella typhimurium TA100 than on TA98 (59).

Black tea, green tea, and Japanese roasted tea showed mutagenic activity toward Salmonella typhimurium TA100 without S9 mix (60). The mutagenic potencies of these teas prepared in the ordinary way varied from 1.7×10^4 to 3.8×10^4 revertants of TA100 per cup, and the mutagenic activity was abolished by incubation with S9 mix. Black tea and green tea were also mutagenic to TA98 in the presence of S9 mix after treatment with the glycosidase hesperidinase from Aspergillus niger (60,92). The mutagens to TA98 probably exist in the form of glycoside(s) in teas and they are probably glycoside(s) of a flavonoid such as quercetin or kaempferol (60,92).

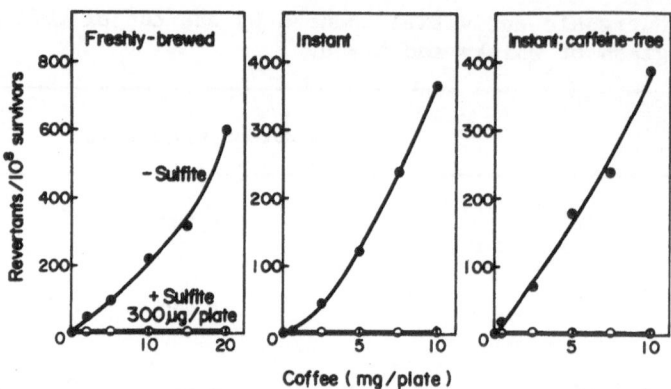

Fig. 4.   Inactivation of the mutagenicity of coffees by sulfite.
Mutagenicity was assayed by S. typhimurium TA100 without
S9 mix.

Red wines are mutagenic to TA98 after treatment with fecalase
from human intestine (85). Orange juice is also known to contain a
similar mutagen(s) (48). These compounds may also be flavonol
glycosides (48).

Various spices have been tested for mutagenic activity. Among
them dill weed was shown to contain much mutagen toward Salmonella
typhimurium TA98 (23). The mutagenic components in spices were
identified as quercetin-3-sulfate and isorhamnetin-3-sulfate
(23). S9 mix was absolutely necessary to convert sulfate esters of
flavonols to free flavonols. Sumac was also mutagenic to TA98, and
the mutagenic component was purified and characterized as a free
flavonoid, quercetin (70).

We found that pickles from Linhsien county in China, where
there is a high incidence of esophageal cancer, contained mutagens
(52,84). A kind of Japanese pickles that is similar in appearance
to Linhsien pickles was found to contain one sixth of the mutagenic
activity of the Chinese pickles and the main mutagenic component
was identified as kaempferol, with isorhamnetin as a minor component (84).

Many flavonoids are mutagenic (8,58). The most widely distributed flavonols in agricultural products are quercetin and its
glycoside, rutin and kaempferol and its glycoside, astragalin.
Kaempferol requires S9 mix for mutagenic activity but quercetin is
mutagenic even without S9 mix although its mutagenicity is enhanced
by S9 mix (58).

Various vegetables and edible plants contain mutagens and
carcinogens. The most well known example is bracken fern
(19,22,36). Diet containing bracken induces tumors of the large

intestine and urinary bladder in rodents (19,36), but the active
carcinogenic principle has not yet been determined. Carcinogenic
pyrrolizidine alkaloids are present in edible plants such as colts-
foot (Petasites japonicus Maxim. and Tussialago farfara L.) and
comfrey (Symphytum officinale L.), which are eaten by Japanese
people (13,35). Feeding of these plants to rats resulted in development of hepatocellular carcinomas and hemoangioendothelial
sarcomas of the liver (35). Fukinotoxin (petasitenine) from colts-
foot and symphytine from comfrey are carcinogenic pyrrolizidine
alkaloids and have been demonstrated to be mutagenic to Salmonella
typhimurium TA100 in the presence of S9 mix by the preincubation
method (105).

    Some beans, such as Vicia fava, are mutagenic after incubation
with nitrite under weakly acidic conditions (66). This means that
the beans contain substances that can be nitrosated and the
nitrosated compounds are mutagenic. The chemical structures of
these mutagens have not yet been established, but the presence of
precursors of nitroso compounds with mutagenicity should not be
overlooked.

    Flavonoids are mutagens found ubiquitously in plants and it is
very important to determine their carcinogenicity. In most cases,
when mutagenic substances are purified from mutagenic extracts of
plants, most of the mutagenicity is found to be due to flavonoids. The most frequently found flavonols, quercetin and
kaempferol, are the most highly mutagenic (58). Quercetin also has
other genotoxic properties: It produced mutations (2,51), chromosomal aberrations (110), and sister chromatid exchanges (110) in
mammalian cells cultured in vitro. Moreover, oral or intraperitoneal injection of quercetin is reported to induce micronulei
in rodents (68), although we could not confirm this. We tested the
in vivo carcinogenicity of quercetin in mice (69), rats (37), and
hamsters (55) and also that of rutin in rats (37) and hamsters
(55), but have not so far demonstrated the carcinogenicities of
these compounds. However, there is one report that diet containing
quercetin results in the formation of neoplasmas in the large intestine and urinary bladder of rats (65). Since most typical carcinogens are mutagenic, it is reasonable to expect that quercetin
is carcinogenic in vivo. Quercetin is active not only in the
microbial mutation test but also in cultured mammalian cell
systems, but at present, results on its carcinogenicity are contradictory and further experiments are required on this subject.
Quercetin is also reported to suppress the hepatocarcinogenicity of
DAB in rats (61), and it inhibits the activity of arylhydrocarbon
hydroxylase (9,98). Thus it may suppress the activity of P-450 in
metabolic activation of quercetin. But the metabolic enhancement
of quercetin mutagenicity by S9 mix depends on the supernatant
fraction, not microsomal enzymes. Recently quercetin was discovered to inhibit the biological activities of the tumor promoter,
12-0-tetradecanoylphorbol-13-acetate (TPA) such as its stimulation
of phospholipid metabolism. These effects of quercetin may explain

why it is not carcinogenic to animals when given at a relatively
high concentration.

IMPORTANCE OF TUMOR PROMOTERS

Mutagens in the environment have two hazardous effects on
humans. One is an effect on germ cells and the other is an effect
on somatic cells. The latter effect is important since mutation of
certain genes of somatic cells is closely related to the step of
initiation in carcinogenesis. Carcinogenesis is completed by the
step of promotion, for which tumor promoters are necessary. This
two-step process, first demonstrated in mouse skin (5), is now
considered to be common to carcinogenesis in various organs.

The presence of tumor promoters in agricultural products
should be investigated like that of mutagens, namely tumor initiators. However, no efficient method of screening for environmental
tumor promoters has yet been established. Many compounds have been
tested by a four-step test; 1) irritancy to mouse ear, 2) induction
of ornithine decarboxylase (ODC) in mouse skin, 3) induction of
adhesion of cultured human leukemic cells (HL-60), and 4) a long-
term two-step carcinogenesis test on mouse skin (21). Many food
stuffs, such as oil, and materials related to foods have also been
tested, and results by these four sequential steps are summarized
in Table 7. Of 270 compounds tested, 3 were shown to be tumor
promoters, namely teleocidin (20,21,76) from a fungus Streptomyces
mediocidicus, lyngbyatoxin (20,21) from a seaweed Lyngbya
majuscula, and aplysiatoxin (21) from another variety of Lyngbya
majuscula. The structures of these new tumor promoters are given
in Figure 5. Before the discovery of these new tumor promoters,
TPA was the only strong tumor promoter known (31,93). TPA was
isolated from croton oil, oil of the seeds of Croton tiglium L.
Phorbol esters and ingenol esters were found as contaminants in
honey (32,91) and it has been reported that leaves of trees used as
tea in Curacao island contain phorbol esters (97). There is a case
report of stomatitis in humans after ingestion of lyngbyatoxin (71)
and molds in food may produce tumor promoters such as teleocidin
formed by Streptomyces.

Large amounts of oral saccharin (33) and tryptophan (11) may
act as tumor promoters in the urinary bladder. It is extremely
important also to investigate the components of foods that act as
tumor promoters in various organs, although unlike TPA and
teleocidin, they may not individually be highly active.

MUTAGENS IN FOOD DETECTED BY DIPHTHERIA TOXIN RESISTANT MUTATION OF
CHINESE HAMSTER LUNG CELLS

Ames' test using Salmonella typhimurium and S9 mix is the most
widely used test for environmental mutagens (3). This test is

simple and reproducible. The <u>Salmonella</u> <u>typhimurium</u> used requires
histidine and reverse mutation to a histidine prototroph occurs in
characteristic base sequences rich in G/C pairs. Transduction with
plasmids converts the original strains TA1535 and TA1538 to the
more sensitive strains TA100 and TA98, respectively (50). Ames'
method is very useful for detecting mutagens in our environment, as
demonstrated in other sessions of this symposium and with this
method alone, we could discover many new heterocyclic amines. But
before subjecting new environmental chemicals to <u>in vivo</u> long-term
animal tests for carcinogenicity, we thought it appropriate to use
another short-term mutation test, if possible, a forward mutation
test using cultured mammalian cells to which S9 mix could easily be
added. For this purpose we established a system for diphtheria
toxin resistant mutation of Chinese hamster lung cells (87). Cells
were exposed to test chemicals with or without S9 mix for 3 hours,
and then washed, replated in fresh medium and grown for an
expression time. Then the cells were replated in medium containing
0.1 Lf per ml of diphtheria toxin and incubated for 7-8 days.
Simultaneously cells were plated in medium without diphtheria toxin
and colonies were counted to determine the plating efficiency.
There are less than 20 spontaneous mutants per 2.5 x 10^5 cells in
this system.

Table 7.   Number of compounds proved positive at each step of the
           four-step test for tumor promoters

Step	Number
Total	270
Irritancy to mouse ear	43
ODC induction	15
Adhesion of HL-60	5
Carcinogenesis <u>in vivo</u>	3

Elongation factor 2 for protein synthesis has a particular
amino acid, diphthamide, which is formed post-translationally from
a certain histidine moiety in the polypeptide chain (54,94).
Diphtheria toxin catalyzes enzymatic ADP-ribosylation of
diphthamide (12,54,94) and thus ADP-ribosylated elongation factor 2
loses its catalytic activity for protein synthesis, resulting in
eventual cell death. Diphtheria toxin resistance of Chinese
hamster lung cells is due to a defect produced by mutation in post-
translational formation of diphthamide from histidine. Since
diphthamide is not present, ADP-ribosylation by diphtheria toxin
cannot take place and thus elongation factor 2 does not lose its
catalytic function. Mutation assay by measuring diphtheria toxin
resistance has also been performed with human fibroblasts (25,26)
and Chinese hamster ovary cells (27). Our results on the
mutagenicities of several new heterocyclic amines and quercetin are
given in Table 8 with those on MNNG and MNU for comparison.

Typical mutagens in food, namely heterocyclic amines and
quercetin which we originally discovered in mutation tests on
Salmonella, were found to be mutagenic to Chinese hamster lung
cells. However, the mutagenic activity of these heterocyclic
amines toward Chinese hamster lung cells is less than that of MNNG,
and that of flavonoid is also weaker than that of MNU.

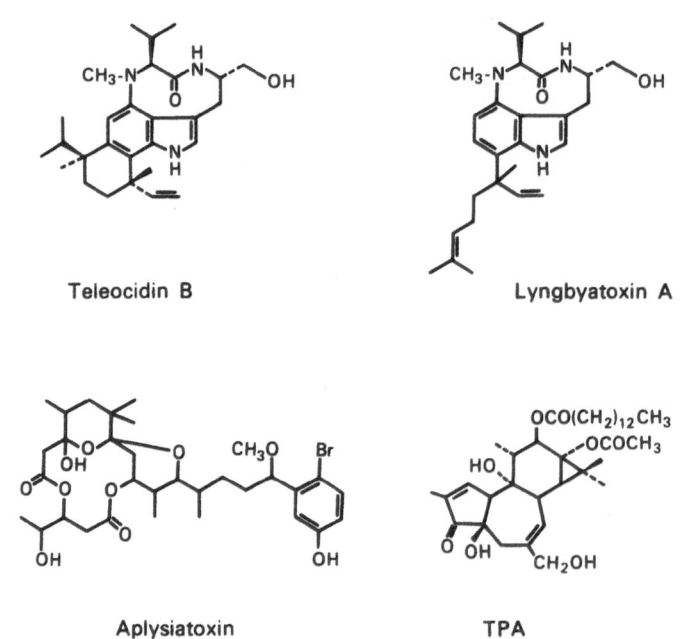

Teleocidin B   Lyngbyatoxin A

Aplysiatoxin   TPA

Fig. 5. Structures of newly-found tumor promoters and TPA.

PROBLEMS OF CANCER RISK FOR FUTURE STUDY

Experiments in our laboratory revealed the presence of highly mutagenic heterocyclic amines in pyrolysates of amino acids, protein and proteinous foods. Some of these compounds were shown to be carcinogenic in in vivo long-term animal tests. Vegetables have been found to contain mutagenic-carcinogenic alkaloids, such as pyrrolizidine alkaloid, that were demonstrated to be carcinogenic in vivo in long-term animal tests. Various other mutagens have also been found in foods, of which carcinogenic mycotoxins such as aflatoxin B_1 and nitrosamines such as dimethyl-nitrosamine have been well investigated. Many foods also contain as yet unidentified mutagens.

Table 8. Mutagenicity of heterocyclic amines and other compounds assayed by diphtheria toxin resistant mutation of Chinese hamster lung cells

Compounds	DT^r mutants/10^6 survivors induced by 1 μg/ml
MNNG	3,300
Trp-P-2	160
IQ	40
Trp-P-1	33
MNU	18
Quercetin	2

MNU: N-methyl-N-nitrosourea

Fruit juice, spices, pickles, coffee, whiskies, and brandies
are mutagenic, and some of them were shown to contain flavonoids,
such as quercetin and kaempferol. Quercetin and kaempferol are
ubiquitious in plants and are definitely mutagenic although their
carcinogenicity is still controversial. Similarly there is no
doubt about the presence of many mutagens in coffee and alcoholic
beverages, but this does not necessarily mean that coffee and
alcoholic beverages contain carcinogens. Mutagenic substances must
be isolated and identified and then tested in time-consuming in
vivo long-term animal experiments.

Before these long-term animal tests, other short-term tests
than the microbial mutation test are useful. In our laboratory,
diphtheria toxin resistant mutation of Chinese hamster lung cells
is routinely used as a short-term test. Newly discovered
heterocyclic amines are mutagenic to Chinese hamster lung cells and
so is a flavonoid. Coffee is also mutagenic to this cell line.
However, judging from the case of flavonoid, definite assessment of
carcinogenicity must still depend on long-term in vivo tests.

Recently we have been studying analbuminemic rats (62). These
rats have almost no serum albumin, but the colloidal osmotic
pressure of their serum is normal owing to compensatory increases
in the concentrations of other serum proteins, such as transferrin
and γ-globulin (16). We found that mRNA for albumin is not present
in the cytoplasm (15) but that there is a mRNA sequence hybridizing
with cDNA to albumin in the nuclei of the liver of this rat (18).
This finding suggests an abnormality in maturation of mRNA for
albumin. Later we cloned genomic DNA of albumin from this rat
mutant and found that it was deficient in seven bases in the intron
after exon H (17). Base pairs were missing from the 5th base from
the junction of the exon H and adjacent downstream intron. An even
more interesting finding was the presence of a very few cells
giving a positive reaction to anti-albumin antibody in the liver of
analbuminemic rats. The number of these cells synthesizing albumin
increased slightly with age and increased remarkably after
administration of a carcinogenic azo dye. These increases may be
due to a new mechanism of reversion of mutated albumin-minus to
albumin-positive cells in vivo, although it is not yet sure what
molecular model for this type of somatic cell mutation is
realistic. Since the mutated site is located in the intron close
to the exon-intron junction, reversion may involve restoration of
the capacity for the normal splicing mechanism which is disturbed
in the original mutant cells. This in vivo restoration of albumin
synthetic capacity in hepatocytes may be a convenient system to use
in tests for substances producing in vivo somatic cell mutation.
Various assay methods should be devised for prediction of the
carcinogenicity of mutagens in foods and the above system could be
useful as one of them.

It is also important to detect tumor promoters in food. Furthermore, mutagens in foods must be tested in combination with tumor promoters to assess their real carcinogenic risk, since our foods contain both mutagens and tumor promoters.

A quantitative chemical assay method for mutagens in foods must be established, and this method must be relatively simple and reproducible. When quantitative data are available the real risks of various foods could be determined. Administration of two different classes of chemical carcinogens results in the enhanced cancer production and a change in the target organs (63). This makes it almost impossible to use data obtained in animals given a single carcinogen to estimate human risk. Thus we still need more data obtained in laborious animal experiments.

It is also important to mention here that the effects of mutagens in foods can be counteracted by various agents by various mechanisms. It is well know that vitamin C prevents the formation of nitrosamines from amines and nitrite (53). Flavonoid can also inhibit metabolic activation leading to the formation of ultimate carcinogens from procarcinogens (9,98). Moreover vitamin A inhibits the carcinogenic process, probably at the step of tumor promotion (7,72). Because foods contain many complex components, experiments not only on single compounds but also on combinations of compounds are very important in evaluation of the risk or safety of foods.

REFERENCES

1. H.U. Aeschbacher, C. Chappuis, and H.P. Würzner, Mutagenicity testing of coffee: A study of problems encountered with the Ames Salmonella test system, Fd. Cosmet. Toxicol. 18:605 (1980).
2. D.E. Amacher, S.C. Paillet, C.N. Turner, V.A. Ray, and D.S. Salsburg, Point mutations at the thymidine kinase locus in L5178Y mouse lymphoma cells, Mutation Res. 72:447 (1980).
3. B.N. Ames, J. McCann, and E. Yamasaki, Methods for detecting carcinogens and mutagens with the Salmonella/mammalian-microsome mutagenicity test, Mutation Res. 31:347 (1975).
4. B. Armstrong and R. Doll, Environmental factors and cancer incidence and mortality in different countries, with special reference to dietary practices, Int. J. Cancer 15:617 (1975).
5. I. Berenblum, The mechanism of cocarcinogenesis: A study of the significance of cocarcinogenic action and related phenomena, Cancer Res. 1:807 (1941).
6. L.F. Bjeldanes and H. Chew, Mutagenicity of 1,2-dicarbonyl compounds: Maltol, kojic acid, diacetyl and related substances, Mutation Res. 67:367 (1979).

7. W. Bollag, Therapy of chemically induced skin tumors of mice
    with vitamin A palmitate and vitamin A acid, Experientia
    27:90 (1971).

8. J.P. Brown, P.S. Dietrich, and R.T. Brown, Frameshift
    mutagenicity of certain naturally occurring phenolic
    compounds in the "Salmonella/microsome" test: Activation of
    anthraquinone and flavonol glycosides by gut bacterial
    enzymes, Biochem. Soc. Trans. 5:1489 (1977).

9. M.K. Buening, R.L. Chang, M.T. Huang, J.G. Fortner, A.W.
    Wood, and A.H. Conney, Activation and inhibition of
    benzo(a)pyrene and aflatoxin B$_1$ metabolism in human liver
    microsomes by naturally occurring flavonoids, Cancer Res.
    41:67 (1981).

10. K.K. Carrol, Experimental evidence of dietary factors and
    hormone-dependent cancers, Cancer Res. 35:3374 (1975).

11. S.M. Cohen, M. Arai, J.B. Jacobs, and G.H. Friedell,
    Promotion effect of saccharin and DL-tryptophan in urinary
    bladder carcinogenesis, Cancer Res. 39:1207 (1979).

12. R.J. Collier, Diphtheria toxin: Mode of action and
    structure, Bacteriol. Rev. 39:54 (1975).

13. C.C.J. Culvenor, J.A. Edgar, L.W. Smith, and I. Hirono, The
    occurrence of senkirkine in Tussilago farfara, Aust. J. Chem.
    29:229 (1976).

14. R. Doll, Strategy for detection of cancer hazards to man,
    Nature 265:589 (1977).

15. H. Esumi, M. Okui, S. Sato, T. Sugimura, and S. Nagase,
    Absence of albumin mRNA in the liver of analbuminemic rats,
    Proc. Natl. Acad. Sci. USA 77:3215 (1980).

16. H. Esumi, S. Sato, M. Okui, T. Sugimura, and S. Nagase,
    Turnover of serum proteins in rats with analbuminemia,
    Biochem. Biophys. Res. Commun. 87:1191 (1979).

17. H. Esumi, S. Sato, Y. Takahashi, S. Nagase, and T. Sugimura,
    A seven base pair deletion in an intron blocks albumin mRNA
    processing, in: "Primary and Tertiary Structure of Nucleic
    Acids and Cancer Research", M. Miwa, S. Nishimura, A. Rich,
    D. Söll, and T. Sugimura, eds., Japan Sci. Soc. Press, Tokyo,
    in press.

18. H. Esumi, Y. Takahashi, T. Sekiya, S. Sato, S. Nagase, and T.
    Sugimura, Presence of nuclear albumin mRNA precursors in
    analbuminemic rat liver lacking cytoplasmic albumin mRNA,
    Proc. Natl. Acad. Sci. USA, 79:734 (1982).

19. I.A. Evans and J. Mason, Carcinogenic activity of bracken,
    Nature(London) 208:913 (1965).

20. H. Fujiki, M. Mori, M. Nakayasu, M. Terada, T. Sugimura, and
    R.E. Moore, Indole alkaloids: Dihydroteleocidin B,
    teleocidin, and lygnbyatoxin A as members of a new class of
    tumor promoters, Proc. Natl. Acad. Sci. USA 78:3872 (1981).

21. H. Fujiki, T. Sugimura, and R.E. Moore, New classes of
    environmental tumor promoters: Indole alkaloids and
    polyacetate, in: "Abstract of International Symposium on
    Health Effects of Tumor Promotion" (1981) p. 14.

22. M. Fukuoka, M. Kuroyanagi, K. Yoshihira, S. Natori, M. Nagao, Y. Takahashi, and T. Sugimura, Chemical and toxicological studies on bracken fern, Pteridium aquilinum var. Latiusculum. IV. Surveys on bracken constituents by mutagenicity test, J. Pharm. Dyn. 1:324 (1978).
23. M. Fukuoka, K. Yoshihira, S. Natori, K. Sakamoto, S. Iwahara, S. Hosaka, and I. Hirono, Characterization of mutagenic principles and carcinogenicity of dill weed and seeds, J. Pharm. Dyn. 3:236 (1980).
24. M.A. Gianturco, A.S. Giammarino, and P. Friedel, Volatile constituents of coffee-V, Nature 210:1358 (1966).
25. T.W. Glover, C.-C. Chang, J.E. Trosko, and S.S.-L. Li, Ultraviolet light induction of diphtheria toxin-resistant mutants in normal and xeroderma pigmentosum human fibroblasts, Proc. Natl. Acad. Sci. USA 76:3982 (1979).
26. R.S. Gupta and S. Goldstein, Diphtheria toxin resistance in human fibroblast cell strains from normal and cancer-prone individuals, Mutation Res. 73:331 (1980).
27. R.S. Gupta and L. Siminovitch, Genetic markers for quantitative mutagenesis studies in Chinese hamster ovary cells, Mutation Res. 69:113 (1980).
28. Y. Hashimoto, K. Shudo, and T. Okamoto, Structural identification of a modified base in DNA covalently bound with mutagenic 3-amino-1-methyl-5H-pyrido[4,3-b] indole. Chem. Pharm. Bull. 27:1058 (1979).
29. Y. Hashimoto, K. Shudo, and T. Okamoto, Metabolic activation of a mutagen, 2-amino-6-methyldipyrido[1,2-a:3;,2;-d]-imidazole and its reaction with DNA, Biochem. Biophys. Res. Commun. 92:971 (1980).
30. Y. Hasimoto, K. Shudo, and T. Okamoto, Activation of a mutagen, 3-amino-1-methyl-5H-pyrido[4,3-b]indole. Identification of 3-hydroxyamino-1-methyl-5H-pyrido[4,3-b]indole and its reaction with DNA, Biochem. Biophys. Res. Commun. 96:355 (1980).
31. E. Hecker, Phorbol esters from croton oil, chemical nature and biological activities, Naturwissenschaften 54:282 (1967).
32. E. Hecker, Cocarcinogenesis and tumor promoters of the diterpene ester type as possible carcinogenic risk factors, J. Cancer Res. Clin. Oncol. 99:103 (1981).
33. R.M. Hicks, J.St.J. Wakefield, and J. Chowaniec, Evaluation of a new model to detect bladder carcinogens or co-carcinogens; results obtained with saccharin, cyclamate and cyclophosphamide, Chem.-biol. Interact. 11:225 (1975).
34. T. Hirohata, Shift in cancer mortality from 1920 to 1970 among various ethnic groups in Hawaii, in: "Genetic and Environmental Factors in Experimental and Human Cancer", H.V. Gelboin, B. MacMahon, T. Matsushima, T. Sugimura, S. Takayama, and H. Takebe, eds. Japan Sci. Soc. Press, Tokyo (1979) pp. 341-350.
35. I. Hirono, H. Mori, M. Haga, M. Fujii, K. Yamada, Y. Hirata, H. Takanashi, E. Uchida, S. Hosaka, I. Ueno, T. Matsushima,

K. Umezawa, and A. Shirai, Edible plants containing
carcinogenic pyrrolizidine alkaloids in Japan, in: "Naturally
Occurring Carcinogens-Mutagens and Modulators of
Carcinogenesis", E.C. Miller, J.A. Miller, I. Hirono, T.
Sugimura, and S. Takayama, eds., Japan Sci. Soc. Press, Tokyo
(1979) pp. 79-87.

36. I. Hirono, I. Sasaoka, C. Shibuya, M. Shimizu, K. Fushimi, H.
     Mori, K. Kato, and M. Haga, Natural carcinogenic products of
     plant origin, Gann Monogr. Cancer Res. 17:205 (1975).

37. I. Hirono, I. Ueno, S. Hosaka, H. Takanashi, T. Matsushima,
     T. Sugimura, and S. Natori, Carcinogenicity examination of
     quercetin and rutin in ACI rats, Cancer Lett. 13:15 (1981).

38. D.P. Hsieh, Z.A. Wong, J.J. Wong, C. Michans, and B.H.
     Ruebner, Comparative metabolism of aflatoxin, in: "Mycotoxins
     in Human and Animal Health," J.V. Rodricks, C.W. Hesseltine,
     and M.A. Mehlman, eds., Pathodox, Park Forest South (1977)
     pp. 37-50.

39. K. Ishii, Y. Yamazoe, T. Kamataki, and R. Kato, Metabolic
     activation of glutamic acid pyrolysis products, 2-amino-6-
     methyldipyrido[1,2-a:3',2'-d]imidazole and 2-aminodipyrido-
     [1,2-a:3',2'-d]imidazole, by purified cytochrome P-450,
     Chem.-biol. Interact. 38:1 (1981).

40. H. Kasai, Z. Yamaizumi, S. Nishimura, K. Wakabayashi, M.
     Nagao, T. Sugimura, N.E. Spingarn, J.H. Weisburger, S.
     Yokoyama, and T. Miyazawa, A potent mutagen in broiled
     fish. Part 1. 2-Amino-3-methyl-3H-imidazo[4,5-f]quinoline,
     J. Chem. Soc. Perkin I:2290 (1981).

41. H. Kasai, Z. Yamaizumi, T. Shiomi, S. Yokoyama, T. Miyazawa,
     K. Wakabayashi, M. Nagao, T. Sugimura, and S. Nishimura,
     Structure of a potent mutagen isolated from fried beef, Chem.
     Lett. 485 (1981).

42. H. Kasai, Z. Yamaizumi, K. Wakabayashi, M. Nagao, T.
     Sugimura, S. Yokoyama, T. Miyazawa, and S. Nishimura,
     Structure and chemical synthesis of Me-IQ, a potent mutagen
     isolated from broiled fish. Chem. Lett. 1391 (1980).

43. T. Kawachi, M. Nagao, T. Yahagi, Y. Takahashi, T. Sugimura,
     T. Matsushima, T. Kawakami, and M. Ishidate, Our view on the
     relation between mutagens and carcinogens in: "Naturally
     Occurring Carcinogens-Mutagens and Modulators of
     Carcinogenesis", E.C. Miller, J.A. Miller, I. Hirono, T.
     Sugimura, and S. Takayama, eds., Japan Sci. Soc. Press, Tokyo
     (1979) pp. 337-344.

44. W. Lijinsky and P. Shubik, Benzo[a]pyrene and other
     polynuclear hydrocarbons in charcoal-broiled meat, Science
     145:53 (1964).

45. B. MacMahon, S. Yen, D. Trichopoulos, K. Warren, and G.
     Nardi, Coffee and cancer of the pancreas, N. Engl. J. Med.
     304:630 (1981).

46. N. Matsukura, T. Kawachi, K. Morino, H. Ohgaki, T. Sugimura,
     and S. Takayama, Carcinogenicity in mice of mutagenic

---

compounds from a tryptophan pyrolyzate, Science 213:346 (1981).

47. T. Matsumoto, D. Yoshida, and H. Tomita, Determination of mutagens, amino-α-carbolines in grilled foods and cigarette smoke condensate, Cancer Lett. 12:105 (1981).

48. M. Mazaki, T. Ishii, and M. Uyeta, Mutagenicity of hydrolysates of citrus fruit juices, Mutation Res., in press.

49. J. McCann and B.N. Ames, Detection of carcinogens as mutagens in the Salmonella/microsome test: Assay of 300 chemicals: Discussion, Proc. Natl. Acad. Sci. USA 73:950 (1976).

50. J. McCann, N.E. Spingarn, J. Kobori, and B.N. Ames, Detection of carcinogens as mutagens: bacterial tester strains with R factor plasmids, Proc. Natl. Acad. Sci. USA 72:979 (1975).

51. M.L. Meltz and J.T. MacGregor, Activity of the plant flavanol quercetin in the mouse lymphoma 15178Y $TK^{+/-}$ mutation, DNA single-strand break, and Balb/c 3T3 chemical transformation assays. Mutation Res. 88:317 (1981).

52. R.W. Miller, Epidemiology, in: "Cancer in China, Section 3, Etiology", H.S. Kaplan and P.J. Tsuchitani, eds., Liss, New York (1978) pp. 39-57.

53. S.S. Mirvish, L. Wallcave, M. Eagan, and P. Shubik, Ascorbate nitrite reaction: Possible means of blocking the formation of carcinogenic N-nitroso compounds, Science 177:65 (1972).

54. J.A. Moehring, T.J. Moehring, and D.E. Danley, Postranslational modification of elongation factor 2 in diphtheria-toxin-resistant mutants of CHO-K1 cells, Proc. Natl. Acad. Sci. USA 77:1010 (1980).

55. K. Morino, N. Matsukura, H. Ohgaki, T. Kawachi, T. Sugimura, and I. Hirono, Carcinogenicity test of quercetin and rutin in golden hamsters by oral administration, Carcinogenesis, 3:93 (1982).

56. M. Nagao, M. Honda, Y. Seino, T. Yahagi, T. Kawachi, and T. Sugimura, Mutagenicities of protein pyrolysates, Cancer Lett. 2:335 (1977).

57. M. Nagao, M. Honda, Y. Seino, T. Yahagi, and T. Sugimura, Mutagenicities of smoke condensates and the charred surface of fish and meat, Cancer Lett. 2:221 (1977).

58. M. Nagao, N. Morita, T. Yahagi, M. Shimizu, M. Kuroyanagi, M. Fukuoka, K. Yoshihira, S. Natori, T. Fujino, and T. Sugimura, Mutagenicities of 61 flavonoids and 11 related compounds, Env. Mutagen 3:401 (1981).

59. M. Nagao, Y. Takahashi, K. Wakabayashi, and T. Sugimura, Mutagenicity of alcoholic beverages, Mutation Res. 88:147 (1981).

60. M. Nagao, Y. Takahashi, H. Yamanaka, and T. Sugimura, Mutagens in coffee and tea, Mutation Res. 68:101 (1979).

61. S. Nagase, C. Fujimaki, and H. Isaka, Effect of administration of quercetin on the production of experimental liver cancers in rats fed p-dimethylaminoazobenzene, Proc. Japan Cancer Assoc. 23rd Meeting (1964) pp. 26-27.

62. S. Nagase, K. Shimamune, and S. Shumiya, Albumin-deficient
    rat mutant, Science 205:590 (1979).
63. P.M. Newberne and M. Connor, Effects of sequential exposure
    to aflatoxin B_1 and diethylnitrosamine on vascular and
    stomach tissue and additional target organs in rats, Cancer
    Res. 40:4037 (1980).
64. A. Nomura, G.N. Stemmermann and L.K. Heilbrum, Coffee and
    pancreatic cancer, Lancet 474 (1981).
65. A.M. Pamukcu, S. Yalciner, J.F. Hatcher, and G.T. Bryan,
    Quercetin, a rat intestinal and bladder carcinogen present in
    bracken fern (Pteridium aquilinum), Cancer Res. 40:3468
    (1980).
66. B.G. Piacek-Llanes, D.E.G. Shuker, and S.R. Tannenbaum, N-
    Nitrosamides of natural origin, in: "Proceeding of 7th
    International Meeting on Analysis and Formation of N-Nitroso
    Compounds", Int. Agency Res. Cancer, Lyon, in press.
67. I.F.H. Purchase, E. Longstaff, J. Ashby, J.A. Styles, D.
    Anderson, P.A. Lefevre, and F.R. Westwood, Evaluation of six
    short term tests for detecting organic chemical carcinogens
    and recommendations for their use, Nature 264:624 (1976).
68. R.K. Sahu, R. Basu, and A. Sharma, Genetic toxicological
    testing of some plant flavonoids by the micronuleus test,
    Mutation Res. 89:69 (1981).
69. D. Saito, A. Shirai, T. Matsushima, T. Sugimura, and I.
    Hirono, Test of carcinogenicity of quercetin, a widely
    distributed mutagen in food, Teratogen. Carcinogen. Mutagen.
    1:213 (1980).
70. Y. Seino, M. Nagao, T. Yahagi, T. Sugimura, T. Yashuda, and
    S. Nishimura, Identification of a mutagenic substance in a
    spice, sumac, as quercetin, Mutation Res. 58:225 (1978).
71. J.K. Sims and R.D.Z. Van Rilland, Escharotic stomatitis
    caused by the "Stinging seaweed" Microcolens lyngbyaceus
    (formerly Lyngbya majuscula), Hawaii Med. J. 40:243 (1981).
72. M.B. Sporn, N.M. Dunlop, D.L. Newton, and J.M. Smith,
    Prevention of chemical carcinogenesis by vitamin A and its
    synthetic analogs (retinoids), Fed. Proc. 35:1332 (1976).
73. H.F. Stich, W. Stich, and M.P. Rosin, and W.D. Powrie,
    Clastogenic activity of caramel and caramelized sugars,
    Mutation Res. 91:129 (1981).
74. T. Sugimura, Let's be scientific about the problem of
    mutagens in cooked food, Mutation Res. 55:149 (1978).
75. T. Sugimura, The Ernst W. Bertner Memorial Award Lecture:
    Tumor initiators and promoters associated with ordinary
    foods, in: "Molecular Interrelations of Nutrition and
    Cancer", M.S. Arnott, J. van Eys, and Y.-M. Wang eds., Raven
    Press, New York, (1982) pp. 3-24.
76. T. Sugimura, H. Fujiki, M. Mori, M. Nakayasu, M. Terada, K.
    Umezawa, and R.E. Moore, Teleocidin: New naturally occurring

tumor promoter, in: "Carcinogenesis, vol. 7", E. Hecker, N. Fuseing, F. Marks, and W. Kunz, eds., Raven Press, New York (1982) pp. 69-73.

77. T. Sugimura, T. Kawachi, M. Nagao, T. Yahagi, Y. Seino, T. Okamoto, K. Shudo, T. Kosuge, K. Tsuji, K. Wakabayashi, T. Iitaka, and A. Itai, Mutagenic principle(s) in tryptophan and phenylalanine pyrolysis products, Proc. Jpn Acad. 53:58 (1977).

78. T. Sugimura and M. Nagao, Mutagenic factors in cooked foods, CRC Critical Rev. Toxicol. 6:189 (1979).

79. T. Sugimura, M. Nagao, T. Kawachi, M. Honda, T. Yahagi, Y. Seino, S. Sato, N. Matsukura, T. Matsushima, A. Shirai, M. Sawamura, and H. Matsumoto, Mutagen-carcinogens in food, with special reference to highly mutagenic pyrolytic products in broiled food, in: "Origins of Human Cancer, Book C", H.H. Hiatt, J.D. Watson, and J.A. Winsten, eds., Cold Spring Harbor Laboratory, New York (1977) pp. 1561-1576.

80. T. Sugimura, M. Nagao, and K. Wakabayashi, Mutagenic heterocyclic amines in cooked foods, in: "Environmental Carcinogens-Selected Methods of Analysis, vol. 4. Some Aromatic Amines and Azo Dyes in the General and Industrial Environment," IARC Scientific Publications No. 40, H. Egan, L. Fishbein, M. Castegnaro, I.K. O'Neill, H. Bartsch, and W. Davis, eds., International Agency for Research on Cancer, Lyon (1981) pp. 251-267.

81. T. Sugimura, S. Sato, M. Nagao, T. Yahagi, T. Matsushima, Y. Seino, M. Takeuchi, and T. Kawachi, Overlapping of carcinogens and mutagens, in: "Fundamentals in Cancer Prevention", P.N. Magee, S. Takayama, T. Sugimura, and T. Matsushima, eds., Japan Scientific Societies Press, Tokyo/University Park Press, Baltimore (1976) pp. 191-215.

82. Y. Suwa, M. Nagao, K. Wakabayshi, A. Kosugi, and T. Sugimura, Inactivation of mutagens in coffee by sulfite, in: "Abstacts of Third International Conference on Environmental Mutagens (Tokyo)" (1981) p. 83.

83. M. Tada, Metabolism fo 4-nitroquinoline 1-oxide and related compounds, in: "Carcinogenesis, vol. 6", T. Sugimura, ed., Raven Press, New York (1981) pp. 25-45.

84. Y. Takahashi, M. Nagao, T. Fujino, Z. Yamaizumi, and T. Sugimura, Mutagens in Japanese pickle identified as flavonoids, Mutation Res. 68:117 (1979).

85. G. Tamura, C. Gold, A. Ferro-Luzzi, and B.N. Ames, Fecalase: A model for activation of dietary glycosides to mutagens by intestinal flora, Proc. Natl. Acad. Sci. USA 77:4961 (1980).

86. A. Tannenbaum and H. Silverstone, Nutrition in relation to cancer, Advances in Cancer Res. 1:451 (1953).

87. M. Terada, M. Nakayasu, H. Sakamoto, K. Wakabayashi, M. Nagao, H.S. Rosenkranz, and T. Sugimura, Mutagenic activity of nitropyrenes and heterocyclic amines on Chinese hamster

cells with diphtheria toxin resistance as a marker, in:
"Abstracts of Third International Conference on Environmental
Mutagens (Tokyo)" (1981) p. 128.

88. M. Tsuda, M. Nagao, T. Hirayama, and T. Sugimura, Nitrite
     converts 2-amino-α-carboline, an indirect mutagen, into 2-
     hydroxy-α-carboline, a non-mutagen and 2-hydroxy-3-nitroso-α-
     carboline, a direct mutagen, Mutation Res. 83:61 (1981).

89. M. Tsuda, Y. Takahashi, M. Nagao, T. Hirayama, and T.
     Sugimura, Inactivation of mutagens from pyrolysates of
     tryptophan and glutamic acid by nitrite in acidic solution,
     Mutation Res. 78:331 (1980).

90. M. Tsuda, K. Wakabayashi, T. Hirayama, T. Kawachi, and T.
     Sugimura, Inactivation of the pyrolysate mutagens Trp-P-2,
     Glu-P-1 and IQ by treatment with chlorinated tap water, in:
     "Abstract of Third International Conference on Environmental
     Mutagens (Tokyo)" (1981) p. 121.

91. R.R. Upadhyay, S. Islampanah, and A. Davoodi, Presence of a
     tumor-promoting factor in honey, Gann 71:557 (1980).

92. M. Uyeta, S. Taue, and M. Mazaki, Mutagenicity of
     hydrolysates of tea infusions, Mutation Res. 88:233 (1981).

93. B.L. Van Duuren, Tumor-promoting agents in two-stage
     carcinogenesis, Prog. Exp. Tumor Res. 11:31 (1969).

94. B.G. Van Ness, J.B. Howard, and J.W. Bodley, ADP-ribosylation
     of elongation factor 2 by diphtheria toxin. NMR spectra and
     proposed structures of ribosyl-diphthamide and its hydrolysis
     products, J. Biol. Chem. 255:10710 (1980).

95. K. Wakabayashi, K. Tsuji, T. Kosuge, K. Takeda, K. Yamaguchi,
     K. Shudo, T. Iitaka, T. Okamoto, T. Yahagi, M. Nagao, and T.
     Sugimura, Isolation and structure determination of a
     mutagenic substance in L-lysine pyrolysate, Proc. Jpn Acad.
     54B:569 (1978).

96. E.A. Walker, L. Griciute, M. Castegnaro, M. Börzsönyi, and W.
     Davis, eds., "N-Nitroso Compounds: Analysis, Formation and
     Occurrence", IARC Scientific Publications No. 31,
     International Agency for Research on Cancer, Lyon (1980).

97. J. Weber and E. Hecker, Cocarcinogens of the diterpene ester
     type from Croton flavens L. and esophageal cancer in Curacao,
     Experientia 34:679 (1978).

98. F.J. Wiebel, H.V. Gelboin, N.P. Buu-Hoi, M.G. Stout, and W.S.
     Burnham, Flavones and polycyclic hydrocarbons as modulators
     of aryl hydrocarbon [benzo(a)pyrene] hydrolase, in: "The
     Biochemistry of Disease, vol. 4, Chemical Carcinogenesis,
     Part A", P.O.P. Ts'o and J.A. DiPaolo, eds., Marcel Dekker,
     Inc., New York (1974) pp. 249-270.

99. H.P. Würzmer, E. Lindström, and L. Vuatz, A 2-year feeding
     of instant coffees in rats. II. Incidence and types of
     neoplasms, Fd Cosmet. Toxicol. 15:289 (1977).

100. E.L. Wynder and G.B. Gori, The contribution of the
     environment to cancer incidence: An epidemiologic exercise,
     J. Natl. Cancer Inst. 58:825 (1977).

101. K. Yamaguchi, K. Shudo, T. Okamoto, T. Sugimura, and T. Kosuge, Presence of 2-amiodipyrido[1,2-a:3',2'-d]imidazole in broiled cuttlefish, Gann 71:743 (1980).

102. K. Yamaguchi, K. Shudo, T. Okamoto, T. Sugimura, and T. Kosuge, Presence of 3-amino-1,4-dimethyl-5H-pyrido[4,3-b]indole in broiled beef, Gann 71:745 (1980).

103. Z. Yamaizumi, T. Shiomi, H. Kasai, S. Nishimura, Y. Takahashi, M. Nagao, and T. Sugimura, Detection of potent mutagens, Trp-P-1 and Trp-P-2, in broiled fish, Cancer Lett. 9:75 (1980).

104. T. Yamamoto, K. Tsuji, T. Kosuge, T. Okamoto, K. Shudo, K. Takeda, Y. Iitaka, K. Yamaguchi, Y. Seino, T. Yahagi, M. Nagao, and T. Sugimura, Isolation and structure determination of mutagenic substances in L-glutamic acid pyrolysate, Proc. Jpn Acad. 54B:248 (1978).

105. H. Yamanaka, M. Nagao, T. Sugimura, T. Furuya, A. Shirai, and T. Matsushima, Mutagenicity of pyrrolizidine alkaloids in the Salmonella/mammalian-microsome test, Mutation Res. 68:211 (1979).

106. Y. Yamazoe, K. Ishii, T. Kamataki, R. Kato, and T. Sugimura, Isolation and characterization of active metabolites of tryptophan-pyrolysate mutagen, Trp-P-2, formed by rat liver microsomes, Chem.-biol. Interact. 30:125 (1980).

107. Y. Yamazoe, M. Tada, T. Kamataki, and R. Kato, Enhancement of binding of N-hydroxy-Trp-P-2 to DNA by seryl-tRNA synthetase, Biochem. Biophys. Res. Commun. 102:432 (1981).

108. M. Yokota, K. Narita, T. Kosuge, K. Wakabayashi, M. Nagao, T. Sugimura, K. Yamaguchi, K. Shudo, Y. Iitaka, and T. Okamoto, A potent mutagen isolated from a pyrolysate of L-ornithine, Chem. Pharm. Bull. 29:1473 (1981).

109. D. Yoshida, T. Matsumoto, R. Yoshimura, and T. Matsuzaki, Mutagenicity of amino-α-carbolines in pyrolysis products of soybean globulin, Biochem. Biophys. Res. Commun. 83:915 (1978).

110. M. Yoshida, M. Sasaki, K. Sugimura, and T. Kawachi, Cytogenetic effects of quercetin on cultured mammalian cells, Proc. Jpn Acad. 56:443 (1980).

DISCUSSION

Q. STEWARD: Is it possible that quercetin induces its own metabolism and detoxification (e.g. by inducing cytochrome P-448) and that this could explain why it appears to have little carcinogenicity in in vivo tests?

A. SUGIMURA: It is possible but I don't remember any report on quercetin. A report is available that tangeretin, a naturally occurring flavone, was active on the in vivo induction of benzo(a)pyrene hydroxylase in the liver of rat (L.W. Wattenberg et al., Cancer Res. 28:934, 1968).

DETECTION AND EVALUATION OF POTENTIAL HAZARDS TO HUMAN HEALTH

CHAIRMAN'S COMMENTS

James L. Byard

Department of Environmental Toxicology
University of California
Davis, California 95616

This morning our speakers will present several approaches for assessing genetic toxicity, including plant and animal systems. As with any scientific experiment, we should be evaluating each assay system in regard to: the adequacy of controls, the statistical validity of the effects, the completeness of metabolism by activating systems, the relevance of the genotoxic endpoints to germinal or somatic mutation, and the relevance of the biological system and genotoxic endpoints to mutation in humans.

While some assay systems may be intended as general screens for genotoxic chemicals, others have a narrower range of response but offer more relevant or more specific information. In the time remaining for my introductory comments, I would like to discuss one such system which we've been studying here at Davis; namely, primary hepatocyte cultures.

The hepatocytes are prepared by an in situ or biopsy perfusion of liver with collagenase. Adult liver parenchymal cells are cultured without serum on collagen-coated dishes in culture medium supplemented with hormones. Stable monolayers are obtained within 24 hours and can be maintained for up to 10 days. The hormone supplement maintains in vivo levels of cytochrome P-450, a critical component of mixed function oxygenases responsible for activation of many promutagens. Viable cultures from mice, rats, guinea pigs, rabbits, dogs, monkeys, and humans have been prepared.

The hepatocyte cultures have been used to bioassay cytotoxicity and genotoxicity, which should be predictive for hepatic necrosis and hepatocarcinogenicity, respectively. Metabolism studies have revealed the rate of metabolism and extent

271

of covalent binding to total macromolecules and to specific
macromolecules, such as DNA. Comparative metabolism, cytotoxicity
and genotoxicity studies are providing a means of extrapolating
toxicity data from laboratory animals to humans.

Chemicals under study include aflatoxin B_1, aflatoxin M_1 (both
provided by Dr. Dennis Hsieh); senecionine (provided by Dr. Henry
Segall); TCDD, 2-acetylaminofluorene; and benzene. Aflatoxin B_1
was completely metabolized within ten hours. The profile of
metabolites was comparable to the in vivo profile. Twenty times as
much aflatoxin B_1 was covalently bound to macromolecules in rat
compared to mouse hepatocytes, consistent with the much greater
susceptibility of the rat to aflatoxin B_1 hepatocarcinogenesis.
Rabbit and human hepatocytes convalently bound aflatoxin B_1 to
macromolecules at levels intermediate between the mouse and rat,
but closer to the rat than the mouse, suggesting an intermediate
susceptibility to hepatocarcinogenesis. Both aflatoxin B_1 and M_1
were potent genotoxins in rat hepatocyte cultures, detected as a
stimulation of DNA repair. At low doses, aflatoxin B_1 was about 10
times more potent than aflatoxin M_1, paralleling the ratios for
covalent binding to macromolecules.

Senecionine was a moderately potent cytotoxin and genotoxin.
A single dose was metabolized by rat hepatocytes in 10 hours
resulting in 1.5% of the dose covalently bound to macromolecules.
Cytotoxicity was measured by LDH leakage into the culture medium
and loss of cells from the collagen substratum. Human hepatocyte
cultures metabolized senecionine slower than rat hepatocyte
cultures but produced the same levels of covalent binding.
Senecionine produced a marked stimulation of DNA repair in rat
hepatocyte cultures. Senecionine has not been assayed in vivo, but
the hepatocyte data suggest that it is hepatocarcinogenic.

TCDD was a potent inducer of benzopyrene metabolism in rat
hepatocyte cultures. Significant induction could be measured in
the low Fmole/culture range. This system should be an excellent
bioassay of TCDD and its structural analogs in complex
environmental samples. Guinea pig hepatocyte cultures were not
induced by TCDD even at Nmole/culture levels, emphasizing again the
striking species variation, not only in metabolic activation, but
also in the induction of metabolism.

Pretreatment of rats with phenobarbital or butylated-
hydroxytoluene (BHT) reduced the covalent binding of aflatoxin B_1
to macromolecules in hepatocyte cultures. Both chemicals protected
against cytotoxicity. Phenobarbital reduced covalent binding of
aflatoxin B_1 to DNA and produced a parallel decrease in stimulation
of DNA repair. This protective effect of phenobarbital in
hepatocyte cultures is consistent with its protective effect in
vivo, in contrast to the increase in mutagenicity obtained in the
Ames assay with S-9 from rats pretreated with phenobarbital.

Our recent development of a method of culturing hepatocytes on glass permits the assessment of metabolism, cytotoxicity, and genotoxicity of volatile and gaseous chemicals. We listened with interest to Dr. Blair's report of increased leukemia in the rural population. We are presently studying the comparative metabolism of benzene, a chemical that is suspected of producing leukemia. Although benzene acts on the bone marrow, available data indicates that it is activated in the liver. In primary hepatocyte cultures, benzene is metabolized at a much slower rate in rats and mice compared to humans, perhaps explaining the inability of various investigators to produce leukemia with benzene in these rodents. We are now assessing the metabolism of benzene in hepatocyte cultures from other species to identify an appropriate model for humans.

STUDY OF PESTICIDE GENOTOXICITY

Michael D. Waters,[1] Shahbeg S. Sandhu,[1]
Vincent F. Simmon,[2] Kristien E. Mortelmans,[2]
Ann D. Mitchell,[2] Ted A. Jorgenson,[2] David C.L. Jones,[2]
Ruby Valencia,[3] and Neil E. Garrett[4]

[1]Genetic Toxicology Division
U.S. Environmental Protection Agency
Research Triangle Park, NC

[2]SRI International
Menlo Park, CA

[3]WARF Institute, Inc.
Madison, WI

[4]Northrop Services, Inc.
Research Triangle Park, NC

INTRODUCTION

With a limited supply of arable land supporting an ever-increasing human population, the threat of crop loss to agricultural pests becomes continually more acute. Thus pesticides have become an essential component of modern agriculture. As competing organisms evolve resistance to commonly used agents, new and more effective poisons and repellants must constantly be developed. The fundamental problem in pesticide development is to produce chemicals that act specifically against certain organisms without adversely affecting others. Because of the similarities in the structural, metabolic and genetic components of all life forms, absolute species specificity is frequently difficult to attain. Furthermore, such toxic chemicals improperly used may engender biological effects beyond those for which they were originally manufactured.

Genotoxic effects are considered among the most serious of the possible side effects of agricultural chemicals. These effects include heritable genetic diseases, carcinogenesis, reproductive dysfunction, and birth defects. Carcinogenesis and mutagenesis are of special concern because of the irreversible nature of the processes and the long latency associated with their manifestation. This concern focuses special attention on inherently toxic substances applied to crops or soil, where there is a possibility of direct entry into the food cycle.

Because of its regulatory responsibilities, the U.S. Environmental Protection Agency (EPA) established a research effort (originally under the Substitute Chemicals Program) to evaluate the genotoxicity of a variety of pesticides. These agents represented differing biological activities and diverse chemical classes, and, therefore, offered the opportunity to gain considerable knowledge regarding test system performance and the genetic specificity of the effects observed. The short-term bioassays employed assessed three basic types of genetic damage: 1) gene or point mutations, 2) primary DNA damage and repair, and 3) chromosomal alterations. Point or gene mutation assays detect changes in the DNA sequence of a gene. These changes are usually brought about through insertions, deletions or substitutions of single DNA base pairs. DNA damage and repair assays measure the response of cells to test chemicals that alter DNA directly or affect those processes that synthesize or repair DNA. Chromosomal alterations involve changes in number or structure of entire chromosomes and may include breakage, nondisjunction, translocations and other forms of structural change. Such changes may be observed microscopically and provide direct evidence that a chemical can alter organized genetic material. Since some chemicals exhibit genotoxic effects only after metabolic conversion to active intermediates (15), most of the in vitro bioassays incorporated exogenous metabolic activation systems prepared from rat liver homogenates.

The specific objectives of the study were to:

1) Compare the abilities of selected in vitro and in vivo bioassays to detect or confirm genetic activities of pesticide chemicals.

2) Examine the spectrum of genetic activity displayed by these agents in order to facilitate interpretation of the test results.

3) Examine the test results in relation to other biological and chemical features of the pesticides.

The results of this study may suggest a sensitive battery of short-term tests that would enhance the probability of detection

of relevant genetic activity while minimizing the time and expense
involved in the screening process. Another possible result of
this and similar studies is a correlation of genotoxic effects
with structural features of the chemicals under evaluation.

In this paper are described the bioassays employed, pesticides
examined and preliminary conclusions drawn from the study. A
total of 65 pesticides have been examined according to a sequential
or phased testing strategy (24) involving up to 14 bioassays for
each chemical evaluated. A total of 494 bioassays have been
performed to date, including 299 in vitro tests both with and
without metabolic activation.

PESTICIDES

Battelle Memorial Laboratories, Columbus, Ohio, obtained the
pesticides from the manufacturers and subsequently provided samples
to SRI International, Menlo Park, California, or WARF Institute,
Inc., Madison, Wisconsin, for the studies reported here. A few of
the chemicals were obtained from the manufacturers by the EPA
Office of Pesticide Programs, Washington, D.C. Each pesticide was
a "technical grade" product or equivalent. Product information is
available from the first author. Monocrotophos was tested as a
formulated product, Azodrin 5 (Shell). Mancozeb was tested as two
different products: Dithane M-45 (Rohm and Haas) and Manzate 200
(du Pont). Maneb was also tested as two different products:
Dithane M-22 (Rohm and Haas) and Manzate D (du Pont). All pesticides are listed alphabetically in Table 1 by their common names
and are further described according to one of three general classes
of action (insecticide, herbicide or fungicide) and by chemical
class. Reference is provided to subsequent tables containing
qualitative test data. Nearly a third of the compounds examined
are organophosphate insecticides; other classes examined include
carbamates, chlorinated hydrocarbons, halogenated aromatics,
arsenic compounds, urea derivatives and natural plant products or
synthetic derivatives. The modes of action of these compounds
range from general contact and systemic poisons to specific pre-
and post-emergence herbicides.

BIOASSAYS

All bioassays, except 29 of the Drosophila sex-linked recessive
lethal tests, were performed by SRI International, Menlo Park,
California, under contract to the U.S. Environmental Protection
Agency. The Drosophila assays mentioned above were performed by
WARF Institute, Inc., Madison, Wisconsin. Table 2 lists the 14
bioassays used in this study, divided into three classes of genetic
damage and further divided according to the phylogenetic level of

Table 1.   Pesticides Assayed for Genotoxic Effects

Name (action)	Chemical Class	Table No. for Results
Acephate (I)	thio/dithiophosphoramidate	3, 7
Allethrin (I)	pyrethroid	3, 10
Aspon (I)	organothio/dithiophosphate	3
Azinphos-methyl (I)	organothio/dithiophosphate	3, 8
Benomyl (F)	carbamate	5, 8
Biphenyl (F)	aromatic	5
Bromacil (H)	diazine	4, 9
Cacodylic acid (H)	organoarsenical	4, 8
Captan (F)	phthalimide	5, 7
Carbofuran (I)	carbamate	3
Chlordimeform (I)	haloaromatic amidate	3
Chlorpyrifos (I)	organothio/dithiophosphate	3, 11
Chrysanthemic acid (I)	pyrethroid	3, 11
Crotoxyphos (I)	organothio/dithiophosphate	3, 8
Cypermethrin (I)	pyrethroid	3
Demeton (I)	organothio/dithiophosphate	3, 7
Diallate (H)	thiocarbamate	4, 7
Diazinon (I)	organothio/dithiophosphate	3
Dicamba (H)	halophenoxy	4, 11
Dichloran (F)	chlorinated nitroaniline	5
m-dichlorobenzene (I)	haloaromatic	3, 11
o-dichlorobenzene (I)	haloaromatic	3, 11
p-dichlorobenzene (I)	haloaromatic	3
Dinoseb (H)	dinitrophenol	4, 11
Disulfoton (I)	organothio/dithiophosphate	3, 8
DSMA (H)	organoarsenical	4
Endrin (I)	chlorinated hydrocarbon	3
Ethion (I)	organothio/dithiophosphate	3
Ethyl chrysanthemate (I)	pyrethroid	3, 12
Fensulfothion (I)	organothio/dithiophosphate	3
Fenthion (I)	organothio/dithiophosphate	3
Folpet (F)	phthalimide	5, 7
Fonofos (I)	phosphonate/thiophosphorate	3
Formetanate (I)	carbamate	3
Malathion (I)	organothio/dithiophosphate	3
Mancozeb (F)	ethylenebisdithiocarbamate	5, 12
Maneb (F)	ethylenebisdithiocarbamate	5, 12
Methomyl (I)	carbamate	3
Methoxychlor (I)	chlorinated hydrocarbon	3
Methyl-parathion (I)	organothio/dithiophosphate	3, 8
Monocrotophos (I)	organophosphate	3, 7

Table 1 (continued)

Name (action)	Chemical Class	Table No. for Results
Monuron (H)	urea	4, 8
MSMA (H)	organic arsenical	4
Parathion (I)	organothio/dithiophosphate	3
PCNB (F)	haloaromatic	5
Pentachlorophenol (H)	haloaromatic	4, 12
Permethrin (I)	pyrethroid	3
Phorate (I)	organothio/dithiophosphate	3
Polyram (F)	ethylenebisdithiocarbamate	5
Propanil (H)	haloaromatic	4, 11
Resmethrin (I)	pyrethroid	3
Rotenone (I)	hydrocarbon	3
sec butylamine (F)	aliphatic amine	5, 11
sec butylamine H_3PO_4 (F)	aliphatic amine	5
Siduron (H)	urea	4
Simazine (H)	triazine	4, 9
Sulfallate (H)	thio/dithiocarbamate	4, 10
Sumithrin (I)	pyrethroid	3
Triallate (H)	thio/dithiocarbamate	4, 7
Trichlorfon (I)	phosphonate/thiophosphonate	3, 7
Trifluralin (H)	nitroaromatic	4
Zineb (F)	ethylenebisdithiocarbamate	5, 12
2,4-D (H)	halophenoxy	4, 11
2,4-DB (H)	halophenoxy	4, 11
2,4,5-T (H)	halophenoxy	4, 11

organization of the test organism (prokaryote or eukaryote). The latter distinction is significant in view of the substantial differences in cell structure, metabolism and genetic replicative processes between the two classes of organisms. Each bioassay is denoted by a three-character descriptor, in accordance with the EPA GENE-TOX Program (8, 23) nomenclature, to facilitate computerized tabulation of test results. "YE3" and "SAR" represent enhanced mitotic recombination in S. cerevisiae D3 and differential toxicity assay in S. typhimurium (to be described later). These two code words are not employed in the GENE-TOX data file. Below are brief descriptions of each of the bioassay systems and, where applicable, the associated metabolic activation systems. Also described are the criteria used for judging whether a test chemical yields a genotoxic effect in a particular test. In general a result must be observed repeatedly for a test chemical to be considered

Table 2. Genotoxicity Bioassays Employed

Descriptor	Organism	Property Examined	Reference
Point/Gene Mutations in Prokaryotes			
SAL*	S. typhimurium (5 strains)	Reverse mutation	(1)
WPU*	E. coli WP2 uvrA	Reverse mutation	(2)
Point/Gene Mutations in Eukaryotes			
YER	S. cerevisiae D7	Reverse mutation	(27)
L5T	Mouse lymphoma L5178Y cells	Forward mutation	(5)
SRL	D. melanogaster	Recessive lethality	(25)
Primary DNA Damage in Prokaryotes			
REP*	E. coli polA	Differential toxicity	(21)
REW*	B. subtilis rec	Differential toxicity	(13)
SAR	S. typhimurium uvrB, rec	Differential toxicity	(1)
Primary DNA Damage in Eukaryotes			
YE3*	S. cerevisiae D3	Enhanced mitotic recombination	(4)
YEH	S. cerevisiae D7	Gene conversion and crossing-over	(28)
UDH*	Human lung fibroblasts WI-38	Unscheduled DNA synthesis	(19)
Chromosomal Effects			
SCC	Chinese hamster ovary cells	Sister-chromatid exchange	(16, 22)
MNM	Mouse bone marrow and cardiac blood	Chromosome breakage (micronuclei)	(17)
DLM	Mouse	Dominant lethality	(18)

*A bioassay from the initial battery of screening tests.

"positive" or "negative" for genotoxicity in a bioassay, while mixed or ambiguous results are termed "no test".

The bioassays are also classified as "initial" or "confirmatory"; these designations refer to the sequence in which they were performed. In the initial stage of this study a battery of six bioassays (SAL, WPU, REP, REW, YE3 and UDH) was used to evaluate most of the pesticides discussed here; many of the compounds that exhibited some positive genotoxic effect in the initial tests, or that were suspected of having genotoxic potential from other information available, were later subjected to more extensive testing in confirmatory bioassay systems.

Metabolic Activation

The following mutation bioassays were carried out both in the presence and absence of an Aroclor-1254 induced metabolic activation system: SAL, WPU, YER, L5T, YE3, YEH, UDH and SCC. Adult male Sprague-Dawley rats weighing 250 to 300 g were obtained from Simonsen Laboratories for use in preparing liver homogenates for the metabolic activation systems.

POINT/GENE MUTATIONS IN PROKARYOTES

Salmonella typhimurium Plate Incorporation Assay (SAL)

The S. typhimurium strains used in this test were histidine auxotrophs by virtue of mutations in the histidine operon. When these histidine-dependent cells are grown in minimal media with a trace of histidine, only those cells that revert to histidine independence ($\underline{his}^+$) are able to form colonies. The spontaneous mutation frequency of each strain is relatively constant, but when a mutagen is added to the agar medium, the reversion frequency increases, usually in relation to the amount of the added mutagen. The tester strains used, TA1535, TA1537, TA1538, TA98 and TA100, were obtained from Dr. Bruce Ames of the University of California at Berkeley. Procedures used with these strains have been described by Ames, McCann and Yamasaki (1). All the indicator strains have a mutation ($\underline{rfa}^-$) that leads to a defective lipopolysaccharide coat; they also have a deletion that covers genes involved in the synthesis of biotin ($\underline{bio}^-$) and in the repair of ultraviolet-induced DNA damage ($\underline{uvrB}^-$). The uvrB mutation causes decreased repair of some types of chemically or physically damaged DNA and thereby enhances the strain's sensitivity to some mutagenic agents. Strain TA100 is derived from TA1535 by the introduction of the resistance transfer factor pKM101. Strain TA98 is derived from TA1538 by the addition of plasmid pKM101, which also increases sensitivity to some mutagens.

Each chemical was usually tested at a minimum of six concentrations, with the highest non-toxic concentration tested being 10 mg/plate unless specific solubility dictated a lower amount. The concentrations tested were reduced appropriately for toxic chemicals. Ideally at least four nontoxic concentrations were tested for each chemical.

A mutagenic response was defined as a dose-related increase in the number of histidine-independent colonies per plate. A compound was considered positive when it produced a dose-related increase in the number or revertants in at least one strain for at least three concentration levels. A compound was considered negative when no dose-related increase in the number of revertants was observed in at least two independent experiments. When a compound could not be identified clearly as either positive or negative, the results were classified as inconclusive or "no test".

E. coli Reverse Mutation Assay (WPU)

E. coli strain WP2 is a tryptophan auxotroph (trp^-) by virtue of a base-pair substitution in the tryptophan operon. In addition, it is deficient in the repair of some physically or chemically induced DNA damage ($uvrA^-$), which makes the strain more sensitive to certain mutagens. The procedure used for this bioassay has been described by Bridges (2). Concurrent positive (known mutagen) and negative (solvent) control tests were run with each test. The positive control chemicals were 2-(2-furyl)-3-(5-nitro-2-furyl)-acrylamide (AF-2) without metabolic activation and 2-aminoanthracene with metabolic activation. Each test chemical was assayed at a minimum of six concentrations, with the highest nontoxic concentration tested being 10 mg/ plate (or lower for more toxic chemicals). The criteria for judgement of mutagenicity are the same as for the S. typhimurium bioassay.

POINT/GENE MUTATIONS IN EUKARYOTES

S. cerevisiae D7 Reverse Mutation Assay (YER)

The yeast strain S. cerevisiae D7 is homozygous at the ilvi92/ilvi92 gene locus and requires isoleucine for growth. The isoleucine requirement caused by the homozygous condition can be alleviated by true reverse mutation and by allele-nonspecific suppressor mutation. Mutation induction can be followed by the appearance of colonies not requiring isoleucine on selective media. When the test material is plated on medium that lacks isoleucine, only the mutants are capable of growing. The frequency of reverse mutation can therefore be measured by counting the numbers of revertant

colonies on agar plates that lack isoleucine. The S. cerevisiae
D7 strain used was originally obtained from Dr. F.K. Zimmerman,
who has described the procedures for use of this strain (27).
Solvent was used as the negative control sample. The positive
control agent was 1,2,3,4-diepoxybutane. Five concentrations of
the test chemical were bioassayed both with and without metabolic
activation. For toxic compounds, the concentration range was
decreased until about 50% final toxicity was obtained. A dose-
response relationship in revertant colony formation must have been
observed repeatedly for the test substance to be judged positive.
Otherwise the criteria for interpretation of results were the same
as for SAL.

Mouse Lymphoma Forward Mutation Assay (L5T)

Most mammalian cells possess two metabolic pathways for
production of thymidine triphosphate: the major pathway includes
the enzyme thymidine synthetase, and a second, "salvage" pathway
utilizes the enzyme thymidine kinase to process exogenous thymidine
or thymidine derived from DNA degradation. The thymidine analogue
trifluorothymidine (TFT) is lethal to cells that have the salvage
pathway, as TFT is incorporated into the cells, then irreversibly
binds to and inhibits a key enzyme for DNA synthesis. Thus, cells
possessing thymidine kinase will die while thymidine-kinase deficient
($TK^{-/-}$) cells survive. In the L5178 mouse lymphoma cell mutagenesis
assay (5), cells heterozygous for thymidine kinase ($TK^{+/-}$) were
incubated with the test chemical and subsequently cloned in the
presence of trifluorothymidine; surviving colonies indicated
mutation to homozygous $TK^{-/-}$ cells. The test results were considered
positive if the mutation frequency of at least one concentration
tested was at least twice the background mutation frequency and if
there was a concentration-related increase in the mutation frequency.
Results were considered negative if none of the treated samples
showed a mutation frequency more than double the background rate
and if there was no indication of a concentration-related response
in the mutation frequency. Results were considered inconclusive
if the compound showed limited or no cytotoxicity at the highest
concentrations tested or if there was a lack of reproducibility in
repeated experiments.

Drosophila melanogaster Sex-Linked Recessive Lethal Assay (SRL)

The sex-linked recessive lethality test using the fruit fly
D. melanogaster can detect lethal point mutations and small deletions on the X-chromosomes, which constitutes about 20% of the
Drosophila genome. The sex-linked recessive lethal test used by
WARF Inc. has been described (24). The sex-linked recessive
lethal test used by SRI International was a modification of the
yellow-Bar test described by Würgler et al. (25). In this system,
males that carry the genes BAR (B) and yellow (y) on the X chromosome

plus two minute secondary translocations of the X-chromosome, bearing the wild-type allele (y^+), one on each arm of the Y-chromosome, were exposed to the test chemical. The exposed males were crossed to females carrying the Inscy X-chromosome in homozygous condition; this doubly inverted X is marked with y and scute (sc). The male and female progeny of this mating (F_1 generation) were in turn mated with each other and the resulting progeny (F_2 generation) were examined. Absence of the treated male phenotype in the F_2 generation was considered evidence of recessive lethal mutation.

Cultures of the F_2 generation were examined under a dissecting microscope approximately two weeks after initiation of the brood. If at least two Bar-eyed males were present, the culture was scored as nonlethal. If there were at least 20 progeny and no Bar-eyed males, the culture was retested for confirmation of lethality, as were cultures with less than 20 progeny and a low ratio of Bar-eyed males to Bar-eyed females. In the retest, three F_2 females of the yellow-Bar phenotype were mated with their F_2 male siblings, and their progeny (the F_3 generation) were examined. If no Bar-eyed males occurred among more than 20 offspring, the culture was scored as lethal. If some F_2 females tested lethal and some nonlethal, their gonads were mosaic for a sex-linked recessive lethal mutation and this group was also scored as lethal. If less than 20 progeny emerged from all the F_3 cultures, this test was eliminated from final scoring calculations. On completion of the scoring of all the test results, the tabulated results were subjected to statistical analysis to determine an overall mutation frequency. A compound that induced an increase in the background mutation rate of at least 0.2% at the 95% statistical confidence level was considered to elicit a positive response. Compounds that were tested with a sample population sufficient to permit detection at the 95% statistical confidence level but did not elicit a 0.2% increase in mutation rate over the background level were classified as negative. Compounds tested in insufficient numbers to permit detection of a 0.2% increase in mutation rate over the background rate at the 95% confidence level were rated as inconclusively tested..

PRIMARY DNA DAMAGE IN PROKARYOTES

E. coli polA Differential Toxicity Assay (REP)

E. coli strain p3478 is a DNA polymerase I deficient (polA⁻) derivative of strain W3110 (6). The enzyme DNA polymerase I is involved in resynthesizing DNA segments that have been damaged and excised. Bacterial strains deficient in DNA polymerase I are thus more sensitive to DNA damage, and will exhibit diminished growth in the presence of DNA-damaging agents in comparison with the

parent strain. Therefore, test compounds that are more toxic to
p3478 than to W3100 may be assumed to react with DNA.

The two E. coli strains were obtained from Dr. H. Rosenkranz,
who has described the test procedure (21). To determine a test
compound's relative toxicity to the two bacterial strains, a disk
of filter paper inoculated with the test substance was placed on
the surfaces of two agar plates, each containing nutrient broth
and one of the bacterial strains used for the assay. After the
plates have been incubated for a day, the zone of inhibition of
growth of bacteria by the test compound was measured. Comparison
of the diameters of the zones of growth inhibition for the polA
and normal strains allowed determination of whether the test compound gave rise to DNA damage. The positive control compound in
this assay was methyl methanesulfonate, and the negative controls
were ampicillin, kanamycin or chloramphenicol, which induce equal
zones of toxicity because their toxic effects are not due to DNA
damage. A positive response was indicated by a larger zone of inhibition on the repair-deficient strain than on the normal strain,
while a negative response is indicated by equal zones of growth on
both plates. A result was considered inconclusive when no growth
inhibition was observed on either of the test plates. At least
two concentration levels of test compound were used, and final
testing consisted of two repetitions of the experiments performed on
separate days.

B. subtilis recA Differential Toxicity Assay (REW)

B. subtilis strain M45 is a recombination-deficient (recA⁻)
derivative of strain H17; both strains were obtained from Dr. T.
Kada. Recombination is required for repair of damaged DNA. Except
for the difference in test strains, the method of testing (13)
and criteria for interpretation were the same as for the REP assay.

S. typhimurium SL4525 (rec⁺)/SL4700(rec⁻) Differential Toxicity Assay (SAR)

S. typhimurium strain SL4700 is a recombination-deficient
derivative of strain SL4525; both strains were obtained from
Dr. Bruce Stocker of Stanford University. These two strains also
have an rfa⁻ mutation that leads to a defective lipopolysaccharide
coat, which makes them more permeable to larger molecules and thus
more suitable for testing of possible mutagens. A second pair of
Salmonella strains, also containing the rfa⁻ mutation, are strains
TA1978 and TA1538, obtained from Dr. Bruce Ames of the University
of California. Strain TA1538 lacks the uvrB gene, which is involved
in the repair of DNA damage caused by exposure to ultraviolet
light. The methods for testing and evaluating the ability of
pesticides to induce DNA damage by use of these pairs of bacterial
strains (1) were similar to those described in the REP assay.

PRIMARY DNA DAMAGE IN EUKARYOTES

S. cerevisiae D3 Assay (YE3)

The yeast S. cerevisiae D3 is a diploid microorganism heterozygous for a mutation leading to a defective enzyme in the adenine-metabolizing pathway. When grown on a medium containing adenine, cells homozygous for this mutation produce a red pigment. These homozygous mutants can be generated from the heterozygotes by mitotic recombination. The frequency of this recombinational event is increased by incubation in the presence of recombinogenic agents. The recombinogenic activity of a compound or its metabolites was determined from the number of red-pigmented colonies appearing on test plates, as described by Brusick and Mayer (4). Five concentrations of the test chemical were tested both with and without metabolic activation. For toxic compounds the concentration range was lowered until approximately 50% toxicity was reached. A positive response in this assay was indicated by dose-related increases of more than threefold in the absolute number of mitotic recombinants per milliliter and in the relative number of mitotic recombinants per 10^5 survivors. A negative response was indicated by no recombinogenic activity in any of the assays. When positive results were not dose-related, the test was considered inconclusive.

S. cerevisiae D7 Gene Conversion and Mitotic Crossing-Over Assays (YEH)

S. cerevisiae D7 is heterozygous for a mutation leading to a defective enzyme in the adenine-metabolizing pathway. When grown on a medium containing adenine, cells homozygous for this mutation produce pink and red twin-sectored colonies of the genotype ade2-40/ade2-40 (deep red) and ade2-119/ade2-119 (pink) from the original heteroallelic condition ade2-40/ ade2-119, which forms white colonies. These homozygous mutants can be generated from heterozygotes by mitotic crossing-over, and the frequency of this event is determined by counting the numbers of twin-sectored colonies appearing on the plates. The methods used for testing with this strain have been described by Zimmerman (28).

Also detected by this strain that is heteroallelic for ade2-40/ade2-119 are colonies that are pink, red, white and pink, and red and white. These additional colonies appear more frequently than the twin-sectored colonies and may result from a variety of events such as point mutation, gene conversion, chromosomal deletions, and aneuploidy. No effort was made to distinguish the different phenotypic aberrants or their causes - they were all grouped as total aberrants.

$\underline{S}$. $\underline{\text{cerevisiae}}$ is also heterozygous for a mutation leading to
a specific growth requirement. The heterozygous condition $\underline{\text{trp5-12}}$/
$\underline{\text{trp5-27}}$ leads to the requirement for exogenous tryptophan for
growth. Transfer of the intact region of one mutant allele to
replace the defective nucleotide sequence in the other mutant
allele (gene crossover) will restore a true wild-type genotype
that allows growth in the absence of tryptophan. Thus plating the
test substance on medium that lacks tryptophan allows determination
of the frequency of mitotic gene conversion from the number of
colonies appearing on the selective media plates.

The number of mitotic recombinants and the number of total
aberrants per 10^5 survivors, and the number of gene convertants
per 10^6 survivors, were calculated. Positive responses for mitotic
crossing-over and for mitotic gene conversion were indicated by
dose-related increases in the numbers of aberrant or convertant
colonies. Negative responses were indicated when no dose-related
increases in aberration or conversion were observed, and inconclusive results were indicated when responses were not unequivocally
positive or negative.

Human Lung Fibroblast Unscheduled DNA Synthesis Assay (UDH)

Unscheduled DNA synthesis (UDS) is the incorporation of
nucleotides into the DNA of cells during repair of damage induced
by physical or chemical agents. In this test, the incorporation
of tritiated thymidine, $[^3H]$-dT, into human lung fibroblast cells
(strain WI-38) was monitored by liquid scintillation counting.
The methods used were a variation of those described by Simmon
(19). The cells are grown in synchronous culture so that the
assay was conducted only when the cells were not in the synthetic
(S) phase, when normal DNA synthesis would have overwhelmed any
measurement of DNA repair synthesis. Cells were incubated with
the test chemical and $[^3H]$-dT, with or without a metabolic activation
system, for a few hours, then their DNA was extracted and the
$[^3H]$-dT content measured by liquid scintillation counting. Positive
controls were 4-nitroquinoline-N-oxide, which induces unscheduled
DNA synthesis in the absence of metabolic activation, and
dimethylnitrosamine, which induces UDS only with metabolic activation. The negative control was DMSO in culture medium. Preliminary
studies were performed to select an appropriate concentration
range. Testing was conducted with five concentrations of test
compound for each assay, with six replicate samples for each
concentration to facilitate statistical analysis of the results.
A test material was considered positive if there was a significant
concentration-related increase in thymidine incorporation in test
cells compared to the negative controls, negative if no significant
increase in thymidine incorporation was observed, and inconclusive
if neither of the above criteria was met.

CHROMOSOMAL EFFECTS

Sister-Chromatid Exchange (SCC)

The induction of DNA lesions by chemical mutagens leads to the formation of sister-chromatid exchanges (SCEs), which may be related to a recombinational or postreplicative repair of DNA damage. Exchanges between two chromatids of a chromosome are observed in cells that have been grown in the presence of bromodeoxyuridine (BrdU) for two rounds of replication. Because of semiconservative DNA replication, such chromosomes possess one chromatid that is half BrdU-substituted and one that is fully substituted. These chromatids are differentially stained by the fluorescence-plus-Giemsa technique; hence exposure to a chromosome-damaging material results in an increased frequency of SCEs, revealed by the "harlequin" pattern of dark and light stained chromatid segments.

The Chinese hamster ovary (CHO) cells used in this assay were obtained from the American Type Culture Collection (ATCC-CCL-61). Procedures for the maintenance of these cells and for demonstration of SCEs have been described by Perry and Evans (16) and by Stetka and Wolff (22). The positive control compounds were ethyl methanesulfonate, which induces SCEs in the absence of a metabolic activation system, and dimethyl-nitrosamine, which induces SCEs only with metabolic activation. Since chemicals may affect the duration of the cell cycle and since treated cells must divide twice to be evaluated for SCE induction, a series of five dilutions of the compound and positive and negative controls were used with and without metabolic activation. For each test, two cytogeneticists analyzed duplicate coded samples of at least three concentrations of the test compound and the controls. Each observer analyzed 25 cells per sample for the total number of SCEs per cell and for the number of chromosomes per cell. A test compound was considered positive if both cytogeneticists agreed that it induced at least twice the baseline SCE frequencies or that at least three concentrations showed a progressive increase in SCE frequencies, with at least one value being significant at a p level less than 0.001. A compound was considered negative if both cytogeneticists agreed that the above criteria were not met, and an inconclusive result was recorded if only one observer judged the positive criteria to have been fulfilled.

Mouse Micronucleus Assay (MNM)

The micronucleus test is a rapid, in vivo assay based on the observation that cells with chromosome breaks and/or exchanges often have disturbances in the distribution of chromatin during cell division. After division, the daughter cells contain this displaced chromatin as distinct micronuclei in the cytoplasm. The

cell population examined consisted of erythrocytes taken from bone
marrow or peripheral blood smears of mice. Since erythrocytes
normally do not contain DNA, the presence of micronuclei in these
cells was considered evidence of chromosomal breakage.

     Test compounds were administered according to the method of
Schmid (17). The test compound was dissolved in an appropriate
solvent and administered by oral gavage or intraperitoneal injection
to a group of male Swiss-Webster mice. Trimethylphosphate (TMP)
was the positive control agent, and solvent was the negative
control. Eight mice were selected randomly from each treatment
group, sacrificed, and cardiac blood and bone marrow were extracted
from each animal and smeared on slides. The slides were stained
with Giemsa stain, and the number of micronucleated cells per 500
polychromatophilic cells was recorded for each slide. The tabulated results were analyzed according to the statistical methods
of Mackey and MacGregor (14) to determine whether a dose group was
positive or negative.

Mouse Dominant Lethal Assay (DLM)

     A final test for chromosomal effects of chemicals was the
mouse dominant lethal assay, in which male mice were fed the test
compound and mated with fertile females. Pregnant females were
sacrificed and sectioned at midterm, and the numbers of corpora
lutea, dead and live fetuses were counted. Comparison of these
mice with those impregnated by untreated males allowed judgement
of whether genotoxic effects of the test chemical affected the
sperm. The methodology for this test followed that of Simmon
(18).

     Adult ICR/SIM mice from a closed, random-bred colony were
used to determine the acute toxicity and maximum tolerated dose as
well as for the dominant lethal assay. The mice were supplied by
Simonsen Laboratories, Gilroy, California. The males were 3- to
4-month-old proven breeders, and the females were 10- to 12-week-old
virgin stock.

     Each pesticide to be tested was dissolved or suspended in
corn oil. The compound-oil concentrate then was added at a level
of 3% to a finely ground commercial diet of known composition.
Untreated control animals were given a diet containing 3% corn
oil. Positive controls were administered a single intraperitoneal
injection of 0.2 mg/kg of triethylenemelamine (TEM) two hours
before the first mating. Treated animals were given diets containing the maximum tolerated dose (or 5 g/kg, whichever was
lower), one-half and one-quarter of the maximum dose. For this
work, a maximum tolerated dose was defined as that dietary level
which may produce up to a 20% weight loss, mild but transient

clinical signs, no inhibition of breeding performance, and no
mortality.

Each control and experimental test group contained 20 adult
male mice. The treatment and control diets were administered for
seven weeks. At the end of the treatment period, each male was
allowed to breed with two virgin females over a period of seven
days. Females were replaced weekly for eight weeks.

Females were sacrificed at midterm of pregnancy. A complete
autopsy was performed to determine if infection was present; such
a condition can induce preimplantation loss and early fetal deaths.
At sacrifice, each female was scored for early fetal deaths, late
fetal deaths, and living fetuses (all of which provided a total
implant score). The index of dead implants per total implants was
analyzed statistically by the t-test on angular transformed data
(8). A result was judged positive only if the level of mortality
increase of implants was statistically significant.

RESULTS AND DISCUSSION

The qualitative test results obtained in each system for each
chemical are presented in Tables 3, 4, and 5 for insecticides,
herbicides and fungicides, respectively. Results are scored as +
for positive responses, - for negative responses, and NT, "no
test," for ambiguous results. In vitro tests that elicited positive
responses only with addition of a metabolic activation preparation
are denoted by asterisks. The data revealed that 35 of the 65
chemicals were positive in one or more test systems: 19 of the 35
caused point/gene mutations, 29 caused DNA damage, and 9 caused
chromosomal effects. Although testing is not yet complete, 11 of
the chemicals produced a positive response in only one test system.

Detection and Confirmation of Genetic Activity

An analysis of the individual test systems for sensitivity is
presented in Table 6. Six tests (SAL, WPU, REP, REW, YE3 and UDH)
were performed with 51 or more of the pesticides. Five of the
test systems, (YER, L5T, YEH, SCC and MNM) were used as confirmatory
tests on pesticides found positive in the initial test battery.
Only a fraction of the 35 positive pesticides was detected in any
one of the tests in the initial battery.

Among the 6 tests applied initially, YE3 detected the largest
number of positive chemicals and WPU the smallest. Of the chemicals
positive in one or more tests in the initial test battery, the
prokaryotic systems REW, SAL, REP and WPU detected 11/32 (34%),
10/34 (29%), 9/32 (28%), and 4/34 (12%), respectively. One tester
strain in the SAL assay, TA100, detected all 10 of the chemicals

Table 3. Genotoxicity Bioassay Results for Insecticides

| Compound | Point/Gene Mutation | | | | | DNA Damage | | | | | | Chromosomal Effects | | |
| | Prokaryote | | Eukaryote | | | Prokaryote | | | Eukaryote | | | | | |
	SAL	WPU	YER	L5T	SRL	REP	REW	SAR	YE3	YEH	UDH	SCC	MNM	DLM
Acephate	+	-	+*	+	-	NT	NT	-	+	+	+	+	-	-
Allethrin	+*	-				NT	-		-	-	-	-		
Aspon	-	-			-	NT	NT		-				-	
Azinphos-methyl	-	-	-	+*	-	NT	NT	-	+		-	-	-	-
Carbofuran	-	-			-	NT	NT		-		-			
Chlordimeform	-	-				NT	-		-		-			
Chlorpyrifos	-	-			-	+	+	+	-		-			
Chrysanthemic acid	-	-				-	+		-					
Crotoxyphos	-	-		+	-	NT	NT	-	+	-		-	-	
Cypermethrin	-	-			-	NT	NT		-		-			
Demeton	+	+	+	+		-	+	-	+	+	+	+	-	
Diazinon	-	-				NT	NT		-		-			
m-dichlorobenzene	-	-				+	-		+					
o-dichlorobenzene	-	-				+	-		-					
p-dichlorobenzene	-	-				-	-		-					
Disulfoton	-	-	-	+	-	NT	NT	-	-	-	+	+*	-	
Endrin	-	-				-	-		-		-			
Ethion	-	-				-	-		-		-			

Table 3 (continued)

Compound	Point/Gene Mutation					DNA Damage						Chromosomal Effects		
	Prokaryote		Eukaryote			Prokaryote			Eukaryote					
	SAL	WPU	YER	L5T	SRL	REP	REW	SAR	YE3	YEH	UDH	SCC	MNM	DLM
Ethyl chrysanthemate	-	-				-					-			
Fensulfothion	-	-				-	-		+		-			
Fenthion	-	-				NT	NT		-		-			
Fonofos	-	-			-	NT	NT		-		-			
Formetanate	-	-				-			-					
Malathion	-	-			-	-	-		-		-			-
Methomyl	-	-			-	-	-		-		-			
Methoxychlor	-	-			-	NT	NT		-		-			
Methyl-parathion	-	-	-	+	-	NT	NT	-	+	-	-	+*		-
Monocrotophos	+	-	+	+	-	NT	NT	+	+	+	+*	+	-	-
Parathion	-	-			-	-	-		-		-			-
Permethrin	-	-				NT	NT		-		-			
Phorate	-	-			-	-	-		-		-			
Resmethrin	-	-				NT	NT		-		-			-
Rotenone														
Sumithrin	-	-				NT	NT		-		-		-	
Trichlorfon	+	+	+	+	-	NT	NT	+	+	+	+	+	-	-

Table 4. Genotoxicity Bioassay Results for Herbicides

| Compound | Point/Gene Mutation | | | | | DNA Damage | | | | | | Chromosomal Effects | | |
| | Prokaryote | | Eukaryote | | | Prokaryote | | | Eukaryote | | | | | |
	SAL	WPU	YER	L5T	SRL	REP	REW	SAR	YE3	YEH	UDH	SCC	MNM	DLM
Bromacil	-	-	-	+	+	-	-	-	-	-	-	-	-	-
Cacodylic acid	-	-	+	+	-	NT	NT	-	+	+	-	-	+	
Diallate	+*	-	-	+	+		+		+*	-	-			
Dicamba	-	-				+	+	-	-		-			
Dinoseb	-	-			-	+	+	+	-		-			
DSMA	-	-				-	-		-		-			
Monuron	-	-	+	+		-	-		-	-	-	+*	+	
MSMA	-	-			-	-	-		-		-			
Pentachlorophenol	-	-				-	+	+	+		-			
Propanil	-	-				-	+	+	-		-			
Siduron	-	-			-	NT	NT	-	-		-			
Simazine	-	-	-	+*	+	NT	NT		-	-	-	-	-	
Sulfallate	+*	-				-	-		-					
Triallate	+*	-	-	+	-				+*	-				
Trifluralin	-	-			-	-	-	-	-		-			
2,4-D	-	-				-	+	-	-		-			
2,4-DB	-	-				+	-	-	-		-			
2,4,5-T	-	-				-	+		-		-			

Table 5. Genotoxicity Bioassay Results for Fungicides

Compound	Point/Gene Mutation					DNA Damage						Chromosomal Effects		
	Prokaryote		Eukaryote			Prokaryote			Eukaryote					
	SAL	WPU	YER	L5T	SRL	REP	REW	SAR	YE3	YEH	UDH	SCC	MNM	DLM
Benomyl												+	+	
Biphenyl	−	−		+		NT	NT	−	−		−			
Captan	+	+		+	+	+	+	+	+		−			
Dichloran	−	−				−	−		−					−
Folpet	+	+		+	+	+	+	+	+		−			−
Mancozeb	−	−				−	−	+	+		+[a]			
Maneb	−	−				−	−	+	+		+[b]			
PCNB	−	−			−	NT	NT		−		−			−
Polyram	−	−				−	−		−		−			
sec-butylamine	−	−				+	−		−		−			
sec-butylamine H₃PO₄	−	−				−	−							
Zineb	−	−				−	−		+		−			

[a] Dithane M-45: negative; Manzate 200: positive without metabolic activation, negative with metabolic activation.

[b] Dithane M-22: negative; Manzate D: positive without metabolic activation, negative with metabolic activation.

Table 6.   Summary of Positive Results for Pesticide Bioassays

Test System	Positive Responses				Total Tested
	Insecticide	Herbicide	Fungicide	Total	
Initial Battery					
YE3	9	4	5	18	63
REW	3	6	2	11	61
SAL	5	3	2	10	63
REP	3	3	3	9	61
UDH	5	0	2	7	51
WPU	2	0	2	4	63
Subsequent Tests					
L5T*	8	6	3	17	17
SCC*	6	1	1	8	13
SAR	3	2	2	7	19
YER	4	1		5	14
YEH	4	1		5	14
SRL	0	3	2	5	31
MNM	0	2	1	3	13
DLM	0	0	0	0	10

*Employed as confirmatory bioassay on chemicals showing genetic activity in another system.

positive in this system. The eukaryotic systems in the initial test battery, YE3 and UDH detected 18/34 (53%) and 7/31 (23%), respectively. Confirmation of initial test results was highest with the L5T assay (17/17, or 100%) and lowest with the MNM test (3/13, or 23%). When the test results were considered independently according to the functional classes of the pesticides, it was seen that of the initial tests YE3 detected the largest numbers of the positive insecticides and fungicides, 8/14 and 5/6, respectively.

Of the 18 pesticides positive in YE3, 12 were subsequently shown to be positive in L5T. (Six pesticides positive in YE3 have not yet been tested in L5T.) Hence, it appears that L5T confirms the genetic activity of many of the chemicals detected in YE3. Of 10 pesticides positive in SAL, 8 were positive in YE3 and these 8 were also positive in L5T. (Two pesticides positive in SAL have not yet been tested in L5T.) Thus, it appears that L5T also confirms the genetic activity of many pesticides detected by SAL. On the other hand, it appears that SAL may miss some genetically

active chemicals: of 10 pesticides negative in SAL, all were
positive in YE3 and four of these were subsequently shown positive
in L5T (six have not been tested in L5T.) Furthermore, of 34
pesticides positive in the initial test battery, 24 were negative
in SAL.

Clearly, no single test of the initial battery was sufficiently
sensitive to detect all genetically active pesticides. The results
underscore the need for a battery of screening tests to detect the
various kinds of genetic activity displayed by pesticide chemicals.

The present data are not complete enough to enable selection
of the most appropriate battery of assays for pesticide genotoxicity.
However, the results do indicate that a battery composed of SAL,
REP, REW, YE3, and L5T detected 35/35 of the positive chemicals;
five of these pesticides were detected only in the L5T system and
confirmed in another eukaryotic system. A test battery consisting
of SAL, YE3, and L5T detected 25 of the 35 positive pesticides (this
excludes 10 chemicals positive only for DNA damage in prokaryotic
systems); 20 of these 25 chemicals were positive in the SAL and YE3
test systems. Three tests, SAL, YE3, and L5T were required to
detect all pesticides active in the eukaryotic systems studied.

In 13 of the 100 in vitro tests scored positive, metabolic
activation was required. Only two compounds tested displayed an
absolute requirement for metabolic activation to produce genotoxicity (allethrin and sulfallate). In seven other instances
activity was observed without metabolic activation but not in the
presence of the activation system; these were azinphos-methyl in
YE3, demeton in L5T, and acephate, disulfoton, mancozeb, maneb and
trichlorfon, all in UDH.

Categories of Genetic Damage

We shall now examine in more detail the positive chemicals
with respect to the specific bioassays involved, the categories of
genetic damage observed, and the diversity of genetic activity
displayed by certain groups of chemicals.

Point/Gene Mutation. The 19 pesticides that caused point/gene
mutation as a major category of genetic damage may be further
subgrouped according to their genetic activities. Eight of these
compounds, as shown in Table 7, were positive for point/gene
mutation in prokaryotic and in eukaryotic systems and caused DNA
damage in eukaryotes. Acephate, demeton, monocrotophos, trichlorfon,
diallate, triallate, captan, and folpet all were positive in the
SAL and YE3 test systems of the initial test battery. In addition,
diallate, captan, and folpet were positive germ cell mutagens in
the Drosophila SRL test. Since the fungicides captan and folpet
had already been thoroughly evaluated in previous studies (3) and

Table 7. Pesticides Positive for Point/Gene Mutations in Pro- and Eukaryotic Systems and for DNA Damage in Eukaryotic Systems

| Compound | Point/Gene Mutation | | | | | DNA Damage | | | | | | Chromosomal Effects | | |
| | Prokaryote | | Eukaryote | | | Prokaryote | | | Eukaryote | | | | | |
	SAL	WPU	YER	L5T	SRL	REP	REW	SAR	YE3	YEH	UDH	SCC	MNM	DLM
Acephate (I)	+	-	+*	+	-	NT	NT	-	+	+	+	+	-	-
Demeton (I)	+	+	+	+	-	-	+	-	+	+	+	+	-	-
Monocrotophos (I)	+	-	+	+	-	NT	NT	+	+	+	+*	+	-	-
Trichlorfon (I)	+	+	+	+	-	NT	NT	+	+	+	+	+	-	-
Diallate (H)	+*	-	-	+	+				+*	-				
Triallate (H)	+*	-	-	+	-				+*	-				
Captan (F)	+	+	+	+	+	+	+	+	+	+	-			-
Folpet (F)	+	+	+	+	+	+	+	+	+	+	-			-

the herbicides diallate and triallate have recently been the
subject of additional testing (7), confirmatory tests were performed
only with the insecticides acephate, demeton, monocrotophos, and
trichlorfon. All four were positive in the YER, L5T, YEH, and SCC
test systems, providing strong confirmation of the initial test
results. These four insecticides are phosphoric/phosphonic acid
esters distinguished by side chains without ring structures
(Figure 1).

     Diallate and triallate (Figure 2) exerted similar genetic
effects in the battery of bioassays performed with each. Interestingly, these thiocarbamate compounds, which differ in structure
by only one chlorine atom, apparently differ in their abilities to
cause genetic damage in the Drosophila sex-linked recessive lethal
test. Sulfallate, a structurally similar thiocarbamate (Figure 2)
that is considered a carcinogen (9), has not been evaluated in the
L5T and SRL systems. The chemical structures of captan and folpet,
structually similar phthalimide fungicides, are shown in Figure 3.
Both of these compounds were highly active and virtually identical
in their bioassay responses.

     An additional group of seven pesticides were positive for
gene mutation and DNA damage or chromosomal effects only in
eukaryotic systems (Table 8). The genetic activities of azinphos-
methyl, crotoxyphos, methyl-parathion and cacodylic acid were
detected initially in the YE3 system, and that of disulfoton in
the UDH test. Monuron and benomyl were evaluated as a result of
other reports of genotoxic effects. All these chemicals except
benomyl were tested thoroughly in prokaryotic systems with negative
results. Despite the positive results for these compounds in
eukaryotic systems, there is no evidence that they cause germ cell
damage, as the Drosophila sex-linked recessive lethal tests were
negative. However, the positive mouse micronucleus tests for
cacodylic acid, monuron and benomyl do suggest that these compounds
can cause chromosomal damage in vivo.

     The chemical structures of the insecticides represented in
Table 8 (azinphos-methyl, crotoxyphos, disulfoton, and methyl-
parathion) are shown in Figure 4. These four compounds are
organophosphate or organothio/dithiophosphate ester insecticides.
Crotoxyphos is a phosphoric acid ester and methyl-parathion is a
thiophosphoric acid ester. Most of the thiophosphoric acid insecticides were negative or had little activity in the initial test
battery. The structures of some of these compounds are shown in
Figure 5. These particular thiophosphoric acid compounds differ
in one respect from the highly active insecticides (Figure 1), namely
by the presence of bulky side chain units often containing aromatic
rings. The activity of methyl-parathion in L5T, YE3, and SCC is
quite interesting in that parathion itself was negative in eight

Table 8. Pesticides Positive for Gene Mutation and DNA Damage or Chromosomal Effects only in Eukaryotic Systems

| Compound | Point/Gene Mutation | | | | | DNA Damage | | | | | | Chromosomal Effects | | |
| | Prokaryote | | Eukaryote | | | Prokaryote | | | Eukaryote | | | | | |
	SAL	WPU	YER	L5T	SRL	REP	REW	SAR	YE3	YEH	UDH	SCC	MNM	DLM
Azinphos-methyl (I)	-	-	-	+*	-	NT	NT	-	+	-	-	-	-	-
Crotoxyphos (I)	-	-	-	+	-	NT	NT	-	+	-	-	-	-	
Disulfoton (I)	-	-	-	+	-	NT	NT	-	-	-	+	+*	-	
Methyl-parathion (I)	-	-	-	+	-	NT	NT	-	+	-	-	+*	-	-
Cacodylic acid (H)	-	-	+	+	-	NT	NT	-	+	+	-	-	+	
Monuron (H)	-	-	-	+	-	-	-	-	-	-	-	+*	+	
Benomyl (F)				+								+	+	

Acephate

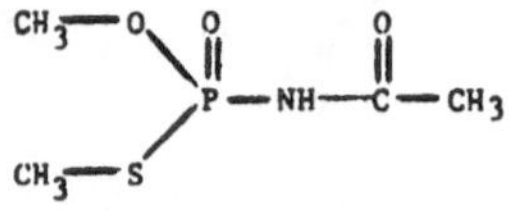

SAL, YER, L5T, YE3, YEH, UDH, SCC

Demeton

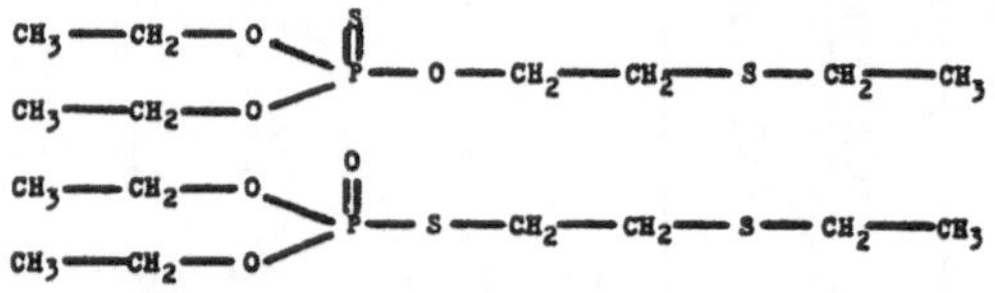

SAL, WPU, YER, L5T, REW, YE3, YEH, UDH, SCC

Monocrotophos

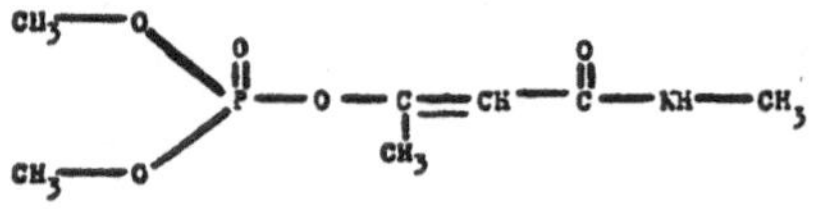

SAL, YER, L5T, SAR, YE3, YEH, UDH, SCC

Trichlorfon

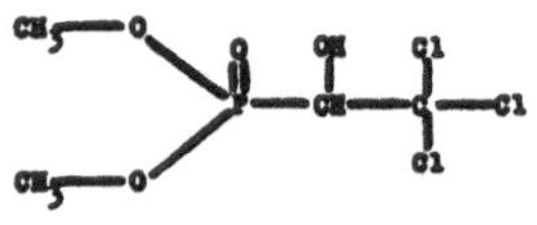

SAL, WPU, YER, L5T, SAR, YE3, YEH, UDH, SCC

Fig. 1.   Four organophosphate insecticides that displayed
extensive genotoxic activity.

Diallate

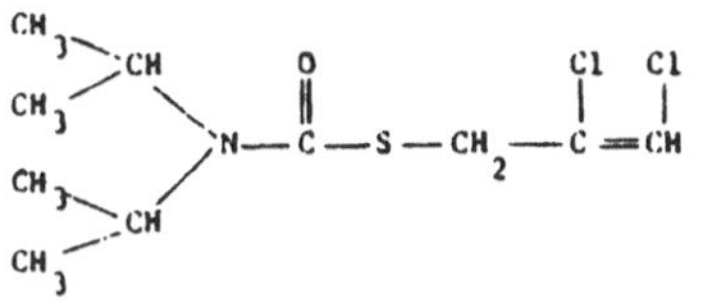

SAL, L5T, SRL, YE3

Triallate

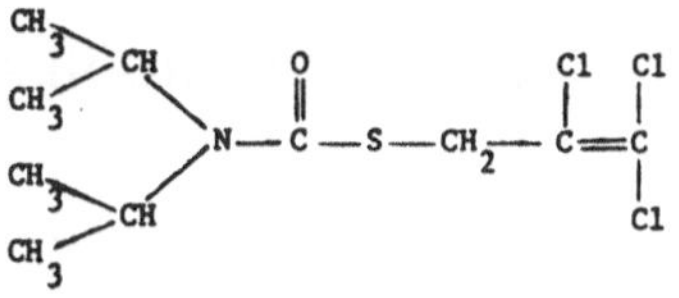

SAL, L5T, YE3

Sulfallate

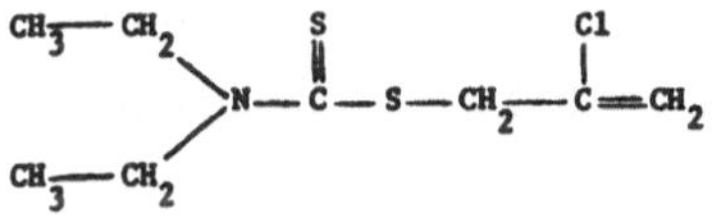

SAL

Fig. 2. Three thiocarbamate herbicides that displayed differing genotoxic effects.

Captan

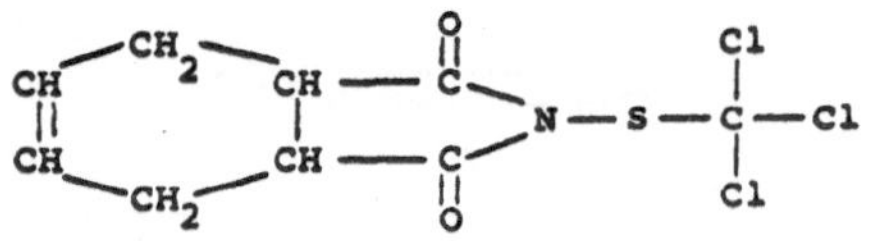

SAL, WPU, L5T, SRL, REP, REW, SAR, YE3

Folpet

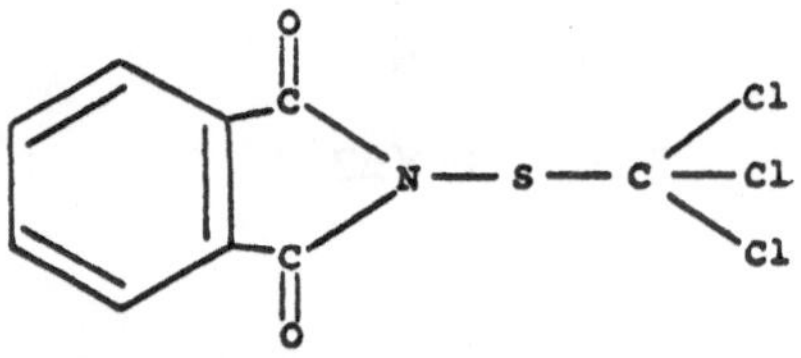

SAL, WPU, L5T, SRL, REP, REW, SAR, YE3

Fig. 3. Two phthalimide fungicides that exhibited extensive
genotoxic activity.

Azinphos-methyl

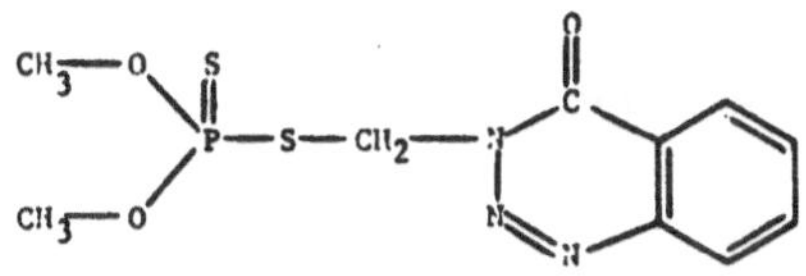

L5T, YE3

Crotoxyphos

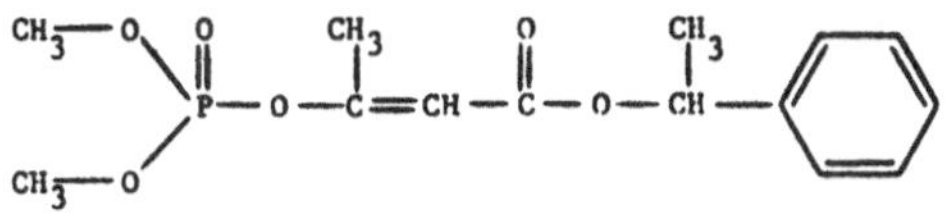

L5T, YE3

Disulfoton

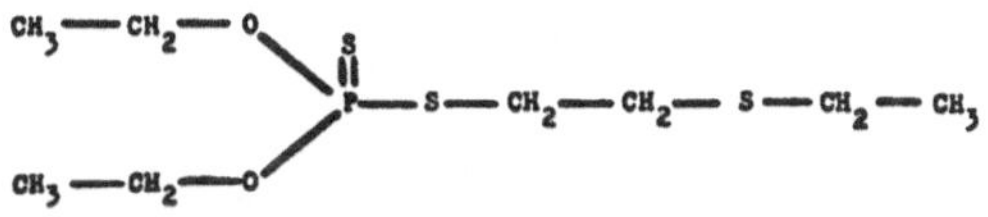

L5T, UDH, SCC

Methyl-Parathion

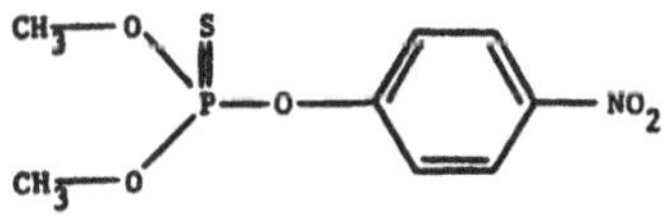

L5T, YE3, SCC

Fig. 4. Four organophosphate insecticides that displayed genotoxic effects only in eukaryotes.

Methyl-Parathion

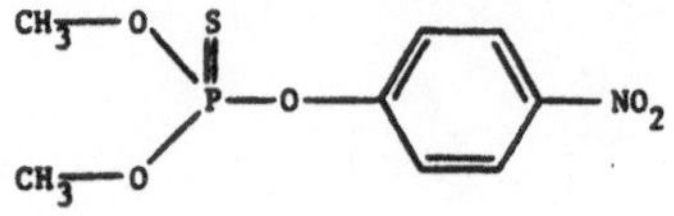

L5T, YE3, SCC

Chlorpyrifos

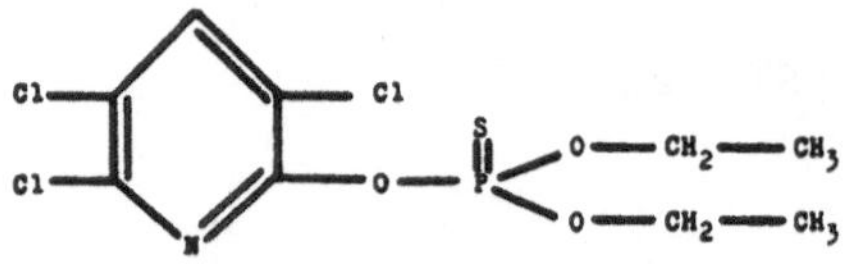

REP, REW, SAR

Aspon

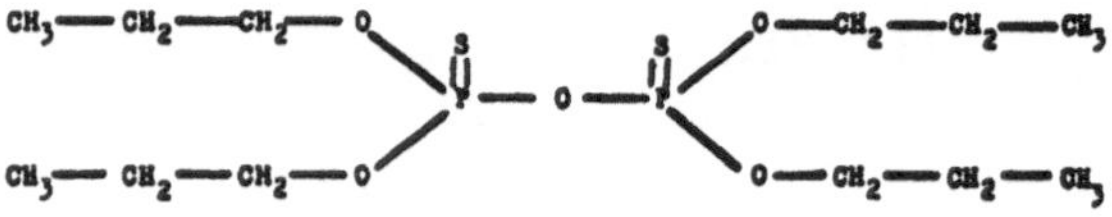

Diazinon

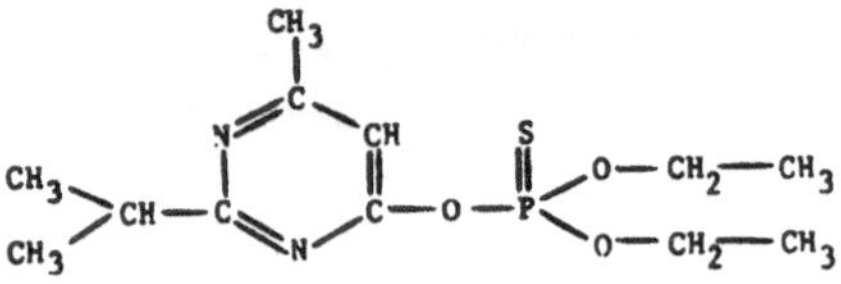

Fensulfothion

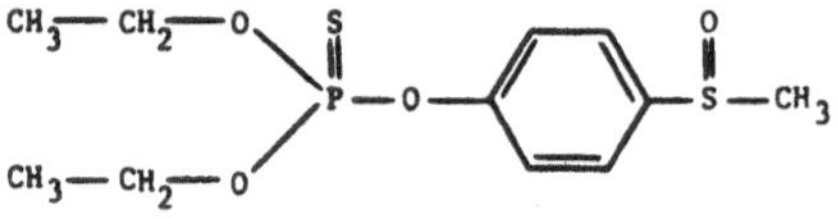

Fenthion

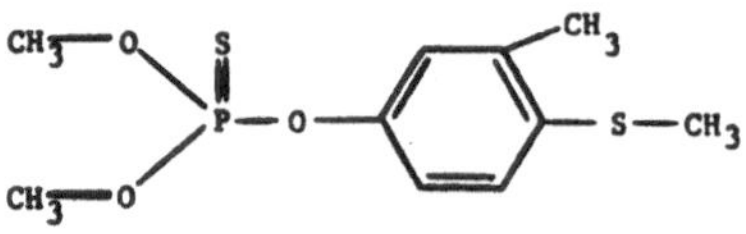

Parathion

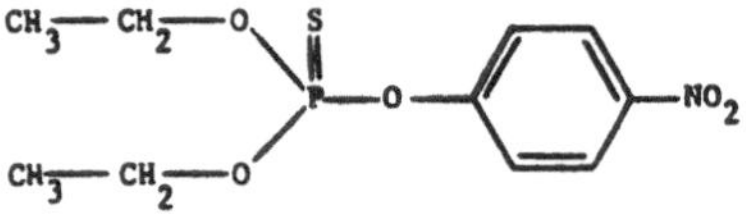

Fig. 5.   Seven thiophosphoric acid insecticides.

test systems. Thus parathion should be evaluated further in the
SCC and L5T systems.

The two other positive insecticides in Table 8, azinphos-
methyl and disulfoton, are dithiophosphate esters. Several compounds in this general category were evaluated and most were
negative (Figure 6). In fact, no dithiophosphoric acid ester
insecticides were present in the group of strongly genotoxic
insecticides. Disulfoton exhibited the most diverse activity
pattern of the dithiophosphate prototypes tested since the compound
elicited gene mutation, primary DNA damage and chromosomal effects.
Interestingly, disulfoton and the structurally similar compound
phorate (which was negative in the initial test battery) resemble
the highly active agents that are distinguished by unbranched side
chains without ring structures. Phorate has not been tested in
two (L5T and SCC) of the three assays for which disulfoton was
positive.

Cacodylic acid, monuron, and benomyl were also positive only
in eukaryotic systems (Table 8). The chemical structures of these
compounds are shown in Figure 7. Cacodylic acid, an organoarsenical,
caused gene mutation, DNA damage, and chromosomal damage, while
the last two compounds produced gene mutation and chromosomal
aberration. In contrast to the previous examples of similar
chemicals eliciting similar genetic effects, Figure 7 illustrates
that structurally diverse chemicals can produce similar genotoxic
effects.

Two chemicals were positive only in eukaryotic gene mutation
assays (Table 9). The genotoxic activities of bromacil and simazine
(Figure 8) were originally detected in the SRL test and were
subsequently confirmed in the L5T system. These are noteworthy
findings, since the results of the initial battery were negative.
It is unlikely that further testing would have been performed had
the SRL assay not been applied to selected chemicals simultaneously
with the initial test battery. These chemicals may be gene mutagens
only and may not cause detectable chromosomal damage. Bromacil is
formed by substitution of the diazine uracil, and simazine, a
triazine, is somewhat similar in structure. It is possible that
these compounds or their metabolites could serve as DNA base
analogues and thus induce point mutations.

Two pesticides, allethrin and sulfallate, were positive only
for point/gene mutation in a prokaryotic system (Table 10); however,
testing of these compounds is incomplete. Allethrin is a member
of a group of pyrethroids that were generally negative in the
initial test battery. The pyrethroids are natural plant products
or their analogues; the complex structures of several of these
compounds are shown in Figure 9.

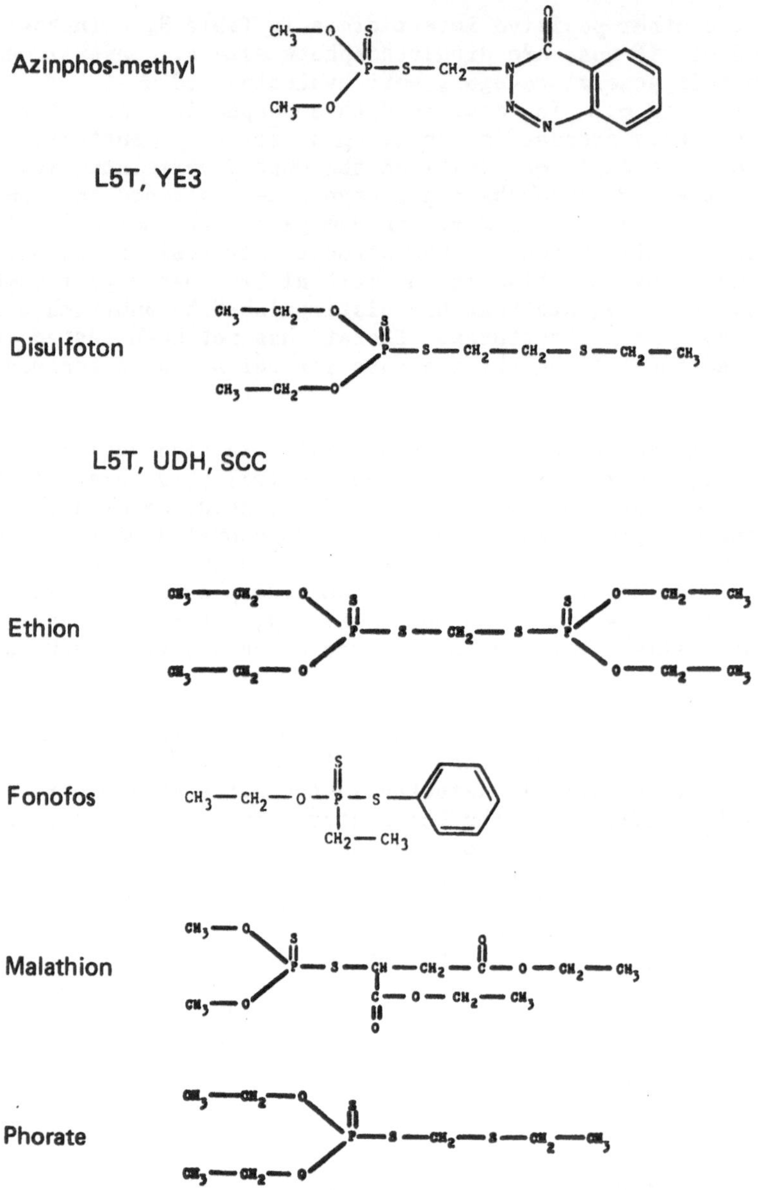

Azinphos-methyl

L5T, YE3

Disulfoton

L5T, UDH, SCC

Ethion

Fonofos

Malathion

Phorate

Fig. 6.   Six dithiophosphate ester insecticides.

Cacodylic acid (H)

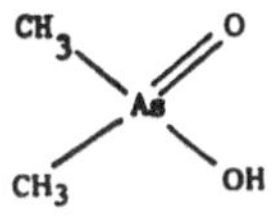

YER, L5T, YE3, YEH, MNM

Monuron (H)

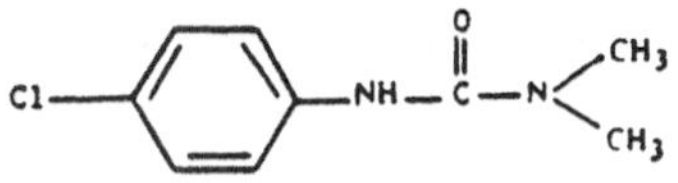

L5T, SCC, MNM

Benomyl (F)

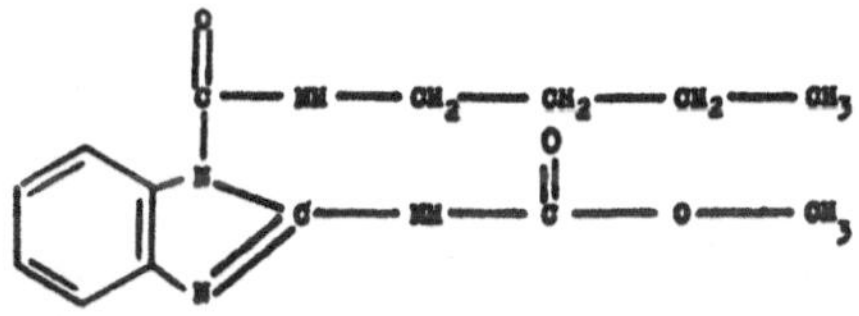

L5T, SCC, MNM

Fig. 7. Three structurally diverse pesticides that displayed
genotoxic effects only in eukaryotes.

Table 9. Pesticides Positive only for Gene Mutation in Eukaryotic Systems

| Compound | Point/Gene Mutation | | | | | DNA Damage | | | | | | Chromosomal Effects | | |
| | Prokaryote | | Eukaryote | | | Prokaryote | | | Eukaryote | | | | | |
	SAL	WPU	YER	L5T	SRL	REP	REW	SAR	YE3	YEH	UDH	SCC	MNM	DLM
Bromacil (H)	-	-	-	+	+	-	-	-	-	-	-	-	-	-
Simazine (H)	-	-	-	+*	+	NT	NT	-	-	-	-	-	-	

Table 10. Pesticides Positive only for Point Mutation in a Prokaryotic System

| Compound | Point/Gene Mutation | | | | | DNA Damage | | | | | |
| | Prokaryote | | Eukaryote | | | Prokaryote | | | Eukaryote | | |
	SAL	WPU	YER	L5T	SRL	REP	REW	SAR	YE3	YEH	UDH
Allethrin (I)*	+*	-				NT		-	-		-
Sulfallate (H)	+*	-				-		-	-		-

Bromacil

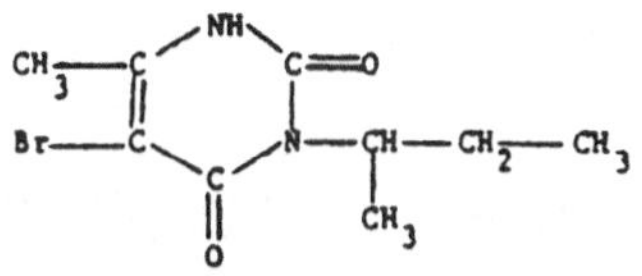

L5T, SRL

Simazine

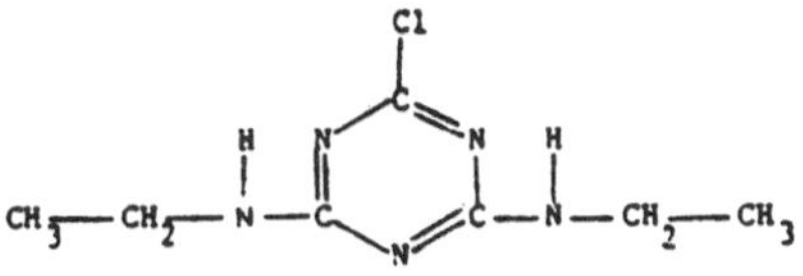

L5T, SRL

Fig. 8. Bromacil and simazine, two genotoxic agents whose activities were detected only in confirmatory bioassays.

Allethrin

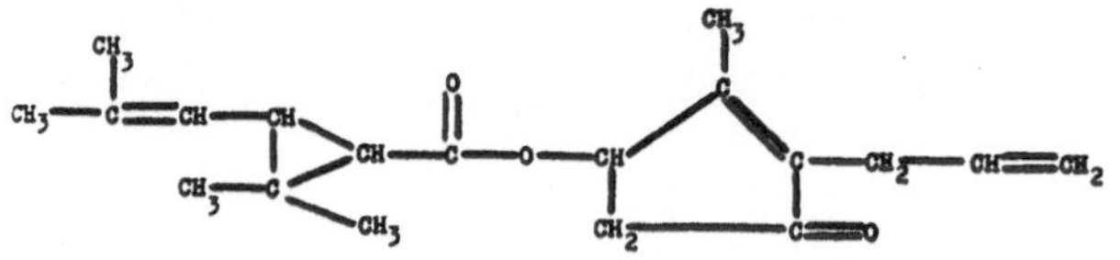

SAL

Ethyl Chrysanthemumate

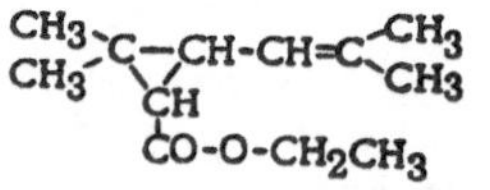

YE3

Permethrin

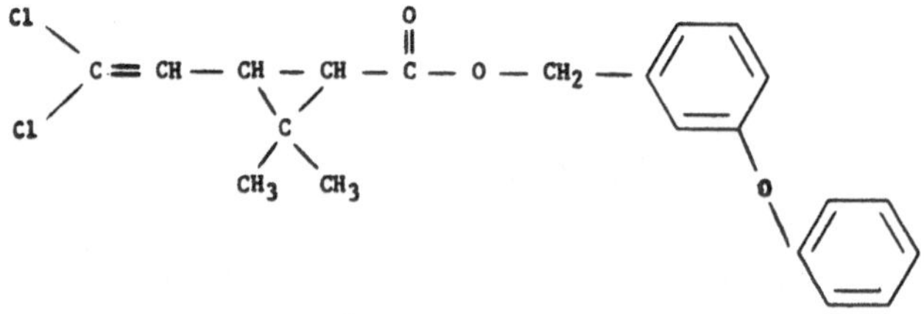

Resmethrin

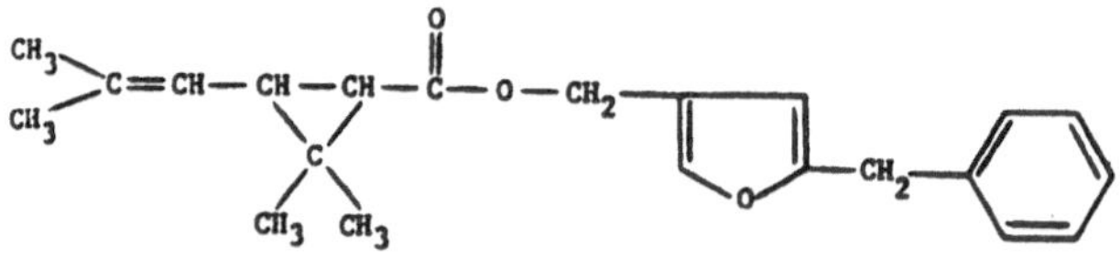

Fig. 9. Two pyrethroid insecticides that displayed limited genotoxic activity and two that were negative.

Primary DNA Damage. Although 29 of the 35 positive pesticides caused primary DNA damage only 16 caused primary DNA damage but not point/gene mutation. A unique group of 10 pesticides was found that caused DNA damage only in prokaryotic systems (Table 11); however, testing for gene mutation and chromosomal damage by these compounds is not complete. A large number of these compounds are chlorinated aromatics (Figure 10). The halophenoxy herbicides 2,4-D, 2,4-DB and 2,4,5-T (Figure 11) form a subgroup of chlorinated compounds; evidence of positive eukaryotic activity for the phenoxy herbicides has been presented elsewhere (26).

Although testing is incomplete, m-dichlorobenzene and pentachlorophenol were positive only for DNA damage in a prokaryotic and a eukaryotic system, and four pesticides (ethyl chrysanthemate, mancozeb, maneb, and zineb) were positive only for DNA damage in eukaryotic systems (Table 12). The last three chemicals in this group have similar structures (Figure 12) and are classified as ethylenebisdithiocarbamate fungicides. Since the data in Tables 7 and 8 suggest that the positive results obtained in the S. cerevisiae D3 assay (YE3) may be confirmed in the L5T system, the five chemicals in Table 12 should be evaluated further for gene mutation in eukaryotes.

Chromosomal Damage. Although the initial test battery did not include tests for chromosomal damage, nine pesticides (Tables 7 and 8) were observed to display this effect. Eight of these chemicals caused a positive response for sister-chromatid exchange in CHO cells (SCC) but only three, cacodylic acid, monuron, and benomyl, caused micronuclei formation in developing erythrocytes of the mouse (MNM). Each of these compounds also caused point/gene mutations or DNA damage, or both. The active gene mutagens, acephate, demeton, monocrotophos, and trichlorfon, were positive in eukaryotic gene mutation and primary DNA damage assay systems except SRL. The five other compounds, disulfoton, methyl-parathion, cacodylic acid, monuron, and benomyl, were positive in eukaryotic gene or DNA damage assays but were negative (or were not tested) in the prokaryotic point/gene assays. All nine of these chromosome-damaging compounds were positive in the L5T system. Negative results were obtained for ten pesticides evaluated in the mouse dominant lethal test. Six of these compounds were positive in at least two eukaryotic assays. The six are the insecticides azinphos-methyl, methyl-parathion, and monocrotophos, the herbicide bromacil, and the fungicides captan and folpet.

Comparison of Bioassay and Carcinogenicity Data

A comparison of the genotoxicity test results with carcino-genicity studies of 15 pesticides is shown in Table 13. Four herbicides (diallate, monuron, sulfallate, and trifluralin) and one fungicide (captan) evaluated in the present study cause tumors in

Table 11. Pesticides Positive only for DNA Damage in Prokaryotic Systems

| | Point/Gene Mutation | | | | | DNA Damage | | | | | |
| | Prokaryote | | Eukaryote | | | Prokaryote | | | Eukaryote | | |
Compound	SAL	WPU	YER	L5T	SRL	REP	REW	SAR	YE3	YEH	UDH
Chlorpyrifos (I)	-	-			-	+	+	+	-	-	-
Chrysanthemic acid (I)	-	-				-	+	+	-		
o-dichlorobenzene (I)	-	-				+	+	-	-		
2,4-D (H)	-	-				-	+	-	-		
2,4-DB (H)	-	-				+	-	-	-		
Dicamba (H)	-	-			-	+	+	-	-		
Dinoseb (H)	-	-			-	+	+	+	-		
Propanil (H)	-	-				-	+	+	-		
2,4,5-T (H)	-	-				-	+	-			
sec-butylamine (F)	-	-				+	-	-	-		

Chlorpyrifos

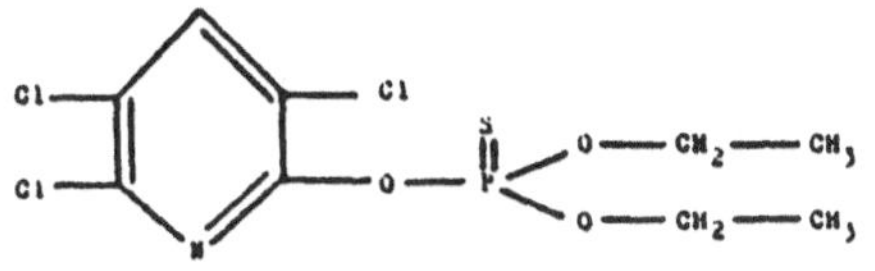

REP, REW, SAR

o-Dichlorobenzene

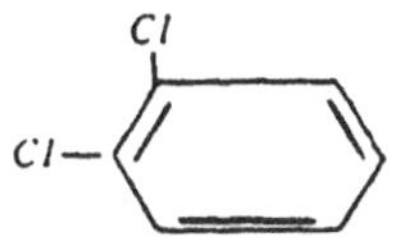

REP

Dicamba

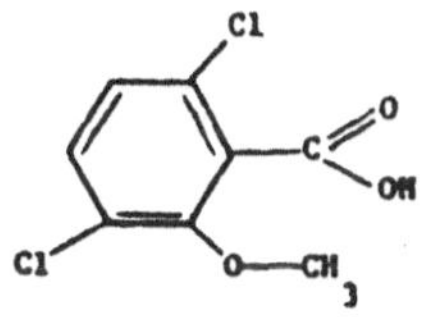

REP, REW

Propanil

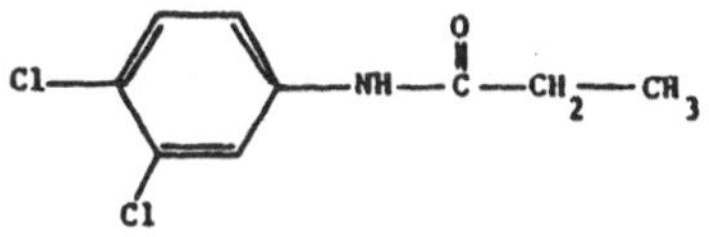

REW, SAR

Fig. 10. Four halogenated aromatic compounds that elicited prokaryotic DNA damage.

2, 4-D Acid

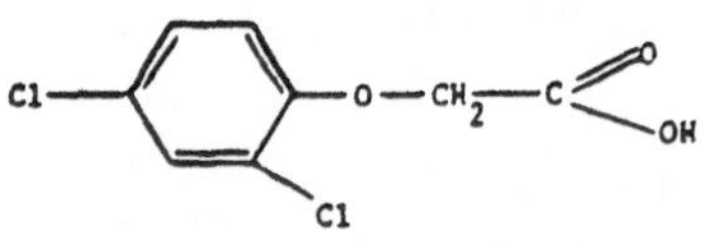

REW

2, 4-DB Acid

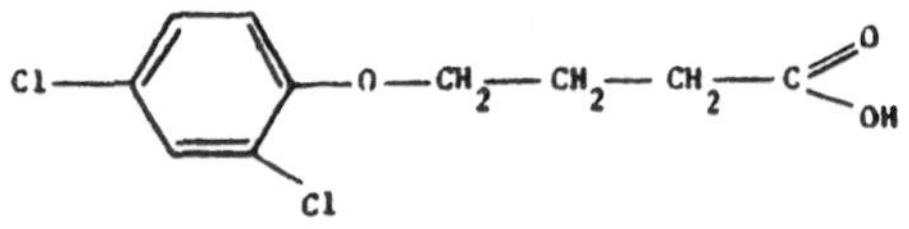

REP

2, 4, 5-T

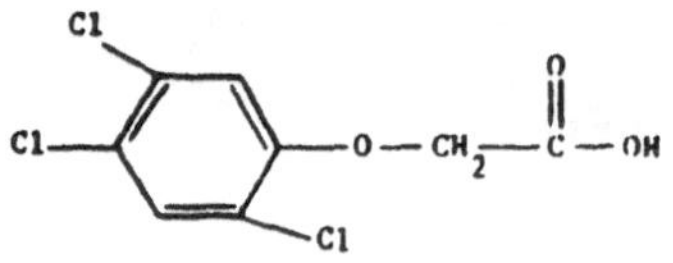

REW

Fig. 11.   Three phenoxy herbicides that elicited prokaryotic DNA damage.

Table 12. Pesticides Positive only for DNA Damage in a Eukaryotic System or only for DNA Damage in a Prokaryotic and a Eukaryotic System

Compound	Point/Gene Mutation					DNA Damage					
	Prokaryote		Eukaryote			Prokaryote			Eukaryote		
	SAL	WPU	YER	L5T	SRL	REP	REW	SAR	YE3	YEH	UDH
Ethyl chrysanthemate (I)	-	-				-	-		+		-
Pentachlorophenol (H)	-	-				-	+		+		
m-dichlorobenzene (F)	-	-				+	-		+		
Mancozeb (F)	-	-				-	-		+		+
Maneb (F)	-	-				-	-		+		+
Zineb (F)	-	-				-	-		+		-

Fig. 12. Three ethylenebisdithiocarbamate fungicides.

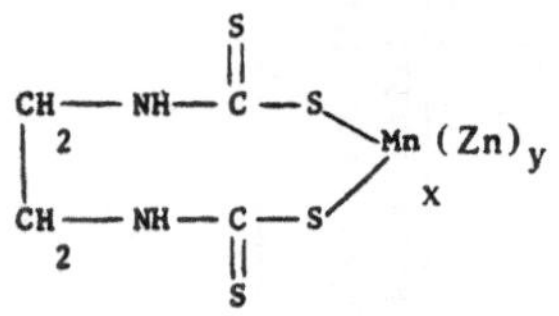

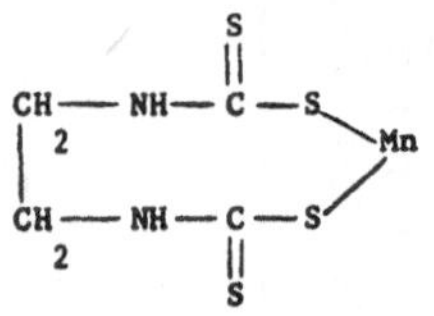

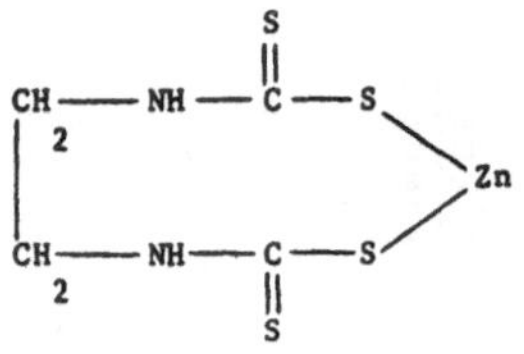

rodents (9, 10). One of these compounds, trifluralin, was shown to be contaminated with dipropyl nitrosamine in the National Cancer Institute carcinogenesis bioassay (24). Three insecticides (azinphos-methyl, fenthion, and parathion) show equivocal evidence of carcinogenicity (9). A stronger relationship between genetic bioassays and carcinogenicity is apparent for the eukaryotic tests, i.e., for the L5T, YE3, SRL and to a lesser extent for the SCC, MNM, and UDH systems. Moreover, sulfallate has not been evaluated in the L5T and YE3 systems, in which the closely related analogues diallate and triallate have been shown to be positive. Diallate is also positive in the SRL test. Parathion has exhibited equivocal evidence of carcinogenicity (9), and although the genotoxicity test results are negative, the insecticide was not evaluated in the L5T, SCC, or MNM systems. A closely related analogue, methyl-parathion, is positive in the L5T, YE3, and SCC tests. Although methyl-parathion has not been shown to be carcinogenic in rodents, these results indicate that additional eukaryotic genotoxicity tests should be performed with parathion before a final judgement is made concerning other carcinogenicity testing. The data for negative carcinogens is generally concordant with the genotoxicity test results.

Comparison with Gross Toxicity

It seems that no correlation is apparent between the in vivo toxicity of the pesticides studied and their potential for genetic damage in short-term tests. Table 14 lists the animal toxicities for 13 pesticides that were positive in at least three different genotoxicity bioassays; the toxicities of these compounds vary by nearly four orders of magnitude, with no correlation between toxicity and bioassay results. Indeed, the two compounds with the highest numbers of positive responses in the genotoxicity bioassays, demeton and folpet, are respectively the strongest and weakest toxicants in the list.

SUMMARY AND CONCLUSIONS

The general problem addressed by this research was the classification of pesticide chemicals according to their DNA-damaging or genotoxic effects. Genotoxicity was assessed in this study by prokaryotic and eukaryotic test systems that measure gene mutation, DNA damage, or chromosomal effects. The chemicals studied can be divided into two groups: those that display no genotoxic response and require little further testing, and those that display some positive response and require further evaluation. The chemicals that elicit positive responses in several kinds of genetic bioassays are of greatest concern, particularly as regards their potential effects on humans.

Table 13. Comparison of Genotoxicity and Carcinogenicity Test
Results

Pesticides	Genotoxicity	Carcinogenicity		
		Mice m/f	Rats m/f	Ref.
Positive Carcinogenicity				
Captan (F)	+: SAL, WPU, L5T, SRL, REP, REW, SAR, YE3 -: UDH, DLM	+/±	-/-	(9)
Diallate (H)	+: SAL, L5T, SRL, YE3 -: WPU, YER, YEH	+/+	±/±	(10)
Monuron (H)	+: L5T, SCC, MNM -: 9 tests	+	±	(11)
Sulfallate (H) (mutagenicity testing incomplete)	+: SAL -: 4 tests	+/+	+/+	(9)
Trifluralin (H)	-: 7 tests	-/+	-/-	(9)
Possible Carcinogenicity				
Azinphos-methyl (I)	+: L5T, YE3 -: 10 tests	-/-	±/±	(9)
Fenthion (I)	-: 5 tests	±/-	-/-	(9)
Parathion (I)	-: 8 tests	-/-	±/±	(9)
Negative Carcinogenicity				
Diazinon (I)	-: 4 tests	-/-	-/-	(9)
Endrin (I)	-: 6 tests	-/-	-/-	(9)
Malathion (I)	-: 8 tests	-/-	-/-	(9)
Methoxychlor (I)	-: 5 tests	-/-	-/-	(9)
Methyl-parathion (I)	+: L5T, YE3, SCC -: 8 tests	-/-	-/-	(9)
PCNB (F)	-: 6 tests	-/-	-/-	(9)
2,4-D and esters (H)	+: REW, REP -: 5 tests	-	-	(12)

+ = positive response, ± = equivocal, - = negative response (under
conditions of bioassay; not necessarily non-carcinogenic).

Table 14. Relative Animal Toxicities of Compounds Positive in Three or More Different Genotoxicity Bioassays

Chemical	LD_{50} (mg/kg in Rats)
Insecticides	
Demeton	2.5
Disulfoton	2.6
Monocrotophos	5.0
Methyl-parathion	9.0
Trichlorfon	450
Acephate	866
Herbicides	
Cacodylic acid	830
Diallate	395
Triallate	1,675
Monuron	3,600
Fungicides	
Captan	9,000
Benomyl	> 9,590
Folpet	> 10,000

Attempts to relate results of in vitro and in vivo bioassays to potential human health hazards lead naturally to a more specific classification or ranking of individual chemicals. The present assessment falls short of a definitive ranking of the chemicals studied for several reasons:

1) In most cases technical grade chemicals were used. While this level of purity is most relevant to the commercial products, it is possible that genotoxic activity of the technical grade chemicals may be related to the presence of contaminants.

2) The data base is incomplete. Not all chemicals were evaluated in all test systems, which introduces considerable bias into any assessment of the present data.

3) The quantitative dose-response data which exist for
    each chemical in each test have been used only to
    establish whether the test was positive or negative,
    not to establish any level of effect for a given
    test.

4) No dosimetry studies have been performed to determine
    the quantity of active chemical or metabolites that
    actually reaches the DNA of the target cells in the
    treated organism; only the quantity of chemical to
    which the organism was exposed has been recorded.

Despite these and other shortcomings, a great deal of preliminary information has been gleaned from this examination of the
qualitative data, and undoubtedly much more can be gained from
careful analysis of the quantitative data which are available from
the first author.

Thirty-five of the 65 pesticide chemicals examined in this
report were positive in one or more of the 14 test systems employed.
These 35 positive chemicals could be divided into two major categories representing the genetic damage observed: 19 agents causing
gene mutation, and 16 agents causing primary DNA damage but not
measurable gene mutation. Nine additional pesticides could be
classified as producing chromosomal effects; however, they also
caused gene mutation or primary DNA damage and relatively few
tests for chromosomal effects were performed. Thus, the placement
of pesticides in these broad categories of genetic damage is
somewhat arbitrary. After division into a major category of
genetic effect, the pesticides were further classified with respect
to their activity in prokaryotic or eukaryotic systems and with
respect to specific combinations of the major classes of genotoxic
damage. The members of these groupings of chemicals were thought
to exhibit a similar spectrum of genetic damage. Examination of
these groupings of pesticides revealed that many of them display
similar chemical structures. Notable dissimilarities were also
apparent, and both kinds of observations were discussed.

The Ames test, SAL, detected only 10 of the 34 pesticides
that were positive in the initial test battery. This fact should
serve as a caution against using only this test as a preliminary
screen.

The L5T test confirmed the genetic activity of positive
chemicals from the initial test battery in every case (17 out of
17). This result suggests that this test should be used to evaluate
other suspected agents and, equally importantly, other reputedly
inactive compounds to verify that the test is not overly sensitive.

Eight insecticides that displayed positive genetic activity
in two or more eukaryotic system (Tables 7 and 8) were negative in
SRL and a total of 17 insecticides evaluated were negative in the
test. Not surprisingly, these results indicate that this very
important assay for germ cell damage may not be very useful for
the evaluation of insecticides.

The low rates of detection of positive agents by individual
bioassays of the initial battery provide evidence of the diversity
and organism-dependence of genotoxic effects. This in turn supports
the contention that reliable assessment of genotoxic potential
requires the use of several different bioassays in different
organisms. The three-test battery SAL, YE3, and L5T that detected
all 24 of the compounds positive in eukaryotic systems may be
especially useful in the evaluation of pesticide chemicals. These
tests should perhaps be considered as components of a core battery
of tests for evaluation of pesticides.

Twelve chemicals evaluated in this study may be of particular
concern, because they displayed genotoxic activity in three or
more eukaryotic bioassay systems. These compounds are the insecticides acephate, demeton, disulfoton, methyl-parathion, monocrotophos,
and trichlorfon, the herbicides cacodylic acid, diallate, and
monuron, and the fungicides benomyl, captan, and folpet. Three of
these compounds (cacodylic acid, monuron and benomyl) were shown
to cause chromosomal damage in the in vivo mouse micronucleus
test. On the other hand, four of these agents (methyl-parathion,
monocrotophos, captan and folpet) were negative in the relatively
insensitive mouse dominant lethal test. It is quite possible that
with further testing other pesticides may also show similar effects;
nonetheless these twelve compounds, because of their diverse
genotoxic activities, should be assessed carefully.

Five compounds elicited positive responses in the Drosophila
sex-linked recessive lethal test. All were also positive in the
L5T assay. These compounds are the herbicides bromacil, diallate,
and simazine and the fungicides captan and folpet. Because the
SRL assay measures the ability of a chemical to affect germ cells
directly, these chemicals warrant careful attention.

A relationship was found between bioassay responses and
existing carcinogenesis assay results in rodents. About one-half
of the pesticides that appear to cause tumors in rodents are
positive in the bioassays. It appeared that a better correspondence
with carcinogenicity was demonstrated for eukaryotic tests, particularly L5T, YE3, and SRL, although the data are obviously meager.
The results showed that chemicals which do not produce tumors are
generally negative in the bioassays. Two (L5T and YE3) of the
three eukaryotic tests well correlated with carcinogenicity were

components of the battery of three tests, SAL, YE3, and L5T, mentioned previously.

Although testing is incomplete, ten of the chemicals studied have thus far produced positive results in only one test system. Ten chemicals have thus far produced positive responses only in prokaryotic systems. In contrast, eight pesticides that have been well tested were positive only in eukaryotic bioassays. These results suggest the need for appropriate criteria for the classification of genetic bioassay data in the evaluation of the potential health hazards of pesticides and other toxic chemicals. Agents with positive responses in only one detection system and negative effects in others may be of little concern as presumptive carcinogens or as somatic or germ cell mutagens. Conversely, it is important to understand why some chemicals that are positive as germ cell mutagens appear to have been missed in tests used as detection systems. The results of this study, when added to the much larger data base of genotoxic chemicals currently being assembled by the EPA GENE-TOX Program (8, 23), should permit development of more formal methods for classification and evaluation of genotoxic chemicals. These would include: 1) methods for selection of a sensitive minimal battery of short-term genetic bioassays, 2) techniques to facilitate ranking and prediction of the hazard potential of toxic chemicals, and 3) procedures to study the correlation between genetic toxicity and chemical structure.

ACKNOWLEDGEMENTS

The diversity of disciplines and efforts required for this project are reflected by the scientific and technical personnel who contributed their talents and dedication. The project was first administered by Dr. Gordon W. Newell, who directed the Toxicology Laboratory of SRI International during the initial contract period.

The microbial testing was performed by Edward S. Riccio, Gregory F. Shepherd, Mary V. Peirce and Anne L. Pomeroy. Mary M. Jotz conducted the mouse lymphoma testing, assisted by Douglas E. Rundle, Ronald L. Coleman and Lynn S. Beckhart. Douglas E. Robinson performed the unscheduled DNA synthesis tests, assisted by Martha L. Hay-Kaufman. Dr. Elizabeth L. Evans conducted the sister-chromatid assays, assisted by Marjorie L. Fong, Karen K. Yamamoto, Patricia A. McAfee and Barbara L. Stewart, and supervised the Drosophila testing at SRI, assisted by Jennifer L. White and G. Ann Snyder. Barbara A. Kirkhart conducted the micronucleus tests. Mr. H. Frank Stack and Mr. Barry E. Howard performed computer programming and analysis. Dr. Charles J. Alden, Dr. Stephen Nesnow, and Linda J. Jones assisted in the preparation of the manuscript.

REFERENCES

1. Ames, B.N., J. McCann, and E. Yamasaki, 1975, Methods for
    detecting carcinogens and mutagens with the Salmonella/
    mammalian-microsome mutagenicity test, Mutat. Res., 31:347.
2. Bridges, B.A., 1972, Simple bacterial systems for detecting
    mutagenic agents, Lab. Pract., 21:413.
3. Bridges, B.A., 1975, Mutagenicity of captan and related
    fungicides, Mutat. Res., 32:3.
4. Brusick, D.J., and V.W. Mayer, 1973, New developments in
    mutagenicity screening techniques with yeast, Environ. Health
    Perspect., 6:83.
5. Clive, D., K.O. Johnson, J.F.S. Spector, A.G. Batson, and
    M.M.M. Brown, 1979, Validation and characterization of the
    L5178Y/TK$^{+/-}$ mouse lymphoma mutagen assay system, Mutat.
    Res., 59:61.
6. DeLucia, P., and J. Cairns, 1969, Isolation of an E. coli strain
    with a mutation affecting DNA polymerase, Nature, 224:1164.
7. Douglas, G.R., E.R. Nestmann, C.E. Grant, R.D.L. Bell, J.M.
    Wytsma, and D.J. Kowbel, in press, Mutagenic activity of
    diallate and triallate determined by a battery of in vitro
    mammalian and microbial tests, Mutat. Res.
8. Green, S., and A. Auletta, 1980, Editorial Introduction to
    the Reports of "The Gene-Tox Program." An Evaluation of
    Bioassays in Genetic Toxicology, Mutat. Res., 76:165.
9. Griesemer, R.A., and C. Cueto, Jr., 1981, Toward a classi-
    fication scheme for degrees of experimental evidence for the
    carcinogenicity of chemicals for animals, in: "IARC Monographs
    on the Evaluation of the Carcinogenic Risk of Chemicals to
    Man," Vol. 27, IARC, Lyon, France.
10. Innes, J.R.M., B.M. Ulland, M.G. Valerio, L. Petrucelli,
    L. Fishbein, E.R. Hart, A.J. Pallotta, R.R. Bates, H.L. Falk,
    J.J. Gart, M. Klein, I. Mitchel, and J. Peters, 1969, Bioassay
    of pesticides and industrial chemicals for tumorigenicity in
    mice: a preliminary note, J. Natl. Cancer Inst., 42:1101.
11. International Agency for Research on Cancer, 1976, Monuron,
    in: "IARC Monographs on the Evaluation of the Carcinogenic
    Risk of Chemicals to Man: Some Carbamates, Thiocarbamates,
    and Carbazines," Vol. 12, IARC, Lyon, France.
12. International Agency for Research on Cancer, 1977, 2,4-D and
    esters, in: "IARC Monographs on the Evaluation of the Carcino-
    genic Risk of Chemicals to Man: Some Fumigants, the Herbicides
    2,4-D and 2,4,5-T, Chlorinated Dibenzodioxin and Miscellaneous
    Industrial Chemicals," Vol. 15, IARC, Lyon, France.
13. Kada, T., 1973, Mutagenicity testing of chemicals in microbial
    systems, in: "New Methods in Experimental Chemistry and
    Toxicology," F. Coulston, F. Corte, and M. Coto, eds.,
    International Academic Printing, Tokyo.
14. Mackey, B., and J. MacGregor, 1979, The micronucleus test:
    statistical design and analysis, Mutat. Res., 64:195.

15. Miller, E.C., and J.A. Miller, 1976, The metabolism of chemical carcinogens to reactive electrophiles and their possible mechanisms of action in carcinogenesis, in: "Chemical Carcinogens," C. Searle, ed., ACS Monograph 173, American Chemical Society, Washington, D.C.

16. Perry, P., and H.J. Evans, 1975, Cytological detection of mutagen-carcinogen exposure by sister chromatid exchange, Nature, 158:121.

17. Schmid, W., 1976, The micronucleus test for cytogenetic analysis, in: "Chemical Mutagens," Vol. 4, A. Hollaender, ed., Plenum Press, New York.

18. Simmon, V.F., 1978, In vivo and in vitro mutagenicity assays of selected pesticides, in: "A Rational Evaluation of Pesticidal vs. Mutagenic/Carcinogenic Action," R.W. Hart, H.F. Kraybill, and F.J. de Serres, eds., DHEW Publication No. (NIH) 78-1306.

19. Simmon, V.F., 1978, In vitro microbiological mutagenicity and unscheduled DNA synthesis studies of eighteen pesticides, Final Report on Contract #68-01-2458, U.S. Environmental Protection Agency.

20. Simmon, V.F., A.D. Mitchell, and T.A. Jorgenson, 1977, Evaluation of selected pesticides as chemical mutagens. In vitro and in vivo studies, U.S. Environmental Protection Agency Document EPA-600/1-77-028.

21. Slater, E.E., M.D. Anderson, and H.S. Rosenkranz, 1971, Rapid detection of mutagens and carcinogens, Cancer Res. 31:970.

22. Stetka, D.G., and S. Wolff, 1976, Sister chromatid exchanges as an assay for genetic damage induced by mutagens/carcinogens. Part II. In vitro test for compound requiring metabolic activation, Mutat. Res., 41:343.

23. Waters, M.D., and A. Auletta, 1980, The GENE-TOX program: Genetic activity evaluation, J. Chem. Inf. Comput. Sci., 21:35.

24. Waters, M.D., V.F. Simmon, A.D. Mitchell, T.A. Jorgenson, and R. Valencia, 1980, An overview of short-term tests for the mutagenic and carcinogenic potential of pesticides, J. Environ. Sci. Health, B15:867.

25. Wurgler, F.E., F.H. Sobels, and E. Vogel, 1977, Drosophila as assay system for detecting genetic changes, in: "Handbook of Mutagenicity Test Procedures," B.J. Kilbey, M. Legator, W. Nichols, and C. Ramel, eds., Elsevier/North Holland Biomedical Press, Amsterdam.

26. Zetterberg, G., 1977, Genetic effects of phenoxy acids on microorganisms, Ecol. Bull. (Stockholm), 27:193.

27. Zimmerman, F.K., 1975, Procedures used in the induction of mitotic recombination and mutation in the yeast Saccharomyces cerevisiae, Mutat. Res., 31:71.

28. Zimmerman, F.K., 1975, A yeast strain for simultaneous detection of induced mitotic crossing over, mitotic gene conversion, and reverse mutation, Mutat. Res., 28:381.

DISCUSSION

Q. BYARD: One is not confident of the negative results in these
    in vitro genotoxicity assays since we don't know if the
    chemicals are metabolized. Even slowly metabolized chemicals,
    such as endrin, persist in the body and may slowly produce
    genetic injury, while in a brief in vitro assay they may not be
    significantly activated.

A. WATERS: Yes, this is a problem with the S-9 activation systems
    employed with many genetic bioassays in vitro. It is possible
    that newer activation methods involving co-cultivation of
    metabolically active whole cells with appropriate mutagenesis
    "indicator cells" will enable us to detect certain compounds
    now missed using S-9 activation.

Q. EL-SEBAE: I would like to clarify the point dealing with
    chlordimeform. It was documented by EPA as causing adverse
    effects due to its carcinogenicity to mice and rats. This was
    revealed by the producers, mainly Ciba-Geigy, through the
    process of re-registration. This is why the Company decided to
    withdraw the compound. Then they re-introduced it in 1978
    under amended label, but it was put on the RPAR list and I
    think this hazard should be considered by regulatory agencies
    in evaluation of the status of a compound.

A. WATERS: I am sorry, but I have no knowledge of this specific
    case. In general, all available information is considered in
    the RPAR process.

Q. NEWELL: Do you plan to attempt structure/activity evaluations
    of the pesticides, according to grouped test results? If not
    now, perhaps later when the data base is larger?

A. WATERS: Yes, we do. The data developed on these chemicals in
    Saccharomyces cerevisiae D3 is being evaluated for structure-
    activity relationships using several computer-assisted pattern
    recognition models. This work is being performed by Dr. Peter
    Jurs and his associates at the Pennsylvania State University.
    Other bioassays and groups of bioassays will be added as the
    data base grows.

Q. GENTILE: Could the discrepancy between the Salmonella data and
    yeast data for several agents be due to a metabolic activation
    of these compounds by the yeast cells rather than solely due to
    the intrinsic genetic constitutional variances between
    prokaryotes and eukaryotes?

A. WATERS: That is a difficult question to answer. The pattern
    of responses suggests that most of the compounds do not require

exogenous metabolic activation. However, they could be metabolic endogenously by the eukaryotic cells and not by the prokaryotic organisms.

Q. BADR: Captan being shown as positive in sex linked recessive lethal tests in <u>D. melanogaster,</u> I think that it is important to point out how and at what developmental stage the chemical was administered to the organism. Whether we get positive or negative results, this is important to know.

A. WATERS: Dr. Valencia treated adult males by feeding which also involves contact (since the flies walk on their food) and possibly some vaporization.

PLANT DEPENDENT MUTATION ASSAYS

James M. Gentile[1] and Michael J. Plewa[2]

[1]Department of Biology
Hope College
Holland, Michigan 49423

[2]Institute for Environmental Studies
University of Illinois
Urbana, Illinois 61801

INTRODUCTION

Considering the involvement of chemical pesticides in modern agricultural practice, the determination of the compatibility of these agents with the environment and the public health is exceedingly important. During the last decade a new environmental hazard has been recognized. This hazard is that of environmental mutagens. These physical or chemical agents, that have the ability to alter the genetic material or the proper functioning of the genetic material, pose a serious long-term threat to man and other living organisms. A new branch of toxicology, genetic toxicology, has evolved to detect, investigate, manage, and define the risks due to human exposure to environmental mutagens. Depending upon the ontogenetic stage of an individual when exposed, an environmental mutagen can exert teratogenic effects, cause mutations involving germinal cells, induce coronary artery disease, affect the aging process, or induce mutations of somatic cells that may become neoplastic. As geneticists we are alarmed that there may be large amounts of agents released into our environment that can be deleterious not only to an individual but also to his progeny, generation upon generation. We anticipate that adverse genetic effects can be created in the human species by inadvertent exposure to mutagens. It is, therefore, obvious that the induction of genetic damage by the use of mutagens applied to the environment should be avoided.

In this paper, we review the phenomenon of the plant activation of agriculturally related promutagens and the integration of

327

this phenomenon with laboratory and in situ screening for genotoxins present in the agricultural arena.

ACTIVATION OF PROMUTAGENS BY PLANTS

Although plants have been extensively used in the investigation of the genetic effects of chemical and physical agents (13,
39), the activation of promutagens into mutagens by plants is a
relatively new topic in environmental mutagenesis. Since many crop
plants are treated with chemicals, the demonstration that plants
can activate innocuous chemicals into mutagens is a concern.

The term "plant activation" connotes the processes by which a
non-mutagenic chemical is transformed by the biological action of a
plant into a mutagen (44). These processes are analogous to the
familiar mammalian microsome activation system that is routinely
employed in many short-term microbial assays. To prove that a
chemical is a plant promutagen, one must be able to separate the
activation process from the genetic endpoint used to assay for
mutagenicity. This criterion is met, for example, by subjecting
one organism to the test chemical and then using an extract from
the treated organism to test for mutagenicity in a different organism. A positive mutagenic response in a plant assay that does not
meet the above criterion indicates only that the test chemical is
mutagenic under the conditions of the assay.

The two general procedures used in studies of plant activation
are the in vivo and the in vitro methods. In the in vivo method
the test agent is introduced into intact living plants whereas in
the in vitro method the test agent is introduced into a sterile
plant homogenate or coincubated with plant tissue culture cells.
In both methods a plant extract is subsequently assayed with a
microbial indicator organism for genotoxic properties.

In Vivo Plant Activation

The primary advantage of in vivo methods of plant activation
is the use of intact plants to mimic the conditions encountered in
modern agriculture. This approach is flexible and can accommodate
field samples. The disadvantages of in vivo methodologies include
microbial contamination of the plant material, artifacts in microbial assays induced by nutrients in the samples, dosimetry problems
inherent in treating intact plants and possible modification of
metabolites or induction of chemical reactions during the homogen-
ization, extraction, and concentration of samples. Additionally,
one must always consider the possibility of the presence of naturally occurring genotoxins such as certain flavonoids in plant extracts. A summary of studies in which in vivo plant activation was
used to evaluate chemicals for their mutagenic properties is presented in Table 1.

The s-triazine herbicide atrazine (2-chloro-4-(ethylamino)-6-isopropylamino-s-triazine) was the first chemical identified as genotoxic to a microorganism following plant activation (19,20,42,43). The objective of these studies was to resolve the dichotomy that this herbicide was mutagenic in intact plants but not mutagenic when assayed directly on microbial indicator organisms. The hypothesis was that it was a plant promutagen. In these studies Zea mays (maize) seedlings were exposed to atrazine for several weeks thus allowing the chemical to be absorbed, translocated, and metabolized. A homogenate of the plant was prepared, fibers and cellular debris were removed by centrifugation, and the supernatant fluid was concentrated by lyophilization. The lyophilized material was resuspended in ethanol, diluted with buffer, and tested for genetic activity on Saccharomyces cerevisiae. The lyophilized material from treated plants induced gene conversion at the trp-5 and ade-2 loci of S. cerevisiae strain D4 (43) and reversion at the ade locus of S. cerevisiae strain H201.24.4 (42). S. Rogers and G. Warren (Montana State University, 1976, 1977, personal communication) used an identical protocol and found mutagenic responses in Escherichia coli and Salmonella typhimurium although Bakshi et al. (4) using a modified protocol indicated that extracts from field-grown, mature plants treated with atrazine showed no increased genotoxicity. However, a more recent study by Singh et al. (50), using crude extracts from corn plants treated with varying concentrations of atrazine, demonstrated dose-dependent convertogenic activity to S. cerevisiae strain D4 following fractional analysis by high pressure liquid chromatography and recovery in 50% methanol.

Thirty-two pesticides (field formulations and technical grades) and combinations of pesticides were tested for their ability to be activated into mutagens by maize under an in vivo protocol (44). Homogenates were made from seedlings treated and grown in plant growth chambers. The preparation of plant extracts was identical to those previously described (43). Standard procedures for the mutation assays in S. typhimurium and for gene conversion in S. cerevisiae (56) were followed. Rat liver preparations (S-9) were prepared according to the methods of Ames et al. (3). Herbicides that were demonstrated to be plant activated were cyanazine (2-chloro-4-(1-cyano-1-methyl-ethylamino)-6-(ethylamino)-s-triazine), procyazine (2-[4-chloro-6-(cyclopropylamino)-s-triazine-2yl] amino-2-methyl propanenitrile), alachlor (2-chloro-2',6'-diethyl-N-(methoxymethyl)acetanilide), propachlor (2-chloro-N-isopropylacetanilide), and SD50093 which is a commercial formulation of atrazine and cyanazine. The combination of propachlor and cyanazine was also plant activated. Other scientists have demonstrated that extracts of cyanazine-treated plants were mutagenic in S. typhimurium (S. Rogers and G. Warren, Montana State University, 1977, personal communication and ref. 35). The insecticides chlordane (1,2,3,4,6,7,8,8-octachloro-2,3,3a,4,7,7a-hexahydro-4,7-methanoindene) and heptachlor

Table 1. Summary of Chemicals Assayed for Mutagenicity
Incorporating in vivo Plant Activation

Chemical	Genetic Indicator Organism	Response Direct[a]	S-9[b]	Plant[c]	Reference
2-chloro-4-(ethylamino)-6-isopropylamino-s-triazine	S. typhimurium	-[d]	-	+[e]	g
	S. typhimurium	-	-	-	4
	E. coli	-	0[f]	+	g
	S. cerevisiae	-	-	+	42,43
3,6-dichloro-0-anisic acid	S. typhimurium	+	-	-	22,44
	S. cerevisiae	-	-	-	22,44
2-chloro-4-(1-cyano-1-methylethylamino)-6-(ethylamino)-s-triazine	S. typhimurium	-	-	+	22,44
	S. cerevisiae	-	-	-	22,44
2((4-chloro-6-(cyclopropyl-amino)-s-triazine-2-yl) amino)-2-methyl propanenitrile	S. typhimurium	-	+	+	22,44
	S. cerevisiae	-	-	-	22,44
2-chloro-N-(2-ethyl-6-methyl-phenyl)-N-(2-methoxyl-1-methyl-ethyl)acetamide	S. typhimurium	-	-	-	22,44
	S. cerevisiae	-	-	-	22,44
S-ethyl dipropylthiocarbamate + N,N-diallyl-2,2-dichloro-acetamide	S. typhimurium	-	-	-	22,44
	S. cerevisiae	-	-	+	22,44
2-chloro-2',6'-diethyl-N-(methoxymethyl) acetanilide	S. typhimurium	-	-	-	22,44
	S. cerevisiae	-	-	+	22,44
2-chloro-N-isopropylacetanilide	S. typhimurium	-	-	-	22,44
	S. cerevisiae	-	-	+	22,44
Methyl 5-(2,4-dichlorophenoxy)-2-nitrobenzoate	S. typhimurium	-	-	-	22,44
	S. cerevisiae	-	-	-	22,44

(1,4,5,6,7,8,8-heptachloro-3a,4,7,7a-tetrahydro-4,7-methanindene)
were the only insecticides plant activated in the in vivo protocol.

    Sodium azide is mutagenic in several plant systems
(32,37,38,46) mammalian cells in culture (47) bacteria (31) and
yeast (49). It can also be metabolized by plants into a mutagen
(41). Owais et al. (41) isolated and partially characterized a
plant metabolite of sodium azide which was mutagenic to S.
typhimurium. Barley seeds were germinated and treated with sodium
azide. Embryos isolated from the seeds were homogenized and
centrifuged. The supernatant fluid was collected, dialyzed and
evaporated, and the residue was mutagenic to S. typhimurium strain
TA1530. Veleminsky et al. (53), using similar procedures,

Table 1. Continued

Chemical	Genetic Indicator Organism	Response			Reference
		Direct[a]	S-9[b]	Plant[c]	
SD50093	S. typhimurium	-	-	+	22,44
	S. cerevisiae	-	-	+	22,44
1,2,4,5,6,7,8,8-octachlor-2,3,3a,4,7,7a-hexahydro-4,-7-methanoindane	S. typhimurium	-	-	-	22,24,44
	S. cerevisiae	-	-	-	22,24,44
S-[[(1,1-dimethylethyl)thio]methyl] O,O-diethylphosphorodithioate	S. typhimurium	-	-	-	22,44
	S. cerevisiae	-	-	-	22.44
O-ethyl-S-phenylethyl-phosphonodithioate	S. typhimurium	-	+	-	22,44
	S. cerevisiae	-	-	-	22,44
2,3-dihydro-2,2-dimethyl-7-benzofuranyl methylcarbamate	S. typhimurium	-	-	-	22,44
	S. cerevisiae	-	-	-	22,44
1,4,5,6,7,8-heptachloro-3a,4,7,7a-tetrahydro-4,7-methano-idene	S. typhimurium	-	-	-	22,24,44
	S. cerevisiae	-	-	-	22,24,44
O-ethyl-S,S-dipropyl phosphorodiothioate	S. typhimurium	-	-	-	22,44
	S. cerevisiae	-	-	-	22,44
O,O-diethyl S-(ethylthio-methyl) phosphorodiothioate	S. typhimurium	-	-	-	22,44
	S. cerevisiae	-	-	-	22,44
sodium azide	S. typhimurium	+	0	+	41
	S. cerevisiae	+	0	+	49,53

(a) Direct test-chemical assayed for mutagenicity without biological activation.
(b) S-9-in vitro mammalian microsomal activation system.
(c) Plant-in vivo plant activation system explained in text.
(d) Negative response.
(e) Positive response.
(f) Not tested.
(g) Rogers and Warren, personal communication.

demonstrated that a concentrated dialysate of an extract prepared from barley seeds treated with sodium azide was mutagenic and recombinogenic to S. cerevisiae.

In Vitro Plant Activation

Several in vitro plant activation methods have recently been developed. In these systems plant cell cultures or cell-free homo-

genates are exposed to a test chemical and assayed for mutagenicity
in microbial indicator organisms or mammalian tissue cell
cultures. The salient feature of these methods is that the plant-
dependent process required for activation is distinct from the
genetic endpoint.

Although a number of agents are activated by both plants and
animals, some appear to be activated only by plants. The incorporation of plant and animal activation protocols into standard microbial assays will provide a broad data base on the biological activation of promutagens. Presumably, a large number of the molecular
transformations that occur in animal activation occur in plants,
and the most convenient method to compare plant and animal activation is with an in vitro protocol. One important area being
studied is the existence of photosynthetic-dependent plant promutagens (23).

A summary of in vitro plant activation studies is presented in
Table 2. Benigni et al. (5) developed an in vitro method of plant
activation using Nicotiana alata cell cultures. The test chemicals
were coincubated with N. alata cells, the cells were homogenized,
and extracts were assayed for mutagenicity on the genetic indicator
organism, Aspergillus nidulans. The control groups of the
experiment included the test chemical plus the tissue culture
medium and the cells plus the tissue culture medium. Five pesticides were tested: atrazine, dichlorvos (phosphoric acid, 2,2-
dichlorovinyl dimethyl ester), tetrachlorvinphos (2-chloro-1-[2,
4,5 trichlorophenyl]-vinyl dimethyl phosphate), Keleven (1-[5'-
(ethyl-4'-okopentanoate)] decachlorooctahydro-1,3,4 metheno-2H,5H-
cyclobuta[cd]pentalen-1-ol), and maleic hydrazide (6-hydroxy-3-
(2H)-pyridazinone). The authors suggested that this method
simulates the metabolism of the whole plant. One pesticide, atrazine, was plant activated and induced point mutations and somatic
segregation in A. nidulans.

The haloalkane 1,2-dibromoethane (EDB) widely used as a pesticide, fumigant, and gasoline additive, was plant activated into a
mutagen of greater potency (48). Crude homogenates from plants of
Tradescantia clone 4430 were prepared and coincubated with EDB and
E. coli or A. nidulans. The plant homogenate increased the mutagenicity of EDB. This process was apparently energy-dependent
because when NADPH was omitted from the plant homogenate and chemical mixture there was no increase in the mutagenicity of EDB.

In the procedure using potato tubers, the s-triazine herbicide
atrazine was tested for mutagenicity (1,33,34). After plant activation, atrazine was mutagenic to Schizosaccharomyces pombe, Streptomyces coelicolor, A. nidulans, chinese hamster ovary (CHO) V-79
cells, recombinogenic to A. nidulans, and induced unscheduled DNA
synthesis in EUE human cells. Atrazine alone or following in vitro

mammalian activation was negative in the above tests. However, atrazine induced chromosome aberrations in mouse bone marrow cells and dominant lethal mutations in mice. Higashi et al. (26) have used a similar procedure with Jerusalem artichoke tubers (Helianthus tuberosus L.). The use of S-9 preparations from induced tubers hydroxylated benzo(a)pyrene into several genotoxic metabolites.

We (Gentile and Plewa, see ref. 22) used an in vitro protocol where maize seedlings at the three-leaf stage of development were harvested, surface sterilized, homogenized in water, and centrifuged at 1000 x g at 4°C for 20 min. This supernatant fluid (S1) plus cofactors was incorporated in the top agar portion of the standard Ames Salmonella test protocol. The S1 fraction was added to the top agar with bacteria alone or with bacteria and a test chemical. Maize S1 and standard rat liver S-9 preparations activated aflatoxin B_1 into a mutagen to S. typhimurium strain TA98. More revertants were found when S-9 was incorporated with aflatoxin than when S1 was used. However, the concentration of protein in S1 preparations was below 10 mg/ml. The reduced efficiency of the S1 preparations in activating aflatoxin B_1 may be due in part to their lower concentration of protein.

We studied the in vitro plant and animal activation of maleic hydrazide because it is a potent mutagen in higher plants but not in animals (25,52). Fischnich et al. (18) observed a decrease in rat fertility when the animals were fed a diet including potato tubers from plants sprayed with maleic hydrazide prior to harvest. No reduction in fertility was noted when rats were fed tubers sprayed after harvest. These findings suggest that maleic hydrazide was metabolized by green plant tissues into a toxin. We tested maleic hydrazide directly and with the incorporation of S-9 or S1 fractions in the Salmonella assay. Preliminary results suggest that S-9 tissue preparations from rat liver did not activate maleic hydrazide into a mutagen whereas S1 preparations from maize tissues activated this agent. However, Benigni et al. (5) found that maleic hydrazide was not activated by N. alata cell cultures. Recently S1 preparations from wheat (Triticum aestivum) were found to activate pentac (pentachloro[2,4 cyclopentradiene]-yl) into a form weakly mutagenic to S. typhimurium (Gentile, unpublished data).

DEACTIVATION OF MUTAGENS BY PLANTS

In addition to activation of promutagens by plants, data are available on the deactivation of mutagens by plant tissue preparations. Kada et al. (28) and Morita et al. (36) demonstrated that tissue preparations from various plant materials were capable of deactivating the mutagenicity of tryptophan pyrolysis products.

Table 2. Summary of Chemicals Assayed for Mutagenicity Incorporating _in vitro_ Plant Activation

Chemical	Plant Activation System	Genetic Indicator Organism	Response			Reference
			Direct[a]	S-9[b]	Plant[c]	
2-Chloro-4-ethylamino-6-isopropyl-amino-s-triazine	N. alata cells	A. nidulans	-[d]	0[e]	+[f]	5
	N. alata cells	A. nidulans	-	0	+	5
	S. tuberosum	S. typhimurium	-	-	-	34
	S. tuberosum	S. pombe	-	+	+	1,33,34
	S. tuberosum	S. coelicolor	-	-	+	1,33,34
	S. tuberosum	V79 cells (CHO)	-	0	+	1,33,34
	S. tuberosum	S. cerevisiae	-	-	-	34
	S. tuberosum	EUE cells (HUMAN)	-	0	+	1,33,34
Phosphoric acid 2,2-dichloro-vinyl dimethyl ester	N. alata cells	A. nidulans	-	0	-	5
2-Chloro-1-(2,4,5-trichlorophenyl)-vinyl dimethyl phosphate	N. alata cells	A. nidulans	-	0	-	5
Decachloroocta-hydro-1,3,4-metheno-2H-5H-cyclobutal[ed]Pentalen-2-one	N. alata cells	A. nidulans	-	0	-	5
Kelevan	N. alata cells	A. nidulans	-	0	-	5
1,2-Dihydro-3,6-pyridazinedione	N. alata cells	A. nidulans	-	0	-	5
Aflatoxin B_1	Z. mays	S. typhimurium	-	-	+	22,44
	Z. mays	S. typhimurium	-	+	+	22,44

Table 2. Continued

Chemical	Plant Activation System	Genetic Indicator Organism	Response			Reference
			Direct[a]	S-9[b]	Plant[c]	
1,2,Dibromoethane[g]	Tradescantia	A. nidulans	±	0	+	48
	Tradescantia	E. coli	±	0	+	48
benzo(a)pyrene	H. tuberosus L.	S. typhimurium	-	+	+	26
pentachloro[2,4-cylapentradienes]-yl	T. arestivom	S. typhimurium	-	-	+	h

a) direct test - chemical assayed for mutagenicity without biological activation.
b) S-9 - in vitro mammalian microsomal activation system.
c) Plant - in vitro plant activation systems explained in text.
d) Not tested.
e) Positive test.
f) Negative test.
g) EDB is a weak direct mutagen.
h) J. M. Gentile, Unpublished data.

Some of these desmutagenic factors (anti-mutagenic agents) were heat and pronase sensitive suggesting a protein character. Additionally, Yano (55) reported that "vegetable juices" decreased the alkylating activity of N-methyl-N-nitrosourea. Scott et al. (48) showed that the mutagenicity of ethyl methanesulfonate (EMS) to E. coli WP2 was depressed in the presence of Tradescantia tissue preparations. Benigni et al. (5) found dichlorvos not to be mutagenic to A. nidulans after metabolism by N. alata cells. They postulated that the potential mutagenic metabolites of this agent were deactivated by plant tissues. Gentile et al. (21) compared the deactivating potential of plant and animal systems. They found rat liver S-9 preparations reduced the mutagenicity of N-methyl-N'-nitro-N-nitrosoguanadine to S. typhimurium, however, Z. mays tissue preparations had no effect. We observed that the direct acting genotoxic insecticides fonofos (o-ethyl S-phenyl ethylphosphorodithioate) and terbufos (S-(((1, 1-dimethylethyl) thio) methyl) 0,0-diethyl phosphorodithioate) are not genotoxic following plant metabolism, suggesting that some detoxification of these agents occurs in plants (24).

IN SITU EVALUATION OF THE MUTAGENICITY OF PESTICIDES

In the United States, hundreds of millions of kilograms of pesticides are used annually by the agricultural community. While many uses of pesticides are beneficial, we are concerned that a comprehensive understanding of the mutagenic properties of pesticides is lacking. We conducted a research project that integrated the analysis of a group of pesticides for their mutagenic properties on several genetic indicator organisms using both animal and plant activation protocols under both laboratory and field conditions.

This research was designed as a demonstration project to investigate the mutagenic properties of a group of pesticides employed in the production of a significant commercial crop in the United States (Tables 3 and 4). The crop plant we chose was corn, Z. mays because it is a major agricultural commodity, a large number of pesticides are used in commercial corn production and corn is a well defined genetic tool that is amenable as an in situ genetic indicator organism for mutation induction. We employed three genetic indicator organisms, a prokaryote (S. typhimurium), a lower eukaryote (S. cerevisiae), a higher eukaryote (Z. mays) and established a comprehensive data base to resolve a spectrum of genetic damage that a pesticide or combination of pesticides may induce. Finally we introduced the use of an in vivo plant activation protocol to complement the in vitro mammalian microsomal activation system in current use with most microbial genetic assay systems. It was our intention that this project be used to evaluate pesticides for their mutagenic properties under a reasonable set of conditions, one of which is agricultural in nature.

In this section of this paper we concentrate primarily on the in situ maize assay to show how a plant genetic assay may be used to complement the standard microbial assays. A complete description of the data for the insecticides evaluated in this project has been published (24).

ZEA MAYS ASSAY

Indian corn or maize (Z. mays) is an angiosperm plant that is a member of the grass family. Maize is a cultivated grain and a major agricultural product of the United States (27). Maize is a good genetic indicator for genotoxins because more genetic information exists for maize than for any other plant species (9, 45). Z. mays is a higher eukaryote with a diploid number of 2n = 20 chromosomes; its chromosomes are of suitable size for cytogenetic studies and a large body of information exists on maize cytogenetics (8).

THE WAXY LOCUS POLLEN ASSAY

Since the microgametophyte (pollen grain) is a functional haploid, studies can be conducted that measure the mutation rate among germinal cells (as opposed to the mutation rate in developmental somatic cells per locus per generation). The test requires a moderate amount of time because no crosses are required. The advantage of this assay is that the pollen grain is the unit of measurement, therefore, large numbers can be analyzed providing the assay with a high degree of genetic resolution.

The waxy (wx) locus is located in the short arm of chromosome 9 at position 9-59. The wx locus controls the synthesis of the carbohydrate amylose. Genetic studies confirmed that the waxy allele is recessive to starchy (Wx) and wx segregates in the F2 generation as a Mendelian monohybrid (10,11). In waxy kernels, the starch of the endosperm contains only amylopectin, while in kernels possessing the dominant allele, Wx, the endosperms contain starch with a carbohydrate composition of both amylose and amylopectin (51,54). The presence of amylose in kernels with a Wx allele causes a blue-black color when an iodine solution is placed on the endosperm. When an iodine solution is reacted with endosperms of kernels homozygous for wx a light red color is produced. The iodine test also works with pollen grains. A pollen grain carrying a Wx allele can synthesize amylose and this carbohydrate will form part of its starch content. The exposure of a Wx carrying pollen

Table 3.   Pesticides Evaluated For Their Genotoxic Properties

		INSECTICIDES	
Common Name	Trade Name	Chemical Name	CA Reg. No.
Chlordane	Chlordane	1,2,4,5,6,7,8,8-Octachloro-2,3,3a,4,7,7a-hexahydro-4,7-methanoindene and related compounds	57-74-09
Terbufos	Counter	S-(((1, 1-Dimethylethyl) thio) methyl) 0,0-diethyl phosphoro-dithioate	13071-79-9
Fonofos	Dyfonate	0-Ethyl S-phenyl ethyl-phosphonodithioate	944-22-9
Heptachlor	Heptachlor	1,4,5,6,7,8,8-Heptachloro-3a,4,7,7a-tetrahydro-4,7-methanoindene	76-48-8
Carbofuran	Furadan	2,3-Dihydro-2,2-dimethylbenzo-furan-7-yl methylcarbamate	1563-66-2
Chlorpyrifos	Lorsban	0,0-Diethyl 0-(3,5,6-trichloro-2-pyridyl) phosphorothioate	2921-88-2
Ethoprop	Mocap	0-Ethyl S,S,-dipropyl phosphorodithioate	13194-48-4
Phorate	Thimet	0,0-Diethyl-S-((ethylthio) methyl) phosphorodithioate	298-02-2
Curacron	CGA	0-(4-bromo-2-chloro-phenyl)-0-ethyl-S-propyl phosphorothioate	
Metham	SRA	Sodium methyldithiocarbamate	6734-80-1

grain with an iodine solution will cause the pollen grain to appear black.

The starch type of a pollen grain is controlled by the genetic constitution of that pollen grain and not by the parental sporophyte. Therefore, a genetic reversion (back mutation) of wx to Wx can be detected by scoring for pollen grains obtained from sporophytes that are homozygous wx that stain a black color after treatment with an iodine solution. Likewise, forward mutation can also be measured by scoring tan staining wx carrying pollen grains obtained from plants that are homozygous for the Wx allele.

Studies have confirmed that pollen from maize plants treated with ionizing radiation demonstrated a clear dose dependent response in the mutation rate among gametophytes. Although a

Table 4. Pesticides Evaluated For Their Genotoxic Properties

HERBICIDES			
Common Name	Trade Name	Chemical Name	CA Reg. No.
Cyanazine	Bladex	2-[(4-Chloro-6-(ethylamino)-s-triazin-2-yl) amino]-2-methyl-propionitrile	21724-46-2
Eradicane	Eradicane (EPTC)	S-Ethyl dipropyl-thiocarbamate	759-94-4
Alachlor	Lasso	2-Chloro-2',6'-diethyl-N-(methoxymethyl) acetanilide	15972-60-8
Bifenox	Modown	Methyl 5-(2,4-dichlorphenoxy)-2-nitrobenzoate	42576-02-3
Procyazine	Cycle	2-((4-Chloro-6-(cyclopropyl-amino)-1,3,5-triazine-2-yl) amino)-2-methylpropionitrile	32889-48-8
Metolachlor	Dual	2-Chloro-N-(2-ethyl-6-methylphenyl)-N-(2-methoxy-1-methylethyl) acetamide	51218-45-2
Propachlor	Ramrod	2-Chloro-N-isopropyl-acetanilide	1918-16-7
Simazine	Princep	2-Chloro-4,6-bis(ethylamino)-1,3,5-triazine	122-34-9
Atrazine	Aatrex	2-Chloro-4(ethylamino)-6-(iso-propylamino)-1,3,5-triazine	1912-24-9
Butylate	Sutan	S-Ethyl N,N-diisobutylthio-carbamate	2008-41-5
-	SD50093		-
Dicamba	Banvel	2-Methoxy-3,6-dichloro-benzoic acid 3,5-Dichloro-o-anisic acid	1918-00-9

number of studies have reported increased forward mutation rates
after acute and chronic exposure to ionizing radiation (14-17,40)
we shall limit our discussion to reverse mutation at the wx locus
of maize. Briggs and Smith (7) analyzed the effect of X-radiation
on the reversion frequencies of three wx heteroalleles wx-H21, wx-C
and wx-90 and on frequency of intragenic recombination among three
different combinations of heteroalleles. They found an increase in
the reversion frequency of wx-90 to Wx and a significant decrease
in intragenic recombination between wx-C and wx-90. Bianchi and
Tomassini (6) analyzed the effect of increased X-radiation on maize
plants heteroallelic for various wx mutational sites. They
analyzed the effect of increased X-radiation (0 to 1680 R) on

plants heteroallelic for the following genotypes wx-H21/wx-90, wx-C/wx-H21 and wx-90/wx-C. The induction of Wx pollen grains was scored. Only the wx-H21/wx-90 heteroallelic combination showed a significant increase in the frequency of Wx pollen grains. However, a direct dose dependent response for the induction of aborted pollen grains was observed in all genotypes. Of great interest was the fact that in homoallelic plants for wx-C or wx-90 an increase in revertant Wx pollen grains over the spontaneous frequency in controls was demonstrated. For wx-C the exposure of 0, 800 R, and 1,600 R of X rays gave frequencies of revertant pollen grains of 1.2, 7.5, and 5.0 x 10^{-5}, respectively. For wx-90 the same radiation doses induced frequencies of revertant pollen grains of 2.3, 5.6, and 11.5 x 10^{-5}, respectively. Thus, wx-C and wx-90 can revert to the dominant allele after exposure to a mutagen. Amano and Ukai (2) reported that reverse mutation at the wx-R heteroallele was induced by chronic gamma irradiation. At dose rates of from 0 to 12 R/day the increase in average frequency of revertant pollen grains was linear. The lowest dose rate tested was 3.84 R/day and the frequency of mutant pollen grains increased from approximately 3 x 10^{-5} in the controls to 7 x 10^{-5} in the irradiated plants. At dose rates of 12 R/day the average frequency of revertant pollen grains was approximately 19 x 10^{-5}.

EXPERIMENTAL DESIGN

    The plants used throughout this study were inbred W22 homozygous for the wx-C heteroallele. Inbred W22 kernels were originally obtained from the Maize Genetics Cooperation Stock Center at the University of Illinois. The inbred line was propagated in the genetic nursery of M. Plewa. The wx-C heteroallele was reconfirmed by conducting a cis-trans test with a homozygous wx-C line in inbred M14 supplied to us by Dr. O. E. Nelson of the University of Wisconsin, Madison. No intragenic recombination at the wx locus was observed in pollen grains from the F1 progeny. Therefore, we certified that the heteroallele used in the maize wx locus reversion assay was wx-C.

In Situ Test Plots

    The in situ field plots were constructed at the Illinois Natural History Survey and at the South Farms of the Department of Agronomy at the University of Illinois. The in situ test plots for the evaluation of ten insecticides used in commercial corn production were set up at the Natural History Survey. A series of rows were plowed in an experimental field and each evaluation plot measured approximately 2 m x 0.5 m. Five kernels of homozygous wx-C inbred W22 were planted in each plot. Control plots were distributed within the field. A field grade formulation of each insecticide was applied to its assigned test plot prior to the emergence of the maize seedlings. These test plots were instituted during the 1976 growing season. The application rate in equivalent kg/ha is listed below.

Insecticide	Application Rate (kg/ha)
Curacron	2.24
Chlordane	2.24
Chlordane	4.48
Terbufos	2.24
Fonofos	2.24
Carbofuran	2.24
Heptachlor	1.12
Chlorpyrifos	2.24
Ethoprop	2.24
Metham	2.24
Phorate	2.24

The in situ test plots for the evaluation of herbicides were conducted at the South Farms of the University of Illinois. Each plot was approximately 10 m x 3 m and consisted of three parallel 10 m long rows. The outer two rows were planted with a commercial hybrid corn variety while the center row of each plot was planted with inbred W22, wx-C/wx-C kernels. A field grade formulation of each herbicide or combination of herbicides was applied prior to the emergence of the maize seedlings. Since all of the herbicides were not evaluated in a single year and since some of the weaker inbred maize plants did not survive during a season, three separate plantings were conducted. Herbicides were evaluated in situ during the growing seasons of 1976, 1977 and 1978. The 1977 test plots also included the herbicides and combination of herbicides contracted for testing during option two of this program. The herbicides and combinations of herbicides and their appropriate application rate in equivalent kg/ha are listed below.

Herbicides

1976 Test Plots	Application Rate (kg/ha)
Cyanazine	3.58
Procyazine	3.58
Metolachlor	6.00
Eradicane	0.56
Eradicane	3.36
Bifenox	2.24
SD50093	4.48
Cyanazine + Alachlor	2.24 + 2.24
Procyazine + Metolachlor	2.24 + 2.24
Metolachlor + Dicamba	2.24 + 0.56
Alachlor + Dicamba	2.34 + 0.56
Alachlor + Bifenox	2.34 + 1.12
Alachlor + Bifenox	2.24 + 1.68
Propachlor + Cyanazine	3.36 + 2.24

1977 Test Plots

Atrazine	3.84
Cyanazine	4.80
Metolachlor	8.40
Eradicane	7.20
Alachlor	6.00
SD50093	4.80
Simazine	3.84
Butylate	7.20
Metolachlor + Atrazine	3.00 + 2.40
Metolachlor + Dicamba	3.00 + 0.60
Metolachlor + Cyanazine	4.80 + 4.80
Eradicane + Atrazine	3.60 + 1.92
Eradicane + Cyanazine	3.60 + 2.40
Propachlor + Cyanazine	4.80 + 2.24
Butylate + Atrazine	4.80 + 1.92
Butylate + Cyanazine	4.80 + 2.40

1978 Test Plots

Dicamba	0.56
Propachlor	3.36

Control plots were uniformly distributed within the in situ experimental field for each year. The control plots were identical to the treatment plots except that no herbicide was applied to them. The control and treatment plots were cultivated by hand throughout the growing season and each plant was individually labeled with an experiment number.

Collection and Storage of Tassels

The plants were allowed to grow until early anthesis. This ontogenetic stage is marked by the flowering of the tassel and the extrusion of the anthers from the florets. A tassel was harvested when only a few anthers were dehisced and the majority of florets were unopened. Each tassel was labeled with the experiment number of the parental sporophyte immediately after its removal. The tassels were dehydrated in a tank of 70 percent ethanol for two days. After such time the tassels were placed in labeled 1 liter jars filled with 70 percent ethanol. Tassels may be stored in ethanol indefinitely. The advantage of the wx locus assay is that the samples can be collected and the genetic endpoint analyzed at the convenient time.

Preparation of Pollen Slides

Each tassel was removed from its storage jar and agitated in clean 70 percent ethanol to remove any contaminant field corn pollen grains from the surface of the tassel. Approximately 15 unopened florets were removed from the tassel and agitated in a petri dish filled with 70 percent ethanol. The anthers were dissected from unopened florets and placed in a stainless steel cup of a Vir-Tis microhomogenizer containing 0.6 ml of a gelatin-iodine stain. The gelatin-iodine stain was prepared as follows. The stock iodine solution consisted of 25 ml deionized water, 500 mg potassium iodide and 95 mg iodine. The potassium iodide was dissolved in 5 ml of water and the iodine was added before diluting the solution to a volume of 25 ml with water. The stock gelatin solution was prepared by mixing 25 ml of heated deionized water and 1.5 g bacteriological gelatin. Each day a fresh gelatin-iodine stain was made by mixing equal volumes of the stock iodine solution and the stock gelatin solution plus a drop of the detergent "Tween-80." The anthers were minced with scissors and homogenized for 30 sec. The homogenate was strained through cheesecloth onto the surface of a large microscope slide, and a cover slip was placed upon the pollen suspension. An additional 0.4 ml of stain was placed into the stainless steel cup and the anthers were rehomogenized for 20 sec. After the pollen suspension solidified the slide was examined under a dissecting microscope at a magnification of 40 X. The black staining pollen grains were counted. The number of pollen grains per slide was estimated by counting the number of pollen grains within 20 randomly chosen one square mm areas and multiplying this value by an appropriate factor. The random one square mm areas were generated by computer and transcribed onto a glass template. The template was used to estimate the total number of pollen grains per slide. After an appropriate number of slides were analyzed for each plant the frequency of revertant pollen grains was calculated by dividing the total number of Wx pollen grains by the total estimated number of pollen grains.

RESULTS AND DISCUSSION OF THE MAIZE WAXY LOCUS DATA

The results of the in situ maize wx locus assay are presented in Table 5.

Three descriptive statistical parameters were used to determine if a pesticide elicited a positive response. For each pesticide or combination of pesticides the appropriate estimator of the induced mutation rate at the wx locus among gametophytes was compared with a doubling of the appropriate control value. Thus, a twofold increase in the spontaneous mutation rate among gametophytes was considered as one of three indicators of a positive response. The other two measurements were a significant Ø

Table 5.   Maize Summary Table

Treatment	Estimated $\mu-(\times10^{-5})$	Statistical Evaluation		
		2X Control	t	φ
Insecticides 1976				
Control	3.97	NA	NA	NA
Curacron	6.73	-	-	-
Chlordane	9.82	+	+	-
Terbufos	7.30	-	-	-
Fonofos	6.14	-	-	-
Carbofuran	6.15	-	-	-
Heptachlor	10.40	+	+	+
Chlorpyrifos	2.74	-	-	-
Ethoprop	7.92	-	+	+
Metham	6.85	-	-	-
Phorate	4.08	-	-	-
Herbicides 1976				
Control	5.28	NA	NA	NA
Cyanazine	28.26	+	+	+
Procyazine	4.65	-	-	-
Bifenox	9.05	-	+	-
SD50093	39.37	+	+	+
Metolachlor + Dicamba	8.22	-	+	-
Metolachlor + Procyazine	9.84	-	+	-
Alachlor + Dicamba	3.82	-	-	-
Bifenox + Alachlor	6.96	-	-	-
Bifenox + Alachlor	4.29	-	-	-
Herbicides 1977				
Control	4.24	NA	NA	NA
Atrazine	8.53	+	+	+
Cyanazine	14.76	+	+	+
Metolachlor	2.84	-	-	-
Metolachlor	4.06	-	-	-
Eradicane (EPTC)	4.33	-	-	-
Alachlor	4.21	-	-	-
SD50093	16.25	+	+	+
Simazine	10.86	+	+	+
Butylate	5.28	-	-	-
Metolachlor + Atrazine	12.27	+	+	+
Metolachlor + Dicamba	7.31	-	+	-
Metolachlor + Cyanazine	10.84	+	+	+
Eradicane (EPTC) + Atrazine	14.20	+	+	+
Eradicane (EPTC) + Cyanazine	8.61	+	+	+
Propachlor + Cyanazine	6.29	-	-	-
Butylate + Atrazine	8.25	-	+	+
Butylate + Cyanazine	5.89	-	-	-
Herbicides 1978				
Control	2.91	NA	NA	NA
Dicamba	2.44	-	-	-
Propachlor	3.20	-	-	-

test and/or a t-test when the appropriate data from a control distribution and an independent treatment distribution were
compared. For a pesticide treatment to be considered as positive a
twofold increase over the estimated spontaneous mutation rate among
gametophytes or a significant $\emptyset$ test was required plus a
significant t-test. Two of the three statistical parameters must
indicate an increase in the number of mutant pollen grains induced
by a pesticide treatment for the treatment to be determined as
genotoxic.

The insecticide treatments that were determined to be negative
in all three statistical measurements employed with the maize wx
locus assay were curacron, terbufos, fonofos, carbofuran, chlorpyrifos, metham, and phorate. Ethoprop, chlordane and heptachlor
elicited positive responses.

The herbicides or combinations of herbicides that proved negative were procyazine, bifenox, metolachlor plus dicamba,
metolachlor plus procyazine, alachlor plus dicamba, and bifenox
plus alachlor. The herbicides that induced a positive response
were cyanazine and SD50093 (a field grade formulation of atrazine
plus cyanazine). In the 1976 in situ evaluation plots only the s-
triazine herbicides mentioned above demonstrated a positive
response in all three statistical measurements when compared to the
1976 in situ control values.

A second set of in situ evaluation plots were constructed in
1977. The herbicides or combinations of herbicides that were
negative were metolachlor, eradicane, alachlor, butylate,
metolachlor plus dicamba, propachlor plus cyanazine, and butylate
plus cyanazine. The herbicides or combinations of herbicides that
induced a positive response were atrazine, cyanazine, SD50093,
simazine, metolachlor plus atrazine, metolachlor plus cyanazine,
eradicane plus cyanazine, eradicane plus atrazine, and butylate
plus atrazine. Note that all positive cases comprised s-triazine
herbicides when used alone or in conjunction with another
herbicide.

The final set of in situ evaluation plots were constructed in
1978. Only dicamba and propachlor were tested. When compared to
the 1978 control values these herbicides were found not to be
mutagenic.

SUMMARY

The results of the comprehensive analysis of the mutagenic
properties of these pesticides used in commercial corn production
are summarized in Table 6. Each agent was tested directly, after
in vitro mammalian microsome activation or after in vivo plant

Table 6. Summary of Results

Pesticide (Option I)	S. typhimurium D	S. typhimurium S-9	S. typhimurium 1S	S. cerevisiae D	S. cerevisiae S-9	S. cerevisiae 1S	Z. mays wx
Alachlor (C)	-	-	-	+	-	-	-
Alachlor (T)	-	-	-	-	-	+	NT
Bifenox (C)	-	-	-	-	-	-	-
Bifenox (T)	-	-	-	-	-	-	NT
CGA (C)	-	-	-	-	-	-	-
CGA (T)	-	-	-	-	-	-	NT
Carbofuran (C)	-	-	-	-	-	-	-
Carbofuran (T)	-	-	NT	-	-	-	NT
Chlordane (C)	-	-	-	-	+	+	+
Chlordane (T)	-	-	-	-	+	-	NT
Chlorpyrifos (C)	-	-	-	-	-	-	-
Chlorpyrifos (T)	-	-	-	-	-	-	NT
Cyanazine (C)	-	-	+	-	-	-	+
Cyanazine (T)	-	-	+	-	-	NT	NT
Dicamba (C)	+	-	-	-	-	-	-
Dicamba (T)	+	-	+	-	+	-	NT
EPTC (C)	-	-	-	-	-	-	-
EPTC (T)	-	-	-	-	-	-	NT
Ethoprop (C)	NT	NT	NT	NT	NT	NT	+
Ethoprop (T)	NT	NT	NT	NT	NT	NT	NT
Fonofos (C)	-	+	-	-	-	-	-
Fonofos (T)	-	+	-	+	-	-	NT
Heptachlor (C)	-	-	-	-	-	-	+
Heptachlor (T)	-	+	+	-	-	-	NT
Metolachlor (C)	+	+	-	-	+	-	-
Metolachlor (T)	-	-	-	-	-	-	NT
Phorate (C)	-	-	-	-	-	-	-
Phorate (T)	-	-	-	-	-	-	NT
Procyazine (C)	-	-	NT	-	-	NT	-
Procyazine (T)	-	+	+	-	-	-	NT
Propachlor (C)	-	-	-	-	-	+	-
Propachlor (T)	-	-	-	-	-	+	NT
SD50093 (C)	-	-	NT	-	-	NT	+
SD5003 (T)	-	-	NT	-	-	NT	N1
SRA (C)	-	-	-	-	-	-	-
SRA (T)	-	-	-	-	-	-	NT
Terbufos (C)	-	-	-	+	-	-	-
Terbufos (T)	-	-	-	+	+	-	NT
Alachlor + Bifenox		+			-		-
Alachlor + Dicamba		+			-		-
Cyanazine + Alachlor		+			-		-
Cyanazine + Propachlor		+			-		-
Metolachlor + Atrazine		+			-		+
Metolachlor + Dicamba		-			+		-
Procyazine + Metolachlor		-			+		-

activation in both microbial assays. These data were compared with data from the _in situ_ maize pollen assay. For an agent to be considered genotoxic the following criteria were imposed. For the _Salmonella_ assay a test agent with or without activation was appraised as positive if it induced an increase in the number of

Table 6.   Continued

Pesticide (Option II)	Genetic Assays						
	S. typhimurium			S. cerevisiae			Z. mays
	D	S-9	1S	D	S-9	1S	wx
Atrazine							+
Butylate							-
Butylate + Atrazine							+
Butylate + Cyanazine							-
EPTC + Atrazine							+
EPTC + Cyanazine							+
Metolachlor + Atrazine							+
Metolachlor + Cyanazine							+
Simazine							+

revertants per plate that was twice the appropriate control value (3) or indicated a significant θ value (30). In addition the agent had to induce a reproducible dose-dependent response (3,12). For the Saccharomyces assay a test agent was considered as positive if it induced an increase in the number of convertants per 10^5 survivors that was twice the control value (56) or indicated a significant ∅ value (30). Additionally, the agent had to induce a reproducible dose dependent response. For the maize test the agent was appraised as positive if it induced an increase in the mutation rate among gametophytes that was twice the control value or indicated a significant ∅ value (29, 30). In addition a significant t-test was required for each agent.

Of the insecticides assayed, curacron, carbofuran, chlorpyrifos, metham and phorate were negative in all assays. Two insecticides, terbufos and ethoprop were positive in one assay. Chlordane, fonofos and heptachlor were positive in two of the three genetic assays. No insecticide was positive in all three assays.

Of the herbicides assayed under option one of this project, eradicane and bifenox were negative in all assays. Alachlor, propachlor, procyazine and SD50093 were positive in one assay. Cyanazine, dicamba and metolachlor were positive in two assays; no herbicide was found to be positive in all three assays.

The combinations of herbicides tested under option one were assayed under the condition of in vivo plant activation. All the herbicide combinations were positive in one of the three assays except metolachlor plus atrazine which was positive in two assays.

The herbicides and combinations of herbicides tested in option two were evaluated with the maize wx locus assay only. This option was conducted to gather additional information on the genotoxic properties of s-triazine herbicides. Only butylate and the combination of butylate plus cyanazine were negative in the maize assay.

Genetic assays that include plant systems must be employed to insure the construction of a reliable and accurate data base on the mutagenic properties of agricultural chemicals. The development and use of in situ plant assays is an essential component in the attainment of a comprehensive understanding of the genotoxic implications of agricultural agents.

ACKNOWLEDGEMENTS

This research was supported by USEPA Research Contract 68-02-2704 and NIEHS Research Grant ES-02384.

REFERENCES

1. Adler, I. D., A review of the coordinated research effort on the comparison of test systems for the detection of mutagenic effects sponsored by the EEC. Mutation Res. 74: 77-93 (1980).
2. Amano, E. and Y. Ukai, Use of maize pollen to detect genetic effects by radiation. Abstracts of the Third International Conference on Environmental Mutagens, Tokyo/Mishima, Japan. p.44 (1981).
3. Ames, B. N., J. McCann and E. Yamasaki, Methods for detecting carcinogens and mutagens with the Salmonella mammalian-microsome mutagenicity test. Mutation Res. 31: 347-364 (1975).
4. Bakshi, K. S., D. J. Brusick and D. D. Sumner, Mutagenic activity of corn plants grown in untreated and atrazine (AAtrex) treated soil. Environmental Mutagenesis 3: 302 (1981).
5. Benigni, R., M. Bignami, I. Camoni, A. Carere, G. Conti, R. Iachetta, G. Morpurgo and V. A. Ortali, A new in vitro method for testing plant metabolism in mutagenicity studies. J. Tox. Environ. Health, 5: 809-819 (1979).
6. Bianchi, A. and C. Tomassini, Reversion frequency of waxy pollen type in normal and hypoploid maize plants. Mutation Res. 2:352-365 (1965).
7. Briggs, R. W. and H. H. Smith, Effects of X-radiation on intracistron recombination at the waxy locus in maize. J. Heredity 56: 157-162 (1965).
8. Carlson, W. R., The cytogenetics of corn, in G. F. Sprague (ed.) Corn and Corn Improvement, Am. Soc. Agron. Inc., Madison, WI. pp. 225-304 (1977).
9. Coe, E. G. and M. G. Neuffer, The genetics of corn, in G. F. Sprague (ed.) Corn and Corn Improvement, Am. Soc. Agron. Inc., Madison, WI. pp. 111-223 (1977).

10. Collins, G. N. and J. H. Kempton, Inheritance of waxy endosperm in hybrids of Chinese maize. Bull. Bureau Plant Indus. U. S. Dept. Agric. 161: 547-556 (1909).
11. Collins, G. N., A new type of Indian corn from China. Bureau of Plant Indus. U. S. Dept. Bull. 161 (1909).
12. de Serres, F. J. and M. D. Shelby, The Salmonella mutagenicity assay: recommendations. Science 203: 563-565 (1979).
13. Ehrenberg, L., Higher plants in A. Hollaender, ed. Chemical Mutagens: Principles and Methods for Their Detection, Vol. II, Plenum Press, New York. pp. 365-386 (1971).
14. Eriksson, G., Induction of waxy mutants in maize by acute and chronic gamma irradiation, Hereditas 50: 161-178 (1963).
15. Eriksson, G. and E. Tavrin, Variations in radiosensitivity during meiosis of pollen mother cells in maize. Hereditas 54: 156-169 (1965).
16. Eriksson, G., The waxy character. Hereditas 63: 180-204 (1969).
17. Eriksson, G., Variation in radiosensitivity and the dose effect relationship in the low dose region. Hereditas 68: 101-114 (1971).
18. Fischnich, O., C. Patzold and C. Schiller, Wachstumregulatoren in kartoffelbau, Eur. Potato, J. 1: 25-30 (1958).
19. Gentile, J. M. and M. J. Plewa, Plant activation of herbicides into mutagens - the mutagenicity of atrazine metabolites in maize kernels. Mutation Res. 38: 390-391 (1976).
20. Gentile, J. M., E. D. Wagner and M. J. Plewa, The detection of weak recombinogenic activities in the herbicides propachlor and alachlor using a plant-activation bioassay. Mutation Res. 48: 113-116 (1977).
21. Gentile, J. M., L. K. Overton and J. Schubert, Inactivation of N-methyl-N'-nitro-N-nitrosoguanadine in the Ames Salmonella/microsome test. Naturwissenschaften 65: 659-660 (1978).
22. Gentile, J. M. and M. J. Plewa, The activation of promutagens by green plants. Environmental Mutagenesis 2: 312 (1980a).
23. Gentile, J. M.. and M. J. Plewa, In vitro activation of promutagens by green plants. Research Grant NIH I-R01-ES02384-01-TOX (1980b).
24. Gentile, J. M., G. J. Gentile, J. Bultman, R. Sechriest, E. D. Wagner and M. J. Plewa, An evaluation of the genotoxic properties of insecticides following plant and animal activation. Mutation Res. 101: 19-29 (1982).
25. Haley, T. J., Maleic hydrazide: Should the Delaney Amendment apply to its use? J. Toxicol. Environ. Health 2: 1085-1094 (1977).
26. Higashi, K., K. Nakashima, Y. Karasake, M. Fukunaga and Y. Mizuguchi, Activation of benzoapyrene by microsomes of higher plant tissues and their mutagenicity. Biochemistry Inst. 2: 373-380 (1981).

27. Jiler, H., ed., Commodity Year Book 1978. Commodity Research Bureau, Inc., New York (1978).
28. Kada, T., K. Morita and T. Inoue, Anti-mutagenic action of vegetable factor(s) on the mutagenic principle of tryptophane pyrolysate. Mutation Res. 53: 351-353 (1978).
29. Katz, A. J., Design and analysis of experiments on mutagenicity I. minimal sample sizes. Mutation Res. 50: 301-307 (1978).
30. Katz, A. J., Design and analysis of experiments on mutagenicity II. Assays involving microorganisms. Mutation Res. 64: 61-77 (1979).
31. Kleinhofs, A. and J. A. Smith, Effect of excision repair on azide-induced mutagenesis. Mutation Res. 41: 233-240 (1976).
32. Konzak, C. F., M. Niknejad, I. Wickham and E. Donaldson, Mutagenic interaction of sodium azide on mutations induced in barley seeds treated with diethyl sulfate or N-methyl-N-nitrosourea. Mutation Res. 30: 55-62 (1975).
33. Loprieno, N. and I. D. Adler, Cooperative programme of the European Economic Community on short-term assays for mutagenicity, in, R. Montesano, H. Bartsch, and L. Tomatis, eds., Molecular and Cellular Aspects of Carcinogen Screening Tests, IARC Sci. Publ. No. 27, International Agency for Research on Cancer, Lyon, France. pp. 331-341 (1980).
34. Loprieno, N., R. Barale, L. Mariani, S. Presciuttini, A. M. Rossi, I. Sbrana, L. Zaccaro, A. Abbondandolo and S. Bonnatti, Results of mutagenicity tests on the herbicide atrazine. Mutation Res. 74: 250 (1980).
35. Matijesevic, Z., Z. Erceg, R. Denic, V. Bacun and M. Alacevic, Mutagenicity of the herbicide cyanazine: plant activation bioassay. Mutation Res. 74: 212 (1980).
36. Morita, K., M. Hara and T. Kada, Studies on natural desmutagens: Screening for vegetable and fruit factors active in inactivation of mutagenic pyrolysis products from amino acids. Agric. Biol Chem. 42: 1235-1238 (1978).
37. Nilan, R. A., E. G. Sideris, A. Kleinhofs, C. Sander and C. F. Konzak, Azide-a potent mutagen. Mutation Res. 17: 142-144 (1973).
38. Nilan, R. A., A. Kleinhofs and C. Sander, Azide mutagenesis in barley, in H. Gaul, ed., Barley Genetics III, Thiemig, Munich. pp. 113-122 (1976).
39. Nilan, R. A., Potential of plant genetic systems for monitoring and screening mutagens. Environmental Health Persp. 27: 181-196 (1978).
40. Nettancourt, D. D., G. Eriksson, D. Lindgren and K. Puite, Effects of low doses by different types of radiation on the waxy locus using barley and maize. Hereditas 85: 89-100 (1977).
41. Owais, W. M., A. Zarowitz, R. A. Gunovich, A. L. Hodgon, A. Kleinhofs and R. A. Nilan, A mutagenic in vivo metabolite of sodium azide. Mutation Res. 53: 355-358 (1978).

42. Plewa, M. J. and J. M. Gentile, A maize-microbe bioassay for
    the detection of proximal mutagenicity in agricultural
    chemicals. Maize Genetics Coop. Newsl. 49: 40-43 (1975).
43. Plewa, M. J. and J. M. Gentile, The mutagenicity of atrazine:
    a maize-microbe bioassay. Mutation Res. 38: 287-292 (1976).
44. Plewa, M. J. and J. M. Gentile, The activation of chemicals
    into mutagens by green plants in F. J. de Serres and A.
    Hollaender, eds., Chemical Mutagens: Principles and Methods
    for Their Detection, Vol. VII, Plenum Press, New York. pp. 401-
    420 (1982).
45. Plewa, M. J., Specific locus mutation assays in Zea mays.
    Mutation Research (1981). IN PRESS.
46. Sander, C. and F. J. Muehlbauer, Mutagenic effects of sodium
    azide and gamma irradiation in Pisum. Environ. Exp. Bot. 17:
    43-47 (1977).
47. Sander, C., R. A. Nilan, A. Kleinhofs and B. K. Vig, Mutagenic
    and chromosome breaking effects of azide in barley and human
    leukocytes. Mutation Res. 50: 67-75 (1978).
48. Scott, B. R., A. H. Sparrow, S. S. Schwemmer and L. A.
    Schairer, Plant metabolic activation of 1,2-dibromoethane (EDB)
    to a mutagen of greater potency. Mutation Res. 49: 203-212
    (1978).
49. Silhankova, L., V. Smiovska and J. Veleminsky, Sodium azide
    induced mutagenesis in Saccharomyces cerevisiae. Mutation Res.
    61: 191-196 (1979).
50. Singh, I., A. F. Lusby and P. M. McGuire, Mutagenicity of HPLC
    fractions from extracts of herbicide treated corn.
    Environmental Mutagenesis (1982). IN PRESS.
51 Sprague, G. F., B. Brimhall and R. M. Hixon, Some effects of
    the waxy gene in corn on properties of the endosperm starch.
    J. Am. Soc. Agron. 35: 817-822 (1943).
52. Swietlinska, Z. and J. Zuk, Cytotoxic effects of maleic
    hydrazide. Mutation Res. 55: 15-30 (1978).
53. Veleminsky, J., L. Silhankova, V. Smiovska and T. Gichner,
    Mutagenesis of Saccharomyces cerevisiae by sodium azide
    activated in barley. Mutation Res. 61: 197-205 (1979).
54. Weatherwax, P., A rare carbohydrate in waxy maize. Genetics 7:
    568-572 (1922).
55. Yano, K., Effect of vegetable juices and milk on alkylating
    activity of N-methyl-N-nitrosourea. Agric. Food Chem. 27: 456-
    568 (1979).
56. Zimmermann, F. K., Procedures used in the induction of mitotic
    recombination and mutation in the yeast Saccharomyces
    cerevisiae. Mutation Res. 31: 71-86 (1975).

DISCUSSION

Q. SUGIMURA: What is known about P-450's in plants? Is there any
    P-450 in chloroplasts or other particles?

A. GENTILE: The mechanistic features of plant cytochrome P-450
    systems in plants have not been characterized nearly as
    thoroughly as the hepatic microsomal system. Dr. Higashi in
    Japan has characterized some aspects of P-450 dependent
    benzo(a)pyrene activity in Jerusalem artichoke tubers,
    suggesting that some P-450 activity can be observed in plant
    tissues other than those containing active chloroplasts.
    Specifically whether chloroplasts or other particles in plant
    tissues and cells have P-450 activity is a question still to be
    answered.

Q. BROWN: I am very interested in your results with PENTAC. Can
    you tell me what strain of Salmonella gave you the result?
    Also, I would like to point out that PENTAC is used on
    ornamental plants and is not registered for use on food crops.

A. GENTILE: We used strain TA98 in our studies. Additionally, we
    decided to study PENTAC because it worked in our system in
    preliminary experiments and not because the chemical had any
    economic relevance for food crops. We essentially used it in
    our studies as we used 2-aminofluorene or other promutagens.
    We are using all these chemicals as tools to study the
    mechanisms of plant activation.

Q. BADR: Using plant extracts in activating mixtures for
    mutagens, wouldn't you think that the chemical may produce
    genetic effects on the plant itself? It would be easy to check
    for both on the same plant.

A. GENTILE: I completely agree with your comments. It is our
    goal to correlate our in vitro plant activation protocols with
    genetic assays available in plants. Specifically, we would
    like to use the Zea mays waxy locus reversion assay as our
    comparative assay. By using these two approaches we would thus
    have a comprehensive data set to assist us in our understanding
    of plant activation of chemical agents.

CYTOGENETIC STUDIES OF AGRICULTURAL CHEMICALS IN PLANTS

William F. Grant

Genetics Laboratory, Box 282
Macdonald Campus of McGill University
Ste. Anne de Bellevue, Quebec, Canada H9X 1C0

INTRODUCTION

Of the some 1500 chemicals used in agriculture (99), pesticides are the most controversial for their known or potential genotoxicity (mutagenicity-carcinogenicity-teratogenicity) and will
comprise the subject matter of this paper. Pesticides are a large
diverse group of compounds which include fungicides, herbicides,
insecticides, fumigants, growth regulators and inhibitors, acari-
cides, rodenticides, soil nematicides, seed sterilants, soil condi-
tioners, and chemosterilants. In addition, there are emulsifiers
and solvents which are combined with pesticides and which are potential mutagens in their own right (25).

Pesticides are subject to close scrutiny on account of the
large annual volume of chemical used (1.6 billion lbs in up to
50,000 separate products appraised at 3 billion dollars in
1975)(99), the considerable number of individuals which come in
contact with pesticides in their manufacturing and application (the
herbicide trifluralin is estimated to involve 470,000 applicators
and 38,000 field workers) (99), the potential effects on human
health (11,56) and on the flora and fauna (46).

The first cytogenetic study of an agricultural chemical in
higher plants resulted from an observation of reduced seed set of
tobacco and eggplants after they had been fumigated with nicotine
sulfate. In 1931, Kostoff (67) reported many chromosome irregularities in the meiotic cells of these plants and he considered the
nicotine sulfate to be the cause of their partial sterility. Evidence accumulated during the past two decades has confirmed the
observations of Kostoff and emphasized the link between pesticide

exposure, cytogenetic abnormalities and gene mutations both in wild
and cultivated plants.

THE PRODUCTION OF CHROMOSOME ABERRATIONS FOLLOWING PESTICIDE
TREATMENT

    Chromosome aberrations have been detected after pesticide
treatment in embryonic shoot and root tip cells, in pollen mother
cells (meiocytes), as micronuclei resulting from fragments or lagging chromosomes in quartet cells and in pollen tube cells. All of
the common types of chromosome aberrations have been reported in
higher plants after pesticide treatment and these will be briefly
described with examples.

Colchicine Mitosis

    Levan (68), who introduced the now classical Allium test as an
assay system for studying the effects of chemicals on plant chromosomes, described colchicine mitosis as an inactivation of the
spindle followed by a random scattering of the chromosomes over the
cell. Sister chromatids may remain adjacent often forming "star-
metaphases", or they may separate widely throughout the cytoplasm
(31). Such compounds have also been classified as mitotic poisons
or antimitotic agents.

    There are a number of pesticides which are typical C-mitotic
agents (Table 1). It has been reported that some mercury compounds
have a greater C-mitotic activity than colchicine (37,70). Likewise, the carbamates have been so effective as C-mitotic chemicals
that several have been recommended for the artificial induction of
polyploidy (118). Polyploidy has been induced as high as 16-ploid
with the carbamate propham (26). Levan (70) has reported that
organic mercury compounds used as seed dressings have induced polyploid rye plants in field experiments.

    Plant systems have been shown to be sensitive indicators of
cytological aberrations. The studies of Fernandez-Gomez (35) and
Fernandez-Gomez et al. (36) on the C-mitotic effect of the four
isomers (α, β, γ, δ) of hexachlorocyclohexane may be used as an
example. They found that the β isomer had no C-mitotic effect, the
α isomer produced partial C-mitosis, while the γ and δ isomers
produced complete C-mitosis.

    It has been shown that compounds which have a C-mitotic effect
in plant tissue will induce the same effect in animal tissue.
Several pesticides including mercurial compounds (37,38) and
griseofulvin (90) have been shown to have the same C-mitotic effect
in both plant and animal tissues.

Table 1.   Examples of Pesticides Reported With C-Mitotic Activity

Class	Compound	Type*	Species	Reference
Mercurials				
	Phenylmercury acetate	F	Allium cepa	15
	Methylmercury dicyandiamide	F	Tradescantia, Vicia faba	1
	Methyl, ethyl and methoxyethyl mercury chloride; butyl mercury bromide	F	Allium cepa	37
Chlorinated Hydrocarbons				
	Hexachlorocyclohexane	I	16 species	47
	2,4-D	H	9 species	47
	2,4-DB	H	Pisum sativum	83
	2,4,5-T	H	Allium cepa	23,44,89
	DDT	I	Allium cepa	124
	Dieldrin	I	Crepis capillaris	77
Aryl Halide				
	Griseofulvin	F	Allium cepa	39,90
Dinitroaniline	Dichloran	F	Hordeum vulgare	129
	Trifluralin	H	Allium cepa	61
Carbamates	Barban	H	Vicia faba, Allium cepa, Carica papaya	75
	Benomyl	F	Zea mays	114
	Carbaryl	I	Vicia faba	6
	Chloropropham	H	Tradescantia reflexa, Allium fistulosum, Vicia faba; Hordeum vulgare	58,75,101
	Diallate	H	Triticum, Hordeum, Secale, Pisum, Linum, Avena, Zea	82,115
	Propham	H	Allium, Vicia, Hordeum, Secale Zea	26,28,58

*F = fungicide; I = insecticide; H = herbicide

Tripolar and Tetrapolar Anaphases

Partial C-mitosis may lead to abnormal anaphases in which multiple poles are formed so that the chromosomes separate in more than the two normal groups at anaphase. Tripolar and tetrapolar anaphases have been reported from treatment of a number of pesticides such as simazine (121), liro (IPC + diuron) (60) and others (Table 2).

Binucleate, Multinucleate, and Polyploid Cells

Binucleate cells arise as a consequence of the inhibition of cell plate formation. These form a distinct sub-population of easily detected cells. Failure of cell plate formation in already binucleate cells may give rise to the multinucleate condition.

A number of pesticides are known to induce the binucleate or multinucleate condition in plants including gramopol (24), dalapon (101), linuron (127,128), and propham (19,28,34). Other pesticides reported to induce the binucleate or multinucleate condition are given in Table 3. Mitotic irregularities such as incomplete anaphases or unequal distribution of the chromosomes to the daughter cells can result in aneuploid and also euploid cells. Atrazine and chloranil have been reported to induce aneuploid cells in root tips of Sorghum (71) and Vicia faba (131). Univalents in meiotic cells have been reported after treatments with carbaryl (6) and dimethoate (8).

Tetraploid and higher levels of polyploidy have been reported after treatment with some pesticides, for example 2,4-D (62). Other examples are given in Table 4. Endoreduplication in which chromosome duplication occurs without nuclear division has also been reported after 2,4-D (32), 2,4,5-T (18,83) and ferbam treatment (95).

C-Tumors

The phenomenon of C-tumors has been reported in root tips after treatments by herbicides (61). Two types of enlargement have been reported: (a) a complete swelling affecting the major length of the root tip and (b) a complete swelling restricted to an area of the root 2 mm above the tip.

C-tumor is a misnomer as it has been shown that the hypocotyl cells which are non-meristematic swell to form a tumor and the nuclear volume remains constant (61). Consequently, the tumors are not related to C-mitosis or induced polyploidy but are a cellular growth reponse to a chemical.

Table 2. Examples of Pesticides That Induced Spindle Disturbances
Resulting in Tri- and Tetra-polar Anaphases

Pesticide	Type[*]	Species	Reference
Carbaryl	I	Vicia faba	6
Dexon	F	Allium cepa	93
Dimethoate	I	Vicia faba	8
Fenitrothion	I	Allium cepa	93
Leptophos	I	Vicia faba	9
Linuron	H	Hordeum vulgare	127
Methyl parathion	I	Allium cepa	93
Phenylmercury acetate	F	Allium cepa	15

[*]I = insecticide; F = fungicide; H = herbicide.

Fiskesjö (37) has reported a characteristic variant of the C-
tumor reaction called the "crochet-hook" effect (33). After a 24
hour treatment of the root tips of Allium cepa with methoxyethyl
mercury chloride the terminal 3 to 4 mm of the root tips bend up-
wards making each root resemble a hook. With treatment after 24
hours the bending continues for one or more complete turns making
the root form irregular spirals.

Chromosome Stickiness and Clumping

McGill et al. (78) and Klásterská et al. (65) have suggested
that chromosome stickiness arises from improper folding of the
chromosome fibers. As a result there is an intermingling of the
fibers, and the chromosomes become attached to each other by means
of subchromatid bridges.

Chromosome stickiness and clumping have been reported following treatment with a number of pesticides including 2,4-D (23,89),
2,4,5-T (4), demeton (42), isodrin (104), and pentachlorophenol
(3). Other examples are given in Table 5.

Chromosome Haziness or Paling and Dissolution

Haziness or paling of chromosomes probably results from a
partial despiralization of the chromosomes, whereas dissolution

Table 3. Examples of Pesticides Known to Induce the Binucleate
or Multinucleate Condition

Pesticide	Type[*]	Species	Reference
Bromacil	H	Avena sativa	12
Carbaryl	I	Vicia faba	6
Dexon	F	Allium cepa	93
Dinoseb	H	Tradescantia reflexa	101
Fenitrothion	I	Allium cepa	93
Fensulfothion	I	Allium cepa	93
Fenthion	I	Allium cepa	93
Hexachlorocyclohexane	I	Pisum sativum	13
Methyl parathion	I	Allium cepa	93
Nitralin	H	Zea mays	41
Phenylmercury acetate	F	Hordeum vulgare, Pisum sativum	19

[*] H = herbicide; I = insecticide; F = fungicide.

refers to a complete breakdown in chromosome structure arising from
an almost complete despiralization of the chromosome. Haziness or
paling has been reported after treatment with the carbamates,
chlorpropham and propham (57). The long, thin chromatin threads
which characterize chromosome dissolution have been observed in
barley cells after seed treatment with monuron. The threads form
bridges between aggregations of chromosomal material (129).

Interchromatid Connections

Chromatid fibers which connect two chromatids at metaphase
and presumably hold the chromatids together until anaphase have
been termed interchromatic connections (30). Such interchromatid
connections have been observed after treatment of Tradescantia and
Vicia faba root tip cells with a mercurial fungicide (1).

Chromosome Erosion and Fragmentation

Chromosomes characterized by constrictions and a mottled appearance, possibly as a result of chromosome despiralization and
partial breakage of the chromonemata, are said to be eroded. Chro-

Table 4. **Examples of Pesticides Reported to Induce Euploidy –** Tetraploidy, etc.

Pesticide	Type[*]	Species	Reference
Carbaryl	I	Vicia faba	6
Diallate	H	Triticum, Avena, Hordeum, Secale, Pisum, Linum	82
Dimethoate	I	Vicia faba, Allium cepa, Chlorophytum elatum	7,8,118
Hexachlorocyclohexane	I	Pisum, Cicer, Lens, Lathyrus	108
Leptophos	I	Vicia faba	9
Propham	H	Allium, Vicia, Hordeum	26,118

[*]I = insecticide; H = herbicide.

mosome erosion has been reported following treatment of Allium cepa root tips with phenylmercury acetate (15). Partial dissolution of chromosomes resulting in the blurring of the chromosome borderlines has been reported following simazine treatment (60).

Chromosome fragmentation results from multiple breaks of the chromosome in which there is a loss of chromosome integrity. Fragmentation can range from partial to total disintegration of the chromosome. The latter has been termed chromosome pulverization. There is some confusion in the literature reporting chromosome fragmentation as breakage of chromosomes resulting in single fragments must be distinguished from multiple chromosome breakage as defined above. Chromosome fragmentation has been reported after treatment with phenylmercury acetate (15) and ferbam in Allium cepa (95), linuron in Hordeum (127,128), and simazine in Vicia cracca (121).

Chromatin Bodies

Intensely stained micronuclei in interphase which result from multiple chromosome breakage or aberrations have been termed chromatin bodies (80). Chromatin bodies have been observed in root tip cells of Vicia faba from treatment with amitrole and Allium cepa after 2,4-D treatment (80).

Table 5. Examples of Pesticides That Induce Chromosome Stickiness, Clumping, Sticky Bridges, and Lagging Chromosomes

Pesticide	Type[*]	Species	Reference
Asulam	H	Allium cepa	117
Bromacil	H	Vicia faba	129
Carbaryl	I	Vicia faba	6,26,34
Carbicron	I	Vicia faba	43,88
Dalapon	H	Tradescantia reflexa	101
Dimethoate	I	Vicia faba	8
Dithane S-60	F	Triticum, Aegilops	113
Ferbam	F	Allium cepa	95
Fungisol-Z	F	Vicia faba	24
Leptophos	I	Vicia faba	9
Mevinphos	I	Vicia faba	1
Methylmercury dicyandiamide	F	Tradescantia, Vicia	1
Monochloroacetic acid	H	Vicia faba	5
Phenylmercury acetate	F	Allium cepa	15
Trichloroacetic acid	H	Vicia, Tradescantia	5,101

[*]H = herbicide; I = insecticide; F = fungicide

Chiasma Frequency

Sharma et al. (109) have recently shown that the chiasma frequency, which reflects genetic recombination, is a good measure of the action of a potential mutagen. They treated barley seed with three herbicides and found the chiasma frequency to be reduced to different extents (Table 6). The herbicide terbacil reduced the chiasma frequency significantly from the control level of 15.40 to 13.76 and had about the same effect as that of EMS. In the case of lenacil, there was an initial decline but there was no further

Table 6. Chiasma Frequency in Hordeum vulgare After Treatment
With Herbicides Lenacil, Bromacil and Terbacil.
Modified from Sharma et al. (109)

Herbicide	Concentration (ppm)	Mean chiasma frequency per cell
Lenacil	0	15.34
	100	14.34*
	500	14.56
	1000	14.62
	1500	14.52
Bromacil	0	15.46
	100	15.20
	500	15.02
	1000	14.96
	1500	14.72
Terbacil	0	15.40
	100	14.42
	500	14.10*
	1000	14.30*
	1500	13.76**
EMS	0	16.00
	100	15.52
	500	15.54
	1000	15.22
	1500	14.36*

Significant at 5% (*) and 1% (**) levels.

response with increasing dosage. Bromacil had the least effect on
chiasma frequency.

Singh et al. (111) have reported decreased chiasma frequency
at significant levels after treating barley seeds for three hours
with 0.1% concentrations of the following insecticides: cythion,
ambithion, dimecron, citrolane, thimet, counter, furadan and disyston. Grover and Tyagai (54) have also reported in barley a
decrease in chiasma frequency with the pesticides thiodan and kita-
zin.

Table 7. Chromosome Aberrations Induced in Barley Shoot
and Root Tips After Seed Treatment (6 h) With Two
Organophosphorus Insecticides, Trichlorfon and
Dichlorvos. Modified from Panda and Sharma (92)

Insecticide	Concentration (ppm)	Chromosome aberrations (%)	
		Shoot tip[a]	PMC[a]
Trichlorfon	0	0	0.33
	100	1.74	1.33
	500	2.16	1.80
	1000	2.28	4.79[a]
	1500	2.85	4.95[a]
Dichlorvos	0	0.25	0.26
	100	1.91	1.04
	500	2.74[b]	1.72
	1000	3.58[b]	4.84[b]
	1500	3.74	5.34[b]

[a] Bridges, fragments, lagging chromosomes (and non-congression and non-disjunction of bivalents in PMCs).

[b] Chromosome aberrations exceeded those of EMS at equivalent dosage.

A reduction in chiasma frequency by a pesticide may lead to undesirable consequences, such as changes in genetic recombination or increased desynapsis.

Chromosome Breakage and Exchange

Many pesticides are clastogens producing chromosome breaks which may give rise to exchanges, anaphase bridges and fragments both in mitotic and meiotic cells (Table 7). These have been recorded in different categories as (a) chromatid and subchromatid exchanges, (b) chromosome and chromatid breaks, (c) acentric fragments, (d) chromatid gaps (achromatic lesions), (e) sister chromatid exchanges at metaphase, and (f) chromatid, chromosome and side-arm bridges at anaphase. The chromosome breaking efficiency of pesticides may be readily compared (Fig. 1; Table 8) and the effects followed for more than one generation (Table 9).

Reports of chromosome breakage and exchange following pesticide treatment are too numerous to cite here and only a few repre-

sentative examples will be given: leptophos (9), ethephon (17),
monochloroacetic and trichloroacetic acids (5), 2,4-D (80), 2,4,5-T
(48), trichlorfon and dichlorvos (92) and vitavax and dithane
(2,76,113).

Chromosome Aberration Specificity

Certain pesticides have been shown to induce aberrations in
specific regions of the chromosomes forming "hot spots" in contrast
to the more random distribution of chromosome aberrations observed
after irradiation. For example, it has been shown that the growth
retardant chemical maleic hydrazide induces chromosome breakage
largely in heterochromatic regions (79,96). Similarly, Nicoloff
and Gecheff (86) have shown that in barley seeds, following treatment with ethylenimine, the greatest number of aberrations were
located in the region of the centromere. On the other hand, pesticides may produce chromosome number irregularities, but be ineffec-
tive as clastogens. For example, pesticides which interfere with
the spindle mechanism and thus induce C-mitosis, such as phenylmercury acetate (15) and gamma-hexachlorocyclohexane (59), generally possess only a very mild clastogenic effect.

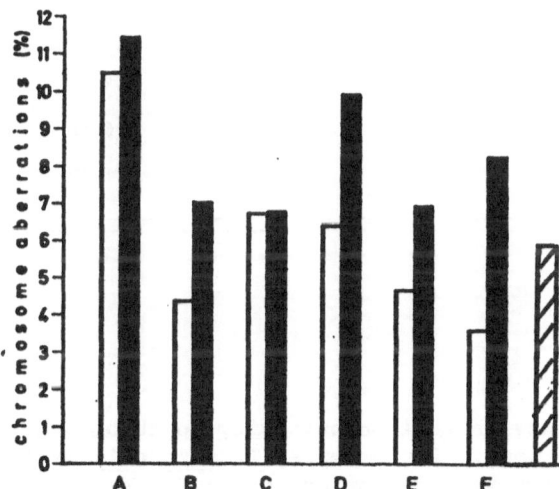

Fig. 1.   Percentage of chromosome aberrations induced by
            herbicides in barley root tips. (A) monolinuron, (B)
            isoproturon, (C) metobromuron, (D) chlorbromuron, (E)
            linuron, (F) methabenzthiazuron. White bar, 6 hour,
            black bar, 12-hour treatment. Cross-hatched bar
            represents a dose of 2.3 X 10^{-3} M ethylenimine, 3 hour-
            treatment, used as a positive control. Dose of positive
            control was calculated not to decrease germination below
            90%. Modified from Pusztai and Végh (97).

Table 8.   Various Herbicides (100 to 800 ppm; 6 or 12 h) Inducing
           Chromosome Aberrations in Root Tips of Barley and the
           Relative Efficiency of Each to Control Given a Value of
           1.0, 2.3 x 10^{-3}M Ethylenimine (EI) and 10 krad γ-Ray.
           Pusztai and Végh (97)

Herbicide	Relative efficiency
Monolinuron	5.57
Chlorbromuron	4.09
Metabromuron	3.39
Methabenzthiazuron	3.18
Linuron	2.93
Isoproturon	2.83
Metoxuron	1.70
Chloroxuron	1.59
Diuron	1.28
EI	3.03
α-rays	6.12
water	1.00

Species vary in their sensitivity to chromosome breakage after
pesticide treatment. For example, Tradescantia is less susceptible
to chromosome breakage following pesticide treatment than Vicia
faba (1), and likewise, Hordeum vulgare is also less sensitive
than Vicia faba (45). The susceptibility of a species to chromosome breakage has been shown to be related to the level of ploidy,
life-form and nuclear volume (81).

POLLEN STERILITY AND LOWERED SEED SET

A number of studies have shown that those pesticides which
induce chromosome aberrations in meiotic cells, such as unequal

Table 9.   Chromosome Aberrations and Mutagenic Activity of 2,4-DB
            in Barley (127)

	Concentration (ppm)	Duration of treatment (h)	C_1 chromosomal aberrations (%)	C_2 chromosomal aberrations (%)	C_2 mutant seedlings (%)
2,4-DB	500	6	1.24		
		12	1.87		
		24	2.26		
	1000	6	1.23		
		12	4.12*	1.44	1.02
		24	4.17*		
	1500	6	2.49		
		12	3.81*		
		24	9.74*		
Negative control, H_2O			0.68	0.00	0.11
X-rays	5500R		9.15*	2.48	3.58

*Significant   from control at 5% level.

exchanges, fragments or lagging chromosomes, in general, cause reduced pollen fertility and a lower seed set. Examples from fungicides include maneb, zineb, and nabam which were sprayed on imma-
ture inflorescences of Allium cepa (76). A 1500 ppm maneb reduced
pollen fertility from 95.85% in the control to 82.28%. Likewise,
seed set was reduced from 88.25% to 52.18%. Seed viability was
also reduced from the control of 95% to 45%. Similar results were
obtained with zineb in which pollen fertility was reduced with a
concentration of 1500 ppm from 95.85% to 75.21%; seed set from
88.25% to 50.12% and seed viability from 95% to 48%. Nabam was
more drastic, reducing pollen fertility from 95.85% to 65.20%; seed
set from 88.25% to 40.25% and seed viability from 95% to 29%.
Singh et al. (111) treated seed of Hordeum vulgare for three hours
with 0.1% solutions of several insecticides. Pollen sterility was
increased two to three times the control level with the insecticides endrin, ambithion, dimecron, citrolane, furadan and disyston.
Amer and Ali (4,5) sprayed plants of Vicia faba when they were 35
days old with several pesticides but found 2,4,5-T to be the only
treatment which significantly reduced pollen viability. Yield expressed as the number of pods and mean weight of seed was signifi-

cantly reduced for plants sprayed with 2,4,5-T at 15 days of age. In second and later generations yield may revert to normal levels or even increase (8). In such cases, chromosome aberrations may be lethal to the cells possessing them and could be eliminated (121).

In general, the initial disruption of the chromosomal apparatus by pesticides may affect the vigor and fertility of the exposed plants and the genetic constitution of the progeny. As has been suggested where seed is being grown for multiplication purposes (elite seed), the question of pesticide treatment of such plots or plants should be carefully considered (127).

SPECIES RESISTANCE

It is well known that species vary in their susceptibility or resistance to pesticides (14,46,51,52). While it is well known that numerous insects have developed resistance to pesticides, considerable documentation now exists on plants which have developed resistance to pesticides, including species of agricultural importance (Table 10). Other species of plants which have developed resistance are listed by Grant (46). Intraspecific and interspecific variation in resistance exists in a number of crop species (51).

Mohandas and Grant (81) studied the responses of 15 weed species to eight auxin herbicides (2,4-D, 2,4-DB, 2,4,5-T, MCPA, MCPB, fenoprop, mecoprop, dicamba) to the level of ploidy, the life form, the nuclear volume and the interphase chromosome volume. The response of any one of the weeds to each herbicide was found to be more or less identical. In general, susceptible weeds had a lower nuclear volume than those showing an intermediate or a resistance response to the herbicides. The interphase chromosome volume, although correlated with radiosensitivity of the plants, did not show any relationship to the sensitivity of the plants to herbicide treatment. Intermediate and resistant plants were mostly perennials, whereas susceptible ones were annuals or biennials.

While resistance to herbicides such as 2,4-D and 2,4,5-T may be less serious to cultivated species, the triazine resistant species would appear more critical to cultivated crops of agricultural importance. Resistance in barley and maize has been shown to be under the control of a single recessive gene, but polygenes may also play a role [for references see Grant (46)].

GENE MUTATIONS IN HIGHER PLANTS FOLLOWING PESTICIDE TREATMENT

Almost 30 years ago Unrau and associates (122,123) showed that the herbicide 2,4-D was an effective agent in inducing chromosomal aberrations in meiotic cells of barley and wheat and produce heritable changes in awning, earliness, and stature. Also in wheat (Triticum aestivum), Suneson and Jones (119) have reported herit-

Table 10. Examples of Species Reported to Have Developed Genetic
Resistance to Pesticides

Pesticide	Species	Reference
Atrazine	Amaranthus retroflexus	51
	Ambrosia artemisiifolia	51
	Brassica campestris	51
	Chenopodium album	51
	Chenopodium strictum	126
	Glycine max	51
	Poa annua	29
	Senecio vulgaris	22
	Zea mays	46
Barban	Hordeum vulgare	46
?,4-D	Daucus carota	51
	Nicotiana sylvestris	51
DDT	Hordeum vulgare	46
Diquat	Zea mays	46
Picloram	Nicotiana tabacum	46
Simazine	Brassica napus	46
	Sinapis alba	46
	Triticum aestivum	46
	Zea mays	46

able morphological changes following the application of the
herbicide dalapon, and later showed that this herbicide produced a
wide spectrum of mutants in barley and oats, as well as wheat
(120).

Several studies have shown that pesticides will induce chlorophyll mutations in Hordeum vulgare (Table 11). The chlorophyll
mutations reported include albina, xantha, viridis, striata, ti-
grina, and maculata (53,80,91,111). Panda and Sharma (91) reported
mostly alboviridis mutants whereas Singh et al. (111) reported
mostly albina and Mohandas and Grant (80) only albina. Gustafsson
(55), in his studies on the effect of X-rays on barley, observed

Table 11. Mutants Observed in the C$_2$ Generation of <u>Hordeum</u>
<u>vulgare</u> after Pesticide Treatment

Pesticide	Concentration	Time (h)	Chlorophyll (%)	Dwarf (%)	Reference
Atrazine	1000 ppm	12	0.57	0.57	127
Carbaryl	1000 ppm	12	0.64	0.21	127
2,4-D	200 ppm	6	1.30	--	80
2,4-DB	1000 ppm	12	0.45	0.45	127
Diazinon	0.8 %	4	4.40	--	53
Dicamba	1000 ppm	12	0.14	0.56	127
Dichloram	1000 ppm	12	0.12	0.58	127
Dichlorvos	1500 ppm	6	0.82	--	91
Dimethoate	0.01-0.05%	4	3.94	--	53
Dursban	0.2-1.0%	4	4.33	--	53
Ekalux	0.5%	6	4.90	--	111
Ekatin	0.5%	6	5.80	--	111
Endrin	1000	12	0.11	0.21	127
Fenitrothion	1500	6	0.20	--	91
Linuron	100	12	1.99	0.44	127
Metasystox	0.5%	6	5.70	--	111
Methyl parathion	0.15-0.75%	4	4.47	--	53
Monocrotophos	1500 ppm	6	0.52	--	91
Monuron	1000 ppm	12	0.56	0.56	127
Naptalam	1000 ppm	12	0.43	--	127
Nuvan	0.5%	6	2.10	--	111
Oxydemeton methyl	1500 ppm	9	0.14	--	91
Phosphamidon	1000 ppm	12	0.11	0.53	127
Phosphamidon	1500 ppm	6	0.52	--	91
Simazine	1000 ppm	12	2.10	0.31	127
Thiodemeton	1500 ppm	6	0.47	--	91
Trichlorfon	1500 ppm	6	0.60	--	91

that <u>albina</u> was the most common type of induced chlorophyll mutation. Grover and Kaur (53) found <u>tigrina</u> to be the most frequent
type and <u>albina</u> to be induced only with methyl parathion. It would
appear that different pesticides induce one type of chlorophyll
mutation more frequently than another.

Singh et al. (111) found the frequency of cholorophyll mutations to depend on the stage in interphase that the pesticide was
applied. The pesticides ekalux and metasystox produced a higher
frequency of mutations when applied in the S phase, whereas the
pesticides ekatin and nuvan were more effective in the G_2 phase.

HIGHER PLANT GENETIC SYSTEMS FOR SCREENING AND MONITORING MUTAGENS

Over 230 higher plants have been used in various aspects of
mutagenesis (110), from studies on the mechanism of mutagenesis to
the production on new mutant cultivars of crop species. In
general, those plants used for screening and monitoring of mutagens
have special features, such as, (a) many gene markers (Hordeum
vulgare, Pisum sativum, Lycopersicon esculentum), (b) relatively
few and large chromosomes (Vicia faba, Allium cepa, Tradescantia,
Lilium, Hordeum vulgare (49,63,127-130), (c) grow in culture media
under defined conditions (Arabidopsis thaliana) (21,98), (d)
somatic crossing over (Glycine max) (125), (e) self-incompatibility
test systems (Oenothera, Nicotiana, Petunia) (85,116), (f) sister
chromatid exchange (Allium, Hordeum, Secale, Zea) (20,64,105,106),
(g) isozyme systems (40,107) and (h) pollen systems (16,84,87,94).

Higher plant screening and monitoring mutagen assay systems
have been in existence for many years, but they are only beginning
to receive the recognition which these sensitive and reliable
systems warrant (27,100). In the area of mutagen in situ
monitoring, there are at present no organisms as useful as the
Tradescantia stamen hair system (72,102,103) and micronucleus test
(73) for the detection of air pollutants, the Osmunda regalis system for the detection of water pollutants (66) and the Zea mays
pollen system for the detection of mutagenic pesticides under agricultural practice (94). Recent studies have shown that for a
specific chemical agent, comparable results in terms of genetic
abnormalities are obtained in higher plant and animal systems, and
specifically plant systems have shown excellent correlations with
mammalian systems (49,50).

ACKNOWLEDGEMENTS

Financial support from the National Sciences and Engineering
Research Council of Canada for studies in genetic toxicity of environmental chemicals is gratefully acknowledged.

REFERENCES

1. Ahmed, M. and W. F. Grant, Cytological effects of the
    pesticides Phosdrin and Bladex on Tradescantia and Vicia
    faba, Can. J. Genet. Cytol. 14: 157-165 (1972).
2. Al-Najjar, N. R. and A. L. Soliman, Cytological effects of
    fungicides. I, Mitotic effects of vitavax-200 and dithane S-

60 on wheat and two related species, Cytologia 45: 163–168 (1980).

3. Amer, S. M., and E. M. Ali, Cytological effects of pesticides. IV. Mitotic effects of some phenols, Cytologia 34: 1–8 (1969).

4. Amer, S. M. and E. M. Ali, Cytological effects of pesticides, V. Effects on Vicia faba, Cytologia 39: 633–643 (1974)

5. Amer, S. M. and E. M. Ali, Cytological effects of pesticides. XI. Meiotic effects of the herbicides monochloracetic and trichloroacetic acids, Cytologia 45: 715–719 (1980).

6. Amer, S. M. and O. R. Farah, Cytological effects of pesticides. III. Meiotic effects of N–methyl-1-naphthyl carbamate "Sevin", Cytologia 33: 337–344 (1968).

7. Amer, S. M. and O. R. Farah, Cytological effects of pesticides. VI. Effects of the insecticide "Rogor" on the mitosis of Vicia faba and Gossypium barbadense, Cytologia 39: 507–514 (1974).

8. Amer, S. M. and O. R. Farah, Cytological effects of pesticides. VIII. Effects of the carbamate pesticides "IPC", "Rogor" and "Duphar" on Vicia faba, Cytologia 41: 597–606 (1976).

9. Amer, S. M. and O. R. Farah, Cytological effects of pesticides. IX. Effects of the phosphonothioate insecticide Leptophos on Vicia faba, Cytologia 44: 907–913 (1979).

10. Amer, S. M. and O. R. Farah, Cytological effects of pesticides X. Meiotic effects of "Phosvel", Cytologia 45: 241–245 (1980).

11. Ames, B. N., Identifying environmental chemicals causing mutations and cancer, Science 204: 587–593 (1979).

12. Ashton, F. M., E. G. Cutter and D. Huffstutter, Growth and structural modifications of oats induced by bromacil, Weed Res. 9: 198–204 (1969).

13. Baquar, S. R. and N. R. Kahn, Effect of γ-hexachloro-cyclohexane (HCCH) on the mitotic cells of Pisum sativum L., Rev. Biol. 7: 195–202 (1971).

14. Bandeen, J. D. and V. S. Machado, Weeds resist triazine, Highlights of Agricultural Research in Ontario 1(2): 1–2 (1978).

15. Bielecki, E., The influence of phenyl mercury acetate on mitosis and chromosome structure in Allium cepa, Acta Biol. Crac. Ser. Bot. 17: 119–132 (1974).

16. Bilderback, D. E., Impatiens pollen germination and tube growth as a bioassay for toxic substances, Environ. Health Perspect. 37: 95–103 (1981).

17. Boyle, W. S., Cytogenic effects of Benlate fungicide on Allium cepa and Secale cereale, J. Hered. 64: 49–50 (1973).

18. Bradley, M. V., J. C. Crane, and N. Marei, Some histological effects of 2,4,5-trichlorophenoxyacetic acid applied to mature apricot leaves, Bot. Gaz (Chicago) 129: 231–238 (1968).

19. Canvin, D. T.and G. Friesen, Cytological effects of CDAA and
     IPC on germinating barley and peas, Weeds 7: 153-156 (1959).

20. Chou, T.-S. and D. F. Weber, Visualization of sister-
     chromatid exchanges in maize mitotic chromosomes utilizing 5-
     bromodeoxyuridine. Maize Genet. Coop. Newslet. 54: 88
     (1980).

21. Christianson, M. L. and M. O. Chiscon, Use of haploid plants
     as bioassays for mutagens, Environ. Health Perspect. 27: 77-
     83 (1978).

22. Conrad, S. G. and S. R. Radosevich, Ecological fitness of
     Senecio vulgaris and Amaranthus retroflexus biotypes
     susceptible or resistant to atrazine, J. Appl. Ecol. 16: 171-
     177 (1979).

23. Croker, B. H., Effects of 2,4-dichlorophenoxyacetic acid and
     2,4,5-trichlorophenoxyacetic acid on mitosis in Allium cepa,
     Bot. Gaz. (Chicago) 114: 274-283 (1953).

24. Patino, J. F. Curtis, Efecto de dos pesticidas agricolas en
     el comportamiento mitotico de los cromosomas de hava (Vicia
     faba L.), Chapingo, Neuva Ecoca 16-17: 11-14 (1979).

25. Dävring, L. and M. Sunner, Late prophase and first metaphase
     in female meiosis of Drosophila melanogaster, Hereditas 85:
     25-32 (1977).

26. Derenne, P., Effets morphologiques, physiologiques et
     cytologiques dus `a l'action de l'isoprophylphénylcarbamate
     sur les genres Allium, Vicia et Hordeum, Bull. Inst. Agron.
     Stn. Rech. Gembloux 21: 37-57 (1953).

27. de Serres, F. J., Introduction: Utilization of higher plant
     systems as monitors of environmental mutagens. Environ.
     Health Perspect. 27: 3-6 (1978).

28. Doxey, D., The effect of isopropyl phenyl carbamate on
     mitosis in rye (Secale cereale) and onion (Allium cepa), Ann.
     Bot. 13: 329-335 (1949).

29. Ducruet, J. M. and J. Gasquez, Observation de la fluorescence
     sur feuille entière et mise en évidence de la résistance
     chloroplastique à l'atrazine chez Chenopodium album et Poa
     annua L., Chemosphere 8: 691-696 (1978).

30. DuPraw, E. J., DNA and Chromosomes, Holt, Rinehart and
     Winston, New York (1970).

31. Dustin, P., Microtubules, Springer-Verlag, New York (1978).

32. Dvorak, J., Endopolyploidy in the roots of rye, Secale
     cereale L., Biol. Plant. 10: 112-117 (1968).

33. Ehrenberg, L., A. Gustafsson, A. Levan, and U. v. Wettstein,
     Radiophosphorus, seedling lethality and chromosome
     disturbances, Hereditas 35: 469-489 (1949).

34. Ennis, W. B., Jr., Some cytological effects of o-isopropyl-N-
     phenyl carbamate upon Avena, Am. J. Bot. 35:15-21 (1949).

35. Fernandez-Gomez, M. E., Alteraciones en el ciclo de division
     celular inducidas por los isomeros del HCCH. I. Isomeros
     alfa, beta y gamma, Genét. Ibé. 19: 103-121 (1967).

36. Fernandez-Gomez, M. E., G. Gimenez-Martin, and J. F. Lopez-
     Saez, Alteraciones en el ciclo de division celular inducidas

por los isomeros del HCCH. II. Isomero delta. Posible
mecanismo de accion del HCCH, Genét. Ibé. 19: 123-142 (1967).

37. Fiskesjö, G., Some results from Allium tests with organic
    mercury halogenides, Hereditas 62: 314-322 (1969).

38. Fiskesjö, G. The effect of two organic mercury compounds on
    human leukocytes in vitro, Hereditas 64: 142-146 (1970).

39. Frank, V., Restoration of mitotic and differentiation
    processes in the root apices of Allium cepa treated with
    cyanein and griseofulvin, Biol. Plant. 16: 28-34 (1974).

40. Freeling, M., Maize Adh 1 as a monitor of environmental
    mutagens, Environ. Health Perspect. 27: 91-97 (1978).

41. Gentner, W. A. and L. G. Burk, Gross morphological and
    cytological effects of nitralin on corn roots, Weed Sci. 16:
    259-260 (1968).

42. Gibson, P. B. and G. Beinhart, Abnormal meiosis in clover
    plants treated with organic phosphate pesticides, Bull. South
    Carolina Acad. Sci. 31: 38 (1969).

43. Gopalan, H. N. B. and G. D. E. Njagi, Cytogenetic studies in
    Vicia faba with some insecticides, fungicides and herbicides,
    Environ. Mutagen. 1: 141-142 (1979).

44. Gori, C. and E. Maugini, Effetti citologici et rizogeni di
    alcune sostanze di crescita, Caryologia 7: 404-414 (1955).

45. Grant, W. F., Cytogenetic factors associated with the evo-
    lution of weeds, Taxon 16: 283-293 (1967).

46. Grant, W. F., Pesticides -- subtle promoters of evolution,
    Symp. Biol. Hung. 12: 43-50 (1972).

47. Grant, W. F., Chromosome aberrations in plants as a moni-
    toring system, Environ. Health Perspect. 27: 37-43 (1978).

48. Grant, W. F., The genotoxic effects of 2,4,5-T, Mutat. Res.
    65: 83-119 (1979).

49. Grant, W. F., Chromosome aberration assays in Allium, Mutat.
    Res. In press (1982).

50. Grant, W. F., A. E. Zinov'eva-Stahevitch, and K. D. Zura,
    Plant genetic test systems for the detection of chemical
    mutagens, in: "Short Term Tests for Chemical Carcinogens",
    H. F. Stich and R. H. C. San, eds., Springer-Verlag, New
    York, pp. 200-216 (1981).

51. Gressel, J., Genetic herbicide resistance: Projections on
    appearance in weeds and breeding for it in crops, in: "Plant
    Regulation and World Agriculture", T. K. Scott, ed., Plenum
    Press, New York (1979).

52. Grignac, P., The evolution of resistance to herbicides in
    weedy species, Agro-Ecosystems 4: 377-385 (1978).

53. Grover, I. S. and P. Kaur, personal communication (1981).

54. Grover, I. S. and P. S. Tyagi, Chromosomal aberrations
    induced by pesticides in meiotic cells of barley, Caryologia
    33: 251-260 (1980).

55. Gustafsson, A., The mutation system of the chlorophyll
    apparatus, Lunds Univ. Arsskr. 36: 1-40 (1940).

56. Heath, C. W., Jr., Environmental pollutants and the epide-
    miology of cancer, Environ. Health Perspect. 27: 7-10 (1978).

57. Herichova, A., Study of the effect of isopropyl-N-phenyl-carbamate and isopropyl-N-(3 chlorophenyl) carbamate on chromosome structure and cytokinesis, Acta F. R. N. Univ. Comen. Physiol. Plant. 1: 147–154 (1970).

58. Herichova, A., Cytological study on the effect of isopropyl-N-(3-chlorophenyl) carbamate on the division and ultra-structure of meristematic cells of barley (Hordeum sativum L. Acta F. R. N. Univ. Comen. Physiol. Plant. 6: 85–107 (1973).

59. Hervas, J. P. and G. Gimenez-Martin, Measurements of multi-polar anaphases production by γ-hexachlorocyclohexane in onion root tip cells, Cytobiologie 9: 233–239 (1974).

60. Jagoda, M., Cytological disturbances in Allium cepa L. root-meristems induced by herbicides, Acta Biolog. Cracov. 22: 189–211 (1980).

61. Kabarity A. and A. Nahas, Induction of polypoloidy and C-tumors after treating Allium cepa with the herbicide 'Tref-lan', Biol. Plant. 21: 253–258 (1979).

62. Kar, S., Cytogenetic effects of 2,4-D on Pisum sativum, Proc. Indian Sci. Congr. Bot. 62: 122 (1975).

63. Kihlman, B. A., Root tips of Vicia faba for the study of the induction of chromosomal aberration, Mutat. Res. 31: 401–412.

64. Kihlman, B. A. and S. Sturelid, Effects of caffeine on the frequencies of chromosomal aberrations and sister chromatid exchanges induced by chemical mutagens in root tips of Vicia faba, Hereditas 88: 35–41 (1978).

65. Klásterská, I., A. T. Natarajan and C. Ramel, An inter-pretation of the origin of subchromatid aberrations and chromosome stickiness as a category of chromatid aberrations, Hereditas 83: 153–162 (1976).

66. Klekowski, E. J., Jr., Detection of mutational damage in fern populations: An in situ bioassay for mutagens in aquatic ecosystems, in: "Chemical mutagens. Principles and Methods for their Detection", vol. 5, A. Hollaender and J. F. de Serres, eds., Plenum Press, New York, pp. 79–99 (1978).

67. Kostoff, D., Heteroploidy in Nicotiana tabacum and Solanum melongena caused by fumigation with nicotine sulfate, Bull. Soc. Bot. Bulgar. 4: 87–92. (Biol. Abstr. 8: 10, 1934) (1931).

68. Levan, A., The effect of colchicine on root mitosis in Allium, Hereditas 24: 471–486 (1938).

69. Levan, A., The influence on chromosomes and mitosis of chemicals, as studied by the Allium test. Proc. 8th Int. Congr. Genet., Stockholm, Hereditas, Suppl. 325–337 (1949).

70. Levan, A., Chemically induced chromosome reactions in Allium cepa and Vicia faba, Cold Spring Harbor Symp. Quant. Biol. 16: 233–244 (1951).

71. Liang, G. H. and Y. T. S. Liang, Effects of atrazine on chromosomal behavior in sorghum, Can. J. Genet. Cytol. 14: 423–427 (1972).

72. Lower, W. R., P. S. Rose and V. K. Drobney, In situ mutagenic and other effects associated with lead smelting, Mutat. Res. 54: 83-93 (1978).

73. Ma, T.-H., Tradescantia micronucleus bioassay and pollen tube chromatid aberration test for in situ monitoring and mutagen screening. Environ. Health Perspect. 27: 85-90 (1981).

74. Mann, J. D. and W. B. Storey, Rapid action of carbamate herbicides upon plant cell nuclei, Cytologia 31: 203-207 (1966).

75. Mann, J. D., L. S. Jordan, and B. E. Day, The effects of carbamate herbicides on polymer synthesis, Weeds 13: 63-66 (1965).

76. Mann, S. K., Cytological and genetical effects of dithane fungicides on Allium cepa, Environ. Exp. Bot. 17: 7-12 (1977).

77. Markaryan, D. S., Effect of dieldrin on the mitosis in Crepis capillaris sprouts, Genetika 3: 55-58 (1967).

78. McGill, M, S. Pathak, and T. C. Hsu, Effects of ethidium bromide on mitosis and chromosomes: A possible material basis for chromosome stickiness, Chromosoma 47: 157-167 (1974).

79. McLeish, J., The action of maleic hydrazide in Vicia, Heredity (Suppl.) 6: 125-147 (1953).

80. Mohandas, T and W. F. Grant, Cytogenetic effects of 2,4-D and amitrole in relation to nuclear volume and DNA content in some higher plants, Can. J. Genet. Cytol. 14: 773-783 (1972).

81. Mohandas, T. and W. F. Grant, A relationship between nuclear volume and response to auxin herbicides for some weed species, Can. J. Bot. 51: 1133-1136 (1973).

82. Morrison, J. W., Cytological effects of the herbicide "Avadex", Can. J. Plant. Sci. 42: 78-81 (1962).

83. Mühling, G. N., J. Van't Hof, G. B. Wilson, and B. H. Grigsby, Cytological effects of herbicidal substituted phenols, Weeds, 8: 173-181 (1960).

84. Mulcahy, D. L., Pollen tetrads in the detection of environmental mutagenesis, Environ. Health Perspect. 37: 91-94 (1981).

85. Mulcahy, D. L. and C. M. Johnson, Self-incompatibility systems as bioassays for mutagens, Environ. Health Perspect. 27: 85-90 (1978).

86. Nicoloff, H. and K. Gecheff, Methods of scoring induced chromosome structural changes in barley, Mutat. Res. 34: 233-244 (1976).

87. Nilan, R. A., J. L. Rosichan, P. Arenaz, A. L. Hodgdon, and A. Kleinhofs, Pollen genetic markers for detection of mutagens in the environment, Environ. Health Perspect. 37: 19-25 (1981).

88. Njagi, G. D. E. and H. N. B. Gopalan, Mutagenicity testing of herbicides, fungicides and insecticides. I. Chromosome aberrations in Vicia faba, Cytologia 46: 169-172 (1981).

89. Nygren, A., Cytological studies of the effects of 2,4-D, MCPA, and 2,4,5-T on Allium cepa, Ann. Roy. Agric. Coll. Sweden 16: 723-728 (1949).

90. Paget, G. E. and A. L. Walpole, Some cytological effects of griseofulvin, Nature (London) 182: 1320-1321 (1958).

91. Panda, B. B. and C. B. S. R. Sharma, Organophosphate induced chlorophyll mutations in Hordeum vulgare, Theor. Appl. Genet. 55: 253-255 (1979).

92. Panda, B. B. and C. B. S. R. Sharma, Cytogenetic hazards from agricultural chemicals 3. Monitoring the cytogenetic activity of trichlorfon and dichlorvos in Hordeum vulgare, Mutat. Res. 78: 341-345 (1980).

93. Panda, B. B., B. W. Behera, and C. B. S. R. Sharma, Mutagenic potential of some insecticides and fungicides in plant systems, in: Nuclear techniques in studies of metabolism effects and degradation of pesticides. Proc. Symp. at Sri Venkateswara Univ. Tirupati, Dept. of Atomic Energy, Govt. of India, pp. 190-203 (1978).

94. Plewa, M. J. and E. D. Wagner, Germinal cell mutagenesis in specially designed maize genotypes, Environ. Health Perspect. 37: 61-73 (1981).

95. Prasad, I. and D. Pramer, Genetics effects of ferbam on Aspergillus niger and Allium cepa, Phytophathology 58: 1188-1189 (1968).

96. Price, M. and S. C. Schank, Chromosomal damage and abnormal seedling development in barley induced by chemical treatment with TIBA, maleic hydrazide and foramide, Proc. Soil and Crop Sci. Soc. Fla. 32: 41-46, Agron. Dept. U. Fla. Gainesville (1973).

97. Pusztia, T. and A. Végh, Mutagenic effects of pesticides. I. Acta Bot. Acad. Sci. Hung. 24: 327-342.

98. Rédei, G. P. and G. Acedo, Biochemical mutants in higher plants, in: "Cell Genetics in Higher Plants", D. Dudits, G. L. Farkas and P. Maliga, eds., Akademiai Kaido, Budapest, p. 39 (1976).

99. Ridgway, R. L., J. C. Tinney, J. T. MacGregor and N. J. Starler, Pesticide use in agriculture, Environ. Health Perspect. 27: 103-112 (1978).

100. Sandhu, S. S., Regulation of environmental pollutants: Introductory remarks, Environ. Health Perspect. 1-3 (1981).

101. Sawamura, S., Cytological studies on the effect of herbicides on plant cells in vivo II. Non-hormonic herbicides, Cytologia 30: 325-348 (1965).

102. Schairer, L. A., J. Van't Hof, C. G. Hayes, R. M. Burton, and F. J. de Serres, Exploratory monitoring of air pollutants for mutagenicity activity with the Tradescantia stamen hair system. Environ. Health Perspect. 27: 51-60 (1978).

103. Schairer, L. A., A. H. Sparrow, and N. R. Tempel, Mobile monitoring vehicle designed to assess the mutagenicity of ambient air in high pollution areas, Mutation Res. 53: 111-112 (1978).

104. Scholes, M. E., The effects of aldrin, dieldrin, isodrin,
      endrin and DDT on mitosis in roots of the onion (Allium cepa
      L.), J. Hortic. Sci. 30: 181-187 (1955).
105. Schubert, I., G. Künzel, H. Bretschneider, R. Rieger, and H.
      Nicoloff, Sister chromatid exchanges in barley, Theoret.
      Appl. Genet. 56: 1-4 (1980).
106. Schvartzman, J. B. and P. Hernandez, Sister chromatid ex-
      changes and chromosomal aberrations in 5-aminouracil-syn-
      chronized cells, Theor. Appl. Genet. 57: 221-224 (1980).
107. Schwartz, D., Adh locus in maize for detection of mutagens in
      the environment, Environ. Health Perspect. 37: 75-77 (1981).
108. Sharma, A. K. and S. Gosh, A comparative study on the effects
      of certain chemical agents on chromosomes, Acta Biol. Acad.
      Sci. Hung. 20: 11-21 (1969).
109. Sharma, C. B. S. R., B. Partra, D. S. S. Raju and K. V.
      Murty, Chiasma variation in Hordeum vulgare after exposure to
      herbicides, Mutation Res. 91: 333-336 (1981).
110. Shelby, M. D. and the Environmental Mutagen Information
      Center Staff, "Chemical Mutagenesis in Plants and Mutageni-
      city of Plant Related Compounds", Oak Ridge National Labo-
      ratory, ORNL/EMIC-7 (1976).
111. Singh, B. D., T. B. Singh, R. M. Singh, Y. Singh and J.
      Singh, Effect of insecticides on germination, early growth
      and cytogenetic behavior of barley (Hordeum vulgare), En-
      viron. Exp. Bot. 19: 127-132 (1979).
112. Singh, R. M., A. K. Singh, R. B. Singh, J. Singh, and B. D.
      Singh, Chlorophyll mutations induced by seed treatment with
      certain insecticides in barley (Hordeum vulgare), Indian J.
      Exp. Biol. 18: 1396-1397 (1980).
113. Soliman, A. S. and N. R. Al-Najjar, Cytological effects of
      fungicides. II. Chromosomal aberrations induced by vitavax-
      200 and dithane S-60 in meiotic cells of wheat and two
      related species, Cytologia 45: 169-175 (1980).
114. Spasojević, V., Effect of fungicide Benlate on the mitosis of
      maize, Arch. Poljopr. Nanke 27 (100): 13-21 (1974).
115. Spasojević, V., Cytogenetical effect of Tuberite on Zea
      mays, Arkiv. Poljopr. Nanke 28: 119-125 (1975).
116. Ramulu, K. Sree, H. Schibilla, and P. Dijkhuis, Self-incom-
      patibility system of Oenothera organesis for the detection of
      genetic effects at low radiation doses, Environ. Health
      Perspect. 37: 43-51 (1981).
117. Sterrett, R. B. and T. A. Fretz, Asulam-induced mitotic
      irregularities in onion root-tips, HortScience 10: 161-162
      (1975).
118. Storey, W. B., L. S. Jordan and J. D. Mann, Carbamate her-
      bicides -- new tools for cytological studies, Calif. Agric.
      22(8): 12-13 (1968).
119. Suneson, C. A. and L. G. Jones, Herbicides may produce
      instability, Agron. J. 52: 120-121 (1960).

120. Suneson, C. A., H. C. Murphy, and F. C. Petr, Fostering the recombination of oats with a mutagen, Crop Sci. 5: 176 (1965).

121. Tomkins, D. J. and W. F. Grant, Monitoring natural vegetation for herbicide-induced chromosomal aberrations. Mutat. Res. 36: 73-84 (1976).

122. Unrau, J., Cytogenetic effects of 2,4-D on cereals, Annu. Rep. Can. Seed Growers' Assoc. 1953-1954: 37-39 (1954).

123. Unrau, J. and E. N. Larter, Cytogenetical reponse of cereals to 2,4-D. I. A study of meiosis of plants treated at various stages of growth, Can. J. Bot. 30: 22-27 (1952).

124. Vaarama, A., Experimental studies on the influence of DDT pesticide upon plant mitosis, Hereditas 33: 191-219 (1947).

125. Vig, B. K., Somatic mosaicism in plants with special reference to somatic crossing over. Environ. Health Perspect. 27: 27-36 (1978)

126. Warwick, S. I., V. Souza Machado, P. B. Marriage, and J. D. Bandeen, Resistance of Chenopodium strictum Roth (late-flowering goosefoot) to atrazine, Can. J. Plant Sci. 59: 269-270 (1979).

127. Wuu, K. D. and W. F. Grant, Morphological and somatic chromosomal aberrations induced by pesticides in barley (Hordeum vulgare), Can. J. Genet. Cytol. 8: 481-501 (1966).

128. Wuu, K. D. and W. F. Grant, Induced abnormal meiotic behavior in a barley plant (Hordeum vulgare L.) with the herbicide Lorox, Phyton, 23: 63-67 (1966).

129. Wuu, K. D. and W. F. Grant, Chromosomal aberrations induced by pesticides in meiotic cells of barley, Cytologia 32: 31-41 (1967).

130. Wuu, K. D. and W. F. Grant, Chromosomal aberrations induced in somatic cells of Vicia faba by pesticides, Nucleus 10: 37-46 (1967).

131. Yakar, N., Mitotic disturbances caused by chloranil, Am. J. Bot. 39: 540-546 (1952).

DISCUSSION

Q. SHAWKY: Don't you think that reading slides for such alterations as chromosome stickiness and faint pigmentation is somewhat subjective, as they are quantitative in nature and they might be slight or intensive? Are there any standard parameters for readings? Or is it only a matter of experience, that varies from one person to another and one laboratory to another?

A. GRANT: Experience plays a major role in all cytological studies and the types of aberrations you mention are subjective and depend on the experience of the investigator. While the degree of these abnormalities is subjective, the presence or absence of the effect is not

except when the effect is very slight. However, normally
such aberrations would merely be noted and qualitative
measurements, such as gaps, exchanges, bridges, fragments,
micronuclei, etc., would be recorded in a cytological
evaluation. A detailed classification system has been
proposed by Savage (J. Med. Genet. 12:103, 1975) and forms
for scoring aberrations are given by Ma in his paper
"Tradescantia Cytogenetic Tests for Environmental Mutagens"
(Mutation Res., in press).

Q.   ZWEIG: Do you believe that plant mutation due to
       environmental mutagens poses an environmental hazard?

A.   GRANT: It has been shown that pesticides will (1) eliminate
       certain species as a result of their extreme susceptibility,
       (2) produce resistant plants as well as insects, (3) induce
       mutations of a nature sufficient for taxonomic recognition
       and (4) affect non-target organisms such as insect
       pollinators depending on a particular species (Grant, Symp.
       Biol. Hung. 12:43-50, 1972). Thus, they are disruptive to
       the environment.

CYTOGENETIC STUDIES IN ANIMALS

R. Julian Preston

Biology Division
Oak Ridge National Laboratory
Oak Ridge, Tennessee 37830

INTRODUCTION

It is clearly impossible to provide a detailed discussion of all the possible areas of research encompassed by the title of this presentation. The intention is to provide some indication of the types of cytogenetic assays that can be performed in order to indicate the clastogenic potential of an agent, whether the data obtained can reasonably be used to estimate the potential genetic or carcinogenic risk to man, and the possible ways in which results can be misinterpreted or over-interpreted.

Specific guidelines for conducting cytogenetic assays will not be presented, because the information is available in the literature. The reports that best reflect the views presented here are those produced by the Committee on Mutagenicity of Chemicals in Food, Consumer Products and the Environment (6) and the U. S. Environmental Protection Agency Gene-Tox Committee (12).

Discussion of Available Cytogenetic Assays

Information on chromosomal abnormalities can be and has been obtained from many different cell types from a wide variety of species. Essentially, studies can be conducted on any cell population that is cycling or that can be induced to enter the cell cycle. This, of course, means that it is possible to study cells treated both in vivo and in vitro. The cell types most commonly used for completely in vivo studies are the cycling cell populations of the bone marrow and testis, and the population of cells in the liver that can be induced to divide by partial hepatectomy. The lymphocyte has to be stimulated to enter the cell

cycle, and so the culturing has to be performed in vitro, following
treatments either in vivo or in vitro. A wide variety of in vitro
cell cultures are also available, and can be established from many
different cell types from any appropriate species. There are
additional assay systems that, because of technical complications,
are used less freqently. These include oocytes, analysed at
metaphase I or II, and embryos analysed either at the first
cleavage division or at subsequent cleavage divisions.

There are clearly many assay systems available to the
cytogeneticist, and the question is which one is the most
appropriate in a specific situation? Such a choice is to a large
extent determined by the particular information that is required.
Three general categories are discussed.

Determination of Clastogenicity. If the assay is to be used
simply to determine whether or not a specific agent is clastogenic,
then clearly the most rapid and economical one should be
utilized. The choice would be to use an in vitro cell culture or
an in vivo bone marrow assay. There are advantages to choosing the
in vivo assay even in this case. In particular, if it has been
indicated that the agent being studied requires metabolic
activation to an active metabolite or is metabolically inactivated,
then it is appropriate to use the in vivo assay when the activation
or inactivation is provided by the animal itself. It is
appreciated that it is possible to add S-9 microsomal fractions of
induced livers to provide in vitro metabolic activation, but this
is a complicating factor, particularly with lymphocytes, and it
seems sensible to avoid it if at all possible.

Assessment of a Potential Genetic Risk. If the problem is
whether or not an agent presents a genetic hazard, then it is
appropriate to study the cytogenetic effects in germ cells. An
analysis of differentiating spermatogonia will determine either the
ability of an agent to reach the testis and/or whether or not the
agent is clastogenetic. However, it is generally not possible when
no induced aberrations are observed to determine whether the
chemical fails to reach the germ cells or that it is non-
clastogenic. The only way to distinguish these is to make direct
measurements of the presence of the agent in the testis, or analyze
germ cells for specific DNA adducts (13). In order to determine
the ability of an agent to reach the female germ cells it is
necessary to treat the female animal, but analyze the first
cleavage division embryos (1). The reasons for this will become
apparent from the later discussion, but suffice it to say that the
first DNA replication phase after treatment will take place after
fertilization, during the first cleavage cycle. Again here, the
possible reasons for a negative result can only be distinguished by
direct measurements of the chemical or specific DNA adducts in
oocytes.

Once it has been established that an agent reaches the germ cells and produces a measurable frequency of chromosome aberrations, several assays can be utilized to determine whether or not aberrations can be recovered in the offspring or treated animals, which is the indication of a genetic risk.

The heritable translocation test can be used to detect reciprocal translocations in the spermatocytes of F_1 individuals, when either the male of female parent is treated. Cytogenetic analysis can be carried out on all F_1 male progeny, or on those F_1 males that are suspected translocation heterozygotes from the fact that they show semi-sterility when mated to normal females (7). The length of time between treatment and mating can be varied, such that the sensitivity of germ cells in the different stages of maturation can be analyzed. It is also important to analyze sterile animals for the presence of reciprocal translocations. This can be performed on spermatocytes, if the sterility does not result in a lack of this stage, or on a somatic cell type, such as peripheral lymphocytes, when meiotic cells are not available. It is also important to note that in some F_1 animals, categorized as semi-sterile, a translocation is not observed, usually as a result of the break points being close to the centromere or the ends of the chromosomes. In such cases, it is also necessary to study somatic cells, utilizing chromosome banding techniques, to determine whether or not the animal is a translocation heterozygote. Again it should be emphasized that not all translocations can be detected even with banding.

If an analysis of all induced chromosome aberration types is required then first cleavage embryos can be studied, following treatment of either male or female parent. Again, by varying the interval between treatment and mating, the sensitivity of the different germ cell stages can be assessed. It is also possible from such studies to estimate the dominant lethality from a particular treatment, since it appears that all, or at least the vast majority of dominant lethals are the result of chromosome aberrations (1, 5, 8, 10).

An assessment of the frequency of aberrations transmitted through several cell division (as opposed to the induced frequency) can be obtained by studying later embryo divisions. However such an assay requires chromosome banding techniques in order for the aberrations to be ascertained, and even then with well less that 100% efficiency.

Thus in general terms it is possible to assay cytogenetic damage directly in germ cells, and also to determine the proportion that is transmitted to the F_1. It is also clear that the only animals readily usable with these types of studies, specifically those involving F_1 analysis, are those that are litter-bearing.

Estimation of a Genetic Risk to Man. If an agent has been
shown to induce chromosome aberrations in germ cells and some
proportion of these can be recovered in the F_1, it is reasonable to
assume that it presents a potential genetic hazard. Therefore, the
question to be asked now is, whether or not the particular agent
represents a genetic hazard to man, and, if· so, is it possible to
estimate this?

It is, of course, not possible to study the induction of
chromosome aberrations in human germ cells, and so an indirect
approach has to be taken. By far the most readily available human
cell type for studies is the peripheral lymphocyte, and so it is
used for comparisons of the sensitivity to aberration induction
between humans and laboratory animals. The approach is to
establish a relationship between the frequencies of aberrations
induced in human lymphocytes in vitro and those in the lymphocytes
of a laboratory animal in vitro and in vivo. It is appreciated
that human populations occupationally or environmentally exposed
can be analyzed, but, with the exception of radiation, information
on exposure is inadequate.

Correlations can then be established between the frequency of
specific aberration types induced in the lymphocytes of laboratory
animals with their frequency induced in different germ cell stages,
or recovered in the F_1. The assumption is made, with rather little
specific evidence, that a similar relationship exists in man. Thus
an estimate can be made of the frequency of specific aberration
types in human germ cells, or that recovered in the F_1, from the
frequency observed in the peripheral lymphocytes. This approach
has been taken in the case of radiation (2), and has in fact been
confirmed to some extent by direct measurements of the frequency of
radiation-induced reciprocal translocations in human spermatocytes
(3). It is considerably more difficult to conduct these
experiments with chemical agents, and to date no reliable estimate
is available for the genetic risk to man from any chemical.

This experimental approach should only be contemplated in
rather specific cases. The anticipated or known exposed population
would need to be large, and the agent had to be established as
being clearly clastogenic, and capable of reaching the germ
cells. In addition, considerable caution should be taken in
interpreting the data, as will become apparent from the discussion
in the following sections.

Factors Affecting the Interpretation of Data from Cytogenetic
Assays

There are many factors that can influence the observed
chromosome aberration frequencies and types of aberrations, some of
which can be controlled and others that cannot, but that have to be
considered when interpreting the results.

Cytogenetic assays are performed with cycling cell populations, either normally cycling ones, or ones that are induced to enter division before or after treatment with a particular agent. This means that the exposed population will either contain cells in all stages of the cell cycle, or, in the case of populations that are induced to cycle, the treated population will probably be synchronous, but will pass through the cell cycle between treatment and observation. There are two specific consequences of this.

Analysis at the First or Subsequent Divisions after Treatment. There are a few agents (e.g. X-rays, streptonigrin and bleomycin) that can induce significant frequencies of aberrations in all stages of the cell cycle -- chromosome-type aberrations in G_1 and chromatid-type in S and G_2. However, the majority of clastogenic chemicals induce only chromatid-type aberrations and then only in cells that pass through the S phase between treatment and observation. Thus in order to obtain a measure of the induced aberration frequency cells have to be analyzed at their first post-treatment metaphase. Failure to do this will result in a frequency less than the induced frequency, since many of the aberrations are cell lethal events, either because of the loss of genetic material in the form of acentric fragments at mitosis, or because of a mechanical interference with division as the result of bridge formation. Furthermore, the aberration type seen in surviving cells at the 2nd mitosis after treatment will be a derived chromosome-type, as the result of segregation and replication of the induced chromatid-type aberration.

In some instances it is not possible to analyze cells at their first post-treatment metaphase. These include chronic exposures, exposures to stem cells when the differentiated cell type (e. g. spermatocyte or lymphocyte) is that which is analyzed, or developing embryos when the male or female parent is treated. The frequency of aberrations observed will be the recovered frequency as opposed to the induced frequency. If the induced aberration-type, the probability of transmission through several cell divisions, and the expected observed aberration types are taken into consideration then the results obtained can be correctly interpreted. Two types of study will exemplify this.

When mice are treated with chemicals that are known to induce chromosome aberrations in differentiating spermatogonia, no induced aberrations, specifically non-lethal reciprocal translocations, are observed in spermatocytes that are derived from treated spermatogonial stem cells (9, 12). This is not due to the fact that the spermatogonial stem cell is insensitive to the induction of translocations, but rather that the majority of such aberrations are lost from the analyzed population between treatment and observation. As mentioned above the aberrations induced will be of

the chromatid-type. The majority of these aberrations are cell
lethal, and thus will not be observed in cells that have passed
through several cell divisions, as is the case for spermatogonial
stem cells progressing to spermatocytes. The symmetrical chromatid
translocations induced will have a probability of 0.25 of being
recovered as a balanced translocation as a result of segregation at
the first cell division after treatment. Also the translocation
will be lost from the analyzed spermatocyte population if it is
present in a cell that also contains a cell-lethal aberration
type. The probability of observing chromosome aberrations in
spermatocytes following spermatogonial stem cell treatment will be
low, particularly at the high doses normally employed where the
probability of inducing translocations is high, but so also is the
probability of inducing other lethal aberration types in the same
cell. The observed result is exactly what would be predicted if
the simple facts of aberration segregation and cell lethality are
taken into account.

The second example of aberration analysis at post-treatment
divisions other than the first is for chronic or sub-acute
exposures. The intention in such studies is to treat cells for
several cell cycles, usually with low doses of the agent. However,
in the vast majority of reported studies of this type the
aberration types recorded are of the chromatid-type. These
aberrations can only have been induced during the last cell cycle
before analysis, since those aberrations induced in earlier cell
cycles of the chronic exposure, albeit induced as chromatid-type
aberrations, will have been converted into derived chromosome-type
aberrations following division and replication. Furthermore, the
expected frequency of observed chromatid-type aberrations will be
low since the exposure during only one cell cycle will be low. The
derived chromosome-type aberrations have to be analyzed by banding
techniques, and their frequency will be low, since many aberrations
are lost from the analyzed population as a result of their being
cell lethal. Thus data that report only chromatid-type aberrations
following chronic or sub-acute exposures should be considered with
caution or disregard.

These considerations also apply to the other cytogenetic
assays discussed, and their influence on the interpretation of data
can be predicted in a similar way.

Analysis of Cells Treated in Different Cell Cycle Stages. As
already mentioned the majority of chemical agents only produce a
significant frequency of aberrations when the treated population
passes through the S phase between treatment and observation, and
that chromatid aberrations are the type induced. The probability
of producing aberrations, therefore, will be related to the amount
of the specific DNA damage that is converted into aberrations that
is present at the time of replication or after replication. It is

not clear whether replication itself or a post-replication event leads to the formation of aberrations. The amount of damage remaining in the DNA at the time of replication will be influenced by several factors: (i) the amount of the initial DNA damage and the rate of its repair; a discussion of which is outside the scope of this paper, but has been considered in another recent paper (11), (ii) the stage of the cell cycle in which the cells are at the time of treatment, and (iii) the relative lengths of the different stages of the cell cycle. A consideration of the assays discussed in the section on "Discussion of Available Cytogenetic Assays" in these terms will demonstrate this.

Bone marrow cells are fairly rapidly cycling, and so, unless the damage converted into aberrations is repaired rapidly, cells in all stages of the cell cycle would be expected to have damage remaining at replication, and thus a finite probability of containing chromatid aberrations. Of course cells close to or in the S phase will have the greatest probability, but all cells have the potential of contributing to the overall category of aberrant cells. The bone marrow cells will be relatively sensitive to aberration induction.

In contrast, spermatogonial stem cells, often considered to be the germ cell at risk from chronic exposures, are very slowly cycling, largely because of a long G_1. This will mean that the majority of treated cells will be in G_1 or, for G_2 cells, will pass through the long G_1 before entering the S phase when aberrations will be produced. The time available for repair before replication for most cells will be long, and the probability of producing an aberration will be low. The probability of aberration production in or close to the S phase would be expected to be the same as for bone marrow cells. However, the proportion of cells contributing to the aberrant cell class will be much lower than for bone marrow cells, and the spermatogonial stem cell population will be rather insensitive to aberration induction, when compared to bone marrow cells.

Peripheral lymphocytes represent a third category of cell cycle, since they are non-cycling cells, in the G_0 or G_1 phase of the cycle. Damage to the DNA of G_0 lymphocytes produced by most chemicals, is probably repaired in the absence of mitogenic stimulation, albeit slowly. If the lymphocytes are stimulated to enter the cell cycle by a mitogen, such as phytohemagglutinin, they still have a long G_1 stage, so that much of the induced damage can be repaired before replication. The probability of producing chromatid aberrations is low, and thus the peripheral lymphocyte is a relatively insensitive cell to the induction of aberrations by chemicals. Of course, it is sensitive to the induction of aberrations by radiation, because aberrations can be induced in all stages of the cycle, including G_0 and G_1, and so the time

relationship between treatment and the S phase is not influential
upon the aberration frequency. This consideration explains why
few, if any, aberrations are induced in G_0 lymphocytes by most
chemical agents, and also why aberrations are not observed in the
lymphocytes of individuals treated with high doses of
chemotherapeutic agents, when some time lapses between the
cessation of treatment and sampling (12).

Similar arguments can be applied to all the assays discussed
in section A, and need to be taken into account when considering
the results obtained with a single assay, or when comparing the
relative sensitivities of two or more assays. There are also other
factors that can influence the interpretation of results on
aberration frequencies, but the ones discussed here are especially
important, because they are essentially not controllable by
experimental design, but rather need to be considered in the design
of experiments.

Cytogenetic Assays, and the Estimation of Mutagenic or Carcinogenic Risk to Man

This section will be short for several valid reasons. The
amount of available data is small, and it is all too common to
over-interpret data in order to establish relevance to man.

It is possible, as discussed earlier in the section of
"Estimation of a Genetic Risk to Man" to make some estimate of the
genetic risk to man by extrapolation from germ cell studies in
laboratory animals, using the analysis of human and animal
lymphocytes as the common cell type by which relative sensitivities
can be obtained. It is not legitimate to draw conclusions about
the potential genetic hazard of a particular agent simply from the
analysis of somatic cells. This is especially applicable to human
population monitoring studies, where the presence of aberrations in
lymphocytes is perhaps an indicator of a possible genetic hazard,
not necessarily to the individual(s) having elevated aberration
frequencies, but rather to the exposed population. However, the
magnitude of the risk cannot be ascertained from such studies,
because of the differences in cell cycle kinetics of lymphocytes
and specific germ cell stages, the different cell selection
processes in somatic and germ cells, the possibility that DNA
repair kinetics are different in the different cell types, and
because of probable differences in the amount of the initial DNA
damage, due to different doses to the peripheral blood and testis
or ovary.

The correlation between mutagenicity and carcinogenicity has
been discussed so much that little need be added here. The
cytogenetic assays, taken as a whole, show about a 70%
effectiveness at detecting carcinogens as clastogens and non-

carcinogens as non-clastogens. This value is about the same as
that for most other assays (4). The percentage detection
efficiency will, of course, be dependent upon the accuracy of
classification of agents as carcinogens and non-carcinogens. It is
usual, however, to assume infallibility to this classification.

It is worth restating here that an increase in chromosome
aberration frequency in the peripheral lymphocytes of exposed or
possibly exposed individuals is not a predictor of an increased
risk of cancer in those individuals. It can be argued that it
might indicate an increased cancer risk in the exposed population
as a whole, and not just to those individuals with an elevated
aberration frequency. It is further possible that chromosome
aberrations themselves are the initial event, or one of the initial
events leading to some tumors, and that the analysis of chromosome
aberrations in specific cell types might be a direct way of
assessing tumor risk, rather than a correlative one. However, this
has clearly not been established at this time, and so any further
discussion would fall into the category of over-interpretation.

Conclusion

In conclusion, cytogenetic assays can be utilized to predict
the genetic risk of chemical agents to man, but only if they are
performed correctly and also only if germ cell studies, and
analysis of F_1 individuals, are included.

The intent of this paper has not been to provide specific
details on how to conduct cytogenetic assays, since these are
already available, but rather to provide information that might aid
in the choice of the right assay to answer the question posed, and
also to indicate how a more detailed understanding of the
particular assay will help in the interpretation of results, and
hopefully how to avoid over-interpretation or mis-interpretation.

ACKNOWLEDGEMENT

Research sponsored by the Office of Health and Environmental
Research, U.S. Department of Energy, under contract W-7405-eng-26
with the Union Carbide Corporation.

REFERENCES

1. Brewen, J. G., H. S. Payne, K. P. Jones, and R. J. Preston,
    1975, Studies on chemically induced dominant lethality. The
    cytogenetic basis of MMS-induced dominant lethality in post-
    meiotic male germ cells, Mutation Res. 33: 239.
2. Brewen, J. G. and R. J. Preston, 1974, Cytogenetic effects of
    environmental mutagens in mammalian cells and the
    extrapolation to man, Mutation Res. 26: 297.

3. Brewen, J. G., R. J. Preston, and N. Gengozian, 1975, Analysis of X-ray-induced chromosomal translocations in human and marmoset spermatogonial stem cells, Nature, 253: 468.
4. Brookes, P. and F. J. de Serres, in: "Progress in Mutation Research. Vol I." F. J. de Serres and J. Ashby, eds. Elsevier/North Holland, Amsterdam, pp. 96-111 (1981).
5. Burki, K. and W. Sheridan, 1978, Expression of TEM-induced damage to post-meiotic stages of spermatogenesis of the mouse during early embryogenesis II. Cytological investigations, Mutation Res., 52: 107.
6. Committee on Mutagenicity of Chemicals in Food, Consumer Products and the Environment," Guidelines for the Testing of Chemicals for Mutagenicity," H. M. S. O., London (1981).
7. Generoso, W. M., J. B. Bishop, D. G. Gosslee, G. W. Newell, C-J. Sheu, and E. von Halle, 1980, Heritable translocation tests in mice, Mutation Res., 76: 191.
8. Generoso, W. M., R. J. Preston, and J. G. Brewen, 1975, 6-mercaptopurine, an inducer of cytogenetic and dominant-lethal effects in premeiotic and early meiotic germ cells of male mice, Mutation Res., 28: 437.
9. Leonard, A., G. DeKnudt, and G. Linden, 1971, Failure to detect meiotic chromosome rearrangements in male mice given chemical mutagens, Mutation Res., 13: 89.
10. Matter, B. E. and I. Jaeger, 1975, Premature chromosome condensation, Structural chromosome aberrations, and micronuclei in early embryos after treatment of paternal post-meiotic germ cells with triethylenemelamine: Possible mechanisms for chemically-induced dominant-lethal mutations, Mutation Res., 33: 251.
11. Preston, R. J. and P. C. Gooch, 1981, The induction of chromosome-type aberrations in G_1 by methyl methanesulfonate and 4-nitroquinoline-N-oxide, and the non-requirement of an S-phase for their production, Mutation Res., 83: 395.
12. Preston, R. J., W. W. Au, M. A. Bender, J. G. Brewen, A. V. Carrano, J. A. Heddle, A. F. McFee, S. Wolff, and J. S. Wassom, In vivo and in vitro cytogenetic assays: A report of the "Gene-Tox" program, Mutation Res. IN PRESS
13. Sega, G. A. and J. G. Owens, 1978, Ethylation of DNA and protamine by ethyl methanesulfonate in the germ cells of male mice and the relevancy of these molecular targets to the induction of dominant-lethal, Mutation Res., 52: 87.

DETECTION AND EVALUTAION OF POTENTIAL HAZARDS TO HUMAN HEALTH
(SECOND SESSION)

CHAIRMAN'S COMMENTS

Keith F. Killam, Jr.

Department of Pharmacology
School of Medicine
University of California
Davis, California 95616

Earlier in the Symposium the perspectives on agricultural imperatives were presented. The world population continues to increase. The food providers and associated technology must respond. Included in the technology is the use of chemical substances to modify the agricultural environment. Under discussion are the implications for human, animal and plant welfare with the use of substances to curtail unwanted competing plant growth and to control pests of a wide variety. In order to move beyond empiricism or to capitalize on the fruits of empiricism, attempts are made to explain the mechanisms of the biological effects induced by the chemicals. Continuing studies relating chemical structure to activity - wanted or unwanted - allow the design of second, third and succeeding generations of chemicals to maximize effectiveness against specific targets while sparing or reducing the consequences to the user or producer populations.

The papers this afternoon examine on the one hand some biological mechanisms and indicators to help define the boundaries for consideration and, on the other hand, the use of toxicological data in a decision-making model. Dr. R. B. Setlow examines the types of damage to DNA, the multiplicity of sites of occurrence of damage and the biological implications of the damage. Included would be the nature of the repair process(es). He relates the ultimate apparent resistance to damage to the effectivenss of the repair processes. Dr. J. Albertini and his coworkers report exciting new methodologies to monitor the occurrence of mutagenesis using both maternal and fetal blood samples. The profile of

389

lymphocytes appears to reflect the incidence of mutagenesis but not causitive factors or mechanisms. Dr. P. J. Gehring and his colleagues review laboratory tests evaluating carcinogenesis based upon genetic and/or non-genetic mechanisms of action. He illustrates the decision-making process for classification of substances and defining limits of exposure safety by comparing the activity of dimethylnitrosamine, chloroform, sodium orthophenyl-phenol and perchloroethylene.

The papers should provide further definition of the boundary conditions that need attention in developing chemicals needed to help realize the agricultural imperative of continued increase of food production.

DOSE RESPONSE RELATIONS: THE EFFECTS OF DNA REPAIR

R. B. Setlow

Biology Department
Brookhaven National Laboratory
Upton, New York 11973

INTRODUCTION

Environmental agents that react with DNA, either directly or indirectly by conversion to reactive intermediates, are potentially harmful to people. The biological effects of concern are cell killing, mutation, and transformation. The magnitude of the potential danger to humans from changes in their DNA depends upon the types of changes made and their lifetimes relative to the times of important cellular processes, such as replication, transcription, and cell division. It should be obvious that we cannot wait for epidemiological data to assess the hazards or the safety of agents that affect DNA. If we did, the harm would have been done and perpetuated before any corrective action could be taken.

We need to know three things about alterations to DNA: 1) what types of damage are made; 2) how many damages are made, and 3) what are the biological effects of individual types of damage (1). The effects of these three quantities are not necessarily independent of one another. If we have identified various types of damage, it would be possible to estimate the numbers of individual types of damage as a function of exposure of cells or an organism to a presumptive deleterious agent. Such determinations require sensitive methods to detect products in DNA, and are made, at present, by using radioactive compounds for animal experiments but they may be extendable to humans by the use of sensitive radio-immunoassays for known products (2,3). Thus, it is probable that we shall be able to construct, at the molecular level, dosimetry scales for humans exposed to environmental agents. The reason it is important to know the various types of damage, and the hazards

from each, is that the major product is not necessarily one with a
major biological importance. For example, there are many
alkylation products in DNA treated with alkylating agents (4). A
relatively minor product is O^6alkylguanine. This product seems to
be the most important for mutation and carcinogenesis (4). On the
other hand, for the best studied environmental carcinogen,
ultraviolet radiation (UV), the major products are pyrimidine
dimers and these products are mutagenic and tumorigenic (5).
Prediction of the number of damages to DNA as a function of
exposure is complicated by two factors — activation and repair.
Many agents need activation and the primary activating tissue is
the liver. Hence, the number of products may vary greatly from
tissue to tissue and depend on the administered dose (6).
Moreover, the repair of damaged DNA, although in many instances a
continuous process, may be inducible, in part, as it seems to be
for the removal of O^6methylguanine, (7,8) and the magnitude of DNA
repair may vary from tissue to tissue as it does for alkylating
agents (9). These complications mean that it is not possible, a
priori, to predict the shape of the curve that relates magnitude of
damage to DNA and exposure. We expect that the shape of such
curves may depend upon the magnitude of DNA repair and also on the
concentration of the agent applied as is indicated in Figure 1.
Since the level of adducts, and hence the biological effects
observed, most probably depend on both concentration and time and
not on the product of the two, the time weighted average of

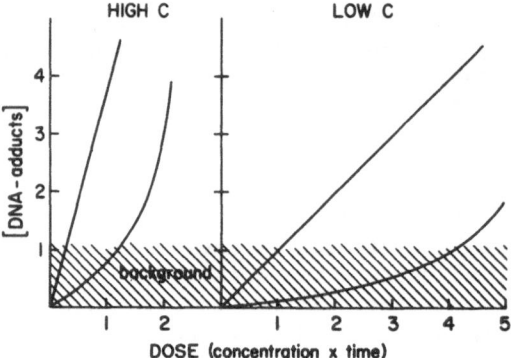

Fig. 1.   Possible dose response curves relating DNA adducts to the
          product of concentration and time. The figure is meant to
          illustrate different possible types of dose curves, that
          the curves depend on more than just concentration
          multiplied by time, and that the curves may also be
          functions of concentration. The hatched area labeled
          background could represent DNA adducts that arise from
          some endogenous metabolic reaction.

concentration is not an appropriate measure to use. The
appropriate measure would weight the concentration proportionately
to the biological effect resulting from a given level of DNA
adducts for known times.

NUCLEOTIDE EXCISION

     One of the better known, but still incompletely understood,
repair systems involves the removal of bulky lesions from DNA by an
attack on the polynucleotide strands. Pyrimidine dimers are the
prototype lesion and have been studied extensively in both prokaryotic and eukaryotic systems (10). UV damage is repaired by
such systems and in mammalian cells is characterized by the fact
that the repair patches are long — approximately 100 nucleotides
— and that individuals with the genetic, sun sensitive, cancer
prone disease xeroderma pigmentosum (XP) are defective in removing
UV damage from their DNA (11). XP cells are also defective in
removing other bulky types of lesions such as those arising from

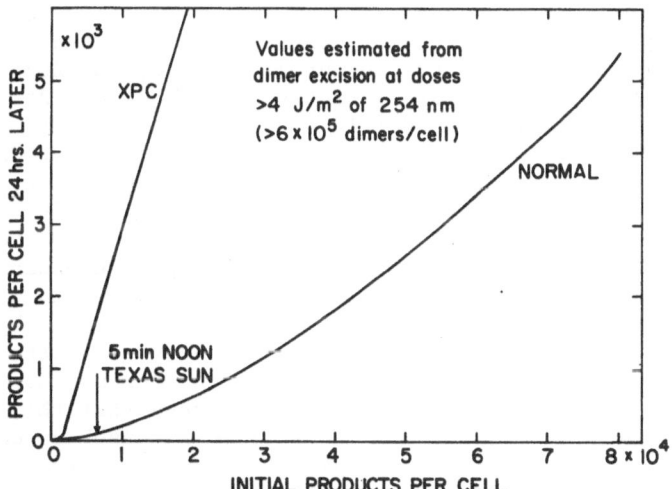

Fig. 2. Estimated relations between the numbers of pyrimidine
         dimers per cell 24 hours after exposure and the initial
         numbers of pyrimidine dimers per cell for normal and XP
         group C fibroblasts (13). Note that for normal cells the
         great majority of the initial numbers of products per cell
         are removed in 24 hours, whereas for the XP cells the
         great majority remain. The estimated numbers from an
         exposure to 5 minutes of Texas sun are obtained from Harm
         (14).

aflatoxin and benzo(a)pyrene (11,12). An XP individual in sunlight
accumulates over a period of time much more damage because of his
low repair capability than does a normal individual. The disease
does not confer an absolute deficiency in repair but there is a
rough correlation between the severity of the disease and the magnitude of the repair defect. Figure 2 shows estimates of the
amount of damage remaining in cellular DNA as a function of the
initial damage resulting from one acute dose. Note that most of
the doses used in laboratory experiments are appreciably greater
than an individual would receive in the outside world, that large
numbers of initial products are tolerated by normal individuals,
and that the shapes of the curves in Figure 2 depend upon repair
capability. The doses normally encountered by normal humans are
far from saturating their repair system (13), but the doses that
might be encountered by XP individuals who go out into the sun
probably do tend to saturate their repair system.

      The sunlight induced cancer incidence in XP individuals is
between 10^3 and 10^4-fold greater than in normal individuals (15).
Epidemiological data on the US population indicate that the incidence of nonmelanoma skin cancer is an exponential function of the
annual UV flux at ground level (16). The existence of such an
exponential relation means that, on the average, there is no
threshold for UV induced nonmelanoma skin cancer. One may use the
observed exponential relationship to estimate that the effective
number of UV induced products in normal skin is 7 to 20-fold less
than in XP skin (15). Repair effectively reduces the dose to
normal individuals by 7 to 20-fold. This change in dose is
accompanied by a 10^3-10^4 decrease in cancer incidence. Hence, it
is reasonable to suppose that small changes in repair capability
might make significant alterations to the susceptibility of
"normal" people to sunlight induced skin cancer. There have been
relatively few experiments on the range of repair capacities of
normal individuals. Data from two of these experiments are in
Table 1 which shows excision repair capability measured by
unscheduled DNA synthesis in peripheral leukocytes. Although a one
to one correlation has not been made between such a measure of
repair and others in other tissues, it is known that the
lymphocytes of XP individuals are defective in unscheduled DNA
synthesis (5,12). The variation among presumably normal
individuals is large and indicates that lifestyle factors--heroin
addiction, for example--may affect DNA nucleotide excision
repair. If the variances shown in Table 1 were to be found in
other tissues as well, they would have important implications for
estimating the susceptibility of populations to sunlight induced
skin cancer.

Table 1. Variations among individuals in unscheduled DNA synthesis
          measured in their leukocytes exposed to UV

Number and Type	Standard Deviation (%)	Reference
40 normal	26	18
90 normal	44	17
38 heroin addicts[*]	100	17

[*]Average unscheduled DNA synthesis was 0.3 of normal.

BASE EXCISION

This repair system is characterized by no initial attack on
the polynucleotide backbone and by the appearance of only small
repair patches (10,11,19)--patches that may represent, as indicated
in Figure 3, an average among patch sizes of 0, 1, and small. The
repair by dealkylation--patch size 0--has been found in E. coli,
mouse, rat, and human cells (20-23). In these systems repair is
stoichiometric, an alkyl group is transferred from 0^6alkylguanine
to the cysteine residue of a protein, and in the process the protein is used up and is not available for subsequent reactions.
Human cells able to accomplish repair of methylation damage are
called Mer^+ and are much more resistant to the action of alkylating
agents than are Mer^- because they can repair 0^6methylguanine (24)
(see Figure 4). Moreover, in Mer^- cells there is a greater
increase in sister chromatid exchanges as a result of treatment
with methylating agents (24). The distribution of demethylating
activity has been measured in extracts of human lymphocytes (23)
and, as for UV repair, shows a wide distribution. For unstimulated
lymphocytes there is a bimodal distribution and for lymphocytes
stimulated to divide there is one broad peak of activity that is at
an approximately 3 times higher level than for unstimulated ones.
If data on other tissues mimic those for lymphocytes, at least as
far as relative values are concerned, one would conclude that there
is a wide variation in repair capacity among the normal
population. There is also a wide variation among individuals in
the ability of their tissues to activate certain carcinogens, such
as the polycyclic aromatic hydrocarbons (25).

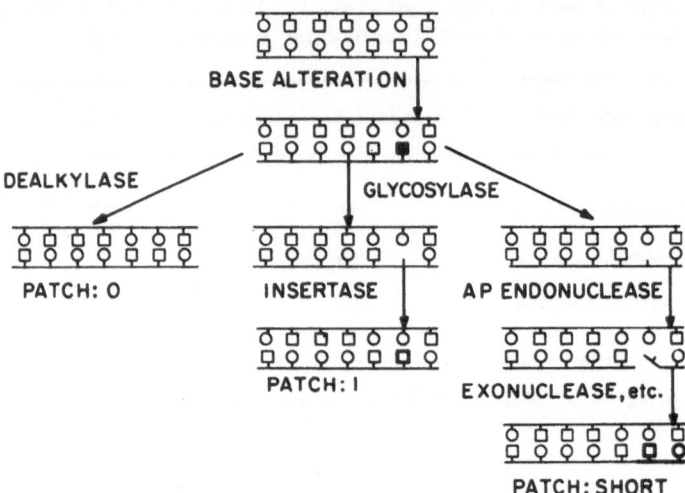

Fig. 3.   Various ways of repairing altered bases in DNA. The
          squares represent purines, the circles pyrimidines, the
          solid squares an altered base, and the outlined symbols
          bases inserted by repair. The assumed base alterations
          are alkylation damage.

     DNA repair in cells irradiated with ionizing radiation is also
of the short patch type (11), although the particular lesions
responsible for the effects of ionizing radiation have not been
identified. Radiation sensitive individuals are known. The
largest group are those with the genetic disease ataxia
telangiectasia (AT) (26). There have been two extensive studies
(27,28) on fibroblasts of normal, AT and other individuals
comparing their sensitivities to ionizing radiations in terms of
the dose that would give 37% survival on an exponential dose-
response curve, the so-called D_o value. The distributions of D_o
values obtained in these studies are shown in Figure 5. The
distributions are broad. It is clear that there exist various
sensitive subsets in the populations, which luckily do not make up
a very large proportion, and that the two surveys although agreeing
qualitatively have different values of D_o for the normal
populations. Thus, the determination of radiation sensitivity by
this parameter has some, as yet, unknown systematic variation from
laboratory to laboratory. It is improbable that the variation is
in the dosimetry.

     The sensitivities in Figure 5 are for the killing of fibro-
blasts. However, whatever the damage is that results in cell
death, it does not seem to be related to mutation and by inference
transformation, since AT cells are hypomutable by X-rays (26), a

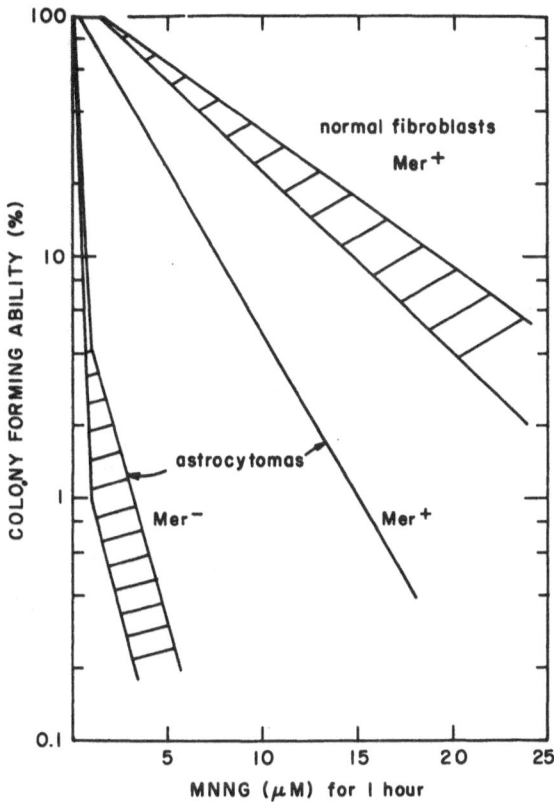

Fig. 4   The colony forming ability of various cell strains as a
         function of exposure for one hour to MNNG. Mer$^+$ refers to
         cells able to remove O^{6}methylguanine, Mer$^-$ refers to cells
         deficient in removal activity. This figure is adapted
         from data in Day et al. (24).

finding that is just the reverse of that for XP cells, since they
are hypermutable by UV (5,12).

CONCLUSIONS

     1) Human cells that are defective in the ability to repair
damage to DNA are more sensitive to the cytotoxic effects of such
damage and, in many instances, are more sensitive to the mutagenic
effects of such damage than are repair proficient cells.
     2) "Normal" individuals show a wide variation in the repair
abilities of fibroblasts and lymphocytes.
     3) In view of the fact that relatively small changes in
repair result in very large changes in cancer incidence, as

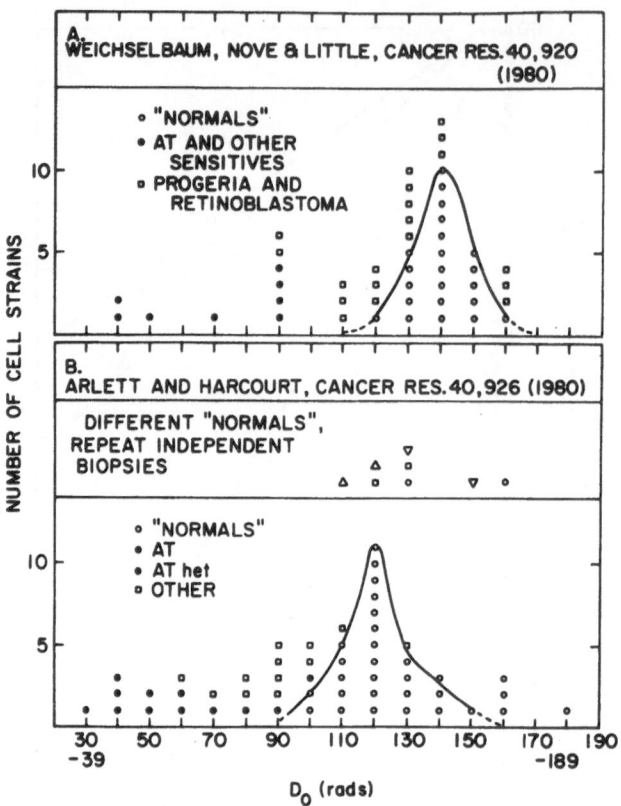

Fig. 5.   The distribution of D_0 values (the dose that gives 37%
          survival) among fibroblast strains used in two inves-
          tigations (27, 28). The shapes of the normal distri-
          butions have been drawn by eye. The widths of the
          distributions appear to be greater than expected from
          repeat biopsies.

indicated by the XP data, it is reasonable to infer that cancer
initiation among "normal" individuals may be in part deterministic
and depend on variations from the mean of repair ability. This
determinism is superimposed on the stochastic nature of the damage
to DNA and other cellular macromolecules resulting from exposure to
physical or environmental agents. We have no knowledge about factors, if any, such as lifestyle or genetic background that control
the inferred deterministic aspect of cancer susceptibility among
"normal" individuals.

ACKNOWLEDGEMENT

     This work was supported by the United States Department of
Energy.

REFERENCES

1. Setlow, R. B., Damages to DNA that result in neoplastic trans-
    formation, Adv. Biol. Med. Phys. 17: 99 (1980).
2. Muller R. and M. F. Rajewsky, Immunological quantification by
    high affinity antibodies of O^6-ethyldeoxyguanosine in DNA
    exposed to N-ethyl-N-nitrosourea, Cancer Res. 40: 887 (1980).
3. Hsu, I.C., M.C. Poirier, S. H. Yuspa, D. Grunberger, I. B.
    Weinstein, R. H. Yolken, and C. C. Harris, Measurement of
    benzo(a)pyrene-DNA adducts by enzyme immunoassays and radioim-
    munoassay, Cancer Res. 41: 1091 (1981).
4. Singer, B., N-nitroso alkylating agents: formation and per-
    sistence of alkyl derivatives in mammalian nucleic acids as
    contributing factors in carcinogenesis, J. Natl. Cancer
    Inst. 62: 1329 (1979).
5. Setlow, R. B., Repair deficient human disorders and cancer,
    Nature, 271: 713 (1978)
6. Pegg, A. E. and W. Perry, Alkylation of nucleic acids and
    metabolism of small doses of dimethylnitrosamine in the rat,
    Cancer Res. 41: 3128 (1981).
7. Schendel, P. F. and P. E. Robbins, Repair of O^6methylguanine
    in adapted Escherichia coli, Proc. Natl. Acad. Sci. 75: 6017
    (1978).
8. Montesano, R., H. Bresil, and G. P. Margison, Increased exci-
    sion of O^6-methylguanine from rat liver DNA after chronic
    administration of dimethylnitrosamine, Cancer Res. 39: 1798
    (1979).
9. Goth, R. and M. F. Rajewsky, Molecular and cellular mechanisms
    associated with pulse carcinogenesis in the rat nervous
    systems: ethylation of nucleic acids and elimination rates of
    ethylated bases from the DNA of different tissues, Zeit.
    Krebsforsch 82: 37 (1974).
10. Hanawalt, P. C., P. K. Cooper, A. K. Ganesan, and C. A. Smith,
    DNA repair in bacteria and mammalian cells, Ann. Rev.
    Biochem. 48: 783 (1979).
11. Regan, J. D. and R. B. Setlow, Two forms of repair in the DNA
    of human cells damaged by chemical carcinogens and mutagens,
    Cancer Res. 34: 3318 (1974).
12. Friedberg, E. C., U. K. Ehmann, and J. I. Williams, Human
    diseases associated with defective DNA repair, Adv. Radiat.
    Biol. 8: 85 (1979).
13. Ahmed, F. E. and R. B. Setlow, Kinetics of DNA repair in
    ultraviolet-irradiated and N-acetoxy-2-acetylaminofluorene-
    treated mammalian cells, Biophys. J. 24: 665 (1978).
14. Harm, W., Biological determination of the germicidal activity
    of sunlight, Radiat. Res. 40: 63 (1969).
15. Setlow, R. B., Different basic mechanisms in DNA repair, Arch.
    Toxicol. Suppl. 3: 217 (1980).

16. Scott, E. L. and M. L. Straf, Ultraviolet radiation as a cause of cancer, in: "Origins of Human Cancer", H. H. Hiatt, J. D. Watson, and J. A. Winsten, eds., Cold Spring Harbor Laboratory (1977).

17. Madden, J. J., A. Falek, D. A. Shafer, and J. H. Glick, Effects of opiates and demographic factors on DNA repair synthesis in human leukocytes, Proc. Natl. Acad. Sci. 76: 5769 (1979).

18. Lambert, B., U. Ringborg, and L. Skoog, Age-related decrease in ultraviolet light-induced DNA repair synthesis in human peripheral leukocytes, Cancer Res. 39: 2792 (1979).

19. Lindahl, T., DNA glycosylases, in "Chromosome Damage and DNA Repair", E. Seeberg and K. Kleppe, eds., Plenum Pub. Co. (1982).

20. Olsson, M. and T. Lindahl, Repair of alkylated DNA in Escherichia coli. Methyl group transfer from 0^6-methylguanine to a protein cysteine residue, J. Biol. Chem. 255: 10569 (1980).

21. Bogden, J. M., A. Eastman, and E. Bresnick, A system in mouse liver for the repair of 0^6-methylguanine lesions in methylated DNA, Nucl. Acid Res. 9: 3089 (1981).

22. Mehta, J. R., D. B. Ludlum, A. Renard, and W. G. Verly, Repair of 0^6-ethylguanine in DNA by a chromatin fraction from rat liver: transfer of the ethyl group to an acceptor protein, Proc. Natl. Acad. Sci. 78: 6766 (1981).

23. Waldstein, E. A., E.-H. Cao, M. A. Bender, and R. B. Setlow, Abilities of extracts of human lymphocytes to remove 0^6methyl-guanine from DNA, Mutat. Res., in press.

24. Day, R. S., III, C. H. J. Ziolkowski, D. A. Scudiero, S. A. Meyer, A. S. Lubiniecki, A. J. Girardi, S. M. Galloway, and G. D. Bynum, Defective repair of alkylated DNA by human tumor and SV40 transformed human cell strains, Nature 288: 724 (1980).

25. Harris, C. C., H. Autrup, R. Connor, L. A. Barrett, E. M. McDowell, and B. F. Trump, Interindividual variation in binding of benzo(a)pyrene to DNA in cultured human bronchi, Science 194: 1067 (1976).

26. Paterson, M. C. and P. J. Smith, Ataxia telangiectasia: an inherited human disorder involving hypersensitivity to ionizing radiation and related DNA-damaging chemicals, Ann. Rev. Genet. 13: 291 (1979).

27. Weichselbaum, R. R., J. Nove, and J. B. Little, X-ray sensitivity of fifty-three diploid fibroblast strains from patients with characteristic genetic disorders, Cancer Res. 40: 920 (1980).

28. Arlett, C. F. and S. Harcourt, Survey of radiosensitivity in a variety of human cell strains, Cancer Res. 40: 926 (1980).

DISCUSSION

Q. KREWSKI: I have two questions concerning the role of DNA repair and DNA damage in determining dose response relationships. First, you indicated that repair efficiencies decrease with increasing dose. Could you comment on the <u>rate</u> at which repair efficiency might be expected to decrease <u>with</u> dose?

Second, is there any evidence that the incidence of tumors induced as a result of DNA damage might be proportional to the amount of such damage?

A. SETLOW: Doses in the laboratory experiment are greater than doses in the outside world. Therefore, inhibition by high doses is not an important consideration for environmental exposure. Your second question has to do with the shape of the dose-response curve. I have no good answer, except for ultraviolet; there does not seem to be a threshhold for the white population of the United States, presumably because everyone is exposed on the average to a large amount of ultraviolet and so are above the threshhold, if one existed.

MUTATION IN VIVO IN HUMAN SOMATIC CELLS: STUDIES USING

PERIPHERAL BLOOD MONONUCLEAR CELLS

Richard J. Albertini,
David L. Sylwester,
Bruce D. Dannenberg,
Elizabeth F. Allen

Department of Medicine and Medical Microbiology
University of Vermont
Burlington, Vermont 05405

INTRODUCTION

We review here our efforts to develop a direct mutagenicity test system for detecting somatic cell mutations occurring in vivo in man. Our specific goal is to provide a useful test for directly quantifying mutant cells in human blood samples.

As outlined elsewhere, direct tests such as those to be described provide unique advantages for human mutagenicity monitoring. Among these are: (i) the ability to assess the effects of metabolic and/or pharmacokinetic factors in chemical mutagenesis, (ii) the identification of possible differences in susceptability to mutagenic influences among humans, and (iii) the determination of genetic effects due to environmental mixtures. However, of most importance, human direct mutagenicity test results in man can be compared with health outcomes, allowing a direct determination of the value of the test result in predicting health risk.

DEVELOPMENT OF THE SYSTEM

Background

The 6-thioguanine resistant (TG^r) peripheral blood lymphocyte (PBL) system is a descendent of the human diploid fibroblast system, which detects somatic cell mutations to TG^r in vitro (1,2). That system has been used widely for in vitro mutagenesis testing with human cells. Because of this close relationship between the systems, and because findings with the lymphocyte system

403

are interpreted in light of the fibroblast system, the rationale
for the earlier method is summarized.

Rationale for Using the Lesch-Nyhan (LN) Mutation as a Prototype for Human Somatic Cell Mutagenesis Assays

The Fibroblast System. The human diploid fibroblast system was
developed so that the induction of specific locus mutations in
diploid human somatic cells in vitro could be studied. It was
intended to provide an in vitro mutagenesis assay that would be
realistic for man in terms of genetic targets. In selecting a
genetic locus for study, certain characteristics of importance were
defined; (i) the locus should not specify a vital function, (ii)
the locus should specify a clear and unambiguous phenotype at the
single cell level, (iii) the locus should exist in the haploid
state to obviate dominance/recessive relationships, (iv) the locus
should specify a detectable gene product, and (v) it should be
possible to devise a selective system to allow quantitation of rare
mutant cells.

In man, the enzyme hypoxanthine-guanine phosphoribosyltransferase (HPRT) is specified by a gene located on the X-chromosome
(HPRT locus) (3,4). Hypoxanthine and guanine are the normal substrates of this enzyme, and are converted to inosine-5'-monophos-
phate, and guanosine-5'-monophosphate, respectively.

Certain naturally occurring mutations in man result in the
clinical disorder known as the Lesch-Nyhan (LN) syndrome (5,6).
The hallmark of this disorder is decreased to absent HPRT activity
in all cells (3,7,8,9). The resultant biochemical aberrations
center about abnormalities in purine intercoversions with gross
systemic overproduction of uric acid. The clinical manifestations
are multiple and bizarre, and are characterized by neurological and
behavioral disorders with mental retardation (10,11). Another form
of natural mutation at the HPRT locus is similar but less extensive
than the LN mutation. HPRT activity is decreased but not absent in
cells of such affected individuals, and the clinical manifestations
are less severe (12,13). Only males are affected in both
disorders.

Several family studies strongly suggest the X-linkage of the
HPRT locus (6,10,12,13). This was confirmed subsequently by the in
vitro demonstration of two populations of cells in females
heterozygous for the LN mutation - those with normal and those with
defective HPRT activity (4,14,15,16,17,18,19). This, of course, is
the consequence of the single active-X principle in mammalian cells
(20,21). Finally, the X-chromosomal location of the HPRT locus was
demonstrated by somatic cell hybridization studies (22).

LN prototype mutations at the HPRT locus result in a characteristic phenotype at the single cell level. Normal cells, possessing HPRT activity, are able to convert purine analog substrates such as 8-azaguanine (AG) and 6-thioguanine (TG) to their respective ribotides (8). The ribotide forms of these analogs inhibit and finally kill normal cells. Since only phosphorylated analogs are inhibitory to cells, LN mutant cells not possessing full enzyme activity are relatively or totally resistant to their effects (1,8,14,23). The growth of LN cells in the presence of purine analogs, then, serves as the prototype for HPRT-deficient cell growth.

LN mutant cells also differ from normal cells in their inability to utilize hypoxanthine for growth. This lack may be demonstrated in a variety of ways (1,17,24,25). Furthermore, LN prototype mutant cells show almost no HPRT activity when biochemical determinations are made. Thus, assessment of the primary gene product of the HPRT locus differentiates LN and normal cells at the somatic level (1,2,26).

The human diploid fibroblast system has been used by several investigators to quantify the mutagenic effects of a variety of physical and chemical agents to cultured human cells in vitro (2,27,28,29). Fibroblasts from individuals with the DNA repair defect Xeroderma Pigmentosum have been shown with the system to be exquisitely senstivie in vitro to the cytotoxicity and mutagenicity of ultraviolet light (27,30). Variant purine analog resistant human fibroblasts arising in vitro in cultures of normal human fibroblasts have been characterized as to HPRT deficiency, purine analog resistance and ability to utilize hypoxanthine for growth (29). They have satisfied several of the critieria necessary to define them as somatic cell mutants (31).

The Lymphocyte System

Although the human fibroblast system provides realism in terms of genetic targets for mutagenicity testing, it has the limitations of an in vitro system. However, the prototype LN mutation is useful also for direct mutagenicity testing. Furthermore, because somatic cell mutation occurs in vitro in human fibroblasts, it seems reasonable to expect that it occurs also in other somatic cells in vivo. The LN phenotype should allow detection in samples obtained directly from the body of mutant somatic cells.

Appropriate cells must be studied in direct mutagenicity tests. The cells should be easily obtainable and polyclonal in origin in order to reflect independent genetic events. There should be a method for demonstrating mutant phenotypes while not allowing mutations to occur in vitro. There should be a method for growing the cells in vitro so that the genetic basis of the altered

phenotypes can be demonstrated. Peripheral blood lymphocytes
(PBL's) were chosen for study for all of these reasons.

Experience with TG^r Variant Lymphocyte Assay

Early Studies. Our early studies showed that the phenotype of
purine analog resistance is expressed in LN PBL's as well as in LN
fibroblasts. This was shown by the resistance of LN PBL's to AG or
TG inhibition of phytohemagglutinin (PHA) stimulated tritiated
thymidine (^{3}HTdr) incorporation in vitro. Our initial studies
quantitated ^{3}HTdr incorporation by scintillation spectrometry which
identified females who were heterozygous for the LN mutation by
their PBL mosaicism (32). Minority populations of LN PBL's
comprising 5 to 10% of the total were found in LN heterozygotes.
This suggested incomplete selection in vivo against LN PBL's in
mosaic individuals, otherwise, in heterozygotes, the mutant cells
should be approximately 50% of the total. These early studies
showed unequivocally that mutant PBL's are detectable in mixed
populations. However a sensitivity greater than that afforded by
scintillation spectrometry is required to detect rare LN-like PBL's
in non-LN individuals.

Subsequently, we developed an autoradiographic assay to
enumerate cells incorporating ^{3}HTdr in vitro (33,34). With this
method, we showed that LN PBL's are resistant to 2×10^{-4} M TG, but
partically sensitive to 2×10^{-3}M. PBL mosaicism in LN
heterozygotes was again demonstrated, this time autoradio-
graphically, with LN PBL's present in such women at frequencies
ranging from 10^{-3} to 5×10^{-2}. Furthermore, rare LN PBLs were
quantitatively detected when artifically mixed with normal cells at
frequencies of 10^{-4} or less.

We then undertook a series of studies to determine TG^r PBL
variant frequencies (V_f's) in non-LN individuals (33,34,35,36).
When tested at 2×10^{-4} M TG, fresh blood samples from healthy
control individuals showed a median TG^r PBL V_f of 1.1×10^{-4}. The
TG^r PBL V_f's were not age related. V_f's were determined also in a
group of cancer patients who were receiving cytotoxic
chemotherapeutic agents, most of which are known to be mutagenic.
The median V_f in this group was 8.5×10^{-4}, and the distribution of
values was such that most values were higher than the highest
values seen in the normal control group. Subsequent studies of
patients with psoriasis or vitiligo who were receiving
photochemotherapy with 8-methoxypsoralen and UV-A light (PUVA) also
showed them to have elevated TG^r PBL V_fs when compared with normals
(35).

However, in all of these studies, we found that some untreated
patients (cancer and psoriasis) had elevated TG^r PBL V_f's, often in
the range of patients receiving the known mutagenic therapies.

Vitiligo patients did not show elevated V_f's except in the treated group, suggesting that PUVA was probably responsible for the elevation. Nonetheless, the magnitude of the V_f's, even in the healthy control individuals, made it difficult to implicate somatic cell mutation in vivo as the sole cause of all TG^r cells detected.

   Phenocopies. Phenocopies are nongenetic variants that mimic cells with specific genotypic changes. They are almost certain to occur for any phenotypic variation. At least three systems that have been suggested as human direct mutagenicity tests in the past have been discarded because of an inability to separate phenocopies from true genetic mutants (37,38). Because of findings as noted, plus large variations over time in TG^r PBL V_f's in normals, we suspected that the TG^r lymphocyte system was detecting a great many phenocopies.

   The presence of phenocopies that mimic TG^r PBL's was suggested by further experiments that studied spontaneous DNA synthesis in PBL's in vitro in cultures not containing PHA (39). Although in the absence of stimulation, only rare PBL's are in the cell cycle and capable of DNA synthesis in vitro, a large fraction of these seem to retain this capability whether or not the purine analog is present. Thus, some PBL's are apparently committed to DNA synthesis when put into culture and cannot be inhibited. These almost certainly are not mutant cells, and constitute a serious source of phenocopies in the PBL system.

   Quite by accident, we found that cryopreservation in dimethylsulfoxide (DMSO) and liquid nitrogen of the mononuclear cell (MNC) fraction of whole blood (containing the PBL's) prior to testing for TG^r PBLs eliminated or greatly reduced V_fs (39). We felt that this might be due to removing the effect of phenocopies. Subsequent findings suggested that cryopreservation (or cooling to 4°C prior to test) does not remove PBL's committed to DNA synthesis (phenocopies), but does appear to synchronize them so that they begin DNA synthesis immediately upon being put into culture. These cells then apparently complete DNA synthesis and do not incorporate ^{3}HTdr when this label is added later in the variant lymphocyte assay, 30 hours after PHA stimulation. Thus, they are not scored as TG^r PBLs (39,40).

   Our most recent studies have been to determine with cryopreserved samples TG^r PBL V_f's in normal, non-LN individuals, and in humans knowingly exposed to mutagens. We now find that V_f's of normals are in the range of 10^{-6} to 10^{-5}, and are only infrequently above this value. Elevated TG^r PBL V_f's are still found in groups of patients receiving mutagenic therapies, but much more modest elevations are now found. Sample results are given in this paper. (See Table I).

Table 1. TG^r PBL V_f's (Cryopreserved MNC's)

SUBJECT NO.	SEX	AGE	STATUS	MUTAGEN	DURATION[1]	TIME SINCE EXPOSURE[2]	LI_c	EVALUATABLE NUCLEI =N	LABELED NUCLEI=M	$V_f \times 10^{-6}$	C.I.
			INDIVIDUAL TESTED						TEST RESULTS		
2	M	40	Chemist	--	--	--	0.18	569,000	15	26.4	15.9,43.9
4	M	25	Normal	--	--	--	0.24	2,793,000	7	2.5	1.0,5.2
6	F	57	Normal	--	--	--	0.03	555,000	3	5.4	1.1,15.6
8	M	28	Normal	--	--	--	0.18	2,133,000	8	3.8	1.6,7.4
23	--	0[3]	Newborn	--	--	--	0.54	1,339,000	24	17.9	12.0,26.8
26	--	0[3]	Newborn	--	--	--	0.49	578,000	280	488.6	433.2,551.2
13	F	70	Skin Ca[4]	--	--	--	0.26	2,387,000	13	5.4	3.2,9.4
17	M	68	Skin Ca[4]	--	--	--	0.05	428,000	5	11.4	3.7,27.3
21	M	19	TX[5]	Imuran[6]	10 days	Continuing	0.14	135,000	7	51.9	20.7,106.7
28	F	58	Cancer	L-pam[7]	7 mos	1.5 mos	0.16	451,000	6	13.3	4.9, 29.0
34	F	70	Cancer	ADR[8] Mit-C	4 mos	1 week	0.21	598,000	32	53.5	37.7,76.0
30	F	23	Cancer	L-pam[7]	5 mos	1.5 mos	0.23	286,000	2	7.0	0.7,25.2

[1]Estimated duration of treatment

[2]Estimated interval since last treatment

[3]Umbilical cord blood sample

[4]Multiple skin cancers - no chemotherapy

[5]Renal transplant recipient

[6]Imuran = Azathioprine: Metabolic conversion in vivo to 6-mercaptopurine

[7]L-phenylalanine mustard (alkylating agent)

[8]Adriamycin; mitomycin C

CURRENT WORK

Method

The method of assay for TG^r PBL's has been described elsewhere in detail (40). Venous blood is obtained in heparinized syringes. Whole blood is fractionated by the Ficoll-Hypaque method and the mononuclear cell (MNC) fraction removed and washed with phosphate buffered saline. MNC's are resuspended in medium RPMI 1640 (GIBCO) with additives (25 mM Hepes, 2 mM glutamine, 100 U penicillin, and 100 mcg streptomycin per ml medium) supplemented with 10% human AB serum and 7.5% dimethylsulfoxide (DMSO) for freezing. MNC's are suspended at 5×10^6 to 10^7/ml and aliquoted at approximately 1 ml/Nunc tube. Freezing is in a Union Carbide biological freezing unit for controlled freezing. Frozen cells are stored in the vapor phase of liquid nitrogen.

For testing, frozen MNC's are rapidly thawed and diluted with warm (37°C) RPMI 1640, centrifuged and resuspended in medium RPMI 1640 containing additives, and supplemented with 20% human AB serum at a final density of approximately 10^6 cells/ml.

Two methods are currently used for culture. For the standard method, MNC suspensions are aliquoted as 1 ml samples into point bottom glass tubes to which are added 0.2 ml PHA-P (Burroughs Wellcome) to achieve a final PHA concentration of 5 mcg/ml. TG (0.1 ml) solution in RPMI 1640 and 0.1 N NaOH is added to give a final TG concentration of 2×10^{-4} M in test cultures. Similarily, 0.1 ml of pH adjusted RPMI 1640 is added in control cultures. Cultures are incubated at 37°C in a 5% CO_2 humidified atmosphere for 30 hours, followed by the addition of 5 µC ^{3}HTdr (New England Nuclear), an additional twelve hours incubation and terminated.

In order to study larger numbers of cells, mass cultures in plastic tissue culture flasks are also used. Ten ml cell suspensions of 10^6 cells/ml, are inoculated into plastic flasks. PHA and either TG or pH adjusted medium are added to achieve the same concentrations as for point bottom tube cultures. Tissue culture flasks are placed on end so that the MNC's settle to the bottom in a loose layer. As for tube cultures, ^{3}HTdr (5µC/ml of culture medium) is added after 30 hours and the cultures incubated for another 12 hours before termination.

Tube cultures are terminated by adding 4 ml of 0.1 M citric acid at 4°C to each tube. Tubes are centrifuged at 600 x G for 10 minutes, washed in 4 ml of methanol-acetic acid fixative (3:1), resuspended in 0.2 ml of fixature and refrigerated for several hours. Flask cultures are terminated by addition of 35 ml of 0.1 M citric acid at 4°C. Then the flask contents are transferred to centrifuge tubes. The remaining steps are identical for the two culture methods.

A 0.02 ml sample of each cell suspension in fixative is counted with an electronic particle counter (Coulter Counter; ZBI model). The cell suspensions in toto are then added in measured volumes to 18 X 18 mm coverslips affixed with permount to microscope slides. A single slide is made from the contents of each tube. The slides are dried, stained with aceto-orcein for 20 seconds and rinsed with water. More recently, slides of cells from TG containing cultures have been autoradiographed without staining.

For autoradiography, slides are dipped into NTB-2 (Eastman Kodak) emulsion, exposed at 4°C for 24 hours and developed according to Kodak instructions. Autoradiographed slides are thus available for control (without TG) and test (containing TG) cultures for each individual.

The TG^r PBL variant frequency (V_f) for each individual is calculated from the labeling index of the control cultures (LI_c):

$$\frac{LI_t}{LI_c} = V_f$$

The LI_t of test cultures is determined by counting all labeled nuclei on all slides made from test cultures and dividing by the total number of cells added to slides, which is determined by Coulter count:

$$\frac{\text{Number of labeled nuclei on all slides}}{\text{Total number of cells on all sides}} = \frac{M}{T} = LI_t$$

Test slides are scanned at low power light microscopy (160X), and the presence of rare labeled nuclei is confirmed with oil immersion viewing (1000X).

The LI_c of control cultures is determined from a random differential count of 5000 nuclei on slides to which have been added nuclei from control, non-TG containing cultures:

$$\frac{\text{Number of labeled nuclei per 5000 nuclei}}{5000} = LI_c$$

The differential counts are usually made under oil emersion microscopy (1000X) on control slides. Therefore,

$$V_f = \frac{LI_t}{LI_c} = \frac{M}{LI_c \cdot T,}$$

Where $LI_c \cdot T = N$ = number of evaluatable cells in the test.

Statistical Analysis

In order to define the precision of V_f determinations as well as the optimum size of experiments, confidence intervals (CI's) for true variant frequency values are calculated by assuming that M is a Poisson variable and LI a binomial fraction. Exact CI's for the true Poisson mean of labeled nuclei are available from tables, using the observed count M. Also, since N is a binomial random variable with parameters T and p (the probability that a nucleus from a control culture will be labeled), it can be shown that the approximate standard deviation of N is:

$$S_n = T\sqrt{\frac{pq}{c}}$$

where q = 1-p and c = number of nuclei evaluated in control cultures = 5000.

Elsewhere we describe in detail methods for defining CI's for true variation frequencies (40).

Sample Results

The Appearance of Labeled Nuclei. The differential count of labeling index slides for control cultures (LI_c) is usually made under oil immersion (1000 x power). Test slides are scanned at low power microscopy and "positive" labeled nuclei are confirmed under oil immersion.

Figure 1a is a photomicrograph of a portion of a slide from which the LI_c was determined, while Figure 1b is a photomicrograph of a portion of a test slides (TG culture) from which the variant frequency was determined for the same individual. Both photomicrograms are shown at 160X. There is a single labeled nucleus shown in Figure 1b. Figures 2a and 2b are photomicrographs of the same portion of slides as seen under oil immersion (1000X). A labeled nucleus on a test slide is scored if it has the same appearance as labeled nuclei on control slides. Figure 3 is a photomicrograph of a non-stained slide, showing the appearance of a rare variant labeled nucleus under oil immersion (1000X). We now find that the scoring of slides made from test cultures is easier if the slides are unstained.

Sensitivity of Cryopreserved MNC's to TG

Figure 4 shows the sensitivity of cryopreserved normal MNC's to TG where the apparent V_f is given on the ordinate ($\log_{10}$) and the TG concentration is shown on the abcissa ($\log_{10}$). The apparent V_f at 10^{-5} M and 10^{-4} M TG is near 10^{-4}, but these determinations were based on finding a single labeled nucleus and few cells tested at both TG concentration, and has very wide 95% confidence intervals. The V_f of 26×10^{-6} determined at 2×10^{-4} M TG is based on large numbers of labeled nuclei scored, and probably

represents a more realistic estimate for all three TG concentrations. This is the TG concentration currently used in the variant
lymphocyte assay.

The insert of Figure 4 shows mitogenesis in PHA stimulated
cultures (LI_c) (ordinate, linear scale) resulting from different
concentrations of PHA-P (abcissa, linear scale) in the final
cultures. The concentration of 5 mcg/ml as used in the variant
lymphocyte assay, provides optimal stimulation.

TG^r PBL V_f Determinations

The results of 39 recent TG^r PBL V_f determinations performed
on cryopreserved MNC samples from 37 individuals are shown
graphically in Figure 5, where the abcissa gives the ages of the
individual tested and the ordinate depicts the V_f's. Both scales
are linear; the scale on the ordinate is broken. Ten of the
individuals tested are normal adults, two of whom have psoriasis.
Eight of the individuals have a history of multiple skin cancers,
none of whom is receiving chemotherapy. Three individuals are
renal transplant recipients, all of whom are receiving azathioprine
continuously, and eleven are patients with various visceral
malignancies, all of whom receive intermittant X-irradiation and/-
or cytotoxic chemotherapy. Six samples were from umbilical cord
blood samples (five individuals), but mutagen exposure histories
are not available.

It is apparent from these results that V_f values do not vary
simply as a result of age. This is consistent with our earlier
observations using fresh blood samples (34). The oldest tested
individual tested (85 years) has a V_f of 5.4 x 10^{-6}, which is comparable to the values of younger individuals.

TG^r PBL V_f values for normal, non-mutagen exposed adults range
from less than 1.1 to 26 x 10^{-6}, with only two being greater than
10 x 10^{-6}. One of these two is employed as a chemist, while the
other is under dermatological care for psoriasis. By contrast,
nine of the eleven cancer patients receiving X-irradiation or
cytotoxic chemotherapy have TG^r PBL V_f values greater than 10 x
10^{-6}. Patients with multiple skin cancers were studied because of
the possibility that these multiple malignancies result from
unusual mutagenic influences in vivo (41). Half of the eight
patients tested had V_f values greater than 10 x 10^{-6}.

Renal transplant recipients receiving azathioprine are individuals in whom there is pharmacolgical selection in vivo for TG^r
cells. TG^r PBL V_f's might rise in such persons as a result of
selection (46), although the degree of increase may be a function
of time. Two of the three transplant recipients showed seemingly
elevated TG^r PBL V_f's -- one at 51.9 and the other at 217.5 x
10^{-6}. It is difficult to recover large numbers of PBL's from such

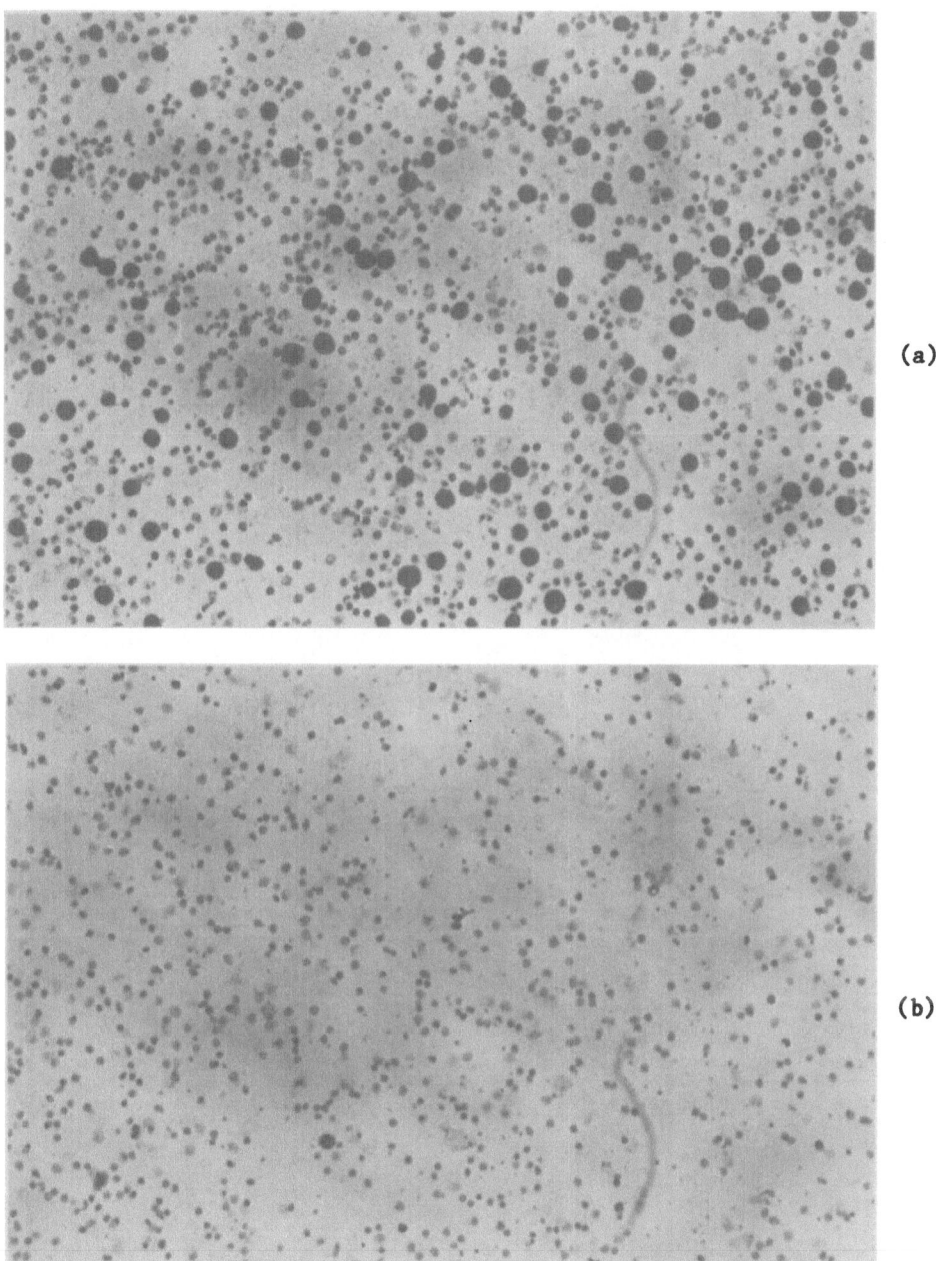

(a)

(b)

Fig. 1.   (a) Appearance of nuclei from a control culture with a
labeling index (LI) of 13% (160X). (b) Appearance of
nuclei from a test culture from the same person as 1a
showing one labeled nucleus (160X). (Both panels reduced 28% for reproduction.)

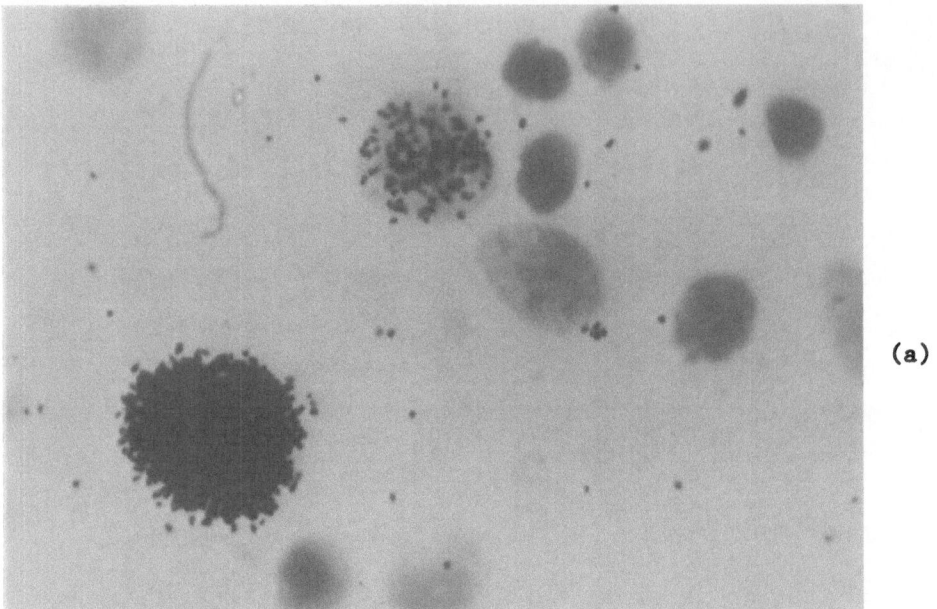

(a)

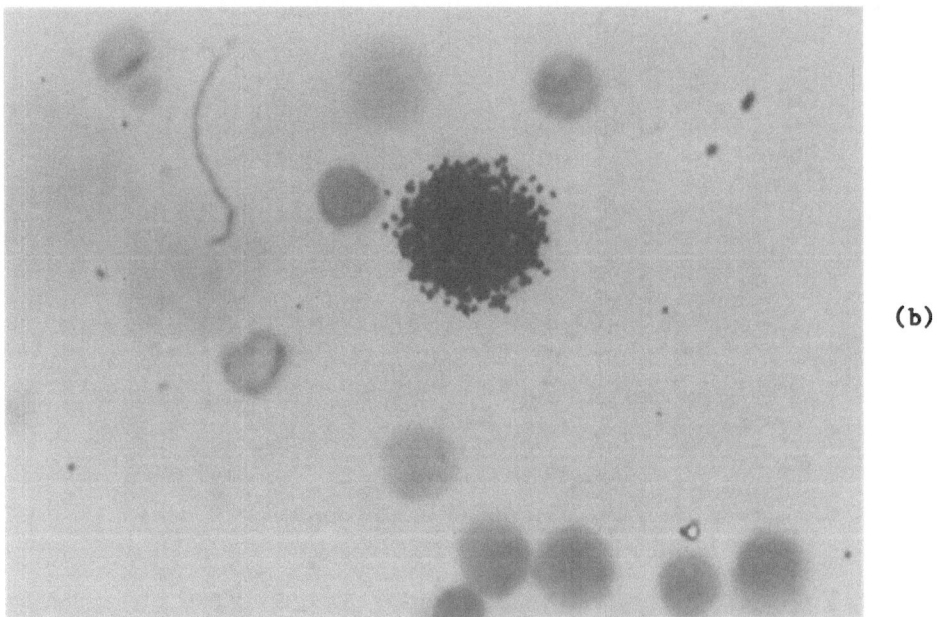

(b)

Fig. 2.   (a) Appearance of nuclei from control culture shown in
            1a with two labeled nuclei (1000X). (b) Appearance of
            nuclei from test culture shown in 1b one labeled nucleus
            (1000X). (Both panels reduced 28% for reproduction.)

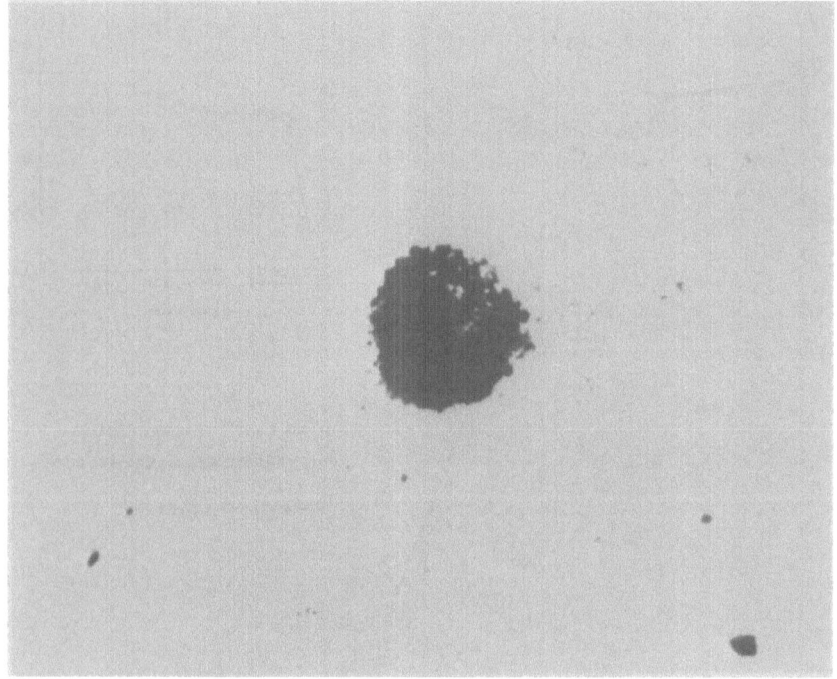

Fig. 3.   Appearance of a labeled nucleus from a test culture.
          Slide was not stained (1000X). (Reduced 28% for re-
          production.)

patients because of the lymphopenia associated with therapy. These
values therefore are based on small numbers of cells evaluated (N)
and small numbers of labeled nuclei scored (M) (7 and 8 respectively).

TG^r PBL V_f values for the six umbilical cord blood samples
range from 6.9 to 489.0 x 10^{-6} and are usually based on large numbers of cells scored. Replicate determinations on a single frozen
sample gave V_f values of 6.9 and 11.2 x 10^{-6}, which provide some
measure of technical variability. Because we have no information
regarding possible mutagen exposures of mothers and fetuses, it is
difficult to speculate on possible interpretations of this range of
values. Umbilical cord lymphocytes may not be comparable to adult
PBL's in several respects, some of which may be important in the
lymphocyte assay.

Table 1 gives results in tabular form for a sample of these
individuals and lists some of the factors which may be important in
determining TG^r PBL V_f values in vivo. Listed also are 95% confidence intervals for the V_f values. It may be noted that many of
the V_f determinations are based on small numbers of labeled nuclei
so that confidence intervals are wide.

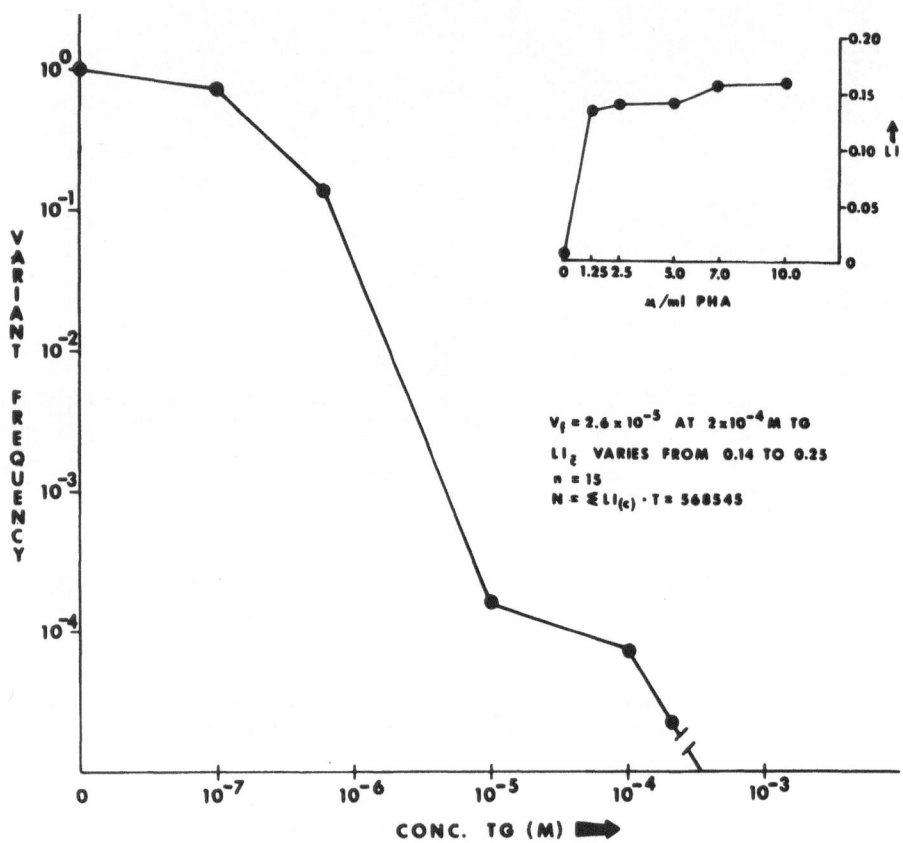

$V_f = 2.6 \times 10^{-5}$ AT 2×10^{-4} M TG

LI_z VARIES FROM 0.14 TO 0.25

$n = 15$

$N = \Sigma LI_{(c)} \cdot T = 568545$

Fig. 4.   Variant frequency (V_f) as a function of thioguanine (TG)
             concentration. The ordinate shows V_f on a $\log_{10}$ scale;
             the abscissa shows molar TG concentration on a $\log_{10}$
             scale. The insert shows labeling index of a control
             culture (LI_c) as a function of phytohemagglutinin (PHA)
             concentration. Both coordinates are on a linear scale.

Relationship of V_f's to LI_c's
_____

     We have reported previously that when fresh samples are
tested, there is no relationship between the LI_c of a control PBL
culture and the V_f determined on its companion test cultures
(34). Thus, the elevated TGr PBL V_f values of cancer patients
receiving chemotherapy are not simply a reflection of lower LI_c's
in this group. Is this true also for cryopreserved MNC samples?
Figure 6 shows graphically the V_f values (ordinate) presented in
Figure 5 and the LI_c's of the respective control cultures

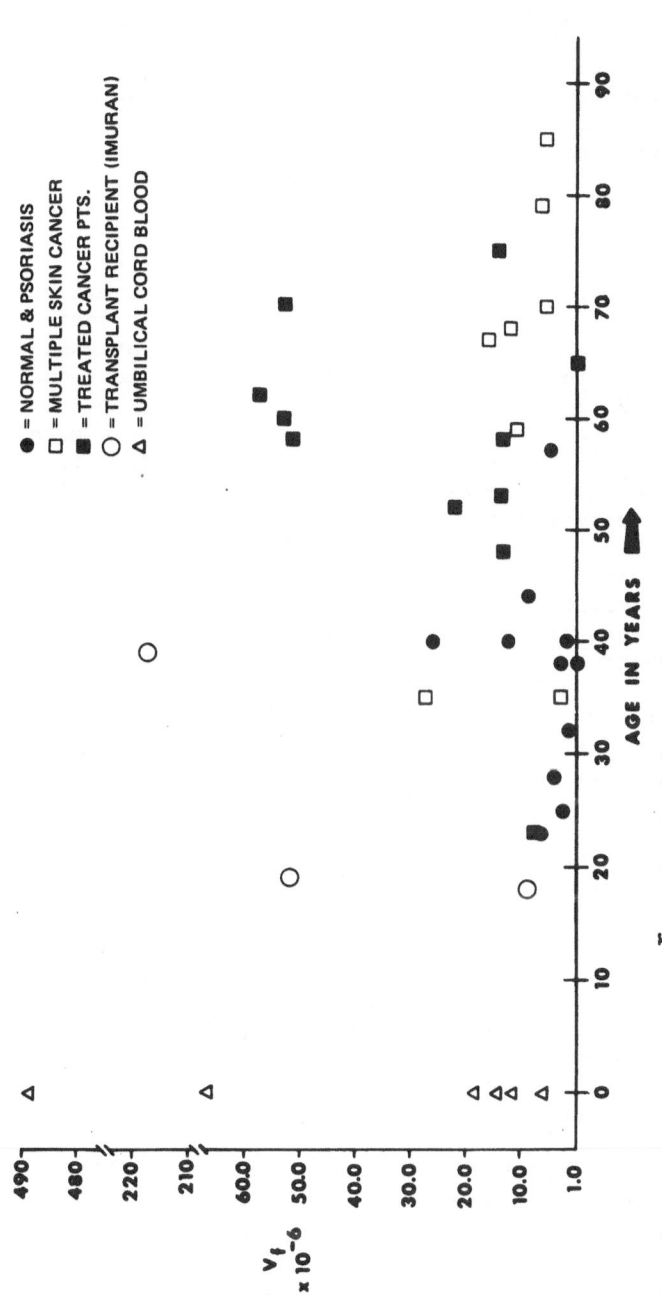

Fig. 5. Frequencies of TG^r PBL's (V_f's) shown by age of the individual. The ordinate shows V_f on a linear scale; the abscissa shows age in years.

(abcissa). Both scales are linear. The LI_c's, range from 0.01 to
0.55, with most being in the range of 0.02 to 0.25. Cultures from
umbilical cord blood samples have the highest LI_c's, with all being
in excess of 0.40. Again, we show that there is no correlation
between LI_c's and V_f's. With the exception of the umbilical cord
samples, the several groups of individuals tested are not distin-
guishable on the basis of LI_c's. Thus, for cryopreserved MNC samples also, an increase in TG^r PBL V_f's in treated cancer patients
is not correlated with a decrease in LI_c's as compared to healthy
controls.

DISCUSSION

    We report again the "LN like" TG variant PBL's are present in
the blood of non-LN individuals. Their frequencies range from 10^{-6}
to 10^{-5} in normal individuals with occasional elevations, and appear to be higher in individuals exposed to known mutagens. Modest
elevations of TG^r PBL V_f's are found in adults who have multiple
skin malignancies -- a sitation which may result from mutagenic
influences in vivo. V_f elevations are seen also in persons receiving therapeutic immunosuppression with azathioprine, a purine analogue that is converted to 6-mercaptopurine in vivo providing
continuous selection for the variant cells. All of these recent
TG^r PBL V_f determinations were made with cryopreserved MNC samples
in order to eliminate or greatly reduce the effects of
phenocopies. Thus, they represent our current and best estimates
of V_f's in adults.

    We report also, for the first time, TG^r PBL V_f's for human
newborns, determined on cryopreserved MNC's obtained from umbilical
cord blood samples. These V_f's are generally higher than those
observed for adults, and show a much wider range -- from 6×10^{-6}
to almost 5×10^{-4}. At present, we do not know the reason for
either the elevation or the wide range of values. Several interpretations are possible, which illustrate current difficulties in
interpreting results of direct mutagenicity tests.

    The different V_f values found in newborns might, in fact, re-
present different rates of somatic cell mutation in the different
pregnancies. Because these were pilot studies, we have no
information regarding possible mutagen exposures of mothers of
these newborns. As we continue to monitor TG^r PBL V_f's in umbilical cord samples, such information will be available.

    Alternatively, although the rate of somatic cell mutation may
have differed in the pregnancies tested, these differences may not
have been nearly as large as the V_f differences measured. The cell
kinetics responsible for amplification of mutations may differ
between the fetus and adult. Selection in vivo against the "LN
like" phenotype, clearly evident in the adult, may be less in the
fetus. Mutations are the events of interest, but are only inferred
through the enumeration of mutants. Non-mutagenic factors may
influence mutant frequencies. This complication, which may be a

factor in the cord blood findings, must be considered for any
direct mutagenicity test.

Finally, phenocopies may be confounding these newborn
results. We have described one source of variant lymphocyte phenocopies in the adult -- that of PBL's that are apparently committed
to DNA synthesis and cannot be inhibited <u>in vitro</u> from incorporating ^{3}HTdr. We have also described a method for removing their
effects, and our current results in testing adult blood samples
suggest that their interference has been largely eliminated. However, other sources of non-mutant "LN like" PBL's may exist in the
fetus. This remains to be demonstrated by further testing.

In the results presented here, we show again that age does not
appear to be a factor in an individual's TG^r PBL V_f, and that there
is no relationship between the degree of mitogenesis in PHA

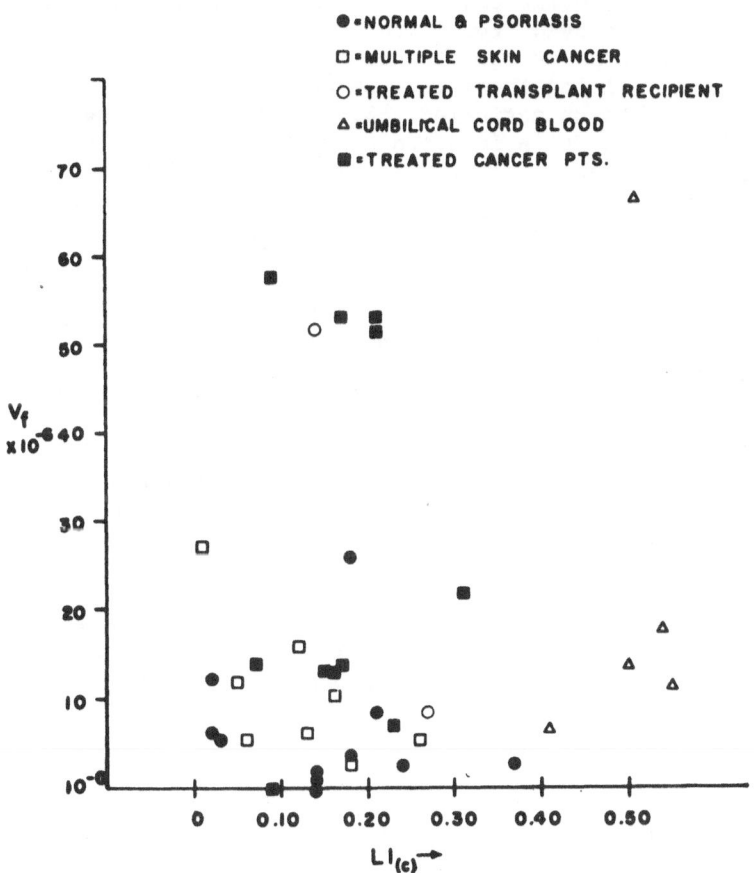

Fig. 6.   Frequencies of TG^r PBL's (V_f) shown by labeling index of
control cultures (LI_c). The ordinate shows V_f on a
linear scale; the abscissa shows labeling index as a
proportion of total cells present.

stimulated cultures as reflected by the labeling index of control cultures (LI_c) and the corresponding V_f value. The variant lymphocyte assay is currently at a point in development where the values determined are reasonable and consistant with a mutational origin of the TG^r cells.

Our evidence on this latter point, however, is still indirect. We can demonstrate that LN PBL's, which are true genetic mutants, behave in the lymphocyte assay as do the cells we measure. LN PBL's can be detected quantitatively in artificial mixtures with normal cells under the conditions used in the assay. Also, with the lymphocyte assay, infrequent mutant LN PBL's are clearly detectable in LN heterozygous females.

PBL's obtained from non-LN azathioprine treated patients with high TG^r PBL V_f's were cultured in vitro directly in TG on two occasions (36). The cultures were lost in both cases before HPRT deficiency in the cells could be demonstrated, and in neither case were the cells removed from TG to ascertain maintenance of the resistant phenotype in the absence of selection. Therefore, the criteria for defining these variant cells as true somatic cell mutants remain to be satisfied. Since methods are now available for cloning human PBL's in vitro using T-cell growth factors (42-45), the demonstration of the genetic basis of TG^r in human PBL's is possible and is a major goal in the development of the lymphocyte system.

If variant lymphocytes are truly genetic mutants, results such as we present here are to be expected, and the test is valuable for human mutagenicity monitoring. However, these results themselves cannot be used to determine the mutational origin of the variant PBL's. The test at present should not be used for uncritical mutagenicity testing.

Direct mutagenicity testing has unique advantages for human mutagenicity monitoring. Perhaps the most important, it may eventually be possible to use the results of such tests in place of affected individuals as realistic indicators of human health hazards and to develop instruments which allow quantitative risk assessments to be made for man. These are the goals of direct mutagenicity testing. The variant lymphocyte assay is presented as a candidate test system, in development.

Full Address:

Richard J. Albertini, M.D., PhD.
Department of Medicine
Given Building E305
University of Vermont
College of Medicine
Burlington, Vermont 05405 USA

Note Added in Proof: TG^r PBL V_f values have been determined for a much larger sample of unbilical cord bloods. The majority of these are in the range of values found for normal non-mutagen exposed adult blood samples.

ACKNOWLEDGEMENT

This work was supported by National Institutes of Health Grant No. PHS RO1 30688-01, Cancer Center Support Grant CA 22435, Genetics Center Support Grant MCH 46-1001-02-0, March of Dimes Grant 15-1.

REFERENCES

1. Albertini, R. J. and R. DeMars, Diploid azaguanine-resistant mutants of cultured fibroblasts, Science 169, 482, 1970.
2. Albertini, R. J. and R. DeMars, Detection and quantification of X-ray induced mutation in cultured, diploid human fibro-blasts, Mutation Res. 18, 199,1973.
3. Seegmiller, J. E, F. M. Rosenbloom and W. N. Kelley, Enzyme defect associated with a sex-linked human neurological disor-der and excessive purine synthesis, Science 155, 1682, 1967.
4. Felix, J. S. and R. DeMars, Purine requirements of cells cul-tured from humans affected with Lesch-Nyhan sydrome (hypoxan-thine-guanine phosphoribosyltransferase deficiency), Proc. Natl. Acad. Sci. US 62, 536-543, 1968.
5. Lesch, M. and W. L. Nyhan, A familial disorder of uric acid metabolism and central nervous system function, Am. J. Med. 36,561-570, 1964.
6. Nyhan, W. L., J. Pesek, L. Sweetman, D. G. Carpenter, and C. H. Carter, Genetics of an X-linked disorder of uric acid meta-bolism and cerebral function, Pediat. Res. 1, 5-13, 1967.
7. Balis, M. E., Enzymology and biochemistry B. Aspects of purine metabolism, Fed. Proc. 27, 1067-1073, 1968.
8. Kelley, N., Enzymology and biochemistry A. HG-PRT deficiency in the Lesch-Nyhan syndrome and gout, Fed. Proc. 27, 1047-1052, 1968.
9. Strauss, M., L. Lubbe, and E. Geissler, HG-PRT structural gene mutation in Lesch-Nyhan syndrome as indicated by antigenic activity and reversion of the enzyme deficiency, Hum. Genet. 57, 185-188, 1981.
10. Nyhan, W. L., Clinical features of the Lesch-Nyhan syndrome. Introduction - clinical and genetic features. Seminars on the Lesch-Nyhan syndrome, Fed. Proc. 27, 1027-1033, 1968.
11. Nyhan, W. L. Clinical features of the Lesch-Nyhan syndrome. Summary of clinical features. Seminars on the Lesch-Nyhan syndrome, Fed. Proc. 27, 1033-1041, 1968.
12. Henderson, J. F., W. N. Kelley, F. M. Rosenbloom and J. E. Seegmiller, Inheritance of purine phosphoribosyl transferase in man, Am. J. Hum. Genet. 21, 61-70, 1969.

13. Kelley, W. N., M. L. Green, F. M. Rosenbloom, J. E. Henderson and J. E. Miller, Review: HG-PRT deficincy in gout, Annals Int. Med. 70, 155-206, 1969.

14. Felix, J. S. and R. DeMars, Detection of females heterozygous for the Lesch-Nyhan mutation by 8-azaguanine resistant growth of cultured fibroblasts, J. Lab. Clin. Med. 27, 596-604, 1971.

15. Fujimoto, W. Y., J. H. Subak-Sherpe, and J. E. Seegmiller, HG-PRT deficiency: Clinical agents selective for mutant or normal cultured fibroblasts in mixed and heterozygous cultures, Proc. Natl. Acad. Sci. US 68, 1516-1519, 1971.

16. Goldstein, J. L., J. F. Marks, and S. M. Gartler, Expression of two X-linked genes in human hair follicles of double heterozygotes, Proc. Natl. Acad. Sci. 68, 1425-1427, 1971.

17. Nigam, B. R., V. M. Der Kaloustian, W. L. Nyhan, W. J. Young, and B. Childs, Hypoxanthine-guanine phosphoribosyltransferase deficiency: heterozygote has two clonal populations, Science 16, 425-427, 1968.

18. Rosenbloom, F. M., W. N. Kelley, J. F. Henderson, and J. E. Seegmiller, Lyon hypotehsis and X-linked disease, Lancet 2, 305-306, 1967.

19. Salzmann, J., R. DeMars, and L. Benke, Single allele expression at X-linked hyperuricemia locus in heterozygous human cells, Proc. Natl. Acad. Sci. 60, 545-552, 1968.

20. Lyon, M. G., Gene action in the X-chromosome of the mouse (Mus musculus L), Nature 190, 372, 1961.

21. Russell, L. B., Mammalian X-Chromosome action: inactivation limited in spread and in region of origin, Science 140, 976, 1963.

22. Nabholz, M., V. Miggiano, and W. Bodmer, Genetic analysis with human-mouse somatic cell hybrids, Nature 223, 358-363, 1969.

23. DeMars, R, Genetic studies of HG-PRT deficiency and the Lesch-Nyhan syndrome with cultured mammalian cells, Fed. Proc. 30, 944-945, 1971.

24. Szybalski, W., E. H. Szybalska, and G. Ragni, Genetic studies with human cell lines, Analytic Cell Culture. National Cancer Institute Monograph No. 7, 75-89, 1962.

25. Littlefield, J. M., The inosinic acid pyrophosphorylase activity of mouse fibroblasts partially resistant to 8-azaguanine, Proc. Natl. Acad. Sci. 50,568-576, 1963.

26. DeMars, R. and K. Held, The spontaneous azaguanine-resistant mutants of diploid human fibroblasts, Humangenetik 16, 87-110, 1972.

27. Maher, V. H., and J. E. Wessel, Mutations to azaguanine resistance in cultured diploid human fibroblasts by the carcinogen N-acetoxy-2-acetylamino fluorene, Mutation Res. 28, 277, 1975.

28. Burger, P. M. and J. W. I. H. Simons, Mutagenicity of 8-methoxypsoralen and long-wave ultraviolet irradiation in diploid human skin fibroblasts: An improved risk estimate in photochemotheraphy, Mutation Res. 63, 371-380, 1979.

29. Jacobs, L. and R. DeMars, Chemical mutagenesis with diploid human fibroblasts in, Handbook of Mutagenicity Test Procedures (B. Kilbey, ed.) Elsevier/N. Holland, Amsterdam, pp. 193-220, 1977.

30. Maher, V. M., L. M. Ouellette, R. D. Curren and J. J. McCormick, Frequency of ultraviolet light-induced mutations is higher in Xeroderma pigmentosum variant cells than in normal human cells, Nature 271, 593. 1976.

31. Chu, E. H. Y. and S. S. Powell, Selective systems in somatic cell genetics, in Advances in Human Genetics, Vol. 7 (Harris and Hirschhorn, eds.), Plenum Press, New York, Chapter 5, 1976.

32. Albertini, R. J. and R. DeMars, Mosaicism of peripheral blood lymphocyte populations in females heterozygous for the Lesch-Nyhan mutation, Biochem. Genet. 11, 397-411, 1974.

33. Strauss, G. H. anmd R. J. Albertini, 6-Thioguanine resistant lymphocytes in human peripheral blood, in Progress in Genetic Toxicology (D. Scott, B. A. Bridges and F.H. Sobels, eds.), Elsevier/N. Holland, New York, pp. 327-336, 1977.

34. Strauss, G. H. and R. J. Albertini, Enumeration of 6-thioguanine resistant peripheral blood lymphocytes in man as a potential test for somatic cell mutation arising in vivo, Mutation Res. 61, 353-379, 1979.

35. Strauss, G. H., R. J. Albertini, P. A. Krusinski, and R. D. Baughman, 6-thioguanine resistant peripheral blood lymphocytes in humans following psoralen long-range UV light therapy, J. Invest. Dermatol. 73, 211-216, 1979.

36. Albertini, R. J., Drug-resistant lymphocytes in man as indicators of somatic cell mutation, Teratogenesis, Carcinogenesis, and Mutagenesis 1, 25-48, 1980.

37. Atwood, K. C. and F. J. Petter, Erythrocyte automosacism in some persons of known genotype, Science 134, 210, 1961.

38. Stamatoyannopoulos, G., Possibilities for demonstrating point mutations in somatic cells, as illustrated by studies of mutant hemoglobins, in, Genetic Damage in Man Caused by Environmental Agents, (K. Berg, ed.) Academic Press, New York, p. 49, 1979.

39. Albertini, R. J., E. F. Allen, A. S. Quinn, and M. R. Albertini, Human somatic cell mutation: In vivo variant lymphocyte frequencies as determined by 6-thioguanine resistance, in Birth Defects Institute Symposium XI, (I. H. Porter and E. B. Hood, eds.) Academic Press, New York, In press.

40. Albertini, R. J., D. L. Sylwester, E. F. Allen, The 6-thioguanine resistant peripheral blood lymphocyte assay for direct mutagenicity testing in man, in Mutagenicity: From Bacteria to Man (J. A. Heddle, ed.), Academic Press, New York, In press.

41. Albertini, R. J. and E. F. Allen, Direct Mutagenicity Testing in Man, in Health Risk Analysis, (P. J. Walsh, C. R. Richmond, and E. D. Copenhaver, eds.) Franklin Institute Press, In press.

42. Gillis, S. M. M. Ferm, W. Ou, and K. A. Smith, T-cell growth
    factor: parameters of production and a quantitative micro-
    assay for activity, J. of Immunol. 120, 2027-2032, 1978.
43. Smith, K. A., T-cell growth factor, Immunol. Rev. 51, 337-357,
    1980.
44. Inouye, H, J. A. Hank, S. Chardonnens, M. Segall, B. J. Alter,
    and F. H. Bach, Cloned primed lymphocytes test reagents in the
    dissection of HLA-D, J. Exp. Med. 152, 143s, 1980.
45. Schendel, D. J. and R. Wank, Production of human T-cell growth
    factor, Human Immunology 2, 325, 1981.

GENETIC VS. NONGENETIC CHEMICAL CARCINOGENESIS AND RISK ASSESSMENT

Richard H. Reitz,
Alan M. Schumann,
Philip G. Watanabe,
Perry J. Gehring

Toxicology Research Laboratory
Dow Chemical USA
1803 Building
Midland, Michigan 48640
Oct. 15, 1981

INTRODUCTION

The fundamental goal of toxicological research is to provide a rational basis for recommending acceptably safe levels of human exposure to potentially harmful agents. Chemically induced cancer is a toxic response that has received primary attention in recent years. The potential lethality of cancer, its generally irreversible nature, and its long latent period have placed carcinogenesis in the forefront of public concern.

Some chemical carcinogens apparently act through direct alteration of DNA (by the induction of somatic mutations). This has led to the speculation that a single molecular event might influence the rate of cancer formation. Such a concept does not allow for the existence of an absolute threshold in carcinogens acting by this mechanism. However, considerations such as the multistage nature of chemical carcinogenesis, the existence of DNA repair systems, immune surveillance mechanisms, and the observation of threshold doses for other pathological responses support a possible

Please address all correspondence concerning this manuscript to:

Dr. Richard H. Reitz
1803 Building
Dow Chemical Co.
Midland, MI 48640
Tel. 517-636-5995

threshold for at least some carcinogenic agents (9). There has been, and continues to be, considerable debate on the subject of thresholds in carcinogenesis.

As important as this question is, it must be realized that the answer is experimentally inaccessible. The existence of a threshold can never be "proven" or "disproven" with a finite number of animals. A more practical question is: how can we make the best possible estimation of carcinogenic risk to human population from exposure to low levels of chemicals, given the data we do have?

The problem of extrapolating an experimentally observable carcinogenic response in laboratory animals to the expected response in humans at low exposure levels is graphically illustrated by Figure 1. The solid line represents the range of observable responses, which decrease with decreasing dose level. As the dose level is further decreased, the response diminishes until it virtually vanishes into the normal background incidence of the lesion. The broken lines of Fig. 1 represent the region into which it is necessary to extrapolate the observed response, and this region is likely to be many orders of magnitude below the observable range. The problem therefore is to choose a mathematical function which accurately predicts the behavior of the dose-response curve as a quantitative function of the dose level.

In order to gain some insight into the choice of models, let us examine what is known about the properties of various chemicals which can increase the incidence of cancer during chronic administration to laboratory animals (so-called "bioassays"). Although the initial assumption was that all such chemicals would probably possess very similar biological properties, it is becoming increasing clear that there are several distinct classes of chemical carcinogens. As pointed out by Weisburger and Williams (26) many of the chemicals which have been classified as carcinogens by bioassy in animals do not appear to interact with genetic material. Consequently, these authors have proposed the subdivision of chemicals into "genotoxic" and "non-genotoxic" classes, depending on whether the predominant mechanisms of carcinogenesis are genetic or epigenetic in nature.

Both genetic and epigenetic processes can lead to the induction of malignant tumors which shorten the lifespan of the affected species. However, although the end point of these processes is the same, there are important differences in their action, with profound implications for risk estimation. To understand why this is so, we need to understand something of how the living cell carries out its activities.

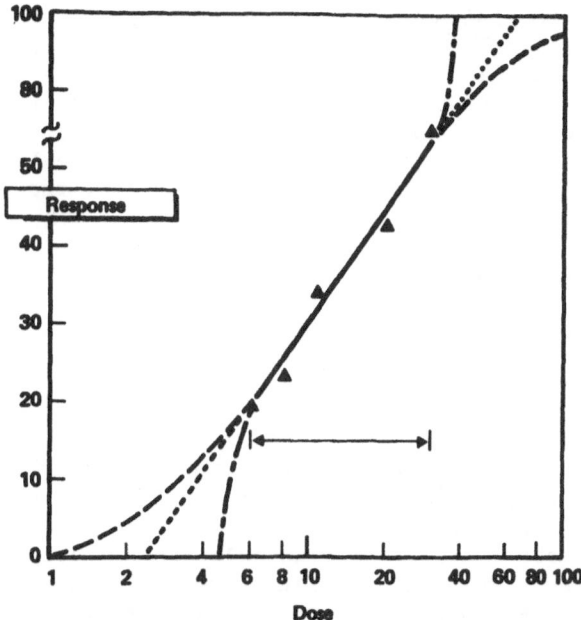

Fig. 1.   Typical Dose-Response Curve. The solid line represents
          the experimentally observable range of toxic response.
          The broken lines at low-dose levels show the region into
          which it is necessary to extrapolate the observed
          response.

        The amount of nuclear DNA in a cell is constant, but the
levels of RNA, protein and protein products vary. New molecules of
RNA, protein, and protein products are constantly being resynthe-
sized according to the instructions contained in DNA as the original molecules of RNA, protein, and enzyme products turn over.
Consequently, destruction of a small portion of the nongenetic
components of the cell has little consequence for the cell since it
is continually replacing those components anyway. Thus there is
very likely to be a threshold in the toxic action of agents acting
through epigenetic mechanisms. That threshold exists in the region
where the rate of destruction of epigenetic components begins to
exceed the rate of their formation. Thus while chemicals acting
through predominantly epigenetic mechanisms can induce cancer at
high doses, one would expect a threshold for the carcinogenicity of
such chemicals at lower doses.

        In contrast, nuclear DNA is not being constantly resynthesiz-
ed. If it is damaged by the action of a toxic chemical, it must be
repaired. Failure to repair the nuclear DNA before cell division
can lead to permanently altered daughter cells which have altered
properties, such as the failure to respond to normal growth
regulation (i.e. cancer).

Therefore, a finite amount of risk is probably associated with exposure to any level of a genotoxic agent. However, the risk from exposure to low levels of such chemicals is probably much less than simple linear extrapolation would indicate because of nonlinearities in DNA repair or pharmacokinetics (9, 10, 19). Consequently, the first step in any risk extrapolation for chemical carcinogenesis should be an attempt to determine whether the predominant mechanisms are genetic or epigenetic in nature.

Experimental Determination of Tumor Mechanisms

Genetic Mechanisms. The genetic mechanism is most simply described as the covalent alteration of sensitive sites in DNA by the test chemical so as to alter the information content of the DNA in a cell.

A number of in vitro systems have been utilized to detect mutagenic (and hence, presumably carcinogenic) potential in test agents. Perhaps the best known of these is the "Ames" test. In this test, materials are mixed with cultures of special strains of bacteria. These strains are unable to multiply in the absence of histidine unless a mutation occurs. These bacteria have been specially selected for their permeability to foreign chemicals. In addition, these bacteria have been altered so that they have lost the ability to repair certain types of DNA damage with DNA repair systems. This system is particularly useful for screening large numbers of chemicals in a short time.

Another in vitro system that has enjoyed considerable popularity is the procedure for measuring unscheduled DNA synthesis (UDS) in rat liver cells growing in tissue culture. This system was developed by Dr. Gary Williams and is based on the fact that DNA synthesis normally does not occur in the nucleus of a cell unless that cell is undergoing division. Consequently the incorporation of 3H-thymidine (a specific precursor of DNA) in cells not undergoing division is an indication that DNA damage has occurred and is being removed by DNA repair systems. This procedure also can be used to screen a large number of chemicals and has the further advantage of giving an endpoint in mammalian rather than bacterial cells.

Additional in vitro systems to indicate mutagenicity include tests such as mutagenicity in Chinese hamster ovary cells and differential killing of DNA repair-deficient E. coli.

In vivo systems for indicating mutagenicity are considerably more complex. Frequently it is as expensive and time-consuming to measure mutagenicity in animals as it is to determine carcinogenicity in animals.

However, Lutz (13) has suggested that the extent of covalent binding of chemicals to DNA in vivo can serve as at least a rough indicator of their potential for genotoxicity. There are many sites where chemicals could bind to DNA, and not all of these would be expected to be equally effective in inducing mutations. Nevertheless, as indicated in Table 1, there appears to be a reasonable correlation between the ability of genotoxic chemicals to bind to DNA in vivo and their potency as carcinogens (13).

An alternate way of measuring genotoxicity in vivo involves the determination of the extent of DNA repair taking place in various organs after exposure to test agents. In this procedure, normal DNA replication is halted by the administration of hydroxyurea, and the amount of DNA repair occurring in response to previous DNA damage is estimated by administering 3H-thymidine.

Epigenetic Mechanisms. As outlined by Weisburger and Williams (26) there are a variety of epigenetic processes which can influence the tumor incidence during an animal bioassay. One such process is the production of recurrent cytotoxicity with concurrent cell death and subsequent cellular regeneration (20, 25). This process is frequently encountered in animal bioassays were maximally "tolerated" doses of chemical are administered in order to increase the chances of detecting a carcinogenic response.

During chronic administration of cytotoxic doses, DNA replication is stimulated in the affected tissues. Since there is a tiny, but still finite chance for error in each replication system, the net effect may be to increase the spontaneous mutation rate and ultimately affect the tumorigenic process.

Another consequence of increasing cell division is that the relative rates of DNA repair and DNA replication are altered. This may be very important because there is evidence that the existing DNA repair systems may fail to recognize DNA alterations once the altered DNA has been copied during replication. Consequently, repair becomes less effective in protecting cells from the consequences of genetic damage after cellular replication. This is shown by the work of Berman et al. (4) who found that momentarily arresting cell division to give added time for DNA repair greatly diminished the mutational action of UV light.

These data stress the role that normal DNA synthesis (occurring during cellular regeneration) plays in converting initially repair-sensitive lesions in DNA into permanent, non-repairable lesions (i.e. mutations).

In vivo correlates of this phenomenon include the report by Belmain and Troll (2) that the inhibition of epidermal hyperplasia by dexamethosone also prevented the tumor-promoting activity of

croton oil in mice. Laroye (12) commented on the frequency with
which tumors arise in chronically inflamed or scarred tissue, and
Berenblum (3) reported the dramatic enhancement of some genetic
carcinogens by the repeated production of physical trauma at the
site of initiation.

Consequently, it has proven vital to determine whether chronic
cellular regeneration is occurring in the target organs during the
bioassay. This may be accomplished by light microscopic examination of various tissues by qualified pathologists. In addition,
the rates of normal (nonrepair) DNA synthesis in organs of treated
and control animals may be established by administration of 3H-
thymidine to animals after exposure to test chemicals.

Specific Examples

In order to demonstrate the principles employed in classifying
chemicals as either predominantly genetic or epigenetic, several
chemicals will be discussed.

Chronic administration of chloroform (by gavage in corn oil)
has been reported to produce hepatocellular tumors in male and
female mice. This agent also produces kidney tumors in male rats
(15).

Similarly, gavage with perchloroethylene (PERC) caused the
development of hepatocellular cancer in mice (16). No tumors were
reported in rats in this study, nor was PERC tumorigenic to rats in
the inhalation study reported by Rampy et al. (18).

Sodium orthophenylphenol (SOPP) has been reported to include
bladder tumors in rats when high levels were present in the diet
(11).

For comparative purposes, dimethylnitrosamine (DMN) will also
be discussed. DMN is a potent genotoxic carcinogen and causes
tumors in a variety of species and sites, including hepatocellular
carcinoma in mice.

In Vitro Results. All four of the selected chemicals have been
tested in the "Ames" test (bacterial mutagenicity in Salmonella
typhimurium). DMN is positive (McCann et al., 1975) but chloroform
(5, 24), PERC (1) and SOPP (7) are all negative in this test.

In addition, DMN has been reported to include mutations in
cells from Chinese hamster ovaries (17).

Chloroform was included in a battery of 42 chemicals selected
for evaluating short term tests for carcinogenesis (8). Conse-

quently, extensive information has been gathered on this chemical. In addition to the negative results in the Ames test, chloroform failed to exhibit differential killing in DNA repair-deficient E. coli, was negative in 6 of 8 yeast assays, and failed to produce unscheduled DNA synthesis, cell transformation, or sister chromatid exchange in a variety of in vitro mammalian cell assays (6).

Toxicity. Chloroform is a strong hepatotoxin in mice at the doses which resulted in tumor formation. Doses of SOPP sufficient to produce urinary tract tumors also induced haematuria in rats. PERC induced hepatocellular swelling in mice when administered at tumorigenic levels.

DMN produces both liver toxicity and tumors at high doses. Lower doses of DMN produce liver tumors but do not produce concurrent liver toxicity (21). In contrast, tumors were not observed after any dose of chloroform, SOPP, or PERC which did not also produce measurable toxicity.

In Vivo Indicators of Mechanisms: DNA Alkylation. Several studies were carried out with these chemicals to determine the degree of DNA alkylation they produced. Since radioactivity covalently bound to DNA served as an indicator of the amount of DNA damage, it was important to eliminate the possibility that some of this radioactivity might have arisen from macromolecules other than DNA. Consequently, the DNA preparations were analyzed for RNA, glycogen, and protein. The final isolates always contained less than 2% RNA, 1% protein, or 1% glycogen by weight. The high purity of the DNA preparations makes it unlikely that contamination was responsible for the radioactivity observed. However, it must be remembered that metabolism of the labeled chemicals in the animals may have produced radioactive fragments in the C-1 pool. Some of the radioactivity in the purified DNA may have arisen from biosynthesis of normal DNA bases rather than alkylation.

Values obtained for the four chemicals studied (as well as alkylation values obtained by other investigators) are summarized in Table 1. For ease of comparison, all values were converted to units of micromoles of chemical bound per mole of DNA when animals were administered a "standard" doses of 1 millimole of test chemical/kg. This calculation produces a Chemical Binding Index (CBI) as suggested by Lutz (13).

The level of DNA alkylation produced by the GENOTOXIC chemicals in Table 1 corresponds roughly to their carcinogenic potency. However, although high frequencies of tumors were observed in the animals exposed to high doses of chloroform, SOPP, and PERC, these materials did not produce appreciable alkylation of

Table 1. Chemical Binding Indexes (CBI) for Binding of Various
Chemicals to DNA In Vivo at a Standard Dose of 1 Millimole
per Kg According to Lutz (13)

Potency Rating	Micromole Chemical/Mole DNA
Strong:	
Aflatoxin	17,000 *
Dimethylnitrosamine	6,000 *
Dimethylnitrosamine	7,430 **
Moderate:	
2-Acetylaminofluorene	560 *
O-Aminoazotoluene	230 *
Weak:	
Urethane	29-90 *
4-Dimethylaminoazobenzene	6 *
Experimental Results for Selected Chemicals	
Chloroform	1.5 (Det. Limit=1)**
Sodium orthophenylphenol	0.0 (Det. Limit=0.3)**
Perchloroethylene	0.0 (Det. Limit=10)**

*Data from Lutz (13)
**Data gathered in Dow Laboratories

DNA. Instead, no alkylation at all was detected for SOPP or PERC,
and the alkylation reported for chloroform was barely above the
detection limit. (The "alkylation" reported for chloroform is an
upper limit and may represent a tiny amount of C-1 incorporation
into normal bases of DNA rather than actual alkylation.) DMN was
reported to have had a CBI of 6,000 (13) and the value from our
laboratory for DMN (CBI = 7,430) was in excellent agreement with
this report (Table 1).

In Vivo Indicators of Mechanisms: DNA Repair. In addition to
the determination of DNA alkylation in vivo, a second procedure was
employed to measure the extent of DNA repair synthesis occurring
after chemical treatment. Replicative DNA synthesis and DNA-repair
synthesis both incorporate the precursor 3H-thymidine into DNA.
Ordinarily, the level of replicative DNA synthesis is such that it
is very difficult to detect DNA-repair synthesis. However, when
hydroxyurea (HU) was co-administered with 3H-thymidine, replicative
synthesis was selectively inhibited. This allows the detection of
DNA repair synthesis as outlined by Reitz et al. (20). When chloroform and DMN were compared for their ability to induce DNA repair
synthesis a dramatic difference was seen. DMN treatment caused a
dramatic increase in the level of HU-resistant 3H-thymidine uptake

(Figure 2). DNA repair synthesis (calculated as outlined in Ref. 20) was elevated more than sevenfold at the highest dose of DMN (20 mg/kg) and declined in a dose-related fashion. In contrast, DNA repair synthesis was less than control in the liver of male B6C3F1 mice receiving the tumorigenic dose of 240 mg/kg chloroform (Figure 2). These results indicate a major difference in the ability of the two chemicals to induce genetic damage recognizable by the DNA repair systems.

In Vivo Indicators of Mechanisms: Histopathology. Chloroform produced severe tissue damage after administration of doses that were carcinogenic in long-term bioassays. This damage occurred in the same organs in which tumors later developed. For example, administration of 277 or 138 mg/kg/day of chloroform produced liver tumors in male B6C3F1 mice (15), but 60 or 15 mg/kg/day of chloroform did not induce liver tumors in four strains of mice used in another study (22). Examination of the livers of mice 48 hrs after a single dose of chloroform indicated that tissue damage was present after 240 but was minimal or absent after 60 or 15 mg/kg (Table 2). Similarly, a small excess of kidney tumors were observed after administration of 60/mg/kg/day of chloroform in one strain of mouse, but kidney tumors were not observed after 15 mg/kg/day of chloroform (22). Again, examination of the mouse tissues indicated that extensive damage had occurred in the kidney after single doses of 240 and 60 mg/kg of chloroform, but was absent following a dose of 15 mg/kg.

Bladder tissue from rats consuming a diet containing 2% by weight SOPP was examined by light microscopy. These tissue sections indicated that a hyperplastic response occurred as early as 3 days. Additional samples were examined at 7, 14, 30, 60 and 90 days. Piling up of epithelial cells increased with the length of time on the diet. Necrosis of bladder cells was not detected.

After gavage with PERC, an accentuated lobular pattern with hepatocellular swelling was observed in mice receiving 100, 250, 500 or 1000 mg/kg/day (23). These tissues were also characterized by altered cytoplasmic staining, microvesiculation, and microvacuolation of the cytoplasm in the centrilobular region. Similar changes were not seen in rats after gavage with PERC, and this species specificity correlates with the report that rats did not develop tumors after chronic administration of PERC.

In Vivo Indicators of Mechanisms: Cellular Regeneration. Cytotoxicity, if sufficient to cause cell death, is generally followed by regeneration of cells within the affected organ. This regeneration may be readily demonstrated in animals by administration of 3H-thymidine, an intermediate in DNA synthesis. 18-48 hrs after chemical treatment, an i.p. injection of 3H-thymidine was given to groups of treated and control animals. This procedure

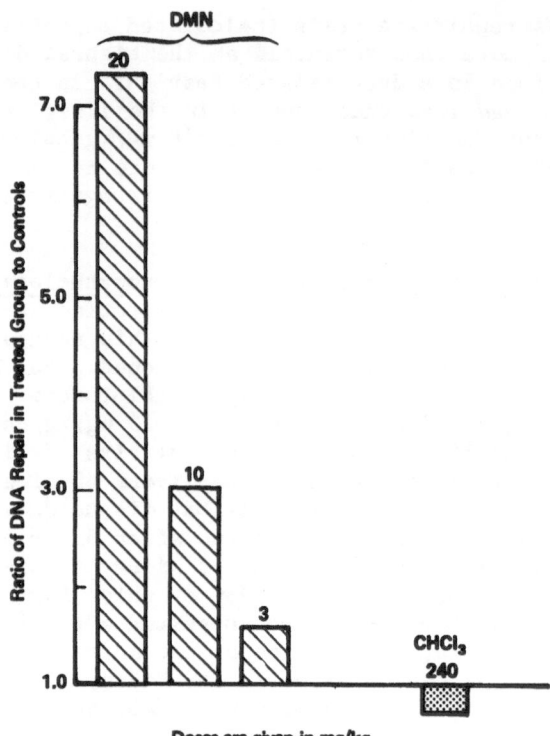

Fig. 2.   DNA Repair in the Liver of Male B6C3F1 Mice Treated with
          Dimethylnitrosamine (DMN) at 20, 10, and 3 mg/kg ip or
          Gavaged with Chloroform at 240 mg/kg. A value of 1.0
          indicates no hydroxyurea resistant 3H-thymidine in excess
          of that expected (i.e. no DNA repair is detected).

differs from that used to measure DNA repair synthesis in two
important respects:

    1.   Hydroxyurea is not used to suppress normal DNA replica-
         tion.

    2.   3H-Thymidine is injected 18-48 hrs after the event
         suspected of causing tissue damage so as to catch the
         cells during the regeneration phase.

     The results of these experiments are summarized in Table 3.
Chloroform induced severe tissue damage, and this is reflected in
the 14 and 25 fold increase in cellular regeneration observed in
the liver and kidney respectively (21).   SOPP induced cellular
hyperplasia in the bladder, and this is reflected in the 2.5 fold
increase in DNA synthesis in the bladders of rats gavaged with 500
mg/kg SOPP (Table 3).

Table 2. Histopathology in Tissues of B6C3F1 Male Mice 48 hr After a Single Gavage Dosage of Chloroform (number of animals affected/number of animals examined)

MICROSCOPIC OBSERVATION	DOSE OF CHLOROFORM (mg/kg)			
	0	15	60	240
Liver				
Individual Hepatocellular Necrosis;				
Inflammatory Cell Infiltration	0/2	0/2	0/2	2/2
Increased Mitosis	0/2	0/2	0/2	2/2
Centralobular Hepatocellular Swelling	0/2	0/2	0/2	2/2
Kidney				
No microscopic changes observable	2/2	2/2	0/2	0/2
Severe diffuse Renal Cortical Necrosis	0/2	0/2	0/2	2/2
Focal Tublar Epithelial Regeneration;				
Corticomedullary Junction	0/2	0/2	2/2	2/2

Similarly, mice gavaged with PERC showed about 2 fold more DNA synthesis than comparable controls (23). It is noteworthy that DNA synthesis was not stimulated in rats gavaged with PERC, and again, this correlates with the failure to observe tumors in rats during the NCI bioassay of PERC. All of these increases were statistically significant at the $p = 0.05$ level (Student's t-test).

In contrast, treatment with a carcinogenic level of DMN (3 mg/kg, i.p.) produced a minimal increase in DNA synthesis (1.14 fold) and this increase was not statistically significant.

CONCLUSION

The experiments described above indicate that genotoxicity produced by agents such as DMN can be readily detected by these types of experimental procedures. However, the results of these experiments are inconsistent with a genotoxic mechanism for induction of tumors following administration of chloroform, SOPP, or PERC. Instead, a pronounced increase in cellular division is produced by each of these agents. This increased division is well correlated with the sensitivity of various organs and species to the tumorigenicity of chloroform, SOPP, and PERC.

Consequently, although exposure to small amounts of DMN may be associated with some finite level of carcinogenic risk, exposure to levels of chloroform, SOPP, or PERC below the cytotoxic threshold should not pose any significant cancer risk.

Table 3. Ratio of Cellular Regeneration (as Measured by
         Incorporation of 3H-Thymidine) in Treated and Control
         Animals After Single Exposure to Chloroform, SOPP, or
         Following Multiple Exposures to PERC

Chemical (Dose)	Liver	Kidney	Bladder
Chloroform (240 mg/kg, po)	14.0	24.8	*
Chloroform (60 mg/kg, po)	2.2	8.2	*
Chloroform (15 mg/kg, po)	0.94	0.79	*
SOPP (500 mg/kg, po)	*	*	2.5
PERC (500 mg/kg, po, 11 doses in 11 days)	1.9	*	*

* Ratio not determined.

The experiments described here are relatively straightforward
to conduct. They provide an objective method for dividing
suspected carcinogens into two classes: (1) those with a significant potential to cause genetic damage and (2) those which apparently lack such potential. Once such a distinction has been made,
it becomes possible to make some intelligent guesses as to which of
the multitude of "suspected carcinogens" actually pose the greatest
risk to human populations. Our limited resources can then be directed to where they will do the most good in removing hazardous
substances from our environment.

REFERENCES

1. Bartsch, H., C. Malaveille, A. Barbin, and G. Planche (1979)
   Mutagenic and alkylating metabolites of halo-ethylenes, chlor-
   obutadienes, and dichlorobutenes by rodent or human liver
   tissues. Arch. Toxicol., 41, 249-277.
2. Belmain, S. and W. Troll (1972) The inhibition of croton oil-
   promoted mouse skin tumorigenesis by steroid hormones. Cancer
   Research 32, 450.
3. Berenblum, I. (1944) Irritation and carcinogenesis. Arch.
   Pathol., 38, 233-244.
4. Berman, J. J., C. Tong, and G. M. Williams (1978) Enhancement
   of mutagenesis during cell replication of cultured liver epithelial cells. Cancer Letters, 4, 277-283.

5. Bridges, B. A., E. Zeiger, and D. B. McGregor (1981) Summary report on the performance of bacterial mutation assays. Prog. Mutation Res., 1, 49-67.

6. Brookes, P. and R. J. Preston (1981) Summary report on the performance in in vitro mammalian assays. Prog. Mutation Res., 1, 77-85.

7. Brusick, D. (1976) Mutagenicity evaluation of orthophenyl-phenol: Final report. Submitted to Dow Chemical USA Ag-Organ-ics Department by Litton Bionetics, Inc., 5516 Nicholson Lane, Kensington, Maryland 20795 as LBI Project No. 2547 (March 31).

8. de Serres, F. J. and J. Ashby, (1981) Selection, preparation and purity of the test chemicals. Prog. Mutation Res., 1, 8-15.

9. Gehring, P. J. and G. E. Blau (1977) "Mechanisms of Carcin-ogenesis: Dose Response" J. Environ. Path. Toxicol., 1, 163-179.

10. Gehring, P. J., P. G. Watanabe, and G. E. Blau (1979) "Risk Assessment of Environmental Carcinogens Utilizing Pharmaco-kinetic Parameters" Annals of the N. Y. Acad. Science, 329, 137-152.

11. Hiraga, K. and T. Fujii (1981) Inductions of tumors of the urinary system in F344 rats by dietary administration of so-dium o-phenylphenate. Food Cosmet. Toxicol., 19, 303-310.

12. Laroye, G. J., (1974) How efficient is immunological sur-veillance against cancer and why does it fail? The Lancet, 1097-1100.

13. Lutz, W. K. (1979) In vivo covalent binding of organic chem-icals to DNA as a quantitative indicator in the process of chemical carcinogenesis. Mutation Research 65, 289-356.

14. Maher, V. M., J. D. Dorney, A. L. Medrala, B. Konze-Thomas, and J. J. McCormick (1979) DNA excision repair processes in human cells can eliminate the cytotoxic and mutagenic conse-quences of ultraviolet irradiation. Mutation Research, 62, 311-323.

15. National Cancer Institute (1976) Carcinogenesis bioassay of chloroform. Nat. Tch. Inf. Service No. PB264018/AS, Bethesda, Maryland, USA (March 1).

16. National Cancer Institute (1977) Bioassay of Tetrachloro-ethylene for possible carcinogenicity. DHEW Publication No. 77-805 Bethesday, Maryland USA.

17. O'Neill, J. P., D. B. Couch, R. Machanoff, J. R. San Sebastian, P. A. Brimer, and A. W. Hsie (1977) A quantita-tive assay of mutation induction at the hypoxanthine-guanine phosphoribosyl transferase locus in Chinese Hamster Ovary cells (CHO/HGPRT system): Utilization with a variety of muta-genic agents. Mutation Res. 45, 103-109.

18. Rampy, L. W., J. F. Quast, B. K. J. Leong, and P. J. Gehring (1978) Results of long-term inhalation toxicity studies on rats of 1,1,1-trichloroethane and perchloroethylene formula-tions. In: Proceedings of the First International Congress on Toxicology (G. L. Plaa and W. A. M. Duncan, eds.) Academic Press, New York.

19. Ramsey, J. C. and R. H. Reitz (1981) "Pharmacokinetics and
     Threshold Concepts" In: The Pesticide Chemist and Modern
     Toxicology (Bandal et al,, ed.) ACS Symposium Series, Pub-
     lished by American Chemical Society, Washington, DC, USA.
20. Reitz, R. H., P. G. Watanabe, M. J. McKenna, J. F. Quast, and
     P. J. Gehring (1980a) Effects of vinylidene chloride on DNA
     synthesis and DNA repair in the rat and mouse; A comparative
     study with dimethylnitrosamine. Toxicol. Appl. Pharmacol.,
     52, 357-370.
21. Reitz, R. H., J. F. Quast, W. T. Stott, P. G. Watanabe, and P.
     J. Gehring (1980b) Pharmacokinetics and macromolecular ef-
     fects of chloroform in rats and mice: Imlications for carcin-
     ogenic risk estimation. In: Water Chlorination: Environmental
     Impact and Health Effects (Jolley et al., eds.) Ann Arbor
     Science Publishers, Inc., Ann Arbor, Michigan 48106.
22. Roe, F. J. C., A. K. Palmer, A. N. Worden (1979) Safety evalu-
     ation of toothpaste containing chloroform I. Long-term
     studies in mice. J. Environ. Pathol. Toxicol., 2, 799-819.
23. Schumann, A. M., J. F. Quast, and P. G. Watanabe (1980) The
     pharmacokinetics and macromolecular interactions of perchloro-
     ethylene in mice and rats as related to oncogenicity.
     Toxicol. Appl. Pharmacol., 55, 207-219.
24. Uehleke, H., T. Werner, H. Greim, and M. Kramer (1977) Meta-
     bolic activation of haloalkanes and tests in vitro for muta-
     genicity. Xenobiotica 7, 393.
25. Watanabe, P. G., R. H. Reitz, A. M. Schumann, M. J. McKenna,
     J. F. Quast, and P. J. Gehring (1980) Implications of the
     mechanisms of tumorigenicity for risk assessment. In: The
     Scientific Basis of Toxicity Assessment (H. Witschi, ed).
     Elsevier/North-Holland Biomedical Press, Amsterdam, The
     Netherlands.
26. Weisburger, J. H. and G. M. Williams (1980) In: Toxicology,
     the Basic Science of Poisons, (Doull et al., ed.) 2nd Ed.
     pp. 84-138, Macmillian Publishing Co., Inc., New York.

AN OVERVIEW OF REGULATORY RESPONSIBILITIES

Burke K. Zimmerman

George Washington University
Washington, DC 20052

A PRIMER ON REGULATORY LAW

Much confusion and misunderstanding of regulations, particularly those concerned with health and safety and the protection of the environment, has resulted from the fact that most laymen, and particularly scientists, do not really understand the structure of the laws that mandate such regulations. Their constitutional basis and distinction between the roles of the Executive, Legislative, and Judicial branches of government in enacting and implementing these laws must be appreciated by those who would take part in shaping such regulations.

Any Federal law must be passed by the Congress as authorized by one or more provisions of the Constitution and so creates an administrative authority within the Executive branch of the Federal government. The law may specify certain requirements explicitly or establish powers and duties to be carried out by an executive agency or department. The authorities so created may have a specified time limit, and may be amended by the Congress at any time with new legislation.

The laws which created the various Federal health regulatory agencies were passed in response to a growing body of data that an array of deleterious agents, mostly chemicals and industrial pollutants, were finding their way into the atmosphere, and our food and water supplies, and posing direct threats to human health, wildlife, and the environment in general. The regulatory laws create the legal means necessary to control them, by granting the authority to promulgate appropriate regulations to a new or exisiting Federal agency.

The first section of most regulatory bills introduced in Congress is usually called "Findings". The Findings usually appear to state the rationale for legislation or regulation, and may include what seem to be editorial opinions, value judgments, etc. The only legal purpose that this section serves, however, is to establish the constitutionality of the proposed legislation. Thus, a properly written bill will include an argument why such regulation is appropriate under the Constitution. Most health and environmental regulatory laws cite the powers granted to Congress by the Constitution pertaining to matters which affect interstate commerce. Other statements may be disregarded, as they would be by a court deciding the constitutionality of the law. The Findings appear in the public law, the version of the bill signed by the President, but once the law is codified (becomes included in the United States Code), the findings are not included, nor can they be found in any compilations of health or environmental law. Laymen often attach undue importance to the Findings of introduced bills.

Of far greater importance is the section of the law concerned with the definitions of terms, generally appearing near the beginning of a bill. The Definitions are thought by some to be of a perfunctory nature, while, in fact, the outcome of a challenge to the law in court may well depend upon precisely how terms such as "safe", "risk", "injury", "hazardous", "adequate", "toxic", "person", etc., are defined.

Closely associated with the definitions are the regulatory standards themselves. While "what" is to be regulated (or "whom") must be explicitly stated, the standards deal with "how" or the criteria according to which regulations will be applied. The legislative or regulatory standards, along with the definitions which back them up, are probably the most important provisions of regulatory laws. The precise way in which the standards are set forth and defined are absolutely crucial to the effectiveness of any regulatory law.

The standards instruct the administrative officer of the regulatory agency whether to set ambient environmental tolerances of toxic substances (e.g., the ambient air quality standards required by the Clean Air Act) or to control the sources of pollutants (such as the authority under the Federal Water Pollution Control Act to set standards for point source emissions). They further specify whether these standards should be based purely upon health risks, and if so, how, or whether other factors should be considered as well, such as costs, benefits, or "best available technology". Thus our regulatory laws are replete with phrases like "unreasonable risk of injury", "adequate protection of health or the environment", "safe under conditions of use", "ample margin of safety", and "shown to cause cancer in animals or man". The last term is an example of a very explicit standard, the basis of the so-called

Delaney clause for food additives. Others allow for considerable
latitude of interpretation, and administrative discretion. Discretion, however, is a double edged sword, which may be used either to
enable a wise and just administrator to adapt regulatory solutions
to the particulars of a given situation, or to permit political
bias and coercion to cloud what should be an objective and rational
process.

      Some of the terms used in such laws are accompanied by lengthy
explanations and interpretations in the legislative history (committee reports, floor debates, conference reports, etc., which
interpret the bills during the legislative process), or have an
extensive history of interpretation in the courts. These are often
called "terms of art", in that their use implies a particular
meaning and interpretation. At times, however, Congress deliberately writes ambiguity into the law, intending the agency to have
a degree of administrative discretion. Of course, additional criteria defining the limits of that discretion may also be included.

      At the opposite end of the spectrum from the specificity of
the Delaney clause are standards like "balance the risks against
the benefits." Regulatory standards based upon incomparable and
subjective values are essentially impossible to define precisely,
and thus are subject to vastly differing interpretations. Even a
requirement to "balance health risks against health benefits" is
essentially calling for an unquantifiable equation. While such
highly open standards may appeal to the legally naive as being the
most flexible way to regulate, the vagueness they impart to the law
only invites litigation and the intrusion of politics, especially
if the object of regulation is a controversial substance, such as
saccharin, 2,4,5,-T, or nitrite. For no matter how the substances
were to be regulated, it can be argued that clearly all the benefits were not taken into account, or that they were far over estimated. If there also exists scientific uncertainty as to the magnitude of the risk presented, as is usually the case, then the
regulatory problems under undefined standards are severe. For
these reasons, the environmental groups have generally lobbied for
more precisely defined standards, while the chemical industry has
fought for the inclusion of costs and benefits in the decision
making process. There is at present no consistency among the
several statutes specifying regulatory standards pertaining to
health or environmental issues.

      In addition to standards and criteria for regulation, every
regulatory law must have certain administrative provisions. These
give an agency the legal authority to act and enforce regulations,
as well as guarantee proper "due process" to citizens and the regulated entities, both in the writing of regulations and in their
implementation.

The Administrative Procedure Act sets forth the process to be followed in the writing of Federal regulations or other administrative practices dealing with rulemaking. Full fledged regulations take approximately one and a half years to promulgate. Public comment periods are required for all such proposed action and provisions are made for hearings, if desired, as well as other mechanisms to ensure fairness and allow any parties affected by the action to have their views taken into account by the agency. Sometimes a law will specify other types of rulemaking, such as "by rule" or "by order on the record." These shorter procedures are usually intended to be used where controversy and challenge is not anticipated.

Other important provisions set forth in regulatory laws concern judicial proceedings. They may specify the level of court in which appeals must first be heard, or define who has standing to sue the government. The Clean Air Act, as amended in 1971, for example, included a precedent setting provision guaranteeing citizens the right to sue the government.

The enforcement of regulations is dependent upon the legislative authority being given the administrative agency to monitor the implementation of regulations, usually through inspection authority. In addition, licensing or registration mechanisms may also be required, both to keep track of who is doing what and to establish the legal basis for prosecution by the government. Thus, the pesticide laws require that each be registered with the Environmental Protection Agency and the label specify instructions for use which will prevent harm to either the user or the environment. The burden of proof of such safe use is on the manufacturer.

Many regulatory laws include a "whistleblowing" provision, which protects the rights of workers to report violations of the laws by their employers. These sections sometimes require that an employer who fires someone for being a good citizen not only will have to restore all lost wages and compensation to the individual, but pay punitive damages as well.

The right to impose penalties for violators must also be established in regulatory laws. These may take many forms, such as license revokation or cancellation of registration, civil or criminal penalties, usually fines, specified as a maximum amount for each day of the violation, or prison sentences. The administrator may levy fines without going to court in some cases. But any criminal proceedings must be handled through the Federal courts, with the United States bringing suit against the particular violater, and the judge determining the nature of the penalty, the limits of which are specified by statute.

Because some regulatory laws require companies to submit to a Federal agency information on a product which may be considered proprietary, special sections may be included to protect against the disclosure of such information. This is a particular concern of the pharmaceutical industry with respect to the drug laws. The Freedom of Information Act (FOIA) specifically states that an agency administrator is not required to disclose any proprietary information under a FOIA request. However, companies are at times concerned that there is no prohibition against disclosure under the FOIA. Another Federal law makes it a criminal offense for any Federal employee to disclose a trade secret.

A final provision that is included in a number of laws pertains to the relationship of the Federal law to state and local laws. In the absence of an explicit provision stating whether or not the Federal law supercedes any state and local laws or whether a state may enact stricter legislation of its own, the law is unclear; there is no well defined legal or Constitutional precedent. In regulatory situations concerning toxic agents, the power of the Congress to regulate matters involved in interstate commerce may be in conflict with the powers guaranteed the states to have jurisdiction over purely internal matters. Thus, if Federal-State conflicts are anticipated, it is best to specify the intent of Congress in statute, subject, of course, to challenges in court on constitutional grounds. Thus, the Clean Air Act permits the stricter performance standards of the State of California.

HISTORICAL PERSPECTIVE

As we emerged from World War II, rapid economic growth and development, along with a preoccupation with technological innovation, dominated the United States and most of those countries involved in the war, whether victors or vanquished. Of particular relevance to this symposium was the chemical revolution, in which thousands of new chemical products - plastics, synthetic fibers, pesticides, antibiotics, drugs, detergents, etc. - gave new meaning to organic chemistry and changed our lives in significant ways.

The mood of the country in those days was generally optimistic; most people were too taken with the fruits of technological "progress" to foresee the dark and more insidious side of better living through chemistry. Although the air in cities and industrial areas began to smell more and more unpleasant, and some anomalous disturbances in fish populations of the Great Lakes and the peregrine falcon in the Northeast were noted, it took many years for the effects of the widespread and indiscriminate use of chemicals to be fully appreciated, even though a considerable body of literature concerning the carcinogenic and other toxic effects of such agents had been accumulating for many years.

The first demonstration of chemical carcinogenesis was reported in 1775 (1). However, the induction of cancer in animals
was not investigated in a systematic way until well into the
twentieth century. By the early 1950's, much was known about the
potential of certain classes of chemicals and ionizing radiation to
induce cancer, both in experimental animals and in humans
(2,3,4). Some epidemiological studies had concluded that lung
cancer was linked to cigarette smoking (5). And even though the
structure of DNA was just being elucidated, it was known that mutations could be induced both by radiation and particular chemical
agents. Thirty years ago, however, there was still little appreciation of the statistical nature of the effects on a population of
low levels of a carcinogen or mutagen, or the fact that the appearance of harmful effects might require as much as twenty years
following the exposure to such an agent. Many scientists believed
that threshold or "safe" levels of carcinogenic or mutagenic substances could exist, and, indeed, there was no good evidence to
prove them wrong.

Early Regulatory Legislation: 1906-1969

Federal authority to regulate toxic agents accumulated rather
slowly and sporadically between the beginning of the twentieth
century and the early 1950's. Virtually all of the early laws were
rather specifically directed and concerned with acute hazards and
toxicity. In 1906, Congress passed the first comprehensive Food
and Drug Act, replacing, under the Constitutional authority to
regulate interstate commerce, a number of inconsistent state laws
and the few rather specific Federal laws which preceded it. The
sections concerning food were generally concerned with adulterated
and misbranded foods. However, the 1906 law did include the predecessor to the very useful general safety clause governing food
additives, but the burden of proof that a substance was injurious
rested with the government. In 1938, the food and drug laws underwent substantial revisions to include premarket testing of new
drugs for safety. Specific amendments were added during the 1940's
pertaining to insulin, penicillin, and finally to antibiotics
generally.

Because of the rapid advances in pesticide development during
World War II and their greatly increased use in agriculture
following the war, Congress passed the Federal Insecticide, Fungicide and Rodenticide Act in 1947. However, the regulatory authority created by this act was limited to the licensing of pesticide
products intended for interstate shipments. The law required adequate labeling directions for safe use and imposed penalties when
improperly labeled or adulterated products were shipped across
state borders. This law thus had many obvious shortcomings. The
only means available to the U.S. Department of Agriculture (USDA)
to control pesticides was to cancel registration, a lengthy and

cumbersome procedure based upon whether the wording on the label provided adequate protection to the user and the environment when the substance was used according to "commonly recognized practice."

In 1954, the food safety laws were amended to give the Food and Drug Administration (FDA) the authority to set tolerances for pesticide residues in "raw agricultural commodities." The FDA has rather broad powers to enforce these provisions. However, even with the cooperation of the Environmental Protection Agency (EPA) and state agencies, it is not possible to monitor all domestically grown and imported fresh fruits and vegetables.

By the late 1950's, the list of chemicals which could be shown to induce cancer in experimental animals was growing longer. Furthermore, the complexity of cancer in comparison with infectious diseases was beginning to emerge. The latent period - the time between exposure to a carcinogen and the appearance of disease - was believed to be as long as twenty years. Promoters were also identified - agents which, while not carcinogenic themselves, greatly enhance the action of primary carcinogens. Many of the carcinogens tested also seemed to be mutagens, at least for microorganisms. Thus, the level of public and, hence, Congressional, concern was increasing.

In 1958, the Food, Drug and Cosmetic Act underwent comprehensive revision. The so-called general safety clause for food additives appeared in its present form in these amendments, with the burden of proof that a particular food additive be "...safe under conditions of use" now placed upon the proponent rather than the government. For the first time in any law, legislative language was directed specifically at the prevention of cancer through the now famous Delaney clause, which amends the general safety clause. It states that no substance shall be considered safe if it has been shown to "cause cancer in animals or man."

The Delaney clause, at present the center of heated controversy, was passed some six years before the first Surgeon General's report Smoking and Health brought before the public the evidence that one of its cherished habits was clearly linked to lung cancer. In that it was offered long before the public preoccupation with cancer that was to follow some years hence, it was ahead of its time, and passed Congress with relatively little concern. Of course carcinogens were bad and should be kept out of food.

However, since it became law, the Delaney clause has been used successfully only twice in its 23 year history, both for relatively unimportant substances. It is the actions proposed recently that have aroused concern, especially concerning saccharin. This and the proposals to ban the use of chloroform, diethylstilbesterol, the nitrofurans, the color additive orange-B and nitrites never

became regulations. It is worth noting that because of the specific way in which the Delaney clause is worded, it cannot be used to
prohibit the use of a <u>suspected</u> carcinogen, nor of a known mutagen,
whereas the general safety clause may be used for this purpose.

By 1960, the perception was held among many scientists that
much of the incidence of cancer was caused by external agents. A
report prepared for Congress by G.B. Mider (6) set forth many of
the aspects of cancer which must be considered in writing regulatory legislation. It included the recognition that a significant
fraction of cancer was probably caused by environmental agents, and
discussed the statistical nature of cancer induction. That is,
unlike the usual cause and effect relationships between acute
toxins and injury, only a small fraction of a population exposed to
a carcinogen may develop cancer, depending on the potency of the
substance and the level of exposure. The report also described the
importance of being aware of the long latent period for most human
cancers, of evaluating the carcinogenic potential of weak carcinogens in the environment, and of the important role of promoters.
The effect of this report was to strengthen the concept that cancer
is largely a preventable disease, and could be controlled to some
degree by limiting carcinogens in the environment. An expert committee assembled by the World Health Organization in 1965 concluded
that at least half of all human cancer could be attributed to the
presence of carcinogenic agents in the environment.

Meanwhile, by the early 1960's, some of the more acute consequences of the chemical revolution were beginning to become obvious. Rachel Carson's <u>Silent Spring</u> (7), published in 1962,
helped to arouse the public's interest in doing something about the
undesirable consequences of the massive use of potent insecticides
over the previous two decades. But these concerns were not directed toward the more subtle effects of agents which might be mutagens
or carcinogens, but rather the fact that the effects of these
chemicals had extended far beyond their target organisms. Not only
had the ecological balance in many areas been disrupted through the
elimination of the insect food supply for many birds and animals,
but stable toxic chemicals were being spread throughout the food
chain, interrupting the reproduction of many species of birds and
fish, even where they escaped the acute toxic effects of direct
exposure. The 1960's, then, saw the growth of citizens' environmental groups, which, by the end of the decade had large consti-
tuencies and began to challenge the large corporations in their
lobbying effectiveness.

Thus, by the late 1960's, there had been a sufficient increase
in public awareness over the quality of the environment to enable
significant evolution of the laws regulating toxic agents to take
place over the next five years. In addition, the rising incidence
of cancer was causing alarm in several quarters. A report by Boy-

land in 1968 (8) concluded that 90% of human cancer is caused by
chemicals, although he went on to note that some of these may not
be of external or environmental origin. Nevertheless, he suggested
that much human cancer could be prevented if carcinogenic agents
could be identified and removed from the environment.

These concerns and fears of a cancer epidemic did play a minor
role in the writing of the new round of environmental laws of the
early 1970's. However, they were principally directed towards
pressuring the government to find a more immediate solution. The
intense and well financed lobbying effort was led by Sidney Farber
and Mary Lasker with the strong backing of the American Cancer
Society, asserting that "...the kind of money and comprehensive
planning that went into putting a man on the moon..." could certainly "...conquer cancer by America's 200th birthday" (9). Thus
in 1970, the Conquest of Cancer Act, sponsored by Edward Kennedy in
the Senate, and the Cancer Attack Act, introduced by Paul Rogers,
were directed at finding a cure for cancer. The White House declared war on cancer. The National Cancer Act, which passed in
1971, greatly increased the authorizations for cancer research
conducted by the National Cancer Institute (NCI). The Act contained scarcely any mention of research to determine the causes of
or to prevent cancer.

At its onset, then, the War on Cancer was to be waged on a
very different battlefield than that within the scope of the regulatory agencies. But, as awareness of the probable causes of cancer increased, pressures were brought to bear upon these agencies
to consider the prevention of cancer (and, eventually, mutations
and teratogenesis) as an important part of their responsibilities. Such considerations eventually received recognition in several of the regulatory laws passed in the 1970's. And while the
naive objective of the National Cancer Act has still not been
achieved, the windfall of new research funds did enable an increase
in research directed toward finding the causes of cancer. A Division of Cancer Cause and Prevention was created within NCI, and by
the mid-1970's the rodent bioassay protocol for animal carcinogenesis which is used today had been developed. To date, tests on more
than 100 suspect chemicals have been completed under this program.

Environmental Regulatory Legislation: 1970 - 1980

Beginning in 1969, a series of actions were taken by Congress
to expand and consolidate regulatory legislation designed to protect the quality of the environment and human health from the effects of toxic agents. While these laws have been continuing
sources of controversy, they provided for the first time Federal
authority which was adequate to take meaningful action toward the
control of toxic agents in the environment, the workplace and consumer goods. These laws are summarized in Table I.

Table 1. Federal Legislation Regulating Toxic Substances

Legislation	Definition of toxic or hazard	Type of regulation	Degree of protection	Burden of proof	Balancing of costs
Clean Air Act (as amended), 1970, 1977	"an air pollutant ... which ... may cause, or contribute to, an increase in mortality or an increase in serious irreversible, or incapacitating reversible, illness" Section 112(a)(1)	Emission standards	"... an ample margin of safety to protect the public health ..." Sec. 112(b)(1)(B)	EPA	No
Federal Water Pollution Control Act (as amended), 1972, 1977	"... pollutants which will ... cause death, disease, behavioral abnormalities, cancer, genetic mutations, physiological malfunctions ... or physical deformations." Sec. 502(13)	Effluent standards, ambient standards	"... ample margin of safety." Sec. 307(a)(4)	EPA	No
Occupational Safety and Health Act, 1970	Not defined	Exposure standards	"adequately assures to the extent feasible that no employee will suffer material impairment of health or functional capacity ..." Sec. 6(b)(5)	OSHA	Yes. Sec. 6(b)(5)
Toxic Substances Control Act, 1976	those substances "... presenting an unreasonable risk of injury to health or the environment ..." Sec. 6(a)	Premarket notification and testing; prohibitions on manufacturing, processing, and distribution; information on chemical components must be supplied to EPA	Not specified	Proponent	Yes. Sec. 2(b)(3)
Federal Food, Drug and Cosmetic Act (as amended) 1958, 1962	Not defined	Labeling; bans on products deemed "unsafe"	"... necessary for the protection of public health ..." Sec. 406[346]	Proponent for drugs and food additives; FDA for cosmetic ingredients	No, in case of food additives; yes, for drugs and cosmetics
Federal Insecticide, Fungicide, and Rodenticide Act and the Federal Environmental Pesticide Control Act, 1972	One which results in "... unreasonable adverse effects on the environment or will involve unreasonable hazard to the survival of a species declared endangered ..." (imminent hazard). Sec. 2(l)	Registration of all pesticides and uses; permits for applicators; cancellation or suspension of specific pesticides or uses	Not specified	Proponent	Yes. Sec. 6(b)(2)
Safe Drinking Water Act, 1974	"... contaminant(s) which ... may have an adverse effect on the health of persons." Sec. 1401(1)(B)	Maximum contaminant standards	"... to the extent feasible ... (taking costs into consideration) ..." Sec. 1412(a)(2)	EPA	Yes. Sec. 1412(a)(2)
Resource Conservation and Recovery Act, 1976	one which "may cause, or significantly contribute to an increase in mortality or an increase in serious irreversible, or incapacitating reversible, illness; or, pose a ... hazard to human health or the environment ..." Sec. 1004(5)(A)(B)	Standards for generators, transporters of hazardous waste; permits for treatment, storage or disposal of hazardous waste	"that necessary to protect human health and the environment ..." Sec. 3002-3004	EPA	No

From Resources, April - July, 1978, published by Resources for the Future

The National Environmental Policy Act of 1969 (NEPA) was
signed into law on New Year's Day, 1970. The purpose of this
legislation was to set forth explicitly what our overall policy
concerning the environment was to be, namely "...to create and
maintain conditions under which man and nature can exist in
productive harmony." The law required specific "action forcing"
procedures to be carried out by the Federal agencies to make sure
that this policy was observed. Of these, the most important by far

has been the requirement that a detailed statement of "environmental impact" be prepared for every proposed major Federal action
which might significantly affect environmental quality, and include
a discussion of alternatives to the proposed action. The statement
must be submitted for comment to other Federal agencies, appropriate state and local governments, and to the public. Since even
large privately financed projects, such as nuclear power plants,
strip mines, and oil and gas development, involve Federal action
through leases, licenses, etc., few such projects escape the
scrutiny of NEPA.

The Council on Environmental Quality (CEQ) was created by the
Act as the focus for environmental issues within the Executive
Office of the President. While Congress was unclear on exactly how
NEPA was to be administered, most of the responsibility for over-
seeing this law has fallen to CEQ, and, of course, for a law as
controversial as NEPA was bound to be, the Federal Courts.

The role of the CEQ, is, thus, somewhat schizophrenic, in that
it is both the overseer of NEPA compliance, and the advisor to the
President on Federal policies which might affect the environment.
In this latter capacity, the CEQ can and has found itself openly
critical of administration policies, including those initiated by
the White House, even though it is itself a White House Office.
Therefore, in practice, the CEQ may fall in or out of grace with
the President and his staff, depending upon the positions it takes
on specific issues. This internal conflict of interest, which is
built into the role of CEQ by law, has, on several occasions since
the passage of NEPA, greatly limited its effectiveness.

The Clean Air Act of 1970 was a comprehensive law directed at
the improvement of air quality, replacing the more limited statutes
passed in 1955, 1963, 1965, and 1967. The 1970 law corrected two
major defects of the earlier laws. First, it defined "air pollution" much more explicitly, rather than leaving the definition to
the discretion of the agency. Second, and most important, it gave
the newly created Environmental Protection Agency the authority to
enforce the law adequately. Previous versions did not require any
abatement of actual pollution unless a court had given "...due
consideration to the practicability of complying with such standards as may be applicable to the physical and economical feasibility of securing abatement of any pollution."

The 1970 law requried the EPA administrator to promulgate
immediately national ambient air quality standards for the major
pollutants, sulfur dioxide (SO_2), total particulates, carbon mon-
oxide (CO), photochemical oxidants, hydrocarbons and nitrogen
oxides (NO_x). It also set forth a policy of preserving clean or
"pristine" areas (the non-deterioration policy), specifically addressed emissions from both stationary and mobile sources, provided

for the direct reduction of certain "hazardous air pollutants"
(which were later specified to include cadmium, mercury, beryllium
and asbestos), and required "new" sources of pollution to observe
more stringent control measures than those which applied to
existing ones. The law also contained an unprecedented feature,
explicitly setting forth the rights of citizens to sue "any person"
alleged to be in violation of the Act. In legal terms, "person"
can also mean a corporation of even the Federal government. A
citizen may also legally compel the EPA Administrator to implement
any requirement or duty specified by the Act.

Predictably, the Clean Air Act, since it affects virtually
every major industry in the United States, has been the basis for
many intense and protracted legal battles. As the provisions were
put into practice, legal weaknesses begin to emerge, as did areas
of the laws which were vulnerable to politics. Therefore, some
provisions of the law were tightened in 1974, and in 1975, Congress
began to consider major amendments. The two year struggle which
followed saw two powerful members of Congress, John Dingell of
Detroit, championing the interests of the automobile industry and
the Union of Automobile Workers, and Paul Rogers of Florida, Chairman of the House Subcommittee on Health and the Environment,
engaged in an historic legislative battle.

Much of the contention over the proposed amendments concerned
specific emission or performance standards written into the law,
and the schedule to be followed in their attainment. The debate
which accompanied consideration of what finally passed as the Clean
Air Act Amendments of 1977 included a discussion of many new
findings which had emerged since the 1970 law was passed. The
increasing acidity of many northern lakes had been demonstrated
years before, but it could not be unequivocally demonstrated that
this phenomenon was due to air pollution. Much more was known
about the action of sunlight on primary air pollutants and the
mutagenic nature of several of the photochemical products had been
demonstrated. The role of fine particulates (one of the principal
photochemical products of heavy concentrations of automobile ex-
hausts) in lung disease had been shown. Yet, the scientific evidence was not yet sufficient to convince the skeptics, who demanded
human epidemiological data before they were willing to believe that
these problems were genuine. Thus, it was extraordinarily difficult for the proponents of strict controls to substantiate their
case, even though their theoretical arguments were sound, and none
of the new findings were recognized in the amendments.

The law which finally passed was a classic exercise in political compromise. In the end, some provisions were strengthened and
others weakened. In the final confrontation on the House floor,
over automobile tailpipe emission standards and when they would
have to be met, the Dingell forces won by 100 votes.

The Occupational Safety and Health Act was also passed in
1970. This law, reflecting growing concern over numerous cases of
specific health problems among particular working populations,
empowered the Department of Labor to set and enforce safety standards covering a wide range of activities, including exposure
standards for toxic agents. The Occupational Safety and Health
Administration (OSHA), the agency created to administer this Act,
has been criticized for focusing too much attention on the seemingly more trivial aspects of worker safety by promulgating volumes of
excessive regulations, specifying the minute details of all sorts
of tools, equipment, clothing, etc., rather than dealing adequately
with those problems which represent significant health risks. For
some classes of toxic chemicals, however, including some mutagens
and carcinogens, OSHA regulations have succeeded in reducing worker
exposure substantially, particularly through requirements for proper storage, ventilation, protective clothing, etc. However, the
enabling legislation has not undergone significant revision since
its original passage in 1970.

The Federal Water Pollution Control Act (FWPCA) of 1972 consists of a comprehensive set of amendments to the then extant water
pollution legislation, dating back to 1948. Like the Clean Air
Act, the FWPCA strengthened weaker statutes to give the EPA authority to set and enforce standards concerning the discharge of pollutants from point sources, especially industrial plants, municipal
sewage treatment plants, and agricultural feedlots; to promulgate
regulations to control the accidental spilling of oil or hazardous
substances; and to provide financial assistance for the construction of sewage treatment plants. This law is noteworthy in the
rather broad but detailed way that it defines "toxic pollutant".
The term includes any substance which is toxic to "any organism",
toxic being defined not only as being capable of causing death, but
"...disease, behavioral abnormalities, cancer, genetic mutations,
physiological malfunctions (including malfunctions in reproduction), or physical malformations." This definition is a milestone
in that it is the first time since the enactment of the Delaney
clause for food additives that "cancer" was mentioned as part of a
legislative standard, and the first ever to specifically include
"mutations". Under this definition, virtually any substance
could be considered toxic, if used in high enough concentration.
However, the way this standard is to be applied is far less
absolute than the Delaney clause, permitting considerable
administrative discretion in the selection of those substances to
be regulated and in the promulgation of standards. The EPA
Administrator is required to publish a list of toxic pollutants
"...for which an effluent standard...will be established under this
section (307a)." In compiling the list, the Administrator "...must
take into account the toxicity of the pollutant, its persistence,
degradability, the usual potential presence of the affected
organisms and the nature and extent of the effect of the
toxic pollutant on such organism." Thus, while the law

overall permits the Administrator some latitude in the regulation
of toxic substances, it establishes criteria which can and have
formed the basis of challenges to the standards, both through administrative proceedings within EPA and in the courts, particularly
if known toxic substances are not regulated, or if the proposed
effluent standards are inadequate in the light of established
data. The FWPCA was amended in 1977 but with no major revisions.

        The Safe Drinking Water Act of 1974 deals primarily with the
contamination of sources of water which may be used to provide
drinking water. While there is some overlap in authority with the
FWPCA, this Act is directed toward the prevention of contamination
of ground water and other sources of water which serve as municipal
drinking water supplies. The FWPCA, on the other hand, is focused
on the pollution of open waterways, and is concerned with the ecology of aquatic wildlife as well as human health. This law places
primary responsibility for the enforcement of Federal drinking
water standards with the States, especially the use of adequate
purification technology to achieve these standards. The EPA, however, does have emergency powers which it may exercise in serious
situations where a water supply is contaminated. In 1977, both the
FWPCA and Safe Drinking Water Act authorities were applicable when
a massive chloroform release into the Ohio River occurred. The EPA
chose to exercise its emergency powers under the Safe Drinking
Water Act. Amendments to the law in 1977 delayed the time required
for certain drinking water standards to be met.

        The Federal regulatory authority which is perhaps of most
concern to this symposium is that concerned with pesticides. In
1972, Congress passed the Federal Environmental Pesticide Control
Act (FEPCA) which amended the Federal Insecticide, Fungicide and
Rodenticide Act (FIFRA), which had not undergone significant
changes since it was first passed in 1947. While it left a number
of legislative problems unsolved, the revised law is a vast improvement over its predecessor. Many of the provisions of that law
deal with the registration of pesticides. The burden of proof that
a pesticide "...will not generally cause unreasonable adverse effects on the environment..." under normal conditions of use rests
with the prospective registrant. The EPA may proceed to cancel the
registration of existing pesticides for which the instructions for
use on the label cannot be shown to prevent unintended harm to man
or the environment. However, the administrative procedures which
must be followed are rather lengthy and prone to delays through
litigation. Cancellation may require as much as two years to become effective, even in the light of incriminating toxicity data.
However, the Administrator may suspend the registration of a pesticide if the EPA determines that it represents an "imminent hazard".

        While this law has provided the vehicle for the cancellation
of registration for most uses of a number of once common and, to

some, notorious, pesticides (DDT, chlordane, heptachlor, aldrin, dieldrin, endrin, and 2,4,5,-T), it contains inherent problems which have only complicated the role of EPA in regulating pesticides. First, the standards are rather poorly defined. As discussed at the beginning of this paper, this only invites litigation, no matter what decisions are made. Second, in part because of the legal fuzziness of the legislation, EPA had dealt with each compound separately, even if the important functional groups are chemically identical, or the toxic contaminant the same (e.g., dioxin, which is responsible for the toxic effects of preparations of 2,4,5-T and related compounds). This practice has greatly increased the red tape involved in regulating pesticides.

Various provisions of the Food, Drug and Cosmetic Act, the FWPCA, the Clean Air Act, and Occupational Safety and Health Act, the Safe Drinking Water Act (1974) and the Poison Prevention Packaging Act (1970) all have sections which can apply to pesticides, sometimes specifically. Some serious regulatory problems still exist, however, such as the exportation of pesticides banned for use in the United States, and their return to U. S. consumers as residues on imported food.

Thus, the regulation of pesticides is more than an illusion of a regulatory morass. Some of the problems have resulted from the sheer size of the EPA and its compartmentalization resulting from the administration of a broad scope of regulatory laws. The following actual case illustrates the kind of problem that can result when an agency grows piecemeal and keeps adding new divisions to implement an increasing burden of statutory authorities.

In 1976, one branch of the EPA had begun proceedings to cancel the registration of endrin at the same time that another branch was proposing and defending an effluent standard for the same substance. For each proposed action, EPA scientists prepare a "criteria document", consisting of a discussion and analysis of all relevant toxicity data for a given chemical. Amazingly, the criteria documents used by these offices had little in common with each other, each using a separate body of data, or nearly so, even though many of the studies were conducted in EPA laboratories. The document upon which cancellation proceedings were based cited the carcinogenicity of endrin, whereas that upon which the proposed effluent standard was based did not, even when the agency was petitioned to include the same body of carcinogenicity data in both documents. Neither document included the results of carcinogenicity tests of endrin in the NCI rodent bioassay system.

This incident not only illustrated the inefficiency which can plague any large bureaucracy, but the problem of information sharing, which still greatly reduces the effectiveness of the EPA and other regulatory agencies in carrying out their statutory function. Mechanisms are clearly needed for the more efficient sharing of toxicity data not only within a Federal agency, such as the EPA, but among all agencies, toxicologists and the public.

The last major legislation to be passed for the control of toxic agents in the environment was the Toxic Substances Control Act (TSCA) in 1976. Originally intended to give the EPA broad and streamlined regulatory powers with which to regulate hazardous chemicals, the battle that raged as it fought its way through the legislative gauntlet left it somewhat battered and swollen, and certainly weaker than when it was first introduced. Both because the implementation of the Act required the addition of several new administrative divisions to the EPA and because of the legislative flaws in the law itself, few of the many provisions of TSCA have been effectively carried out five years after its enactment. But, while TSCA is unlikely to earn a place in history as exemplary regulatory legislation, it does attempt to accomplish some admirable goals.

Specifically, it places the responsibility for showing that the "...manufacture, distribution in commerce, processing, use, or disposal of a chemical substance or mixture,..." does not present "...an unreasonable risk of injury to health or the environment..." upon the manufacturer or other party engaging in any of the activities quoted above. The EPA Administrator may prescribe the test conditions which may (not shall) include "...carcinogenesis, mutagenesis, teratogenesis, behavioral disorders, cumulative or synergistic effects, and any other effect which may present an unreasonable risk of injury to health or the environment.". Thus, while this is the most comprehensive list of specific effects appearing in any environmental law, the key word is "may". The Administrator may, but is not required, to include the above criteria in test conditions. However, he "...must review the adequacy of the standards for the development of data..." at least once every year and make revisions as necessary. But the law also states that this authority should be exercised so as "...not to impede unduly or create unnecessary economic barriers to techno- logical innovation...." Thus, with so many legal hedges written into the law, its effectiveness is dependent entirely on how it is administered by EPA and how it is enforced. The legislative lan- guage cited above also opens the door to legal challenge, regard- less of how the law is administered.

A recent addition to EPA's authority was inspired by the Love Canal episode, and the emerging knowledge that hundreds of other toxic waste dumping sites may pose a serious threat to public health in the surrounding areas. This is the "superfund" legisla- tion whereby EPA will supervise the cleaning up of the worst of these dump sites. This particular task is of monumental propor- tions and extraordinarily difficult. At present, funds permit the cleaning of only around a hundred of the more than a thousand sites identified as extremely hazardous. The selection of the specific sites to be cleaned has generated controversy.

A discussion of the regulatory authorities pertaining to the control of ionizing radiation is perhaps out of place in a conference which is primarily focused on chemical toxicology. However, a comparison of regulatory authorities would be incomplete without at least a brief mention of the ways radiation is regulated. Ionizing radiation was known to produce mutations and cancer long before most chemical mutagens were identified, and our data concerning risk from human exposure to radiation is far better than for most toxic chemicals. The regulatory authority for setting exposure standards is dispersed over several agencies. Some of the laws discussed above may be applied to the control of specific radionuclides in the environment. The Nuclear Regulatory Commission is responsible for setting standards of the release of radioactive material from nuclear power plants, and the EPA for setting standards of radiation intensity at the boundaries of such plants. The largest user of radioactive materials, the Department of Defense, sets its own standards for military personnel but these have usually been consistent with those observed by the rest of the Federal government. The occupational exposure standard of five rem per year applies generally. There is at present no mechanism to account for the total radiation exposure to an individual from occupational, medical or environmental sources.

THE ROLE OF SCIENTIFIC EXPERTS

As a practical matter, one of the most important factors in administering regulatory legislation concerning toxic agents is the proper use of scientific data and scientific experts and witnesses. While determining the level of risk that is acceptable to society is a judgment involving many competing values, the determination of risk itself is a purely scientific matter. Considerable uncertainty exists concerning our knowledge of the degree of risk presented by exposure to most toxic agents for any individual or population. There are many reasons for this uncertainty, including a paucity of large enough human populations exposed to sufficiently high levels of a substance, the difficulties in extending animal or microbial data to man, the variation in sensitivity among individuals, the presence of competing and often unidentified toxic agents, and the statistical problems of measuring a small effect against a high background.

It is particularly important that both Congress and the heads of the regulatory agencies accept that this uncertainty is a fact of life, and that scientists who cannot assign a precise risk to a particular chemical are not necessarily dodging the question nor bad scientists. On the other hand, aside from the uncertainty in-

herent in risk assessment, scientific witnesses invited to testify
on the degree of toxicity of a particular agent will often present
widely differing opinions, depending upon whether they were invited
by an environmental group, a chemical company, or the Congressional
committee sponsoring the proposed legislation. Disagreements among
scientists concerning risk estimates generally confuse and slow
down the regulatory process. Laymen with a preconceived bias can
usually find a Ph.D. who will support their bias. Thus the adver-
sarial process that has accompanied many legislative and regulatory
proceedings has often generated more heat than light. Since it is
fair to assume that a single scientific truth characterizes the
actual risk presented by a specific toxic agent, the objective have
no choice but to then question either the scientific competence or
the integrity, or both, of at least some of the expert witnesses.

This dilemma places a considerable burden of responsibility
upon the community of competent and honest scientists to learn the
art of communicating effectively with the lay people who enact our
regulatory laws and carry them out. The precise way a given body
of data is presented can greatly color the listener's perception of
the degree of risk of a toxic substance.

The National Toxicology Program (NTP), created by administrative action in 1979, was established to consolidate and coordinate
toxicological research within the Federal Agencies, particularly
concerning carcinogens. Since the regulatory agencies will be
somewhat dependent upon the work of the NTP, the Federal government, and especially the National Institute of Environmental Health
Sciences which administers this program, has an opportunity and a
responsibility to provide the lawmakers and regulators not only
with needed data on specific agents, free from the bias of special
interests, but with a clear understanding of the methods of
scientific risk assessment and especially the statistical nature of
environmental health risks.

CURRENT REGULATORY ISSUES

The two specific laws dealing with the regulation of toxic
agents which have received the most recent attention and for which
major congressional attention is planned are the Clean Air Act and
the food safety portions of the Food, Drug and Cosmetic Act.

The Clean Air Act has probably put the most pressure on industry overall than any other single piece of regulatory legislation, and it remains one of the more controversial environmental
laws. Whether or not it has been effective in improving the
nation's air quality is a matter of debate. A recent Brookings
Institution study (10) concluded that the current law has serious,
major flaws, and that only a major overhaul will make it able to
assure good air quality in the future, particularly in view of a

return to coal and wood as energy sources. The authors attribute
the gains in air quality that have occurred to the voluntary switch
to cleaner fuels by utilities and industry purely for economic
reasons. They stress that Congress should focus more on the attainment of ambient air quality goals and not get so wrapped up in
details and mechanisms. The report recommends that the standards
be updated to reflect current scientific data and distinguish fine
particulates from "total suspended particulates" and to develop
standards for acid sulfates rather than sulfur dioxide. A completely new control strategy is recommended.

But critics of the report claim that while it makes some valid
points, it still represents an oversimplification of the massive
problems of trying to achieve clean air, when industry has continually resisted cooperation with the EPA and paying the costs of
meeting the environmental objectives. Because the issue is loaded
with political overtones, many believe that it is unlikely that a
revised clean air law will pass before the 1982 elections, although
there is likely to be extensive congressional debate over the
issue.

Over the past several years, there have been a number of proposals to revise the food safety laws, and especially since the
furor over the proposed saccharin ban, the Delaney clause. A
series of confidential proposals were developed by the FDA in 1979
and were a major issue that was discussed in Secretary Califano's
office before his removal. Recent attention has been given to the
issue by some members of Congress. A report prepared by the Institute of Medicine (11) in response to a request from Congress at the
time of the saccharin question was debated, is being used to justify a major revision of the food safety laws. The report recommends that the outdated categories of foods that now add much in-
consistency to the law be replaced by grouping all foods (or food
additives) by general risk categories, which may perhaps be designated in the marketplace by a color coded logo. The committee of
scientists preparing the report concluded that the FDA should have
greatly increased discretion in the regulation of potentially harmful substances. The philosophy of the report is captured in the
following excerpt from the report:

"To replace this cumbersome set of categories, the committee
recommends a single standard of risk with several broadly defined
risk categories. Classification under these categories would establish a range of regulatory possibilities among which the regulatory agency could choose in the light of the best scientific
advice, taking into account public attitudes and such benefits as
can be assessed."

In emphasizing discretion, the report states that the
regulatory outcome should include an assessment of the "objective

or perceived benefits so as to weight them against risk." While
most agree that the food safety laws contain vestiges of past times
and are, therefore, in need of modernization, many are disturbed at
the naivety expressed by the National Academy report. While
discretion may represent an attractive solution to the problems
posed by a law that is too rigid, the inclusion of an undefinable
risk-benefit standard as proposed is, for the reasons discussed in
the first part of this paper, inviting trouble. I have discussed
the problems inherent in this approach to regulation at length
elsewhere (12).

In conclusion, I would be remiss in my commitment to present
an accurate picture of Federal regulation if I did not at least
mention what is perhaps the most important determinant in the effectiveness of our regulatory laws. And that is politics, which
is, of course, intimately bound up with economics and the less
tangible attitudes of the public. No matter how well regulatory
laws are written, and how committed to their task the public
servants who are charged with carrying them out, there will always
be a strong political effect, which can be reflected in many ways,
including the priorities given certain programs in the Federal
budget, the susceptibility of key individuals to outside pressures,
the prevailing economic goals and the overall environmental philosophy of the party in power. This symposium is not, however, the
place to expand this point further. A glance at almost any daily
newspaper will clearly illustrate the importance of this
phenomenon.

REFERENCES

1. Potts, P., Chirurgical Observations Relative to the Cataract,
    the Polypus of the Nose, the Cancer of the Scrotum, the
    Different Kinds of Ruptures, and the Mortification of the Toes
    and Feet, Hawes, Clark and Collins, London, 1775.
2. Kennaway, E. L., Experiments on cancer-producing substances,
    British Medical Journal II, 1-4 (1925), and Further experi-
    ments on cancer-producing substances, Biomedical Journal, 24,
    497-504 (1930).
3. Hueper, W. C., and H. D. Wolfe, Experimental production of
    aniline tumors in the bladder of dogs, Am. J. Pathology, 13,
    656-657 (1937).
4. Shubik, P. and J. Sice, Chemical carcinogenesis as chronic
    toxicity test, Cancer Research 16, 728-742 (1956).
5. Office of the Surgeon General of the United States, Smoking
    and Health, U. S. Department of Health, Education and Welfare,
    1964.
6. Mider, E. B., The Role of Certain Chemical and Physical
    Agents in the Causation of Cancers, in hearings before the
    Committee on Interstate and Foreign Commerce, U. S. House of
    Representatives, 86th Congress, 2nd Sess., on H. R. 7624,
    Jan. 26, 1970, pp. 45-60.

7. Carson, Rachel, Silent Spring, 1962.
8. Boyland, E., The correlation of experimental carcinogenesis
    and cancer in man, in: Experimental Tumor Research, F.
    Homburger and S. Marger (eds.), pp. 222-224, Basel, 1969.
9. The New York Times, December 9, 1969, Advertisement.
10. Lave, L. and G. Omenn, Clearing the Air: Reforming the Clean
    Air Act, The Brookings Institution, 1981.
11. National Research Council/Institute of Medicine, Report of the
    Committee for a Study on Saccharin and Food Safety Policy.
    National Academy of Sciences, Washington, D. C., 1979.
12. Zimmerman, Burke K., Risk-benefit analysis: The cop-out of
    governmental regulation, Trial 14, 43-47, (1978).

DISCUSSION

WATERS: Regarding the availability of scientific information
within the EPA, I agree that there are problems in the
exchange of scientific data within the Agency. My impression
is that, in part, this is due to the different legislative
mandates to which the regulatory arms of the Agency respond.
In addition, I believe that this deficiency in EPA is
symptomatic of a larger problem in scientific information
exchange that involves all of us. We have seen in this
meeting that scientific information resides in all three
sectors - government, academia, and industry. This
information should be exchanged more freely. It seems to me
that compounds that are produced by several manufacturers
present candidates for development and exchange of scientific
information. Organizations such as CIIT have been set up to
facilitate research and information exchange under the aegis
of industry. Such organizations could serve as a clearing-
house for distribution of industrial data. Similar clearing-
houses could and should be established in government and
academia.

Within the Office of Research and Development, which I
represent, an effort has been initiated to computerize
pesticide research data. This data has been made available
through the published literature and through EPA reports.
Such a data base could become the repository of additional
scientific data from other sources.

Q. EL-SEBAE: I would like to inquire about the present status of
    regulation for exportation of hazardous, banned compounds
    manufactured in the U.S.A. like chlordane and heptachlor.

A. ZIMMERMAN: Exported pesticides are governed by local
    regulation. Most controls of pesticides abroad are far less
    stringent than in the U.S. as they are written and enforced.
    The registration is for specific uses within the U.S. and the

use of chlordane and heptachlor has been cancelled for
agricultural use. Registration in the U.S. has no bearing on
whether a pesticide is exported since some have been cancelled
for all use in the U.S. but are still manufactured for sale
and distribution abroad.

TOXICOLOGICAL PROCEDURES FOR ASSESSING THE CARCINOGENIC POTENTIAL

OF AGRICULTURAL CHEMICALS

D. Krewski, D. Clayson, B. Collins and I. C. Munro

Food Directorate
Health Protection Branch
Health & Welfare Canada
Ottawa, Ontario, K1A 0L2, Canada

ABSTRACT:

Pesticides and other agricultural chemicals are now widely used throughout the world as a means of improving crop yields in order to meet the increasing demands being placed upon the global food supply. In Canada, the use of such chemicals is controlled through government regulations established jointly by the Department of Agriculture and the Department of National Health & Welfare. Such regulations require a detailed evaluation of the toxicological characteristics of the chemical prior to its being cleared for use. In this paper, procedures for assessing the carcinogenic potential of agricultural and other chemicals are discussed. Consideration is given to both the classical long-term in vivo carcinogen bioassay in rodent or other species and the more recently developed short-term in vitro tests based on genetic alterations in bacterial and other test systems.

1. INTRODUCTION

Pesticides and other agricultural chemicals are an integral and necessary component of the technological world in which we live. Although indiscriminate application of such products cannot be condoned, the judicious use of chemicals is an essential feature of modern agricultural practice. The World Health Organization estimates that 20-30% of food is spoiled world-wide due to insect infestation, molds, or other diseases which can be controlled through the use of chemicals (84). Thus, to feed our ever-increasing world population, we must be prepared to use chemicals to reduce food spoilage and increase production.

461

In Canada, as in most developed nations, legislation exists controlling the use of agricultural chemicals. Pesticides, herbicides, fungicides, and rodenticides must be registered under the Pest Control Products Act administered by the Department of Agriculture prior to their being cleared for use. This legislation requires the manufacturer or petitioner to provide the Department of Agriculture with extensive data regarding the efficacy of the chemical under Canadian conditions of use. This includes a determination as to whether chemical residues exist on food products that may be consumed by humans.

A major portion of the manufacturer's submission for registration involves a detailed examination of the toxicological characteristics of the chemical in question. The usual battery of toxicological tests is applied, including acute, sub-chronic, chronic, reproductive, and teratological studies in at least two animal species. Special biochemical studies on neurotoxicity may also be required. Of particular concern is the chemical nature of plant or animal metabolites; if these differ from the metabolites found in experimental animals, they may themselves require in-depth toxicological evaluation.

In Canada, the safety evaluation of agricultural chemicals is performed by the Department of National Health and Welfare which advises the Minister of Agriculture as to the acceptability of the tests conducted and establishes acceptable human exposure limits for specific chemicals. Under the provisions of the Food and Drugs Act and Regulations, maximum residue limits may be established for those chemicals where residues can occur, providing of course that these can be supported with sound toxicological data. It is possible for pesticides to be registered on a negligible residue basis in cases where the residue on food products is considered to be of no toxicological significance. The Health Protection Branch of the Department of National Health and Welfare also conducts a number of monitoring programs designed to determine the degree of compliance with established tolerances.

Labelling of pesticides with regard to conditions of use, application rates, and special precautions for handling is the responsibility of the Department of Agriculture, although the advice of health officials is sought in the development of safety precautions. In Canada, provincial authorities may license spray operators and restrict pesticide use whenever a potential hazard to either the applicator or by-standers is anticipated.

The Departments of National Health and Welfare and Agriculture play an active role in meetings of the World Health Organization and Food and Agriculture Organization Joint Committee on Pesticide Residues. Through these meetings and those of other international bodies such as the Codex Committee on Pesticide Residues, attempts

are made to harmonize legislation on pesticide residues in food at
the international level, thus alleviating concerns among major
trading partners with respect to the establishment of non-tariff
trade barriers.

In this paper, current toxicological procedures for evaluating
the carcinogenic potential of agricultural and other chemicals are
discussed. Carcinogen bioassay studies using animal models for man
are considered in section 2. At present, this test system occupies
perhaps the most prominent place among the different toxicological
and epidemiological approaches to carcinogenic risk assessment
(63). Because of the commitment of resources required in the
conduct of long-term carcinogenicity studies, a number of less
expensive short-term tests for carcinogenicity have been proposed
in recent years (37). These latter tests are based on the premise
that if certain critical events in the carcinogenic process can be
identified, it should be possible to develop in vitro systems to
test for the occurrence of such events and thus rapidly determine
whether or not a particular chemical is likely to be
carcinogenic. The relationship between long-term in vivo studies
and these short-term in vitro tests is discussed in section 3, with
the role of both test systems in the safety evaluation process as
it is now practiced summarized in section 4.

2. CARCINOGEN BIOASSAY

While protocols for toxicological experiments designed to
evaluate the carcinogenic potential of a test compound have been
the subject of many reviews (24,40,43,63,77,78) there remains no
universal agreement on how such tests should be conducted. Since
cancer is largely a disease of old age, it would seem appropriate,
however, that carcinogenicity tests encompass a significant portion
of the experimental animals' lifespan. While most such tests start
with weanling or young adult animals, considerable attention has
recently been directed toward two-generation bioassays involving
exposure to the parent generation as well as the offspring, thereby
providing for the possibility of transplacentally induced effects
(14,32). The strength of the dose of the test compound to be used
has been the subject of some controversy. While this dose must be
high enough to detect any potential carcinogenic effects in a
relatively small population of test animals, the use of too high a
dose may result in the induction of secondary effects which would
not normally be seen at realistic human exposure levels.

Although the experimentalist is free to choose the animal
species to be employed, practical limitations imposed by space,
time, and cost usually preclude the use of species other than
small rodents such as the rat, mouse, and hamster. It is usually
recommended that the test animals be exposed via the same route as
man, although inhalation studies are sometimes contraindicated

because of their greater cost. Good facilities are essential in
order to prevent the spread of intercurrent disease (25) with a
thorough health monitoring program required in order to capture as
much information as possible on any toxic effects which may be
induced (6).

For purposes of our discussion, it will be helpful to
distinguish between a screening bioassay designed to provide only
qualitative information on the carcinogenic potential of the test
compound and a dose response study intended to define the shape and
nature of the dose response curve as well as provide a basis for
quantitative risk assessment. In the former case, as few as two or
even one dose level may be used (in addition to an unexposed
control group), with the highest dose generally being the maximum
tolerated dose or MTD (59). In the latter case three of more
carefully selected dose levels are generally employed in order to
better define the dose response relationship for the compound under
study.

Qualitative Risk Assessment

A screening bioassay may lead to one of two types of errors
(Figure 1). There is a loss to society if a safe yet effective
agricultural chemical is erroneously declared to be a carcinogen (a
false positive). On the other hand, the failure to identify a
hazardous substance (a false negative) which achieves widespread
use can clearly result in serious health risks.

Because tumor incidence rates in many organs and tissues are
examined in each sex and species of animal tested, it was initially
thought that the large number of statistical tests performed on a
single set of bioassay data would lead to the occurrence of an
inordinate number of false positives (72). Due to the conservative
nature of Fisher's exact text in the presence of low spontaneous
response rates (35), however, this problem does not appear to be as
great as was initially anticipated (22,23). Since the evaluation
of bioassay data is not strictly a statistical decision process,
moreover, a chemical will not automatically be labelled a

EXPERIMENTAL EVIDENCE	CARCINOGEN?	
FOR CARCINOGENICITY?	No	YES
No	CORRECT DECISION	FALSE NEGATIVE
YES	FALSE POSITIVE	CORRECT DECISION

Fig. 1. False Positives and False Negatives in Carcinogenicity
Screens.

Table 1. False Negative Rates for a Simple Carcinogenicity Screen[a]

Excess Over Spontaneous Rate[b] (%)	Spontaneous Rate (%)			
	0	1	5	20
5	90	88	87	90
10	43	49	61	77
15	11	18	34	58
20	2	5	15	36
25	< 1	1	5	19

[a]Based on Fisher's exact test (p < .05) with 50 animals in each of a control and test group and assuming that all animals respond independently.

[b]Difference between the response rates in the test and control groups respectively.

carcinogen without assessing the biological consistency of the results, such as the induction of the same effect in different species (28).

In order to gain some idea of the sensitivity of a screening bioassay, consider a simple experiment in which fifty animals are assigned to both a control and single test group. As indicated in Table 1, the false negative rate for compounds inducing an increase of 25% over background is less than 1% whenever the spontaneous response rate is low. While these results also suggest that a carcinogenic compound tested at a dose level inducing only a 5-10% increase over background might well go undetected, it should be remembered that the use of high doses will tend to maximize the carcinogenic potential of the test compound thereby minimizing the risk of a false negative.

Quantitative Risk Assessment

Traditional toxicological procedures define a safe level of exposure as some arbitrary fraction of that dose level at which no adverse effects are observed in test animals. The use of such uncertainty or safety factors, however, has been criticized on three counts. First, the observed no effect level will depend on the number of animals examined, with response rates of 0/10 and 0/1000 clearly providing different indications of safety. Second, the use of a standard safety factor across the board does not take into account the slope of the dose response curve for the response of interest. (While a modest uncertainty factor may suffice if the dose response curve is relatively steep, a much greater margin of

safety may be required when the dose response curve is relatively
shallow.) Finally, the safety factor approach to tolerance
determination appears to be based on the presumption that a
threshold exists below which no adverse effects will be observed.
In the case of carcinogenesis, however, the existence of such
thresholds remains a subject for debate (81).

In an attempt to overcome these problems, statisticians have
proposed the use of mathematical modelling procedures as a means of
establishing acceptable levels of exposure (48). By fitting a
suitable dose response model to the observed experimental data, it
is in principle possible to estimate a virtually safe dose or VSD
corresponding to some suitably low level of risk (Figure 2).
(Direct estimation of such safe dose levels is generally not
possible since the corresponding response rates are normally well
below the observable response range for experiments employing a
practicable number of animals.)

Mathematical models for quantal response data may be divided
into two general classes (60). Statistical or tolerance
distribution models postulate the existence of a threshold dose for
each individual, with the distribution of thresholds in the
population assumed to follow a certain statistical distribution.

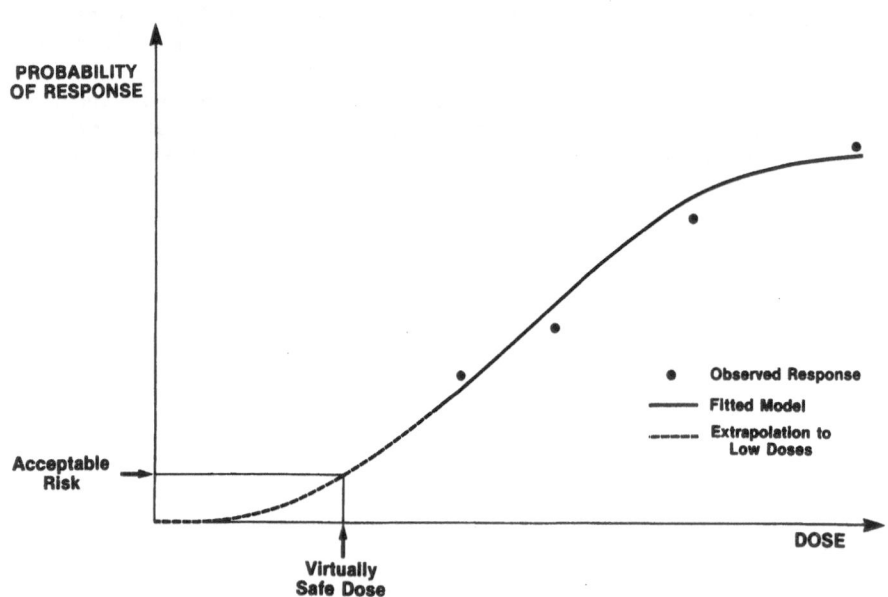

Fig. 2. Estimation of a Virtually Safe Dose by Low Dose
Extrapolation.

Although the selection of such a tolerance distribution is
essentially arbitrary, three commonly encountered statistical
models are the probit, logit, and Weibull. Stochastic or
mechanistic models, on the other hand, are based on the premise
that tumor induction is the result of the occurrence of one or more
random biological events. The one-hit model, for example, requires
only that the target tissue be hit by a single biologically
effective unit or dose. An obvious extention is the multi-hit
model, which stipulates that more than one hit is required for a
response to occur. The multi-stage model requires that a number of
different events or stages must occur, with the hazard rate for
each stage being a linear function of dose. Despite their
biological rationale, these stochastic models must also be
considered somewhat arbitrary until the carcinogenic process is
better understood (57).

Although the mathematical modelling approach to establishing
acceptable levels of exposure takes into account the slope of the
dose response curve and replaces the controversial threshold
concept with that of virtual safety (the effects of increasing
sample size would be reflected in tighter lower confidence limits
on the VSD), point estimates of VSD's obtained using this procedure
remain subject to considerable error. Factors contributing to this
uncertainty include the means by which background reponse is
accommodated, selection of the model to be used for extrapolation,
period of exposure, time to response and the presence of competing
risks, and metabolic activation of the test compound.

   Incorporation of Background Response. In the presence of
spontaneously occuring lesions, a virtually safe level of exposure
may be defined in terms of an acceptable level of added risk over
background. The manner in which spontaneously occurring responses
are accommodated in mathematical modelling procedures, however,
can have a marked impact on estimates of risk at low levels of
exposure. Such responses may be assumed to occur either
independently of those induced by the test chemical or additively
in a mechanistic manner (36). In the case of independence, the
added risk can conceivably be linear, sublinear, or even
supralinear at low doses (60). In the case of additivity, however,
the added risk will quite generally be linear at low doses
(18,64). (It is important to note that this fundamental result
holds even in the case of partial additivity).

   Unfortunately, statistical goodness-of-fit tests are not
sufficiently powerful so as to be able to reliably detect a linear
component in the dose response curve in the low dose region (19).
For example, consider the bioassay data on dieldrin shown in Figure
3 (24). The Weibull models allowing for either independent or
additive background appear to fit these data equally well. The
estimated virtually safe levels of exposure based on additivity

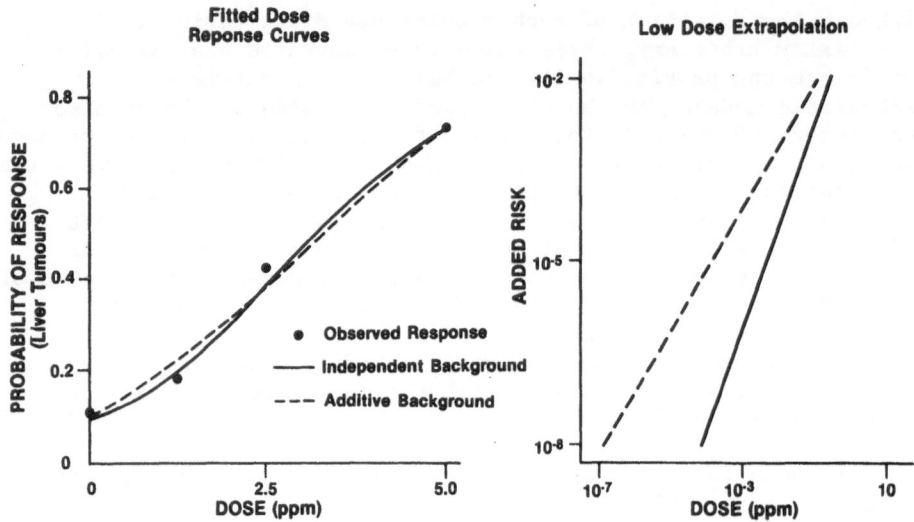

Fig. 3.   Fitted Weibull Dose Response Curves for Dieldrin with
          Independent or Additive Background and Corresponding
          Estimates of Added Risk in the Low Dose Region.

are, however, several orders of magnitude lower than those based on
independence due to the low dose linearity imposed by the
additivity assumption.

     A simple extrapolation procedure which allows for the
possibility of low dose linearity involves fitting a suitable dose
response model to the observed data and then linearly extrapolating
from some point on the fitted curve where the added risk may be
reliably determined, such as the 1% or 10% response rate (82).
Provided that the background rate is reasonably large (say 1% or
more), this linear extrapolation procedure may be expected to lead
to results close to those based on the additivity assumption
discussed above (47).

     Model Specification. Since the estimation of virtually safe
levels of exposure requires extrapolation of the experimental data
well outside the observable range, it is not surprising that
different models can lead to widely divergent results. As an
example, consider the estimates of added risk over background in
the low dose region shown in Figure 4 for the dieldrin data based
on the probit, logit, Weibull, multi-hit, and multi-stage models
with independent background as well as those based on linear
extrapolation from the 1% response rate as determined by the fitted
multi-stage model. The corresponding estimates of the VSD can be
seen to vary over several orders of magnitude, with linear
extrapolation leading to the most conservative results followed by

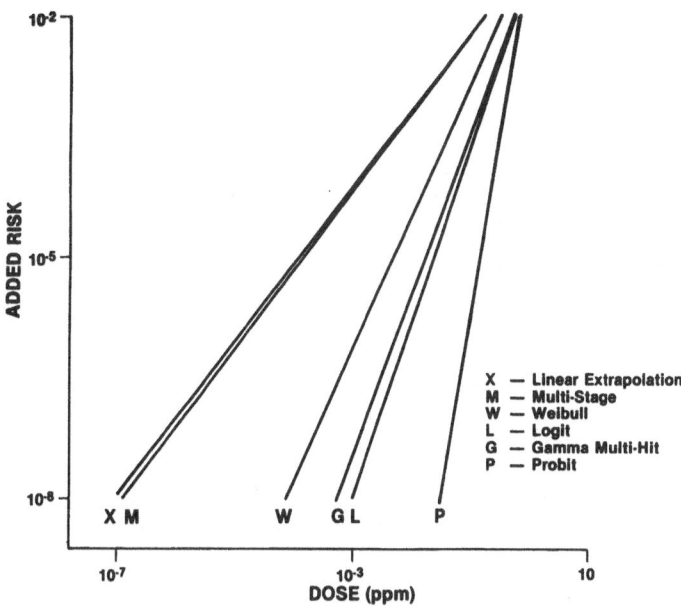

Fig. 4. Estimates of the Added Risk over Background for Dieldrin in the Low Dose Region Based on Six Extrapolation Procedures.

the multi-stage, Weibull, multi-hit, logit, and probit models respectively. Although the magnitude of the differences among models will depend to some extent on the experimental data, the relative ranking of the corresponding VSD's may be expected to be similar to that obtained here whenever the observed dose response curve exhibits some degree of upward curvature (47).

Period of Exposure. Because the risk of tumor development generally increases with time on test, the observed response rates will depend on the period of exposure to the test compound. In the recently completed ED_{01} study with 2-acetylaminofluorene (2-AAF) conducted by the U.S. National Center for Toxicological Research, for example, the incidence of 2-AAF induced liver and bladder tumors increased notably between 18 and 33 months on test (53).

In order to further illustrate this point, consider the hypothetical dose response curves for the general product model shown in Figure 5 (see Appendix A for details). In this case, the steepness of the dose response curve increases with time on test due to the fact that the hazard rate (the rate of occurrence of new tumors among previously unaffected individuals in the population at risk) is increasing linearly with time. Because the slope of the dose response curve is changing with time, the actual VSD also depends somewhat on the period of exposure (Table 2).

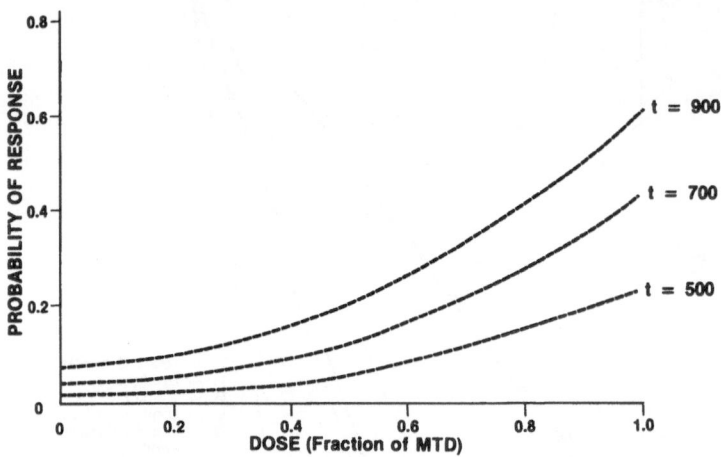

Fig. 5. Hypothetical Dose Response Curves Under the General
         Product Model at t = 500, 700 and 900 Days on Test.

        Time to Response and Competing Risks. In all of the examples
discussed thus far, we have considered only whether or not an
animal developed a tumor by a certain point in time, ignoring any
information on when that tumor may have occurred or on deaths due
to competing risks prior to tumor induction. If such information
is available, statistical techniques for low dose extrapolation
which both utilize individual response times and adjust for the
presence of competing risks may be employed (20,33). Although
these procedures utilize much more of the data available from a
long-term carcinogenicity study, the extent to which the
uncertainty in risk estimation may be reduced through the use of
this additional information remains to be established.

Table 2. Virtually Safe Doses at an Added Risk of 10^{-5} over
          Background for the General Product Model Example

Competing Risks	Exposure Time (Days)	Actual VSD (Fraction of MTD)	Estimates VSD (Fraction of MTD)	
			Time-to-Tumour Data	Observed Incidence
Absent	500	.0089	.0008	a
Absent	700	.0064	.0003	a
Absent	900	.0051	.0002	a
Present	900	.0080	a	.0854

[a]Not applicable.

In order to illustrate how this information is used, however, we simulated a single experimental outcome in which data on both time to tumor and time to death from competing risks was generated (Appendix A). The general product model was fitted to these data in two ways, the first utilizing the data on the time to tumor and the second utilizing only the number of animals which developed tumors by the end of the study (75). In this example, the fitted models approximate the underlying dose response curve quite well (Figure 6) and provide reasonable estimates of the actual VSD (Table 2).

The effects of competing risks on the underlying dose response relationship are also illustrated in Figure 6. The probability of observing a tumor in the presence of competing risks is necessarily lower than in the absence of competing risks due to the fact that many animals will be removed from the population at risk in the former case prior to termination of the study. It is important to recognize that because these two curves in effect measure different endpoints, the corresponding VSD's will also differ somewhat (Table 2).

Metabolic Activation. We have thus far used the administered dose as the dose metameter in our extrapolations of dose response data. It is known, however, that the effective dose at the target tissue may not be directly proportional to the administered dose when one or more steps in the metabolism of the test compound are saturable or rate-limiting (5,30). In such cases, it is important to obtain some measure of internal rather than external dose in order not to distort the shape of the actual dose response relationship.

In order to explore the relationship between the administered and effective dose, consider the simple pharmacokinetic model for metabolic activation depicted in Figure 7a. Here, the initial absorption of the test chemical is proportional to the external dose, as might be expected with inhalation exposure. Once absorbed into the body tissues, the compound may then be immediately eliminated or metabolized to form a reactive metabolite. Under this kinetic model, the metabolite may then be either detoxified or covalently bind with DNA or other macromolecules to form metabolite/macromolecule adducts. Such activated complexes may then lead directly to neoplastic changes in the target tissue.

In this model, elimination, detoxification and adduct formation are all presumed to follow linear or first order kinetics. Metabolic activation, however, is assumed to follow Michaelis-Menten kinetics. In contrast with first order activation, this results in a nonlinear relationship between the effective and administered doses (Figure 8a). Because of the saturability of the metabolic activation process, the fraction of

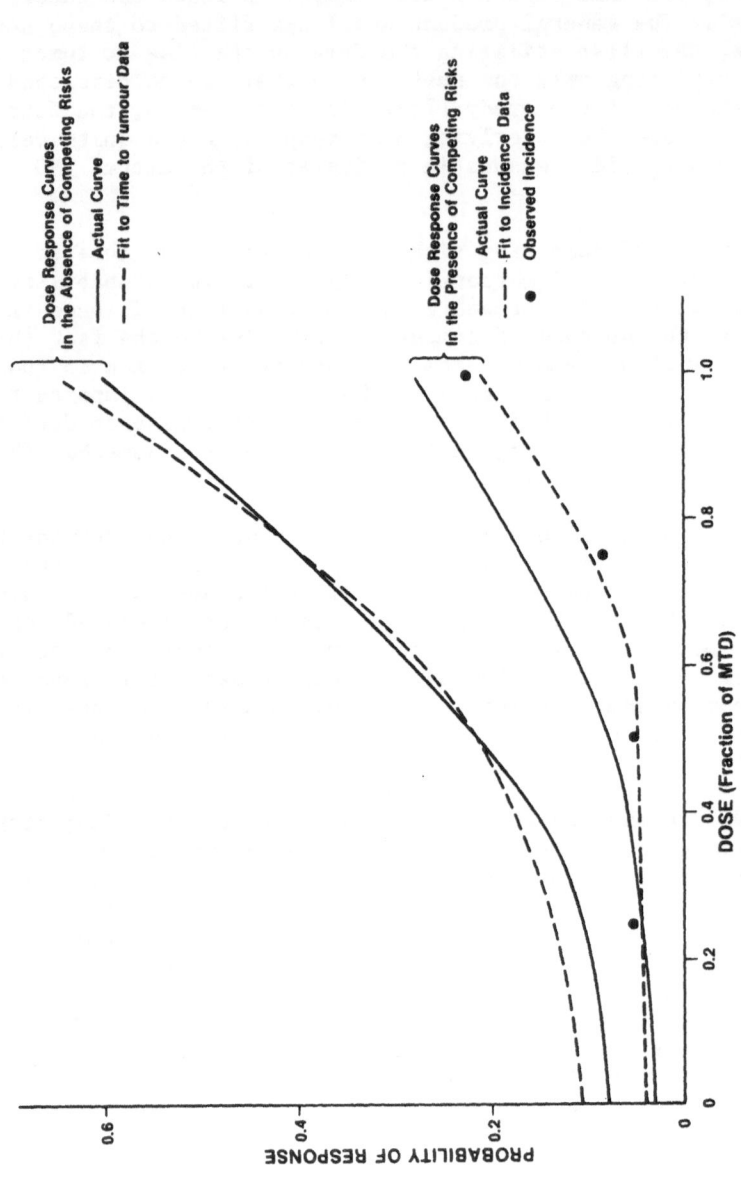

Fig. 6. Hypothetical Dose Response Curves Under the General Product Model and Models Fitted to Simulated Data (t=900 Days on Test).

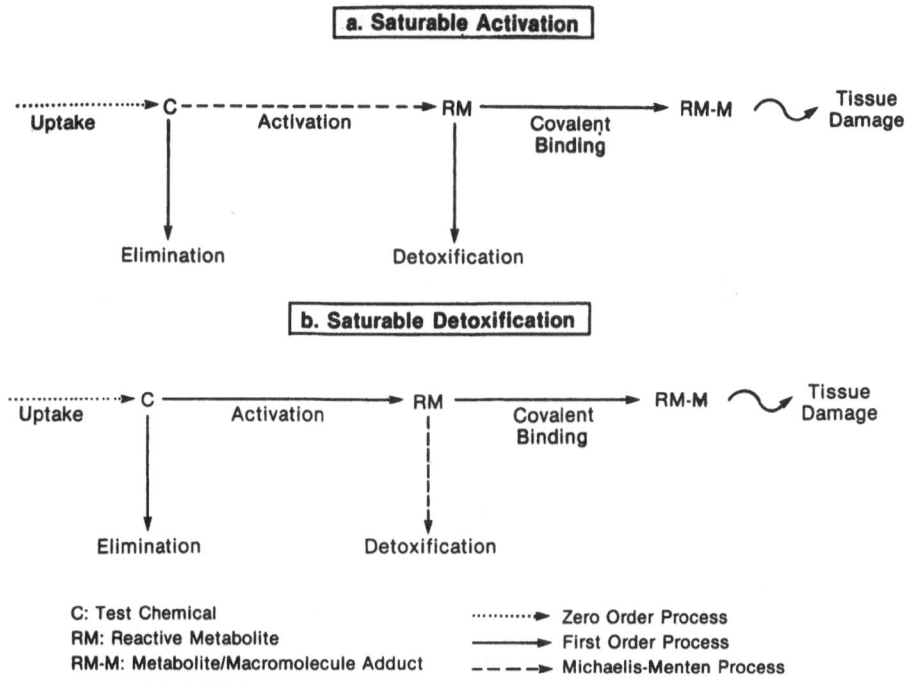

Fig. 7. Two Simple Pharmacokinetic Models for Metabolic Activation.

the absorbed dose converted into the reactive metabolite decreases with increasing dose, resulting in an upper limit on the concentration of the reactive metabolite which may be formed (see Appendix B for details).

Suppose now that metabolic activation is a first order process, but that the detoxification reaction follows Michaelis-Menten kinetics (Figure 7b). In this case, the formation of the reactive metabolite is greater than under first order detoxification (Figure 8b).

Carcinogenic Potency

Because of the difficulties involved in accurately determining virtually safe levels of exposure, several rough yet more robust indices of potency have recently been proposed (15,17). While such measures may provide little quantitative information on actual risks at low levels of exposure, they may be of considerable value in ranking carcinogens with respect to their carcinogenic potential.

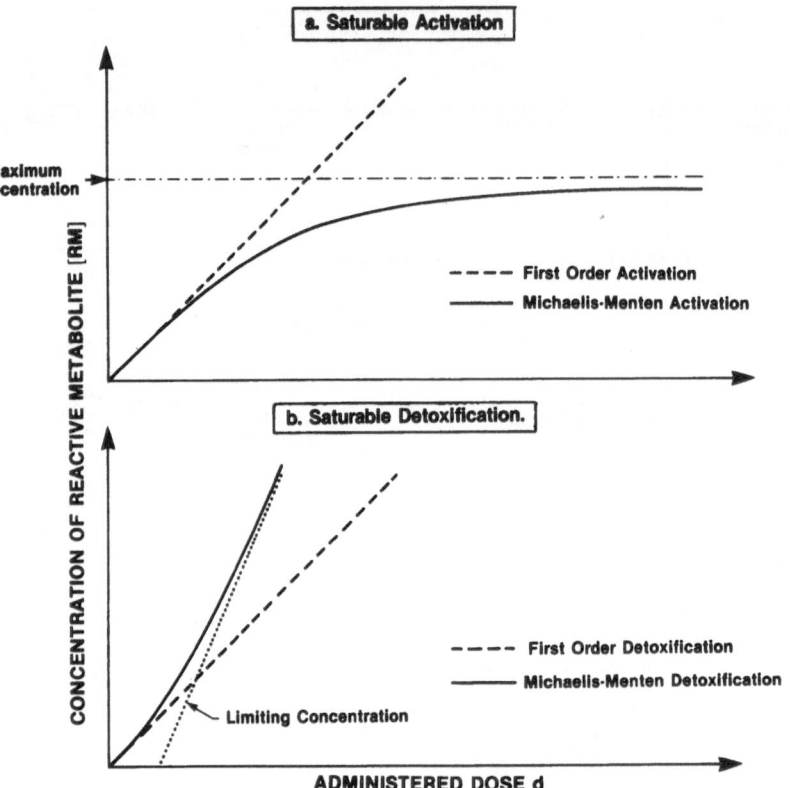

Fig. 8.   Formation of Reactive Metabolite Under Saturable Metabolic
          Activation or Saturable Detoxification.

     Clayson's measure of carcinogenic potency is based on the dose
which induces an added risk over background of 50% in a lifespan
study (ED_{50}). The actual index is defined by:

$$I = C - \log ED_{50},$$

where the ED_{50} is measured in μM/kg body weight/week and C is an
arbitrary constant set equal to 7 in order that the value of I will
be positive. As the dose levels used in actual experiments will
generally not result in precisely 50% added risk, a rough estimate
of ED_{50} may be obtained as:

$$ED_{50} = \frac{d_x}{f_x} \left(\frac{0.5}{P_x}\right),$$

where P_x denotes the observed added risk at dose d_x and f_x denotes
the fraction of the normal lifespan of the test species covered by

the particular experiment. (Provided sufficient data is available, an estimate of the ED_{50} not involving such crude adjustments to the experimental dose and survival rate could be obtained using a suitable mathematical model which provides for nonlinear effects in both dose and time.)

Estimates of carcinogenic potency derived in this manner are shown in Table 3. These results demonstrate that the potency of different compounds can vary by more than seven orders of magnitude.

Inter-Species Extrapolation

Positive results in a carcinogenicity bioassay performed in one species do not necessarily indicate the test agent's ability to induce cancer in another species or in man. As indicated in Table 4, there is considerable variation among species in response to different aromatic amines (12). In contrast, nitrosodiethylamine was an effective carcinogen in all 23 experimental species in which it was tested (73) although, as indicated in Table 5, its potency varies over three orders of magnitude (62).

Differences in potency between species may often be explained in terms of biochemical and metabolic differences (7). For example, the electrophilic theory of chemical carcinogenesis was originally based partly on the fact that 2-AAF was incapable of inducing cancer in guinea pigs because of this species' inability to activate this compound to its N-hydroxy derivative (56,58). Takeishi et al. (80), however, has now shown that the S-9 fraction of guinea pig liver is capable of this activation, suggesting that the resistance of the guinea pig to 2-AAF is a consequence of the ability of intact guinea pig hepatocytes to deactivate this metabolite rather than failure to synthesize it.

Table 3. Potency of Rodent Liver Carcinogens in Lifetime Exposure Studies

Compound	Species	Potency
Aflatoxin	Rat	9.2
NDEA	Rat	6.5
Michler's Ketone	Rat	4.6
2-Aminoanthraquinone	Rat	4.4
Carbon Tetrachloride	Rat	3.9
Trichloroethylene	Mouse	2.1

[a]Based on data summarized by the NAS (1981).

Table 4.   Species Response to Carcinogenic Effect of Occupational
           Bladder Carcinogens

Species	2-Naphthylamine	1-Naphthylamine	Benzidine	4-Aminobiphenyl
Man	Bladder	Bladder[a]	Bladder	Bladder
Dog	Bladder	None	Bladder	Bladder
Monkey	Bladder	b	b	b
Hamsters	Bladder	b	Liver	b
Rat	Bladder	b	Liver, earduct, intestines	Breast, intestines
Mouse	Liver	None	Liver	Liver
Rabbit	None	b	b	Bladder

[a]Contained 4% to 10% 2-naphthylamine.

[b]Not tested.

3.   SHORT-TERM TESTS FOR CARCINOGENICITY

Historical Development

Screening bioassays following the National Cancer Institute
protocol that allows for only two dose levels and a control and
only two rodent species (77) now costs in excess of $500,000 for
each chemical tested and take up to three or more years to
complete. Furthermore, the number of highly trained personnel and
adequate facilities available for the conduct of carcinogen
bioassays are severely limited. Thus, there is a pressing
requirement for less expensive and more rapid ways of identifying
chemical carcinogens.

Table 5.   Carcinogenic Potency of NDEA in Several Species After
           Lifetime Exposure

Species	Strain	Route	Estimated Lifespan (Months)	Target Tissue	Potency
Rat	BDII	Oral	24	Liver	6.5
Mystromys	Albicaudatus	Oral	72	Liver	6.3
Chicken	White Leghorn	i.m.[a]	100	Liver	5.3
Guinea Pig	Hybrid	Oral	84	Liver	4.2
Mouse	MNRI	Oral	18	Liver	4.0
	RF	Oral	18	Liver	3.9
Hamster	Syrian	Oral	18	Trachea	3.7

[a]Intramuscular.

Inexpensive short-term tests for carcinogenicity are currently the focus of considerable research activity (21). As alternative techniques for detecting carcinogenic agents, such tests would appear to have the greatest chance for success if they mimic one or more of the critical events in the carcinogenic process. In 1955, W. J. Burdette reviewed the mutagenic potential of known chemical carcinogens and found that relatively few carcinogens were mutagenic in the assay systems then in use (10). This was partly due to the failure to realize that many mutagens and carcinogens require metabolic activation before they exert their effects on genetic material (56,58). (The organisms used in these systems generally lack the capacity to transform the test compound to the proximate mutagen.)

Considerable progress in correlating mutagenic and carcinogenic effects was made when Malling (54) and Ames et al. (2,3) developed special tester strains of Salmonella typhimurium that lacked the ability to synthesize the essential amino acid, histidine, but reverted to the wild histidine-independent state on mutation. When combined with a tissue brei for metabolic activation (usually the S-9 fraction of rat liver) these organisms appeared to detect carcinogenic agents with a fair degree of accuracy (1,4). Although the original Salmonella-microsome test was somewhat insensitive to certain types of chemicals such as nitrosamines, hydrazines and pyrrolizidine alkaloids (88), modifications of the technique have been proposed to improve its sensitivity. Yahagi et al. (86), for example, resolved the nitrosamine dilemma by pre-incubating the nitrosamines in liquid suspension with the bacteria thereby reducing the possibility of inactivation of labile intermediates by the plate agar (71) and increasing the concentration of both activating enzymes and the test compound during pre-incubation.

At this time more than one hundred short-term tests for carcinogenicity have been described in the literature (38). Although these cannot be detailed here, they fall into several broad categories defined by mutation, cell transformation, DNA adduct formation, DNA repair, and chromosomal or DNA aberrations. Some of these tests are performed entirely in vitro; others may be conducted partially in vivo and thus more accurately reflect the in vivo or host metabolism.

Validation of Short-Term Tests

In order to select those short-term tests which may serve most effectively as predictors of carcinogenic activity, it is necessary to validate individual tests under known conditions (46,67). Such validation studies usually involve applying the test of interest to

a panel of known carcinogens and noncarcinogens.* The utility of
the test may then be measured in terms of its false positive and
false negative rates (Figure 9). The false positive rate may be
considered here to be the proportion $P(M^+|C^-)$ of noncarcinogens
(C^-) in the reference panel which produce positive results (M^+) in
the short-term test system. Similarly, the false negative rate is
given by $P(M^-|C^+)$, where M^- denotes a negative short-term test
result in the presence of a carcinogenic test agent C^+.

Equivalent validation measures are the specificity $P(M^-|C^-)$
and sensitivity $P(M^+|C^+)$ of the test defined by

$$P(M^-|C^-) = 1-P(M^+|C^-)$$
and
$$P(M^+|C^+) = 1-P(M^-|C^+)$$

respectively. Another frequently employed measure is the
predictive value $P(C^+|M^+)$, the probability that a compound is
carcinogenic given that it produced positive short-term test
results. Since

$$P(C^+|M^+) = \frac{P(M^+|C^+)P(C^+)}{[1-P(M^-|C^-)][1-P(C^+)]+P(M^+|C^+)P(C^+)}$$

by Bayes theorem (45, p.157), this measure depends not only on the
specificity $P(M^-|C^-)$ and sensitivity $P(M^+|C^+)$ of the test, but also
on the proportion $P(C^+)$ of carcinogens in the sample. As shown in
Table 6, it is thus possible for a test with only 50% sensitivity
and specificity to have a high predictive value simply because the
panel of test compounds included mostly carcinogens.

The validity of the Ames Salmonella-microsome test has been
the subject of a number of investigations (Table 7). Although many
of these studies have found this system to perform very well in
terms of the measures of validity discussed here, some studies have
also estimated the specificity and sensitivity to be about 50% or
lower.

---

*Since the identification of carcinogens is based on bioassay
results which are in themselves subject to error (section 2), the
effectiveness of validation studies of this type will be influenced
to some extent by the quality of the data base used to establish
the reference panels (31). Similarly, since short-term tests are
also subject to some degree of experimental error, the
reproducibility of the test systems is also an important
determinant in the effectiveness of the validation study.

POSITIVE SHORT-TERM TEST RESULTS?	CARCINOGENICITY?	
	NO(c^-)	YES(c^+)
NO(m^-)	CORRECT DECISION	FALSE NEGATIVE
YES(m^+)	FALSE POSITIVE	CORRECT DECISION

Fig. 9.   Error Rates in Short-term Tests for Carcinogenicity.

The differences among studies in Table 7 may be due to a variety of factors including failure of the in vitro metabolic activation system to reproduce the in vivo situation (13,85) and the fact that certain carcinogens appear to exert their effects by nongenotoxic mechanisms (15,16). In the former case, metabolic processes can differ markedly between species as noted earlier with the activation of 2-AAF in the rat and guinea pig. Perhaps more importantly, the handling involved in the preparation of the S-9 liver fraction in the Salmonella-microsome system results in the disassociation of activating and inactivating enzymes and the destruction of membranes that keep co-factors at appropriate levels in the intact cell. The effect of this in systems employing the S-9 fraction are illustrated by the fact that aflatoxin B_1 is a more potent mutagen in the presence of hamster liver than in the presence of rat liver, whereas this chemical is a much more powerful carcinogen in rats than in hamsters (27). Similarly, Langenbach et al. (51) found that the Ames test placed four nitrosamines in almost inverse order of carcinogenic potency.

The possibility that certain carcinogens may act without affecting the genetic apparatus of the cell is currently the subject of considerable discussion. Some agents may increase tumor yields without necessarily inducing new tumor progenitor cells. For example, they may stimulate the development of tumor progenitor cells initiated by adventitious exposure to traces of other carcinogens (15). Alternatively, the toxic response to an agent may lead to genetic damage such as through the aberrant methylation of DNA (74). Such mechanisms may account for the relative insensitivity of the Ames system in certain classes of chemicals. In this regard, Rinkus & Legator (69) have recently pointed out that only 4 of 12 carcinogenic pesticides were detected using this system.

In order to improve the sensitivity of short-term tests, it has been suggested that a battery of different test systems be employed (83). If a positive result is defined as the induction of mutagenic or other effects in one or more of the component systems, then the sensitivity of the battery will clearly be at least as great as that of any one of the individual tests. Campbell (11),

Table 6. Predictive Value of a Short-term Test as a Fraction of
          the Proportion of Carcinogens in the Population and the
          Sensitivity and Specificity of the Test

Proportion of Carcinogens in Population of Chemicals (%)	Predictive Value (%) Sensitivity/Specificity (%)	
	50/50	90/90
10	10	50
25	25	75
50	50	90
75	75	96
90	90	98

for example, estimated the sensitivity of both the Ames and
mammalian cell transformation systems to be about 91% within a
particular population of chemicals, but found the sensitivity of
these two tests combined to be about 99%.

    Although a battery of short-term tests applied in this fashion
will necessarily result in increased sensitivity, the application
of several tests also leads to decreased specificity. The
magnitude of the tradeoff between sensitivity and specificity
depends on the degree of association among the component tests.
For example, let us consider a simple battery of only two short-

Table 7. Sensitivity and Specificity of the Ames Test[a]

Study	No. of Compounds Tested	Sensitivity (%)	Specificity (%)	Predictive Value (%)	Proportion of Carcinogens (%)
1	300	90	87	92	62
2	120	91	93	93	48
3	60	55	79	68	45
4	146	93	77	89	67
5	51	100	50	81	69
6	26	86	50	90	85
7	25	88	0	65	68
8[b]	86	50	78	89	79
	88	64	74	90	78
9	54	65	81	89	70
10	89	76	57	95	92
11[c]	42	42-68	59-82	-	60
12	21	77	62	77	62
13	87	61	65	85	76

[a]From Purchase (1982).

[b]Not all chemicals tested were classified for carcinogenicity.

[c]Results from 10 investigations on the same 42 chemicals.

term tests. The degree of association between these two tests may be gauged using Yule's measure of concordance Q (see Appendix C), with Q = -1, 0 and +1 indicating complete discordance, no association and complete concordance respectively. As illustrated in Figure 10, the sensitivity of a battery of two unrelated tests (Q=0), each with 80% sensitivity, would be about 95%. The specificity of a battery of two uncorrelated tests each with 80% specificity, on the other hand, would be only about 64%.

Statistical Analysis

Most short-term tests lead to the induction of mutants even in the absence of an external stimulus, i.e., under control conditions. Thus, appropriate statistical tests are necessary to ensure that an increase in the number of mutants in the presence of the test agent is not due to chance alone. Some workers require that the naturally occurring number of mutants be increased by a fixed ratio before the results are considered positive. While this may be a reasonable empirical approach, many of the recently proposed statistical methods for the assessment of short-term test results formally take into account not only the number of mutants formed relative to the controls, but also the relative cytotoxicity in the test and control media, the presence of dose-related effects, and number of test systems utilized (8,42,55,61,76,79).

Future Perspectives

While there is little doubt that the Ames system, or similar microbial assays such as that using E. coli (70), will form the backbone of any modern screening program, such microbial assays need to be supplemented by other tests. In general, it seems

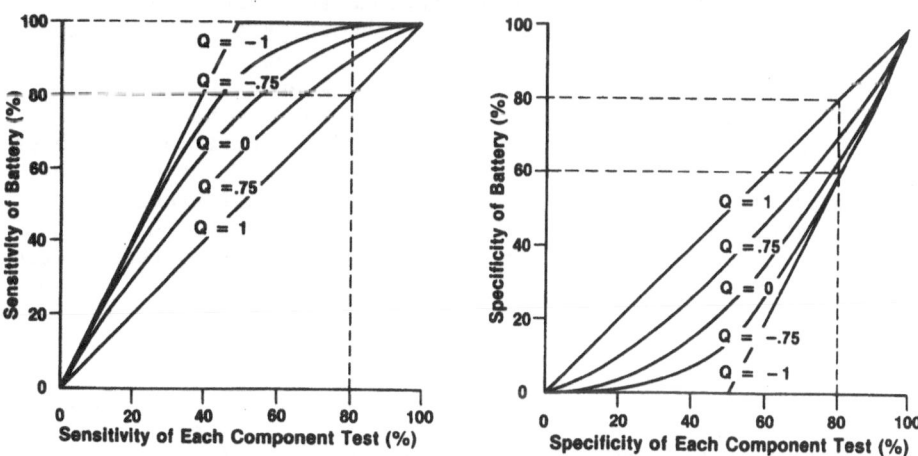

Fig. 10.   Sensitivity and Specificity of a Battery of Two Short-
term Tests (Q=Yule's Measure of Association between the
Two Tests).

reasonable to suggest that the most appropriate short-term tests
will have a precise endpoint, be relatively easy to conduct, and
have a system for metabolic activation closely resembling that in
the whole animal.

Transformation assays (9), for example, may not satisfy these
criteria due to the requirement for skilled differentiation between
colonies in different stages of morphological development as in the
hamster embryo cell technique of Pienta et al. (65) and Pienta
(66). Despite the attractiveness of this approach in producing
transformants that actually grow into tumors in isogenic hosts, it
may pose problems in establishing such an assay in different
laboratories. Similarly, host mediated assays in which the tester
organism is exposed to the test agent as well as metabolites
produced in the host are often relatively insensitive because of
the generally limited recovery of the tester organisms and the
possibly lower degree of metabolic activation in vivo (26).

Thus, although it is possible to define criteria that short-
term carcinogen prescreening tests should fulfill, it is probably
premature at this time to recommend specific tests to be used for
regulatory purposes. On the basis of these criteria, however, the
mammalian cell mediated mammalian cell mutagenesis assay appears to
offer considerable promise for future development. Initially,
Huberman & Sachs (39) co-cultivated Chinese hamster V79 cells with
heavily irradiated fibroblasts to provide metabolic activation.
The endpoints considered were resistance to certain drugs (8-
thioguanine or ouabain) which reflect mutations at specific gene
loci. This sytem was successfully used to detect carcinogens
within a series of nine polycyclic aromatic hydrocarbons. Co-
cultivation of primary explants of unirradiated hepatocytes with
V79 cells differentiated several hepatocarcinogens from
nonhepatocarcinogens (49). While fibroblasts rather than
hepatocytes were required to activate benzo(a)pyrene, the pattern
of activation was reversed with aflatoxin B_1 (50). Several other
tissues, such as transitional cells from the urinary bladder (52),
are also capable of metabolic activation. The recent report by
Jones et al. (44) that 26 nitrosamines showed a striking degree of
correlation between mutagenic and carcinogenic potency using the
rat hepatocyte V79 cell system should provide considerable
encouragement to those who wish to develop this approach. In the
future, the incorporation of isolated human cells into this system
should further improve its predictive value.

4. CONCLUSIONS

In this paper, we have attempted to present an overview of the
currently available techniques for assessing the carcinogenic
potential of pesticides and other agricultural chemicals.
Carcinogenicity bioassays conducted using animal models presently

provide the most widely accepted method of predicting the hazard of specific agents to humans. Since Yamagiwa & Ichikawa's (87) initial observation that coal tar application led to cancer on rabbits' ears, we have accumulated over sixty years of experience with this procedure. Furthermore, the great majority of the 36 agents known or strongly suspected of inducing cancer in man have been shown to induce cancer in experimental animals (41).

Nevertheless, long-term animal bioassays are subject to limitations other than the time and expense involved in their conduct. Rats and mice differ from man in many ways including size and lifespan as well as DNA repair and metabolic capabilities. Such differences lead to the need for trans-species extrapolation in the application of bioassay results to man. In addition, rodent studies are of necessity conducted at high dose levels whereas humans are usually exposed to much lower levels of the agent in question. This results in the need to extrapolate from high to low doses. Thus, while the animal bioassay may serve as an appropriate instrument for the identification of potential human carcinogens, any attempts to quantify human risk on the basis of such studies remain subject to considerable uncertainty.

The role of short-term tests for carcinogenicity in the regulatory process is difficult to assess at this time. On the one hand, those agents that lead to positive results in any reliable test system must be suspected of being able to induce some kind of genetic damage. On the other hand, failure to obtain a positive result does not assure safety since some carcinogens appear to act either by indirect genetic mechanisms or by nongenotoxic pathways. Thus, regulation based only on short-term prescreening tests for carcinogens should not be attempted until these tests are sufficiently improved so as to give much greater confidence in the results. Although Ames (1) found an 80-90% concordance between mutagenicity in the Salmonella-microsome test and carcinogenicity in whole animals, others found the sensitivity and specificity of this test system to be as low as 50% within certain groups of chemicals.

Some degree of quantitative correlation between mutagenicity and carcinogenicity is also needed if risk estimates are eventually to be based on the results of short-term tests. While the mammalian cell mediated mammalian cell mutagenesis assay shows great promise in this respect, much further work is required before this promise can be fulfilled.

APPENDIX A: THE GENERAL PRODUCT MODEL

In this appendix, we describe the general product model used in the examples given in Table 2 and Figures 5 and 6. Under this model, the probability of a tumor occurring by time t and dose d in the absence of competing risks is given by

$$P(t,d) = 1-\exp\{-g(d)H(t)\},\qquad\qquad (A.1)$$

where g(d) and H(t) are positive nondecreasing functions of dose d and time t respectively. The age specific tumor incidence rate is defined by

$$\lambda(t,d) = \frac{-\partial\log\{1-P(t,d)\}}{\partial t} = g(d)h(t),\qquad (A.2)$$

where $h(t) = dH(t)/dt$. Thus, the hazard rate $\lambda(t,d)$ is a product of a function g(d) of dose but not time and a function h(t) of time but not dose. Recently, Hartley, Tolley & Sielken (34) provided two broad biological foundations for this model formulated in terms of a dynamic system of compartmental models or a series of "attacks" on target areas.

Hartley & Sielken (33) employ the parametric forms

$$g(d) = \sum_{i=0}^{a} \alpha_i d^i \text{ and}\qquad\qquad (A.3)$$

$$H(t) = \sum_{j=1}^{b} \beta_j t^j\qquad\qquad (A.4)$$

in (A.1) where α_i and β_j are constrained to be nonnegative with $\Sigma\beta_j=1$. This in effect represents a generalization of the multi-stage model considered by Crump et al. (18), in which H(t) involves only that power of time corresponding to the number of stages in the response process. A similar generalization has been proposed by Daffer et al. (20) in which H(t) is modelled nonparametrically.

In the example presented in this paper, we took

$$\alpha_0 = 0.10294 \times 10^{-6}$$

$$\alpha_1 = 0 \qquad\qquad\qquad\qquad \beta_1 = 0$$

$$\alpha_2 = 0.51414 \times 10^{-6} \qquad\qquad \beta_2 = 1$$

$$\alpha_3 = 0.51414 \times 10^{-6}$$

(a=3, b=2). These values were selected so that (i) the spontaneous response rate P(900, 0) at t=900 days on test would be equal to 8%, (ii) the response rate P(900, 1) at t=900 days on test at the maximum tolerated dose d=1 would be equal to 60%, (iii) the dose response curve P(t,d) at any time t would be sublinear at low doses and exhibit moderate curvature at high doses, and (iv) the hazard rate $\lambda(t,d)$ would increase linearly with time at each dose d.

The time to death after tumor induction was assumed to follow an indepenent Weibull model, with the probability of dying by time t after the occurrence of a tumor given by

$$G(t)=1-\exp(-\exp\{\frac{\log t-\alpha}{\sigma}\}).\qquad\qquad(A.5)$$

Setting α=4.999 and σ=0.35882 in (A.5) results in a median survival time following the onset of a tumor of 130 days.

Deaths due to competing risks were also considered to follow an independent Weibull distribution as in (A.5) with α = 6.3941 and σ = 0.48960. This results in G(500) = 0.50 and G(900) = 0.90. In the presence of such competing risks, some animals may die prior to developing a tumor. Letting t_1 and t_2 denote the time to tumor and time to death from a competing risk respectively, the probability of <u>observing</u> a tumor in any animal dying during the course of the study or killed in the terminal sacrifice at time T is given by

$$P^*(T,d) = \Pr\{t_1 < t_2, t_1 < T\}$$

$$= \int_0^\infty \Pr\{t_1 < t, t_1 < T | t_2 = t\} dG(t)$$

$$= \int_0^T \Pr\{t_1 < t\} dG(t) + \int_T^\infty \Pr\{t_1 < T\} dG(t)$$

$$= \int_0^T P(t,d) dG(t) + P(T,d)\{1-G(T)\},\qquad(A.6)$$

where G denotes the Weibull model for deaths due to competing risks.

In order to illustrate the use of the general product model in the analysis of experimental data, we simulated one experimental outcome using the models discussed above (Table A.1). The experimental design used involved 5 equally spaced dose levels with 48 animals at each dose and a terminal sacrifice at T=900 days. This data was then fitted to the general product model with a=b=4 corresponding to the number of non-zero dose levels assuming that (i) both time to tumor and time to death are observable and (ii) only the number of animals with tumors at the end of the study is observable. The resulting estimates of the VSD defined in terms of either P(t,d) in (A.1) or P*(T,d) in (A.6) are given in Table 2. (Because of the lack of a closed form expression for P*(T,d),

Table A.1. Simulated Experimental Data for the General Product Model Example

Dose (Fraction of MTD)	Cause of Death[a]	Tumour Present (+) or Absent (−) at Necropsy	Number of Animals	Time to Tumour/Time to Death
0.0	S	−	7	900 900 900 900 900 900 900
	C	−	39	494 289 159 854 683 479 156 589 384 580 265 493 164 362 398 708 385 788 701 258 743 544 656 828 360 512 262 27 515 582 756 394 406 816 442 411
0.25	C	+	1	671/707
	T	+	1	336/475
	S	−	5	900 900 900 900 900
	S	+	1	805/900
	C	−	40	787 510 487 850 671 425 380 655 161 565 739 491 395 613 814 753 300 432 305 459 42 618 478 495 419 339 227 453 452 267 622 387 162 512 345 245 318 584 464 146
0.50	T	+	2	180/254 380/556
	S	−	4	900 900 900 900
	C	−	42	129 693 258 219 314 591 190 261 207 46 867 166 813 437 875 900 496 326 418 485 607 482 183 667 875 458 354 616 583 235 566 604 702 299 633 657 530 266 172 44 232 246
0.75	C	+	1	577/708
	T	+	1	185/307
	S	−	3	900 900 900
	C	−	41	618 569 198 468 438 235 422 499 364 739 364 243 238 103 795 598 801 675 228 461 452 417 375 520 721 556 371 876 591 369 340 778 341 225 248 437 576 231 397 259 515
1.00	C	+	1	136/216
	T	+	3	430/653 639/728 337/514
	S	−	1	900
	S	+	1	878/900
	C	−	36	266 454 98 258 824 317 575 349 506 472 471 260 519 393 384 708 666 425 313 83 452 701 725 311 190 216 496 170 442 366 258 193 347 168 421 296
	C	+	4	348/426 239/337 294/315 819/838
	T	+	6	325/466 497/569 240/346 534/706 491/546 598/679

a S = Sacrifice
C = Competing Risk
T = Tumour

calculation of the VSD based on this latter function had to be done
via numerical integration.)

APPENDIX B: PHARMACOKINETIC MODELS FOR METABOLIC ACTIVATION

The purpose of this appendix is to describe some simple
pharmacokinetic models for metabolic activation of the test
agent. To simplify the discussion, details will be presented only
in the case of continuous inhalation exposure involving a constant
concentration of the test chemical in the atmosphere.
(Corresponding results for repeated oral dosing will be
qualitatively similar.) Intake of the test chemical will thus be
assumed to follow zero[th] order kinetics in which the rate of
absorption is directly proportional to the level of exposure. In
this case, the rate of uptake for the absorption process may be
expressed as K_o = pd ($0 < p \leqslant 1$), where d denotes the administered dose
expressed as a concentration in ambient air.

Consider first the kinetic model shown in Figure 7a. Once
absorbed into the body tissues, the test chemical C may then be
eliminated in accordance with linear first order kinetics with rate
coefficient k_a or activated to form a reactive metabolite RM
following nonlinear Michaelis-Menten kinetics with maximum velocity
V_m and "first order" rate coefficient V_m/K_m at low doses (29). The
latter assumption reflects the fact that metabolic activation is
considered to be a rate limiting or saturable process in this
case. The reactive metabolite may then be detoxified or may
covalently bind with macromolecules to form a metabolite/macro-
molecule adduct RM-M. These two kinetic processes are assumed to
follow first order kinetics with rate coefficients k_b and k_c
respectively. The metabolite/macromolecule complex may then
ultimately give rise to tissue damage.

Under this model, the concentration of the test chemical in
the body and its metabolites can be described by the system of
nonlinear differential equations

$$\frac{d[C]}{dt} = K_o - k_a[C] - \frac{V_m[C]}{K_m+[C]}, \qquad (B.1)$$

$$\frac{d[RM]}{dt} = \frac{V_m[C]}{K_m+[C]} - (k_b+k_c)\,[RM], \text{ and} \qquad (B.2)$$

$$\frac{d[RM-M]}{dt} = k_b[RM], \qquad (B.3)$$

where [C], [RM] and [RM-M] denote the concentration of the absorbed
chemical, reactive metabolite and metabolite/macromolecule complex
at time t. Assuming that the system is in steady state, d[C]/dt =
d[RM]/dt = 0. (Although the state of the system during the

approach to steady state thus ignored, the impact of this assumption in long-term studies is expected to be inconsequential for rapidly equilibrating compounds.) In this case

$$[RM-M] = k_b[RM]t, \qquad (B.4)$$

so that [RM-M] is proportional to [RM] at any time t. Thus, in order to determine the pharmacokinetically effective dose, it suffices to determine the concentration of the reactive metabolite [RM]. (Note that although [C] and [RM] are constant in steady state, [RM-M] increases linearly with time t.)

Solving (B.1) for [C] in steady state, substituting the result in (B.2), and solving for [RM] yields

$$[RM] = \frac{\alpha d + \beta - [(\alpha d - \beta)^2 + 4\alpha\beta(1-\gamma)d]^{1/2}}{2\gamma}, \qquad (B.5)$$

where

$$\alpha = \frac{pV_m}{(k_b + k_c)\,(k_a K_m + V_m)}, \qquad (B.6)$$

$$\beta = \frac{V_m}{k_b + k_c}, \text{ and} \qquad (B.7)$$

$$\gamma = \frac{(V_m/K_m)}{(V_m/K_m) + k_a} < 1. \qquad (B.8)$$

Here, α represents the slope of the curve depicting the concentration of the reactive metabolite [RM] formed as a function of the administered dose d in the low dose region in Figure 8a (this corresponds to the slope of the curve which would result in the case of first order activation), β is the limiting value of the concentration of the reactive metabolite which may be formed, and γ denotes the fraction of the absorbed dose which is metabolized at low doses. (We note that as $\gamma \rightarrow 1$, the curve shown in Figure 8a will limit to a curve consisting of two intersecting straight lines. As $\gamma \rightarrow 0$, on the other hand, the curve approaches that defined by [RM] = $\alpha\beta d/(\alpha d + \beta)$.)

An alternative model in which activation is described by first order kinetics and deactivation follows Michaelis-Menten kinetics is shown in Figure 7b. The differential equations which describe this model are

$$\frac{d[C]}{dt} = K_o - (k_a + k_m)\,[C], \qquad (B.9)$$

$$\frac{d[RM]}{dt} = k_m[C] - \frac{V_c[RM]}{K_c+[RM]} - k_b[RM], \text{ and} \qquad (B.10)$$

$$\frac{d[RM-M]}{dt} = k_b [RM], \qquad (B.11)$$

where k_m denotes the rate coefficient for the first order activation process and V_c and K_c denote the Michaelis-Menten parameters governing the detoxification process.

As in the previous model, [RM-M] is proportional to [RM] in steady state so that it suffices to solve for [RM]. Solving (B.9) and (B.10) for [RM] reveals that $[C] = pd/(k_a+k_m)$ and

$$[RM] = \frac{\delta}{2} [d + \frac{\zeta}{(\delta-\epsilon)} + \{[d + \frac{\zeta}{(\delta-\epsilon)}]^2 - 4 \frac{\epsilon \zeta}{\delta(\delta-\epsilon)}\}^{1/2}], \qquad (B.12)$$

where

$$\delta = \frac{pk_m}{(k_m+k_a)k_b}, \qquad (B.13)$$

$$\epsilon = \frac{pk_m}{(k_m+k_a)} \frac{K_c}{V_c+k_bK_c}, \text{ and} \qquad (B.14)$$

$$\zeta = \frac{-V_c}{k_b} . \qquad (B.15)$$

Here, ϵ denotes the slope of the curve depicting [RM] as a function of d in the low dose region in Figure 8b, and δ and ζ denote the slope and intercept respectively of the same curve at high doses.

APPENDIX C: ASSOCIATION BETWEEN TWO SHORT-TERM TESTS

The purpose of this appendix is to describe a quantitative measure of association between two short-term tests. Suppose that the two tests are applied to a population of known chemical carcinogens with the following results.

Test M_2	Test M_1		Total
	M_1^-	M_1^+	
M_2^-	$1-(s_1+s_2)+p$	s_1-p	$1-s_2$
M_2^+	s_2-p	p	s_2
Total	$1-s_1$	s_1	1

Here, $s_i = P(M_1^+|C^+)$ denotes the proportion of carcinogens detected by test $i=1, 2$ (s_i is thus simply the sensitivity of the ith test) and $p = P(M_1^+, M_2^+|C^+)$ denotes the proportion of carcinogens detected by both tests (p is thus the sensitivity of the battery), where

$$\max [0,(s_1+s_2)-1] \leqslant p \leqslant \min [s_1,s_2]. \qquad (C.1)$$

Yule's measure of association Q between the two tests is defined by

$$Q = (w-1)/(w+1) \quad , \; p < \min(s_1,s_2) \qquad (C.2)$$
$$= 1 \qquad\qquad , \; p = \min(s_1,s_2)$$

(45, p. 539), where

$$w = \frac{p[1-(s_1+s_2)+p]}{[s_1-p][s_2-p]} \qquad (C.3)$$

denotes the odds ratio in the above table. It follows from (C.1)-(C.3) that $-1 \leqslant Q \leqslant +1$, with the extreme values occurring when p achieves its upper and lower limits in (C.1). The cases $Q = +1$ and -1 correspond respectively to maximal concordance and discordance between the two tests, while $Q = 0$ implies that the two tests are statistically independent.

As an example, consider the results of the Ames and mammalian cell transformation tests for the 58 carcinogens examined by Purchase et al. (68). (We note that the latter test actually involved the use of human lung, human liver, and baby Syrian hamster kidney cells.)

Mammalian Cell Transformation M_2	Ames Test M_1		Total
	M_1^-	M_1^+	
M_2^-	2/58	3/58	5/58
M_2^+	3/58	50/58	53/58
Total	5/58	53/58	58/58

In this case, we find $w = 11.1$ and $Q = 0.84$.

The value of p corresponding to a given value of Q may be obtained as the root of the quadratic equation

$$2Qp^2 + [1-Q+2Q(s_1+s_2)]p+(Q+1)s_1s_2 = 0 \qquad (C.4)$$

satisfying (C.1). Thus, the sensitivity p of the battery of the two tests may be evaluated as a function of Q using (C.4).

Similar arguments may be used in determining the specificity of the battery as a function of Yule's measure of association for non-carcinogens. We note, however, that the degree of association for noncarcinogens need not correspond to that for carcinogens. For the data on the Ames and mammalian cell transformation tests reported by Purchase et al. (67), we in fact find Q = -1 for the noncarcinogens since these two test never result in simultaneous positive results for any of the 62 compounds examined.

ACKNOWLEDGEMENTS

We would like to thank Dr. R. Sielken for generously providing us with his analysis of the data in Appendix A, Dr. I.F.H. Purchase for his permission to reproduce the results presented in Table 7, Dr. D. Stoltz, Dr. C. T. Miller, Dr. S. Lagakos and Mr. M. Bickis for their most helpful comments on an earlier version of this paper, and Mr. R. Stapley for his assistance in preparing this manuscript.

REFERENCES

1. Ames. B.N. (1977). Environmental chemicals causing cancer and genetic birth defects: Developing a strategy for minimizing human exposure. California Policy Seminar Monographs, Vol. 3, pp. 1-37.
2. Ames, B.N., Durston, W.E., Yamasaki, E. & Lee, F.D. (1973a). Carcinogens are mutagens - A simple test system combining liver homogenates for activation and bacteria for detection. Proceedings of the National Academy of Sciences 70, 2281-2285.
3. Ames, B.N., Lee, F.D. & Durston, W.E. (1973b). An improved bacterial test system for the detection and classification of mutagens and carcinogens. Proceedings of the National Academy of Sciences 70, 782-786.
4. Ames, B.N., Hooper, K., Sawyer, C.B., Friedman, A.D., Peto, R., Havender, W., Gold, L.S. & Haggin, T. (1980). Carcinogenic potency: A progress report. In: Banbury Report 5. Ethylenedibromide: A Potential Health Risk. Cold Spring Harbor Laboratory, Cold Spring Harbor, pp. 55-63.
5. Anderson, M.W., Hoel, D.G. & Kaplan, N.L. (1980). A general scheme for the incorporation of pharmacokinetics in low-dose risk estimation for chemical carcinogenesis: Example - vinyl chloride. Toxicology and Applied Pharmacology 55, 154-161.

6. Arnold, D.L., Charbonneau, S.M., Zawidzka, Z.Z. & Grice, H.C. (1977). Monitoring animal health during chronic toxicity studies. Journal of Environmental Pathology and Toxicology 1, 227-239.

7. ASPET: American Society of Pharmacology and Experimental Therapeutics (1980). Extrapolation of laboratory toxicity and data to man: factors influencing the dose-toxic response relationship. Federation Proceedings 39, 53-82.

8. Bernstein, L., Kaldor, J., McCann, J. & Pike, M.C. (1981). An empirical approach to the statistical analysis of mutagenesis data from the Salmonella Test. Mutation Research. In press.

9. Brookes, P. (1981). Critical assessment of the value of in vivo cell transformation for predicting in vivo carcinogenicity of chemicals. ICPEMC Working Paper 2/4. Mutation Research 86, 233-242.

10. Burdette, W.J. (1955). The significance of mutation in relation to the origin of tumors: A review. Cancer Research 15, 201-226.

11. Campbell, T.C. (1980). Chemical carcinogens and human risk assessment. Federation Proceedings 39, 2467-2484.

12. Clayson, D.B. & Garner, R.C. (1976). Carcinogenic aromatic amines and related compounds. In: Chemical Carcinogens (C.E. Searle, ed.). American Chemical Society Monograph No. 173, American Chemical Society, Washington, D.C., pp. 366-461.

13. Clayson, D.B. (1980). Comparison between in vitro and in vivo tests for carcinogenicity: An overview. ICPEMC Working Paper 2/1. Mutation Research 75, 205-218.

14. Clayson, D.B. (1981a). Carcinogenesis in the developing organism: Could protocols for testing be improved? Biological Research in Pregnancy. In Press.

15. Clayson, D.B. (1981b). Carcinogens and carcinogenesis enhancers. ICPEMC Working Paper 2/3. Mutation Research 86, 217-229.

16. Committee of the Health Council of the Netherlands (1978). The Evaluation of the Carcinogenicity of Chemical Substances. Ministerie van Volksgezond heid en Milieu hygiene, Leidschendam.

17. Crouch, E. & Wilson, R. (1981). Regulation of carcinogens. Risk Analysis 1, 47-57.

18. Crump, K.S., Hoel, D.G., Langley, C.H., Peto, R. (1976). Fundamental carcinogenic processes and their implications for low dose risk assessment. Cancer Research 36, 2973-2979.

19. Crump, K.S., Guess, H. & Deal, K. (1977). Confidence intervals and test of hypotheses concerning dose response relations inferred from animal carcinogenicity data. Biometrics 33, 437-445.

20. Daffer, P.Z., Crump, K.S. & Masterman, M.D. (1980). Asymptotic theory for analyzing dose-response survival data with application to the low-dose extrapolation problem. Mathematical Biosciences 50, 207-230.

21. de Serres, F.J. & Ashby, J. (1981). "Evaluation of Short-Term Tests for Carcinogens". Elsevier-North Holland/Amsterdam.

22. Elashoff, R., Preston, D. & Fears, T. (1979). Comparison and evaluation of some experimental designs for use in carcinogen screening. Journal of the National Cancer Institute 62, 1209-1219.

23. Fears, T., Tarone, R.E. & Chu, K.C. (1977). False-positive and false-negative rates for carcinogenicity screens. Cancer Research 37, 1941-1945.

24. FSC: Food Safety Council (1980). Proposed System for Food Safety Assessment. Food Safety Council, Washington, D.C.

25. Fox, J.G., Thibert, P., Arnold, D.L., Krewski, D.R. & Grice, H.C. (1979). Toxicology studies II. The laboratory animal. Food and Cosmetics Toxicology 17, 661-675.

26. Gabridge, M.G. & Legator, M.S. (1969). A host-mediated microbial assay for the detection of mutagenic compounds. Proceedings of the Society for Experimental Biology and Medicine, 130, 831-834.

27. Garner, R.C., Miller, E.C. & Miller, J.A. (1972). Liver microsomal metabolism of aflatoxin B_1 to a reactive derivative toxic to Salmonella typhimurium TA 1530. Cancer Research 32, 2058-2066.

28. Gart, J.J., Chu, K.C., Tarone, R.E. (1979). Statistical issues in interpretation of chronic bioassay tests for carcinogenicity. Journal of the National Cancer Institute 62, 957-974.

29. Gehring, P.J., Watanabe, P.G. & Blau, G.E. (1976). Pharmacokinetic studies in evaluation of the toxicological and environmental hazard of chemicals. In: Advances in Modern Toxicology, Vol. 1, Part 1. New Concepts in Safety Evaluation. (M.A. Mehlman, R.E. Shapiro & H. Blumenthal, eds.), Hemisphere Publishing, New York, pp. 195-270.

30. Gehring, P.J., Watanabe, P.G. & Park, C.N. (1978). Resolution of dose-response toxicity data for chemicals requiring metabolic activation: Example-vinyl chloride. Toxicology and Applied Pharmacology 44, 581-591.

31. Griesmer, R.A. & Cueto, C. (1980). Toward a classification scheme for degrees of experimental evidence for the carcinogenicity of chemicals for animals. In: Molecular and Cellular Aspects of Carcinogen Screening Tests. (R. Montesano, H. Bartsch & L. Tomatis, eds.). IARC Scientific Publication No. 27, International Agency for Research on Cancer, Lyon, pp. 259-281.

32. Grice, H.C., Munro, I.C., Krewski, D.R. & Blumenthal, H. (1981). In utero exposure in chronic toxicity/carcinogenicity studies. Food and Cosmetics Toxicology 19, 373-379.

33. Hartley, H.O. & Sielken, R.L. (1977). Estimation of "safe doses" in carcinogenic experiments. Biometrics 33, 1-30.

34. Hartley, H.O., Tolley, H.D. & Sielken, R.L. (1981). The
     product form of the hazard rate model in carcinogenic
     testing. In: Statistics and Related Topics (M. Csörgö, D.
     Dawson, J.N.K. Rao and E. Saleh, eds.), North-Holland,
     Amsterdam, pp. 185-200.
35. Haseman, J.K. (1978). Exact sample sizes for use with the
     Fisher-Irwin test for 2x2 Tables. Biometrics 34, 106-109.
36. Hoel, D.G. (1980). Incorporation of background response in
     dose-response models. Federation Proceedings 39, 73-75.
37. Hoffmann, G.R. (1982). Overview of genetic toxicology. This
     volume.
38. Hollstein, M. & McCann, J. (1979). Short-term tests for
     carcinogens and mutagens. Mutation Research 65, 133-226.
39. Huberman, E. & Sachs, L. (1976). Mutability of different
     genetic loci in mammalian cells by metabolically activated
     carcinogenic polycyclic hydrocarbons. Proceedings of the
     National Academy of Sciences 173, 188-192.
40. IARC: International Agency for Research in Cancer (1980a).
     Long-term and Short-term Screening Assays for Carcinogens: A
     Critical Appraisal. IARC Monographs on the Evaluation of the
     Carcinogenic Risk of Chemicals to Humans, Supplement 2, IARC,
     Lyon.
41. IARC: International Agency for Research on Cancer (1980b).
     An evaluation of chemicals and industrial processes associated
     with cancer in humans based on human and animal data: IARC
     monographs, Vol. 1 to 20. Cancer Research 40, 1-12.
42. Irr, J.D. & Snee, R.D. (1980). Statistical evaluation of
     mutagenicity in the CHO/HGPRT system. In: Banbury Report 2
     Mammalian Cell Mutagenesis. Cold Spring Harbor Laboratory,
     Cold Spring Harbor, pp. 263-275.
43. IRLG: Interagency Regulatory Liaison Group (1979).
     Scientific basis for identification of potential carcinogens
     and estimation of risks. Journal of the National Cancer
     Institute 63, 241-268.
44. Jones, C.A., Marlino, P.J., Lijinsky, W. & Huberman, E.
     (1981). The relationship between the carcinogenicity and
     mutagenicity of nitrosamines in a hepatocyte mediated
     mutagenicity assay carcinogenesis. In press.
45. Kendall, M.G. & Stuart, A. (1967). The Advanced Theory of
     Statistics (Vol. 2, Second edition). Hafner, New York.
46. Kretzer, H., Habs, M. & Schmähl, D. (1979). Limitations of in
     vitro short-term tests as prescreening models for
     carcinogenicity in industry: a theoretical approach.
     Toxicology 14, 283-289.
47. Krewski, D.R. & Van Ryzin. J. (1981). Dose response models
     for quantal response toxicity data. In: Statistics and
     Related Topics (M. Csörgö, D. Dawson, J.N.K. Rao & E. Saleh,
     eds.), North Holland, Amsterdam, pp. 201-231.
48. Krewski, D. & Brown, C. (1981). Carcinogenic risk
     assessment: A guide to the literature Biometrics 37, 353-366.

49. Langenbach, R., Freed, H.J., Raveh, D. & Huberman, E. (1978a). Liver cell-mediated mutagenesis of mammalian cells by liver carcinogens. Proceedings of the National Academy of Sciences 75, 2864-2867.

50. Langenbach, R., Freed, H.G., Raveh, D., & Huberman, E. (1978b). Cell specificity in metabolic activation of aflatoxin B_1 and benzo(a)pyrene to mutagens for mammalian cells. Nature 276, 277-280.

51. Langenbach, R., Gingell, R., Kuszynski, C., Walker, B., Hagel, D. & Pour, P. (1980). Mutagenic activities of oxidized derivatives of N-nitroso-dipropylamine in the liver "cell-mediated" and Salmonella typhimurium assays. Cancer Research 40, 3463-3467.

52. Langenbach, R., Malick, L. & Nesnow, S. (1981). Rat bladder cell-mediated mutagenesis of Chinese-hamster V79 cells and metabolism of benzo(a)pyrene. Journal of the National Cancer Institute 66, 913-917.

53. Littlefield, N.A., Farmer, J.H., Gaylor, D.W. & Sheldon, W.G. (1979). Effects of dose and time in a long-term, low-dose carcinogenic study. Journal of Environmental Pathology and Toxicology 3, 17-34.

54. Malling, H.V. (1971). Dimethylnitrosamine: Formation of mutagenic compounds by interaction with mouse liver microsomes. Mutation Research 13, 425-429.

55. Margolin, B.H., Kaplan, H. & Zeiger, E. (1981). Statistical analysis of the Ames Salmonella/microsome test. Proceedings of the National Academy of Sciences 78, 3779-3783.

56. Miller, J.A. (1970). Carcinogenesis by chemicals: An overview. (G.H.A. Clowes Memorial Lecture) Cancer Research 30, 559-576.

57. Miller, E.C. (1978). Some current perspectives on chemical carcinogenesis in humans and experimental animals: President's address. Cancer Research 38, 1479-1496.

58. Miller, E.C. & Miller, J.A. (1976). The metabolism of chemical carcinogens to reactive electrophiles and their possible mechanisms of action in carcinogenesis. In: Chemical Carcinogens (C.E. Searle, ed.). American Chemical Society Monograph No. 173, American Chemical Society, Washington, D.C., pp. 737-762.

59. Munro, I.C. (1977). Considerations in chronic toxicity testing: the chemical, the dose, the design. Journal of Environmental Pathology and Toxicology 1, 183-197.

60. Munro, I.C. & Krewski, D.R. (1981). Risk assessment and regulatory decision making. Food & Cosmetics Toxicology 19, 541-560.

61. Myers, L.E., Sexton, N.H., Southerland, L.I. Wolff, T.J. (1981). Regression analysis of Ames test data. Environmental Mutagenesis 5, 575-586.

62. NAS: National Research Council, National Academy of Sciences (1981). The Health Effects on Nitrate, Nitrite and N-Nitroso Compounds (Part 1). National Academy Press, Washington, D.C.

63. OTA: Office of Technology Assessment (1981). Assessment of Technologies for Determining Cancer Risks from the Environment. U.S. Government Printing Office, Washington, D.C.

64. Peto, R. (1978). Carcinogenic effects of chronic exposure to very low levels of toxic substances. Environmental Health Perspectives 22, 155-159.

65. Pienta, R.J., Poiley, J.A. & Lebherz, W.B. (1977). Morphological transformation of early passage Golden Syrian hamster embryo cells derived from cryopreserved primary cultures as a reliable in vitro bioassay for identifying diverse carcinogens. International Journal of Cancer 19, 642-655.

66. Pienta, R.J. (1979). A hamster embryo cell model system for identifying carcinogens. In: Carcinogens: Identification and Mechanisms of Action (A.C. Griffin & G.R. Shaw, eds.). Raven Press, New York, pp. 121-141.

67. Purchase, I.F.H. (1982). An appraisal of predictive tests for carcinogenicity. In preparation.

68. Purchase, I.F.H., Longstaff, E., Ashby, J., Styles, J.A., Anderson, D., Lefevre, P.A., & Westwood, F.R. (1978). An evaluation of 6 short-term tests for detecting organic chemical carcinogens. British Journal of Cancer 37, 873-959.

69. Rinkus, S.J. & Legator, M.S. (1979). Chemical characterization of 465 known or suspected carcinogens and their correlation with mutagenic activity in the Salmonella typhimurium system. Cancer Research 39, 3289-3318.

70. Rosenkranz, H.S. & Leifer, Z. (1979). Determining the DNA-modifying activity of chemicals using DNA-polymerase-deficient Eichenicia coli. In: Chemical Mutagens: Principles and Procedures for Their Detection, Vol. 6. (A. Hollaender & F. de Serres, eds.). Plenum Press, New York, pp.

71. Rosenkranz, H.S., Karpinsky, G. & McCoy, E.C. (1980). Microbial assays: Evaluation and application to the elucidation of the etiology of colon cancer. In: Short-Term Test Systems for Detecting Carcinogens. (K.H. Norpoth & R.C. Garner, eds.). Springer-Verlag, New York, pp. 19-57.

72. Salsburg, D.S. (1977). Use of statistics when examining lifetime studies in rodents to detect carcinogenicity. Journal of Toxicology and Environmental Health 3, 611-628.

73. Schmähl, D., Habs, M. & Ivankovic, S. (1978). Carcinogenesis of N-nitrosodiethylamine (DENA) in chickens and domestic cats. International Journal of Cancer 22, 552-557.

74. Shank, R.C. & Barrows, L.R. (1981). Toxicity-dependent DNA methylation: Significance to risk assessment In: Health Risk Analysis (C.R. Richmond, P.J. Walsh & E.D. Copenhaver, eds.). Franklin Institute Press, Philadelphia, pp. 225-233.

75. Sielken, R.L. (1981). Re-examination of the ED_{01} study: risk assessment using time. Fundamental and Applied Toxicology 1, 88–123.

76. Snee, R.D. & Irr, J.D. (1981). Design of a statistical method for analysis of mutagenesis of the hypoxanthine-guanine phosphoribosyl transferase locus of cultured Chinese hamster ovary cells. Mutation Research 85, 77–93.

77. Sontag, J.M., Page, N.P. & Saffiotti, U. (1976). Guidelines for carcinogen bioassay in small rodents. National Cancer Institute Carcinogenesis Technical Report Series (NIC-CG-TR-1), U.S. Department of Health, Education & Welfare, Public Health Service, Washington, D.C.

78. Sontag, J.M. (1977). Aspects in carcinogen bioassay. In: Origins of Human Cancer Book C: Human Risk Assessment. (H.H. Hiatt, J.D. Watson & J.A. Winsten eds.), Cold Spring Harbor Laboratory, Cold Spring Harbor, pp. 1327–1338.

79. Stead, A.G., Hasselblad, V., Creason, J.P. & Claxton, L. (1981). Modeling the Ames Test. Mutation Research 85, 13–27.

80. Takeishi, K., Okuno-Kaneda, S. & Seno, T. (1979). Mutagenic activation of 2-acetylaminofluorene by guinea-pig liver homogenates: Essential involvement of cytochrome p450 mixed-function oxidases. Mutation Research 62, 425–437.

81. Truhaut, R. (1979). An overview of the problem of thresholds for chemical carcinogens. In: Carcinogenic Risks/Strategies for Intervention (W. Davis & C. Rosenfeld, eds.), IARC Scientific Publication No. 25, IARC, Lyon, pp. 191–202.

82. Van Ryzin, J. (1980). Quantitative risk assessment. Journal of Occupational Medicine 22, 321–326.

83. Weisburger, J.H. & Williams, G.M. (1981). Carcinogen testing: Current problems and new approaches. Science 214, 401–407.

84. WHO: World Health Organization (1961). Principles governing consumer safety in relation to pesticide residues. Technical Report No. 240, WHO, Geneva.

85. Wright, A.S. (1981). The role of metabolism in chemical mutagenesis and chemical carcinogenesis. ICPEMC Working Paper 2/2. Mutation Research 75, 215–241.

86. Yahagi, T., Nagao, M., Seino, Y., Matsushima, T., Sugimura, T. & Okada, M. (1977). Mutagenicities of N-nitrosamines on Salmonella. Mutation Research 48, 121–129.

87. Yamagiwa, K. & Ichikawa, K. (1918). Experimental study of the pathogenesis of carcinoma. Journal of Cancer Research 3, 1–29.

88. Yamanaka, H., Nagao, M., Sugimura, T., Furuya, T., Shirai, A. & Matsushima, T. (1979). Mutagenicity of pyrrolizidine alkaloids in the Salmonella mammalian-microsome test. Mutation Research 68, 211–216.

MUTAGENS, CARCINOGENS, AND ANTI-CARCINOGENS[*]

Bruce N. Ames

Department of Biochemistry
University of California
Berkeley, California 94720

THE SALMONELLA TEST

Mutagens and carcinogens in the environment represent a potential hazard, and it is important to screen large numbers of compounds and mixtures of compounds to which humans are exposed. However, it is impractical for both technical and monetary reasons to do the bulk of mutagen screening by using mammals. Carcinogenicity testing in mammals is also extremely expensive and takes years for adequate tests. The Salmonella test we have developed, and the other short-term tests that have been developed for testing chemicals for their ability to interact with DNA, or for mutagenicity, are being widely used and should help in solving some of the problems that cannot be adequately approached by human epidemiology or animal cancer tests alone.

The Salmonella/liver test for mutagenicity is in current use in over 3,000 government, industrial, and academic laboratories throughout the world. Most of the major drug and chemical companies in the world are now using the test. The test system is simple, inexpensive, and extremely sensitive, and we believe it will detect a high percentage of the environmental chemicals that cause cancer and mutations in man. The recent improvements we have made on it should make it even more useful, though it has important limitations, such as the lack of detection of many of the halogenated carcinogens. One of its major uses has been the detection of mutagens from complex mixtures, such as energy-

---

[*] This short paper cites a minimum of references. The literature is covered more fully in the references cited.

related pollution, cigarette smoke, water, food, and urine. The
test has also been useful in the development of drugs and
industrial chemicals where large numbers of chemicals must be
screened. In addition, it has become widely used for investigating
the metabolic pathways of carcinogens to their active forms.

The basis for using mutagenicity tests for detecting
carcinogens is the demonstration from our work (and also of others)
that over 80% of carcinogens can be detected as mutagens in our
test, including almost all known organic chemicals causing cancer
in humans (1). Our work, and that of others, has strongly
supported the theory that most carcinogens act by damaging DNA.

There are still several important classes of carcinogens,
however, that are not detected by the test system. We have
discussed (1) the reasons why a few types of carcinogens will never
be detected by the system (e.g., the carcinogen griseofulvin, by
interacting with tubulin, upsets the mitotic apparatus in animal
cells causing chromosome loss: this type of agent must be detected
in a eukaryotic system specially set up for looking at chromosome
abnormalities). There are two classes of carcinogens, however,
that Salmonella does not detect well as mutagens that should, for
theoretical reasons, be detectable, and we have devoted
considerable effort to improving the test for these two classes.

Natural Carcinogens Present as Glycosides: Activation of Carcinogens by Colon Bacteria

There are many glycosides of mutagens present in the human
diet, as these compounds are widespread in plants. Plants often
have blocked forms (usually glycosides) of toxins so that they are
not dangerous to the plant, but are to predators, whose metabolism
liberates the toxin. A compound such as cycasin (the β-D-glucoside
of the mutagen methylazoxymethanol) is negative in the Salmonella
test because neither the rat liver nor the Salmonella split off the
sugar to liberate the mutagen. Cycasin is a carcinogen in animals,
but not in germ-free animals, so it is apparent that the bacteria
in the gut are splitting off the sugar to liberate the mutagen.
Thus, to detect this class of compounds, one needs a model for the
metabolism of the bacteria in the human colon. We have developed
such a model that works quite well for this class of compounds
(2). We have made an enzyme preparation, which we call fecalase,
by sonicating human feces. Feces are almost half bacteria, and
this fecalase preparation appears to be quite a good in vitro model
for the metabolism that occurs in the colon. Fecalase contains a
wide variety of enzymes splitting sugars from glycosides, and many
different glycosides of naturally occurring mutagens (flavonoids
such as quercetin, anthraquinones, cycasin, etc.) now show up as
mutagens in the test in the presence of fecalase (2).

There is an enormous variety of glycosides in nature (and in man's diet) involving hundreds of different sugars and sugar linkages on a large variety of different aglycones. Thus, one cannot use purified enzymes, because, except for β—glucosidase and a few others, these aren't available. Fecalase is a simple solution to this problem.

Using fecalase, tea, red grape juice, and red, but not white, wine are mutagenic (2). This is presumably due to the presence of glycosides of mutagenic flavonols, such as quercetin, known to be present in grape skins, which are used in making red, but not white, wine. The considerable direct mutagenic activity of the red wine in the absence of fecalase may be due to free quercetin formed in the wine during fermentation. The absence of direct-acting activity in red grape juice is consistent with this hypothesis. We discussed (2) some of the conflicting evidence on quercetin carcinogenicity. (It was first found to be a mutagen in our test system by several groups a few years ago.) We also discussed the evidence showing that quercetin is not absorbed appreciably in humans. Recent epidemiological evidence has implicated red wine drinking with stomach cancer in France: an increased risk of about 10—fold for consumption of about a liter of red wine a day (3).

Carcinogens with Short-Lived Active Forms

One major group of "false negatives" are the heavily chlorinated carcinogens, such as dieldrin, hexachlorobenzene, chloroform, and carbon tetrachloride. Another class contains certain dimethylamino chemicals, such as 1,2-dimethylhydrazine and hexamethylphosphoramide. We now think that the cause of this lack of activity is that the test is not detecting active forms of carcinogens with very short half-lives, such as carbanions and free radicals, and that these "false negatives", such as carbon tetrachloride and dimethylhydrazine, are likely to have in common the production of these short half-lived intermediates.

We suspect that for carcinogens yielding free radicals, a good part of the damage to DNA may come from an indirect oxidative damage derived from radical-induced lipid peroxidation (4,5). Some new tester strains that appear to be required for the detection of oxidative damage are discussed below.

New Tester Strains

In the last year we have made progress on a set of new tester strains (M. Hollstein, D. Levin, E. Schwiers, and B. N. Ames, in preparation). Several respond to mutagens causing oxidative damage to DNA. For generating oxidative damage to DNA we have used a mutagen, streptonigrin, which probably causes toxicity through generating a semiquinone which can cycle to form superoxide radicals. Streptonigrin reverts the standard tester strains only slightly. We have now screened about a hundred histidine-requiring mutants and have selected a strain, hisG428, which is the most effective strain for detecting small amounts of streptonigrin as a mutagen. This strain is an ochre mutant and thus has $\frac{-ATT-}{-TAA-}$ in its DNA at the site of the mutation. Our standard base pair substitution mutation, hisG46 (in tester strains TA1535 and TA100), contains a sequence in the DNA of $\frac{-CTC-}{-GAG-}$ that has been mutated to $\frac{-CCC-}{-GGG-}$. To revert it, the mutation must convert a GC pair to an AT pair. (The sequencing of the DNA of the histidine operon has recently been done by Wayne Barnes in St. Louis, and the DNA sequence of the mutation in our tester strains, which we originally knew from the protein sequencing, has been confirmed. In addition, Barnes sequenced the hisG46 mutation.) Thus, we suspect that streptonigrin-produced superoxide is attacking the AT base pair. Dr. Hollstein has recently completed making tester strains from the hisG428 mutation.

A new frameshift tester strain contains a sequence of $\frac{-AAAAA-}{-TTTTT-}$ at the site of a +1 mutation. This strain detects mutagens, such as streptonigrin, hydroperoxides, and malondialdehyde, that the standard frameshift tester strains do not detect well.

With these new strains we have been able to demonstrate that a variety of hydroperoxides are potent mutagens. These include cumene hydroperoxide, t-butyl hydroperoxide, and hydrogen peroxide (which has recently been shown to be a carcinogen in animals). We think these may be very important model compounds for the lipid hydroperoxides which are produced in humans from lipid peroxidation (fat going rancid). We think it likely that lipid peroxidation may be a major source of DNA damage in people (see also refs. 4 and 5). In the processing of oxygen, a certain amount of lipid peroxidation occurs, despite the many defenses against this in the body. Hydroperoxides generated by lipid peroxidation may damage DNA through generating hydroxyl radicals which are also the main active agents in radiation damage to DNA. A variety of compounds of environmental interest cause lipid peroxidation. These include halogenated carcinogens, many metals, quinones, nitro compounds, NO_2 (which is produced in car exhaust and cigarette smoke), and other compounds generating radicals or singlet oxygen.

We hope that these new tester strains will help in detecting some of the carcinogens previously missed that give rise to free radicals generating lipid peroxidation and oxidative damage, though so far the chlorinated carcinogens are still not active, perhaps because of the distance between the microsomes and Salmonella membrane.

Another new frameshift tester strain (6), TA97, contains a sequence of $\frac{-CCCCCC-}{-GGGGGG-}$ at the site of a +1 mutation and is

considerably superior for the mutagens reverting our old frameshift
tester strain TA1537. We recommend that this strain, TA97, replace
TA1537 in mutagen testing. David Levin has cloned and sequenced
the DNA at the site of the mutation.

Relation Between Carcinogens and Mutagens: Validation of the Test Carcinogens as Mutagens and Short-Term Tests

Our original 1975-76 validation of 175 carcinogens tested in
the Salmonella test showed that about 90% of them could be detected
as mutagens in our test. In 1977 we added to this validation by
examining the known human carcinogens and showing that a very high
percentage of the organic chemicals could be detected as
mutagens. We also looked at the mutagenicity of many pairs of
chemicals where only a small change in the molecule would change a
carcinogen to a noncarcinogen and found an excellent agreement
between mutagenicity and carcinogenicity. Our work on mutagenic
impurities clarified a few otherwise anomalous cases. We also
discussed classes of false negatives in the test, particularly the
polyhalogenated carcinogens. Several other extensive reviews have
found roughly the same percentage of carcinogens detected as mutagens, but clearly this percentage could differ somewhat depending
on the particular group of carcinogens chosen. More recently we
have re-examined a group of 275 carcinogens compiled by Rinkus and
Legator and have found that the percentage is about 83% (1).

The predictive value of the test is reinforced by a number of
important environmental chemicals first shown to be mutagens in the
Salmonella system and then later shown to be carcinogens.

CARCINOGENIC POTENCY: OBJECTIVES AND SIGNIFICANCE

Man is exposed to an extremely large number of carcinogens
from a variety of sources: cooking food, natural chemicals in our
diet, inhalation of burnt material, and man-made chemicals. To
improve risk assessments, risk/benefit judgements, and regulatory
policy, an index number of carcinogenic strength (or potency) for
each chemical is desirable to help in setting priorities. Because
quantitative information on the capacity of various chemicals to
cause cancer in man is not available, one must turn to animal bioassays. We have been engaged for several years in creating a
comprehensive data base which incorporates the animal bioassays
reported in the world's literature which are suitable for
determining a potency value (Lois Gold, Kim Hooper, Charles Sawyer,
William Havender, Richard Peto, and Malcolm Pike). We describe
briefly an index of carcinogenic potency, the TD_{50}, and our
progress toward setting up a data base on the estimated potency
values of several thousand cancer tests. The range of carcinogenic
potency is over 10 million-fold. The carcinogenic potency scale
can be used in calibrating short-term tests to show their
limitations and strengths.

MUTAGENS, CARCINOGENS, AND ANTI-CARCINOGENS[*]

Bruce N. Ames

Department of Biochemistry
University of California
Berkeley, California 94720

THE SALMONELLA TEST

Mutagens and carcinogens in the environment represent a potential hazard, and it is important to screen large numbers of compounds and mixtures of compounds to which humans are exposed. However, it is impractical for both technical and monetary reasons to do the bulk of mutagen screening by using mammals. Carcinogenicity testing in mammals is also extremely expensive and takes years for adequate tests. The Salmonella test we have developed, and the other short-term tests that have been developed for testing chemicals for their ability to interact with DNA, or for mutagenicity, are being widely used and should help in solving some of the problems that cannot be adequately approached by human epidemiology or animal cancer tests alone.

The Salmonella/liver test for mutagenicity is in current use in over 3,000 government, industrial, and academic laboratories throughout the world. Most of the major drug and chemical companies in the world are now using the test. The test system is simple, inexpensive, and extremely sensitive, and we believe it will detect a high percentage of the environmental chemicals that cause cancer and mutations in man. The recent improvements we have made on it should make it even more useful, though it has important limitations, such as the lack of detection of many of the halogenated carcinogens. One of its major uses has been the detection of mutagens from complex mixtures, such as energy-

---

[*] This short paper cites a minimum of references. The literature is covered more fully in the references cited.

In the case of a negative (i.e., statistically non-signifi-
cant) bioassay where a TD_{50} cannot be calculated, we still
calculate a lower confidence limit for the TD_{50} which shows the
sensitivity of the bioassay. These sensitivities, which can differ
enormously, depend on the dose levels used and on the experimental
design. A negative test is described as excluding TD_{50}'s below a
certain limit, rather than simply as "negative". Some experiments
have such small numbers of test animals and use such low doses that
they could not have detected any but the most potent carcinogens.
The comparison of research designs and dose levels will sometimes
make it possible to reconcile positive and negative results with
the same compound: for example, if two such tests examined different regions of the dose range, they need not be contradictory.

We have designed a graphic display for presenting the results
of our calculations in a readily comprehensible format. For each
significant site in an experiment the plot provides descriptive
information about sex, strain, species, site and tumor type, length
of exposure, and length of experiment. It also presents the TD_{50}
value, its statistical significance and confidence limits, the
shape of the dose-response relationship, the number of tumors and
of animals at risk for each control and dose group, the
administered dose levels in mg/kg/day, the author's opinion about
tumorigenicity, and the reference. All of the information we use
for the plot is stored in an easily accessible data base. We have
completed our calculations for about 1200 experiments on 250 chemicals and are continuing to process the rest of the literature.

We are just starting on the analysis of the data base. We
have found that carcinogenic potency values (TD_{50}'s) in rodents
vary for different chemicals over a tremendous range -- about 10
million-fold. This great variability in the intrinsic carcinogenic
power of different chemicals is an important aspect of developing a
policy response to chemical hazards for humans. Assessments of
chemical hazards to people need to combine estimates of the extent
and levels of human exposure and estimates of carcinogenic potency
(8,9). We are currently using our data base to secure information
on many issues relevant to human risk assessment, such as the variability of TD_{50} between sexes, strains, and species, and the concordance between different tests on the same chemical (10). We
plan to continue to add tests to the data base and to analyze our
results.

EXTRAPOLATION FROM ANIMAL TESTS TO MAN: OXYGEN RADICALS

Extrapolation from animal tests to man is complicated by such
difficulties as species variation in metabolism and the need to
extrapolate to low doses. These issues have been discussed at
length. We would like to consider here several other difficulties
which relate to oxygen radicals.

Toxicity by oxygen radicals has been suggested as a major cause of cancer, heart disease, and aging (reviewed in 4 and 5). Oxygen radicals and other oxidants appear to be toxic in large part because they initiate the chain reaction of lipid peroxidation (rancidity). Lipid peroxidation generates various reactive species -- such as radicals, hydroperoxides, aldehydes, and epoxides -- with the capability of causing damage to DNA, RNA, proteins, cellular membranes, and cellular organization. Aerobic organisms have an array of protective mechanisms both for preventing the formation of oxidants and lipid peroxidation and for repairing oxidative damage. The protective systems include enzymes, such as superoxide dismutase and selenium-containing glutathione peroxidase, and antioxidants and radical scavengers, such as α-tocopherol (vitamin E) and β-carotene in the lipid portion of the cell and glutathione and ascorbic acid in the aqueous phase. These protective mechanisms are now being recognized as anticarcinogenic and, in some cases, even as life-span extending. Vitamin E, ascorbate, selenium, glutathione, and β-carotene have all been shown to be anticarcinogenic in animal cancer tests.

A marked increase in life-span has occurred in human evolution during the descent from prosimians over the past 60 million years. At the same time an enormous decrease in the age-specific cancer rate has occurred in humans compared to short-lived mammals. It seems likely that a major factor in lengthening life-span and decreasing age-specific cancer rates may have been the evolution of a number of effective protective mechanisms against oxygen radicals (reviewed in ref. 5). We propose (5) that one of these protective systems is plasma uric acid, the level of which increased markedly during primate evolution as a consequence of a series of mutations. Uric acid is a powerful antioxidant and is a scavenger of singlet oxygen and radicals and is about as effective an antioxidant as ascorbate. The plasma urate level in humans (about 300 μM) is considerably higher than the ascorbate level, making it one of the major antioxidants in humans.

We also suspect that damage to membranes from lipid peroxidation may be one of the modes of action of promoters. Promoters are clearly one of the complications in quantitative risk assessment extrapolation.

Thus, differences in antioxidant defense mechanisms and life-span complicate quantitative extrapolation from rodents to man. It is not so clear exactly how to extrapolate from a TD_{50} in mg/kg/day in a short-lived species such as a rat to a long-lived species such as man. In addition, both genetics and nutrition may contribute to human variability in these antioxidants and cause large differences in risk. For example, Hirayama (11) has shown considerable decrease in lung cancers among smokers who eat green and yellow vegetables regularly compared to those who do not. We believe that methods for measuring DNA damage in individual humans and other biochemical approaches to human epidemiology will be needed to help in human risk assessment for environmental mutagens and carcinogens. These methods will complement information from short-term tests, human cancer epidemiology, and quantitative analysis of animal cancer tests.

ACKNOWLEDGEMENTS

This work was supported by DOE contract DE-AT03-76EV70156 to B.N.A., NIEHS Center Grant ES-01896, and NIEHS/DOE Interagency Agreement 222-Y01-AS-10066 through the Lawrence Berkeley Laboratory.

REFERENCES

1. Ames, B. N. and J. McCann, Validation of the Salmonella test: A reply to Rinkus and Legator, Cancer Research 41:4192-4196 (1981).

2. Tamura, G., C. Gold, A. Ferro-Luzzi, and B. N. Ames, Fecalase: A model for activation of dietary glycosides to mutagens by intestinal flora, Proc. Natl. Acad. Sci. USA 77:4961-4965 (1980).

3. Hoey, J., C. Montvernay, and R. Lambert, Wine and tobacco: Risk factors for gastric cancer in France, Am. J. Epid. 113:668-674 (1981).

4. Ames, B. N., M. C. Hollstein, and R. Cathcart, Lipid peroxidation and oxidative damage to DNA, in: "Lipid Peroxide in Biology and Medicine," K. Yagi, ed., Academic Press, New York (1982), in press.

5. Ames, B. N., R. Cathcart, E. Schwiers, and P. Hochstein, Uric acid provides an antioxidant defense in humans against oxidant- and radical-caused aging and cancer: A hypothesis, Proc. Natl. Acad. Sci. USA, 78:6858-6862 (1981).

6. Levin, D., E. Yamasaki, and B. N. Ames, A new Salmonella tester strain, TA97, for the detection of frameshift mutagens: A run of cytosines as a mutational hot-spot, Mutation Research (1982), in press.

7. Ames, B. N., K. Hooper, C. B. Sawyer, A. D. Friedman, R. Peto, W. Havender, L. S. Gold, T. Haggin, R. H. Harris, and M. Rosenfeld, Carcinogenic potency: A progress report, in: "Banbury Report 5. Ethylene Dichloride: A Potential Health Risk?" B. Ames, P. Infante, and R. Reitz, eds., Cold Spring Harbor Laboratory, Cold Spring Harbor, New York (1980).

8. Hooper, K., L. S. Gold, and B. N. Ames, The carcinogenic potency of ethylene dichloride in two animal bioassays: A comparison of inhalation and gavage studies, in: "Banbury Report 5. Ethylene Dichloride: A Potential Health Risk?" B. Ames, P. Infante, and R. Reitz, eds., Cold Spring Harbor Laboratory, Cold Spring Harbor, New York (1980).

9. Gold, L. S., Human exposures to ethylene dichloride, in:
    "Banbury Report 5. Ethylene Dichloride: A Potential Health
    Risk?" B. Ames, P. Infante, and R. Reitz, eds., Cold Spring
    Harbor Laboratory, Cold Spring Harbor, New York (1980).
10. Ames, B. N., L. S. Gold, C. B. Sawyer, and W. Havender,
    Carcinogenic potency, in: "Environmental Mutagens and
    Carcinogens", T. Sugimura, S. Kondo, and H. Takabe, eds.,
    University of Tokyo Press, Tokyo, and Alan R. Liss, Inc., New
    York (1982).
11. Hirayama, T., Diet and Cancer, Nutrition and Cancer, 1:67-81
    (1979).

DISCUSSION

NEWELL: Comment - With regard to the antioxidant
effectiveness of vitamin E, in a study of steatosis in cats,
we found that the free alcohol form must be used if there is
to be effective action.

Q. BYARD: I have personally done experiments to test your
    hypothesis that oxidative reactions mediate the genotoxicity
    of persistent chlorinated hydrocarbons. With mirex, my
    results were negative. Chemicals such as mirex, DDT, TCDD,
    etc. can be cocarcinogens or anticarcinogens by their
    induction of enzymes which activate and inactivate
    initiators. They can also be promoters as a result of their
    hyperplastic effect. However, all available data (Ames assay,
    covalent binding index, etc.) suggest that these chemicals are
    not initiators and are not genotoxic. Their tumorigenesis is
    now thought to result from promotion of the background level
    of initiators in the diet.

A. AMES: I suspect promotion will often be caused by lipid
    peroxidation. TCDD causes lipid peroxidation at very low
    levels.

ROUNDTABLE DISCUSSION

RESEARCH PRIORITIES AND PERSPECTIVES:
INDUSTRY, UNIVERSITIES, GOVERNMENT

Panelists:

Alexander Hollaender, Chairman
Associated Universities, Inc.
Washington, D.C.

Verne A. Ray
Pfizer, Inc.
Groton, CT

Mortimer L. Mendelsohn
Lawrence Livermore Laboratory
Livermore, CA

James Lyons
University of California
Davis, CA

Raymond C. Valentine
University of California
Davis, CA

Robert Colton
National Science Foundation
Washington, D.C.

Richard Rominger
California Department of Food
and Agriculture
Sacramento, CA

The open discussion which followed the individual presentations by
these panelists appears in sequence after their text.

ROUNDTABLE DISCUSSION: RESEARCH PRIORITIES AND PERSPECTIVES--
INDUSTRY, UNIVERSITIES, GOVERNMENT

Alexander Hollaender (Chairman):   We would like to begin the
Roundtable Discussion with some background as to how the planning
for this symposium was initiated a couple years ago.   Dr. Raymond
Valentine and I were at a conference at the Brookhaven National
Laboratory and he brought up the idea that there is an urgent need
to get agriculture much more involved in genetic toxicology re-
search and the new areas which are now developing in the new
biology.   It wasn't easy to get started on the subject.   When I
presented this problem of "Genetic Toxicology: An Agricultural
Perspective", Dr. Michael Waters of the Environmental Protection
Agency immediately gave us a small grant through the Biology
Division of BNL.   We started three workshops.

     At the first workshop, which was held in my office at the
Associated Universities, Inc. in Washington, D.C., representatives
from the Department of Agriculture stated that there is no toxicology problem in agriculture.   However, we had had the same
experience when we started environmental mutagenesis studies
earlier when people from government, industry and the universities
thought that there was not a problem.   You know that it has developed as a very important issue in the protection of the health of
all of us.   At the second workshop, Dr. Gerald Still of the U.S.
Department of Agriculture was present and he saw the point
immediately.   He said that agriculture should be involved in
this.   If it is a problem, what shall we do about it?   Right now, I
am not sure there is any difficulty, but let's take a look at it
and discuss it.   At the third workshop, we finally prepared this
program.

     It is a very important point that when we started studies in
environmental mutagenesis, we got industry involved right at the
beginning and helped us to develop an understanding of this area of
environmental mutagenesis.   It is really industry which, in the
long run, has cooperated to get us started in the consideration of
corporate studies and the application of these new materials for
detecting environmental mutagens.   The program of this symposium
brought up a number of very important questions.   Although we do
not want to overemphasize pesticides, they are really some of the
most important chemical compounds the farmer is handling in a very
extensive way, here in California and elsewhere.   So, in spite of
our plans, the emphasis is on pesticides.

     I would like to give an opportunity to the different repre-
sentatives here, of government, agriculture, medical groups, and
industry, to give their points of view, suggesting how we could
further develop this area and make sure that environmental muta-

genesis does not become a problem in agriculture. And so I would
like to call upon Dr. Verne Ray, a scientist with Pfizer, Inc., who
has been involved in this area from the very beginning. I would
like Dr. Ray to express the ideas that industry sees to help our
colleagues in agriculture to protect themselves against these compounds which, in the long run, may become hazardous.

Verne Ray: It is very clear from the discussions in the last two
days that this interface between genetic toxicology and agriculture
is a very complex one. There are no easy answers to the application of the information that we derive from genetic toxicology
tests. There are concerns however, on both sides of the picture.
Do we consider the fact that one out of every two hundred live
births has chromosomal anomalies is all due to noise in the genetic
system or does it have an environmental component? On the other
side, there are concerns about the need for pesticides and other
agricultural chemicals to maintain our high level of productivity,
recognizing that some of them are indeed genotoxic, others of them
carcinogens. Can we utilize them in such a way as not to produce
undue risk to people in the agricultural community?

    In the chemical industry, the role of genetic toxicology in
the safety evaluation process is to identify the mutagenic and
carcinogenic potential of chemicals, to evaluate this spectrum of
effects and to give an indication of potency relative to known
compounds. If data from compounds of similar structure are available, such comparisons may be instructive. The subsequent hazard
evaluation and risk assessment of chemicals is enhanced by a knowledge of genotoxicity and provides for informed utility of the
genotoxic substance where need or benefit is established and no
suitable non-genotoxic substitute is available. Levels of
exposure, environmental persistance and degree of food or water
contamination which result from the utilization of pesticides or
other agricultural chemicals are evaluations which superimpose on
this knowledge. In my view, the genetic toxicology evaluation
provides an early measure of certain types of toxicity which cannot
be acquired in any other way than long-term animal exposures and
gives perspective to the hazard evaluation and risk assessment
process. Now, having said that, we must face the problems of which
kinds of assays do we use in a routine manner, to be the most beneficial not only in the industrial screening context, but whose
information can be utilized in the process of hazard evaluation and
risk assessment. There is an issue of relevance and it is a difficult one to define. Dr. Albertini has a system in which the
relevance issue is rather well-defined compared to other assays
that we have. Is that the kind of standard we are going to use?
We definitely need a standard for validation purposes. When we do
perform genetic toxicology tests and use carcinogenicity as a
standard, one recognizes the problems we have because of the variability in the carcinogenicity results as obtained in species of

rodents. However, I firmly believe that we need a standard in the
mutagenicity area. Is that standard going to be rodent studies?
If it is, we know we have very well defined problems with the assay
models that are available currently, as Dr. Mendelsohn pointed out
in his paper. We know an assay like the dominant-lethal is not
that suitable. How do we know that? Because, there are a number
of mutagens and carcinogens that are not detected in this assay.
Is this because of the way we apply this system? I think not. I
think it is due to the nature of the assay which measures fetal
wastage. The heritable translocation assay is available to us. It
at least has an explicit genetic end point which the dominant-
lethal does not. But, in both these cases we are dealing with
chromosomal-level end points and we are not measuring gene or point
mutation end points. The animal models available for the latter
are either inadequate, insufficiently documented or impractical.

If one works in an industrial setting and applies a battery of
mutagenicity assays, the utility of the information derived can
have far-reaching consequences. If the industrial organization
decides as a consequence of that information not to continue the
development of a compound, and test results have been overinter-
preted or inappropriate test models applied whose results cannot be
interpreted, then the researcher is doing a marked disservice not
only to the company, but to the population who would benefit from
such a substance. I have felt for some time that those systems
which rely only on prokaryotic cells are inadequate for safety
evaluation purposes.

There has been a considerable degree of criticism of genetic
toxicology because of the number of assays that are available for
use. It is my contention that the number of assays being used by
experienced genetic toxicologists on a routine basis to make
decisions in industry is few indeed. We don't have 135 tests that
are being applied routinely. However, after selecting a well-
defined battery on the basis of detecting the kinds of damage that
chemicals can produce in DNA and building a substantive data base
which gives confidence in utility, one still has a problem when it
comes to extrapolating data in the context of human genetic
disease. The extrapolation usually is toward carcinogenic potential and this has been the main utility of information coming
from genetic toxicology laboratories to date. I would like to use
these comments as a starting point for discussion

Hollaender: At this meeting, very little has been said about a
major effort of the Environmental Protection Agency to evaluate the
usefulness of different methods. We will bring up the very
important survey being conducted under the Gene-Tox Program that,
in a year or so, will give use some very important guidelines for
the testing of chemical compounds.

However, I would like to call upon Dr. Mortimer Mendelsohn to give us a point of view from the medical standpoint.

Mortimer Mendelsohn: That's a good question. The medical point of view is best introduced by recalling something you probably all know but maybe haven't thought of in the context of this meeting. This is the issue of global patterns of cancer. From everywhere that cancer statistics are collected in the world, it is clear that types of cancer occur very much like fingerprints, in distinctive regional patterns. This is true of countries, and in larger countries like our own, it applies to regions within countries. These differences can be dramatic. The most common cancer in one culture may be the least common in another. One could argue that all of this is genetic, but there is convincing evidence that people moving from one country to another take on the new cancer pattern. For some cancers this occurs within years, for others it may require a lifetime. A genetic explanation seems unlikely; rather we must assume that this major disease has a significant local geographic etiology. It must be environmental in the very broadest sense. The effect is too big to be occupational and too big to be genetic, although both factors are probably present. By environmental we must mean everything else, including the kinds of things we have been talking about in this meeting. I don't mean that carcinogenic pesticides are the cause, because the evidence indicates that this also is unlikely to be the case. The cancer patterns have been with us since the turn of the century and probably longer. They are not new, and they are, with few exceptions, surprisingly stable. The cause must be deeper and broader than agricultural chemicals. For example, it might well involve agriculture as a whole: the food we eat, how we grow it, the way we prepare and preserve it, and the way we eat it. It might also include local geology and local meteorology, and what might be called local lifestyle. If food, one way or the other, might be that much a determinant of cancer type in the world, then obviously food needs careful attention, and it needs it in the broadest sense. It needs it at the level of mechanistic understanding, at the level of preventive health, at the level of engineering control and so forth. I would think that the best our society could get out of the attention being given to agricultural environmental mutagenesis is to understand and correct the agricultural environmental causes of cancer patterns. Many of you may be thinking in terms of not letting things get worse, or of avoiding chemical epidemics. But we need not generate new fears; we have enough of an issue already in just dealing with background cancer rates as we find them today.

Hollaender: I would now like to call on Dr. James Lyons of the University of California to present his point of view concerning agriculture. I would like him to tell us what the agricultural sector would like to see us do to make it possible to more

thoroughly develop this area and to make sure that we are on the
right track.

James Lyons: I appreciate the opportunity to be here and you posed
a difficult question. When Dr. Hollaender asked me to represent
agriculture, it certainly assumes a very large responsibility
because agriculture is indeed an enormous area. As I thought about
the topic for this evening, in terms of genetic toxicology as it
relates to chemicals and agriculture, it then quickly relates to
pesticides. It is always easiest to put it into simplistic terms
but as Dr. Ray indicated, everyone is looking for simplistic
answers to many complex questions. As a plant scientist here on
the campus, I teach a freshman class in plant sciences and one of
the things I like to remind the students is the role of agriculture
in producing food and fiber, and to provide a few simple truths
they still need to consider. Number one is that food and population will be balanced. I remind them that we also need to look
at the population that exists and consider the fact that in the 5
million year history of man, up until 1975, we arrived at a population of 4 billion people on the earth's surface. And that
between 1975 and the year 2000-2010, or 25 years, that is going to
go to 8 billion. That says that man must produce as much food
again in this 25 year period as he has in his previous 5 million
year history, and that presents quite a challenge. Much focus must
be placed on food production and providing an adequate food supply
for this population, and certainly agricultural chemicals will play
an important role in that effort. In our early history man's food
supply kept up with increasing populations through exploiting new
lands. That stopped a number of years ago, as most of the lands
became exploited. In recent history increased productivity has
come about through the adoption of new technologies, new varieties,
fertilizers, irrigation, etc. But also in the use of chemicals to
control pests. Pests compete very heavily for that food supply and
always will. I think from an agricultural viewpoint, we would like
to see a balance in terms of understanding the risks and the benefits. People talk about the "natural" ecological balance, but
there really isn't such a thing. As man manipulates anything for
food supply, he disrupts that "natural" balance, and therefore the
real issue is to keep it in as good a balance as possible and to
husband it carefully. I don't believe that agriculturists are
destined to poison the earth. I think that they want to produce
this food supply in a reasonable way with a minimum risk to the
population and the environment. I was interested in Dr.
Mendelsohn's comment about the role of natural products in food and
dietary choices in terms of cancer causing agents. We know very
little relative to other fields about human nutrition and more
emphasis needs to be placed on research in nutrition. One can make
the statement, and there is a validity, that we understand far more
of the nutrition of pets and food animals than we do of humans. Of
course, the goal for animal nutrition is weight-gain and that is
not what we are interested in in the human population.

We recognize the need for having adequate tests identifying
the hazards and risks of the chemicals we use but I think there are
far too many chemicals identified as being problems, when we don't
really have good tests, and as a result of that identification,
there is too great a reaction - an "over reaction" and desire to
ban the use of any chemical. I think the real need is balance and
consideration for the benefits as well as the risks. As we look
forward to the year 2000 and how we are going to feed the world
population and at the same time provide a reasonable quality of
environment to live in, we must be mindful of the risks. Certainly
the development of adequate tests that can be applied and interpreted in a reasonable fashion is a goal we need to strive for.

Hollaender: I would like to now call on Dr. Raymond Valentine of
the UC Davis Plant Growth Laboratory, who got us interested in
planning this symposium. I would like for him to tell us what he
thinks we ought to do to make agricultural practices safer than
they are now. While it is quite safe, with the use of pesticides
and so many other chemicals in agriculture, sooner or later there
will be problems. So, I would like him to tell us what he thinks
we ought to do next.

Raymond Valentine: I'm intrigued with the marriage between
genetics and toxicology, the topic of this meeting. I was de-
lighted to hear Dr. Sugimura's talk last night, in which he
discussed recombinant DNA and genetic engineering. I would like to
continue on that theme for a moment.

I dabble in the field of genetic engineering, as some of you
know. The first question I am always asked after I talk on this
subject is, "What are the first products going to be?" I have a
stock answer for that. I think the first products are going to be
a far deeper understanding of the genetic apparatus. What I am
trying to say is that the first real benefits and use of this re-
volutionary new technology, recombinant DNA and genetic engineering, will be a deeper understanding of the gene and how the
chromosome works. We do need to know a lot more.

How much do we really know about genes and how they interact
with the environment? Perhaps not very much after all. We
sequence genes. We know the flanking sequence of the gene and yet
there are always new horizons. What I'm trying to tell you is,
don't be disappointed, but actually we don't know very much about
the gene. We know ever so much more than was thought possible a
few short years ago, but still we have much more to learn. The new
technology of recombinant DNA offers an important new look at the
chromosome and its interaction with toxic agents. The marriage
between genetics and toxicology will grow stronger. Now as far as
future goals, genetic toxicologists should not be passive in the
sense of merely watching the changing scenery in terms of recom-

binant DNA, but should play a much more active role as catalysts
for increasing activity in using this new technology as a tool to
try to answer many of the questions that have been raised in this
meeting. Indeed there are many fundamental and very exciting and
challenging questions that have been raised.

Hollaender: In all this work, you know we depend very much on what
the federal government will do to encourage us to go ahead and also
what it can do to help us. We all know our country is going
through a serious financial crisis right now, but I have always
found that when things become very difficult, this is the time to
start new ideas and encourage them. Whether it was during the
Depression of the 1930s, or during the Korean War, my experience
was that it is then appropriate to get started in new ideas. So, I
would like to call on Dr. Robert Colton of the National Science
Foundation. What will NSF do to help us develop these new ideas?

Robert Colton: Thank you very much. I am not sure how Dr.
Hollaender arranged the sequence of presentations, but if it was in
accordance with decreasing knowledge of the subject, I am in the
right place. So what I ought to do is what all administrators do
from the bureaucracy, which is to give you a series of one
liners. Your former Governor brings you greetings, and asked me to
come here in his stead. He has some other things to take care of
back at the office. But, seriously, as far as providing you with a
person who could speak authoritatively on genetic toxicology, there
are many other people at the Foundation who I am sure could do a
much better job. I have very little background, if any in the
area. But over the years, I have been involved to a great degree
in examining various kinds of research arrangements, that is,
cooperative arrangements between the government, companies and
universities. I have examined problems such as this and whether it
be in the area of toxicology, or in polymers, or in metal, or in
computers, it appears that there is a certain critial mass of
people to be involved that are necessary to examine, solve and then
implement the solutions to a problem. I have only been here a
short time and really have not made much of an assessment as to
what could be done, what has to be done, or what the National
Science Foundation might do, but I might make some observations as
an engineer as to how I would approach the problem.

At first I would have to see if there was a problem and obviously there appears to be a very serious one from what I heard
today. It also appears that one can point to certain areas that
cause the problem, so that there must be some way to come up with a
solution. One might say that after determining whether there is a
problem and whether it can be solved, one ought to look at where
responsibility lies in solving the problem. That is only a means
to come up with a finite solution, but I think it is important to
resolve some of these responsibility issues. Who the responsible

parties are, not from the standpoint of blame but from the standpoint of concern and involvement is an important issue. Once one
has established that, then one can come up with various roles.
Represented here are the three major parties who can play a part.
It is the government, the university, and industry. As you know
and as Dr. Hollaender has indicated, the government is going
through some soul searching now as to what its role is going to be
in working with industry and universities in various areas of research and development and I suspect that we all have to be re-told
what government's role ought to be. It appears to me that there is
a role for all three partners in this particular area. I think
that it is hard to determine essentially all the causes that we
would like to attribute to these problems, and it also appears that
some of the causes may very well be in the venue of the government
to solve or to support. Certainly industry should play its role
and the university may very well be a source of good technological
innovation and information.

     I think that the situation with the toxicology area, though,
presents a more unique problem than any of the others I have
seen. I think the conditions are quite a bit more sensitive than,
for example, developing a new plastic material. The issues are
extremely delicate and I think the responsibilities may not be
clear at all times. We are dealing with a subject that many people
would like to brush under the rug because it is not a pleasant one,
and in dealing with it we may have suspect complicity, which is not
the kind of thing we would like to have. Therefore, I think that
some very special steps may have to be taken by all of us to solve
this. For instance, it appears that, in general, the role of
government in research and development is going to decrease. The
priorities in government are such now that we feel that by reducing
taxes and eliminating certain regulations the private sector will
achieve tax relief, and thus have more money to spend on such thing
as research and development in areas such as genetic toxicology.
At the same time, it appears that in these reductions we are having
in the federal budget, there may be an effect on university
funds. You all know that there is budget exercise going through
our systems now for reducing the budget an additional 12% and this
12% is primarily aimed at the federal agencies which supply the $5
billion that universities get every year. A simple calculation,
12% x $5 billion, means that there is going to be 600 million dol-
lars less for universities. It may or may not happen, but it
appears that there is a possibility. If it does happen, I would
suspect that genetic toxicology will get its share of reductions.
Reducing taxes and regulations, we hope, will stimulate others in
institutions such as private foundations and the private sector to
pick up where the government left off. But, I think that as
opposed to other areas where it may be more suitable for industry
to do research, as with polymers or computers, it may be a little
more difficult to find ways to get industry to spend more money at

universities in this area. And as such, it may be understandable
from the standpoint--at least from a psychological standpoint--that
there is the potential that if one does research in this area
you're implying that you may be partially responsible for the
problem. I am not going to comment on whether that is true, but I
think it may have a negative effect on private investment. Thus, I
think this is a unique situation and that a clearer picture as to
the shared responsibility for all of this should be painted, so
that no individual organization really is to blame, because this is
a cause that we should all support and it may mean that some of you
will have to provide some very deep soul searching and justifi-
cations to move ahead in supporting this area.

Hollaender: I know that the National Science Foundation has always
been very generous in supporting new ideas, from basic research to
more applied research. I am very sorry that we did not get any
contribution to this conference from NSF, but we are grateful for
the participation of Robert Colton at our symposium.

     From the standpoint of local government, I would like to call
on Dr. Richard Rominger of the California Department of Food and
Agriculture to see what he has to say about our topic.

Richard Rominger: Thank you. I am a user of information that
comes out of the university and other laboratories around the
world. As Director of the California Department of Food and Agriculture it's my responsibility to register and regulate the use of
pesticides in California.

     There has been some advance in the development of biological
controls, but still the chief method for protection of crops is the
use of pesticides. Our Division of Pest Management, Environmental
Protection, and Worker Safety reviews and evaluates the toxicity
data that we get from manufacturers, from EPA and from the
scientific literature before we make a decision on whether or not
to register a product or decide what kind restrictions to put on
that product. We need good data.

     I came here this evening after spending all day at our Medfly
Eradication project in the Santa Clara Valley. Those of you who
have read the newspaper and seen the news on this issue know that
we have had questions raised about the toxicity of the chemicals
used in this eradication project--the first being malathion. Malathion has probably been studied as much as any pesticide, and it
has been in use for many years. You would think that we would have
all the information about it and there wouldn't be much controversy. We found out that was not the case. There is still a lot
of controversy about the use of malathion.

We have, as a result of the Medfly infestation, the requirement of Japan for fumigation of some of our products. Now, we are
using, or the growers and shippers are using, ethylene dibromide to
rid products of any potential Medfly eggs or larvae. Well as you
know, EDB is many times more toxic than malathion. So, here again,
we need good data.

It is our job to take this data and then try to assess the
risks. We have to make judgements on what kind of exposure there
will be. We need information so that we can regulate use to
minimize exposure to these toxic substances. As Jim Lyons said, we
don't aim to ban the use of all of these materials or the more
toxic materials if we can regulate or limit their use in such a way
that the exposure is low enough. We certainly think, in the use of
malathion in the eradication of the Mediterranean Fruit Fly, that
with the dosage being used the exposure is so low it presents no
problem. In fact, the majority of the medical profession concur.
Still, we get into controversy over this kind of issue. EDB is
more serious. EPA has had EDB on an RPAR and a phase-out now for
the past year; it is scheduled to be phased out in a year and a
half. We are very cautious in continuing to use that material.

In making these decisions, it is essential that we have reliable data showing whether or not a product is carcenogenic. Most
times, the evidence on the incidence of cancer in human workers is
not available, or very little is available, so that we have to have
other sources of information. It's been shown that if these
chemicals are mutagenic, they often prove to be carcinogenic.
Therefore, the information on mutagenicity is critical to our
analysis of how we use the chemical. With each application that we
receive to register a pesticide product in California, if there is
a new active ingredient that hasn't been previously registered in
the state, we require that there be submitted three mutagenicity
studies on the active ingredient to detect if there are gene mutations, or chromosomal aberrations, or DNA damage. It's of great
importance to our department that these mutagencity tests have a
high degree of reliability. Research in this field is of great
importance to us.

My plea is for more and better information on the materials
that we need in agriculture. The sooner we have it the better; we
have to make decisions based on this information every day.

Hollaender: And now, before I open this meeting to questions from
the audience, I would like Dr. Michael Waters of the EPA to tell us
a little about the Gene-Tox Program, since it was not discussed
earlier in detail.

Michael Waters: I didn't expect to have this opportunity, Dr.
Hollaender. Thank you very much. GENE-TOX was initiated about two

years ago. It was an idea that came about as a result of a perceived need to systematically evaluate the published literature in the field of genetic toxicology. The information that existed in the literature was in various states of adequacy as well as disarray. In order to evaluate this literature, we felt it necessary to bring together knowledgeable scientists from academia, government, and industry. We accomplished the task using a committee approach; 24 work groups of five to ten scientists each evaluated 39 basic types of bioassays; and assembled data on more than 2,800 chemicals. Work group reports have now been published for several of the bioassay systems in Mutation Research: Reviews in Genetic Toxicology. Others are in press or in final stages of preparation. I think those of you who are in the field have read some of these publications.

The second phase of the GENE-TOX program will be an evaluation of batteries of assay systems as they are used in mutagenesis or carcinogenesis testing and in genetic risk assessment. This is being undertaken at the present time via a Coordinating Committee and a series of Task Groups--each addressing a specific goal in the summary evaluation process. This effort will be completed in approximately six months to one year. One of the major efforts under the GENE-TOX program associated with summary evaluation and assessment will be the computerization of the data base that now exists. This will be made publicly available and will be updated as required by the development of new information. I think that's a brief summary of what the GENE-TOX Program is about.

Hollaender: Now, I would appreciate very much for the audience to tell us about what they visualize as priorities in this field, including what they would like to see being discussed or developed.

James Byard: T.C. Campbell has published a paper in Federation Proceedings in which he points out the limitations of lifetime rodent bioassays for assessing human carcinogenesis. The major limitation being great species variation in carcinogenic susceptibility. He proposes that a battery of genotoxic assays would be as predictive of human carcinogenicity as rodent bioassays. I would be interested in the panel's response to this proposal.

Mendelsohn: I haven't seen the paper, but from your description I would agree that the key issue is prediction. The author is predicting something that is clearly not known. Until we do know the relationship between carcinogenesis and mutagenesis, it seems a bit risky to follow his advice.

Byard: Perhaps I should clarify my question a little. Campbell has compared a number of assays in different species of rodents, and to predict from one species to another and also to predict a human effect, there is as much uncertainty as there is in

predicting from a battery of in vitro bioassays. That's his thesis
and he cites a number of data to support that thesis. I have heard
similar comments made here at this symposium. A battery of in
vitro assays for genotoxicity is not perfect but then there is the
question of the rodent bioassays that we compare them against.
These apparently are not perfect either, but are we in a position
to abandon the rodent bioassays? They are very expensive and time
consuming.

Mendelsohn: I commented on Monday and am perhaps as responsible as
anyone in raising questions about prediction and concordance within
and between these systems. The rodent bioassays were designed to
test for carcinogenesis. They do it directly and convincingly,
although very slowly and expensively. Mutagenicity assays do not
measure carcinogenesis per se, but they have the potential to be an
excellent, cheap, practical surrogate. We cannot discard the bioassays until we can say with assurance that scientifically and
legally the mutagenicity tests are as good as or better than tests
that elicit the cancer endpoint directly. At present, in spite of
its impracticality, the cancer bioassay is the only credible way to
find out if something is carcinogenic. Mutagenicity tests are a
quick and easy way to make an 80-90% prediction; but they are not
definitive proof of carcinogenic activity of a chemical. Maybe
others disagree. I'd like to hear other comments.

Takashi Sugimura: For a long time I have been very very suspicious
about the terminology of carcinogens. Certainly a tumor promoter
is not mutagenic, like a recently discovered indole alkaloid having
very strongly promoting activity. Depending on the conditions, if
we apply such substances, certainly cancer will be developed. But
we should not call those substances carcinogens. I'm quite sure
there are many many classes of such compounds in the environment
which we do not know at this moment yet. So it's really a big
issue. We have, of course, the international commission for
protection against environmental mutagens and carcinogens
(ICPEMC). My personal feeling is that we need one more letter, P,
standing for tumor promoter. With full knowledge of the tumor
promoter, which plays a very important role in carcinogenesis, we
may see a much clearer sky; otherwise we are discussing everything
under a very foggy atmosphere. These are my hypotheses, but I'm
not insisting too much.

Mendelsohn: Well, as usual, Dr. Sugimura is right on target. I
wonder, though. We haven't discussed initiation and promotion.
Does everyone here know what a promoter is? A very simple-minded
interpretation of the distinction between an initiator and a promoter goes somewhat as follows: An initiator begins the cancer
process by inflicting an irreversible lesion on cells in the target
organs. For a tumor to actually develop, a series of evolutionary
steps is required, and it is the promoter that plays the dominant

role in this evolution. Since the classical experiments of
Berenblum, a promoter is characterized as a substance that must be
given chronically, that has a reversible effect, and that works
only after, but any time after, a cell has been initiated. As Dr.
Sugimura suggested, initiators seem generally to be mutagenic,
while promoters are non-mutagenic. Promoters are very complex
agents which have many effects on cells and tissues. A major
current effort in carcinogenesis is to sort out and understand
these effects. From a health viewpoint, we have tended to focus on
initiation and hence mutation, but there is the counter argument
that promotion is the key process; i.e., that we are all initiated
by prevailing environmental mutagens and that it is promotion that
determines who gets clinical cancer and what type it will be. Our
general ignorance about the full catalog of promoters, about how
promoters act, and about how much we should protect ourselves, is a
very real issue in carcinogenesis at the moment.

David Jones: There is an earlier point that we mustn't overlook.
I think the trend toward mutagenesis tests as indicators of carcinogenicity may, in a way, be forced upon us. A year and a half
or so ago, the NCI was proposing to put over 100 compounds on tests
in the bioassay system per annum. The last thing I heard about it,
they are now down to 12 per annum. Maybe that's incorrect, but in
any case it is a small number when compared with the number of
compounds that probably ought to be assessed. In that sense I
think we are going to see a situation where the number of compounds
about which we will get information on the mutagenesis side of the
house in going to vastly exceed the number of compounds about which
we will get information from the carcinogenesis bioassay.
Regardless of the science involved, it is simply a matter of
economics. I can't see the present government increasing the
amount of dollars that are spent in carcinogenesis bioassay.
Inflation has driven the cost of these assays up over several
hundreds of thousands of dollars per compound, and if you can do a
five hundred dollar WP2 test or something, that is the information
that is going to be developed, even if the information is not felt
to be as adequate.

Ray: I think the determination of genotoxicity in a substance
which is shown subsequently to be carcinogenic has a remarkable
impact on the way that substance will be evaluated versus one that
is carcinogenic but not demonstrated to be genotoxic. This has
been the focus of some individuals in regulatory agencies who have
tried to use the information from mutagenicity testing. They have
tried to use knowledge of genotoxicity in the way they approach the
assessment of risk due to carcinogenic agents. This knowledge is
especially useful for assessing agents such as those that we can't
remove from the environment because we need them.

I would like to make one other point, though, to get off carcinogenicity for a moment and return to genetic disease per se.
There is a group of genetic diseases in man which have a source,
numerical chromosomal aberrations. We do not have, at this point
in time, a good assay for measuring the capability of chemicals to
induce numerical aberrations and/or aneuploidy. If there is a
genetic disease burden in man that can be identified well, it is
this one. Disease that orginates from numerical chromosomal aberrations is a public health problem. It is sufficientily well
defined to assess its cost. Yet we do not have a good test to
measure a chemical's ability to produce aneuploidy. We have some
models under development in yeast and other types of cells, but I
am convinced there should be greater priority given to research
activity in this area. I believe that a practical assay for this
purpose would certainly have to rank high on the list of research
priorities.

Gordon Newell: I'd like to echo the comments of Dave Jones and the
basis of our concerns about putting so much emphasis on the long
term bioassays. A study that is currently underway for the
National Toxicology Program at the National Academy of Sciences is
reviewing--attempting to review, if you will in a snapshot manner--
the extent of safety studies that have been done on chemicals to
which man is exposed. The information that has been statistically
evolved from the literature so far indicates that there is a great
paucity of information. In fact, as an example, out of all the
chemicals that are listed in the food additives of the Bureau of
Foods at the Food and Drug Administration, some 65% of those chemicals have absolutely no toxicity data at all. They were taken in
on the basis that they were considered as GRAS, generally recognized as safe. I appreciate the weight is on your shoulders, Dr.
Mendelsohn, considering those 40 chemical that we are going to look
at in a year. At the same time we know there are over a thousand
or more chemicals that are coming into use every year. What are we
doing about those in terms of safety? What about all those cosmetics that people put on their skin and the like? We had a very
difficult time trying to come up with 20 chemicals that even had so
much as eye and skin irritation data, to try to evaluate the information on those. Indeed, it is important to all of us here to
address and try to develop, as rapidly as possible, those kinds of
short term test systems that will provide information, not only
directed towards genotoxic or carcinogenic effects, but the total
battery of concerns adversely affecting health.

I'd like to make one other comment in a slightly different
direction. After listening to the very interesting papers the last
two and a half days, it seems to me that what we have heard is that
the state of the information and the concerns about chemicals used
in agriculture today are not, at the moment at least, shown to be
of great concern. We have studied them quite well. There are

problems, indeed, with many of these and we certainly should be
prepared to look at new materials coming downstream. What I
suggest as an outcome of this program is that we give further
weight to looking at natural materials and their hazards. Perhaps
the types of things that were initiated in Dr. Sugimura's
laboratory, which we are now seeing worked on in this country. But
there are other things, as highlighted through Don Crosby's comments of yesterday, where he talked about natural toxins. Even if
these are not genotoxic, there are suggestions they might be teratogenic. It might be well if we look at the natural materials, the
kinds of foods and the kinds of materials to which we are exposed,
directly as well as indirectly, as related to our state of long-
term health.

William Upholt: May I be the devil's advocate for a minute? I
have been a little bit disappointed in this conference on genetic
toxicology. It seems to me what I have been hearing mostly is
genetic testing as a screening mechanism for carcinogenicity. I
like what Verne Ray said. It seems to me that a much more serious
concern should be genetic disease other than cancer. If I'm not
mistaken, the cancer death rate, age adjusted, has been going down
for the last couple of decades with the exception of four types of
cancer and I think those four types of cancer are not especially
associated with our environmental exposure, though I may be wrong
about that. It seems to me that maybe there has been a little too
much emphasis on cancer and perhaps what we should be concerned
about with all these new chemicals is not so much whether or not
they are carcinogenic, though this is worthwhile, but whether there
are genetic diseases that may be far more important to future
generations. I'm not sure there are, but I would certainly like to
have a group as knowledgeable as this group in genetic toxicology
to reassure me if there are not genetic diseases of major importance, not only to humans but to our environment. And I've heard
very little about this at the conference.

Sugimura: Well I have a little different opinion. Today, one of
four people is dying of cancer. As you know, the atomic bomb
survivors undergo very very careful examination; yet scientists
cannot prove any single evidence that radiation causes genetic or
heritable disease. Of course I am not saying that genetic disease
is not important—it is very important. But in the urgency of
today, tomorrow, the day after tomorrow, we have to worry about the
appearance of the many, many cancers all over the world, with the
order of a million cancer patients appearing annually.

Wylie Burge: With regard to sewage wastes that have been applied
to land, we have looked at the fate of pesticides and pathogens in
the soil, and I would like to ask the panel what they think about
looking at the fate of mutagens in the soil. Are we ready to do
that? Are there tests that are adequate to do that? In my labor-

atory we are working with hazardous wastes and that's one of our
concerns. We have seen that the soil has a way of degrading
pesticides and also trapping and holding pathogens. The soil has
been a buffer or reservoir in which these substances have been held
out of contact with their targets and I was wondering whether it is
also a place where many mutagens may be inactivated. I wonder if
somebody would comment about that.

Michael Plewa: We have been looking at how one investigates
municipal sewage sludges, which our college of agriculture is very
interested in using in soil amendment. We had an incredible dilemma. Municipal sewage sludge from Chicago is mutagenic. It's
mutagenic in Tradescantia, it's mutagenic in the Ames trains, it's
mutagenic in maize. It also gives a positive response in sister
chromatid exchanges. Microbial tests were done with extracts,
Tradescantia and maize were done with the neat sludge. We also
took the sludge in the plots that EPA and USDA were supporting to
encourage the use of municipal sewage sludge. We grew inside two
tests and found dose-response effects. After doing two years of
work on it and having the material presented for publication, I
cannot say whether or not there is a risk there. We find an
effect, but as a scientist I do not know how to weight the benefit
of the fixed nitrogen that is present in the sludge with the risk
of unknown and unquantifiable, in terms of risk, effects on a population that has been exposed to it. In Chicago the use of
municipal sewage sludge has been curtailed by the USEPA, not
because of its mutagenic properties but because crop plants grown
on it can bioconcentrate the cadmium, zinc and nickel to unacceptable levels. So perhaps the presence of the heavy metals has
answered the question for us. But still, there is the problem that
I as a scientist and as a geneticist find very difficult to
approach. We have a mutagen that has some benefit, and now we are
left with the question of what is going to be done with tons of
municipal sewage sludge accumulating in Chicago. Ways of disposing
of this material of course are getting more expensive with time.
It's a natural resource and fixed nitrogen would be very welcome
down on the farm, but the farmers don't want the mutagens nor the
cadmium and nickel. I guess you can call for more research dollars
and look at it, but I don't know how to answer the question.

George Bailey: I would like to address a question to Ray
Valentine. One of the things that we always look for in a
symposium of this kind is the synthesis of some kind of new idea
that will send at least a few researchers off on a new track
perhaps, or a different tangent to an old track. One of the issues
that we all face as experimentalists is that we often see one
system which offers intriguing problems but the ability to answer
those questions may not be answerable in our favorite experimental
model. One example is the growing realization that some viruses,
and I am thinking particularly of hepatitis B, may have some inter-

action with chemicals such as aflatoxin. It would be nice to be
able to investigate that kind of question except that in terms of
an animal model we presently have only the squirrel, and one more
animal, which carry a hepatitis type virus, neither of which forms
a good experimental model in the laboratory. In view of Dr.
Valentine's suggestion that one begin to exploit genetic toxi-
cology--that we might be able to marry genetic engineering and
toxicology questions--has genetic engineering reached the stage
where one can begin to consider the possibility of taking the virus
that you might be interested in and moving it into an animal
species that serves as a convenient model? We know now that you
can move prokaryotic genes in the eukaryotes and the eukaryotic
genes in the prokaryotes. What I'm asking you, do you think it's
possible and perhaps profitable for us to think now of moving some
of the problem sideways. To move a virus from a problematic animal
into one we can conveniently munipulate and examine.

Valentine: The answer is, of course, yes. It is a good point to
discuss and it really mirrors the point that was made earlier--
recombinant DNA has much to offer genetic toxicology. This is a
rapidly advancing field, with new discoveries almost monthly. The
hoof and mouth disease antigen gene has been cloned. A gene for
making the structural protein for hepatitis virus has been cloned
in yeast. Not only was the protein made, but the shell of the
virus also appeared in the yeast. What I'm saying is this human
hepatitis virus gene was not only expressed, but the protein was
able to assemble and make what looks like the ghost of a virus
particle. New ideas are particularly critical at this time. You
can outsmart systems, in a sense of reducing a problem down to its
simplest element, if for no other reason than for economic ones.
Perhaps the next symposium should have a whole section dealing with
questions similar to those you have asked.

R.K. Sharma: I would like to point out an area which I do not
think has received adequate attention in this symposium, the relationship between the mutagens and teratogens. A lot of discussion has been devoted to the relationship between mutagenesis and
carcinogenesis but I don't think the relationship between mutagenesis and teratogenesis is adequately established or studied. As
geneticists, we are responsible for the gene pool, not only in this
generation but the coming generations. I think in addition to Dr.
Sugimura's suggestion of adding a P into ICPEMC, I would like to
add a T for teratogens and would recommend studying the relationship of teratogenesis and mutagenesis in more detail, maybe
studying teratogenesis at a cellular level.

Daniel Krewski: I'd like to suggest that we might want to consider
looking at the relationship between mutagens and mutagens. If the
standard cancer bioassay has been criticized on the grounds that we
look at chemicals one at a time and the reason that is offered for

this is that NTP protocol, calling for a control MTD and a half MTD both sexes of two different species, now costs about a half-million dollars and we just cannot afford to make a more elaborate design which would allow for the assessment of synergism and antagonism of chemical carcinogens. But if we can do mutagenicity studies in the space of a few days, and spend only five hundred dollars doing so, I think that there is no reason why we shouldn't be exploring more the question of synergism among mutagenic compounds.

Irving Putter: I would like to ask a pragmatic question. People speak about loads of insecticides being used for 10 and 20 years and you also hear of people who abuse those insecticides. Perhaps they douse themselves with the formula, and here you have a tremendous reservoir of people who have been abusing insecticides or growth regulants or herbicides. Would it be worthwhile to take some of the funds and examine these people very very carefully. What are their death rates? What are they dying from? Try to follow them up. Look at their chromosomes. Look at their chromosomes with time. Isn't this very very close to the thing you're trying to find out about? This doesn't address new chemicals but is does address those that you've used in the past and those that you are using every year.

Mendelsohn: We have been getting one suggestion after another and by and large they are all reasonable. Yes, yes, yes, we should look at synergism, teratogenesis, chemical waste, and, of course, epidemiology. Two speakers earlier in the program summarized what was known about the epidemiology of farmers, urban-rural contrasts, and workers with pesticides and herbicides. If there are workers with large exposures and they can be identified, then I would certainly encourage your suggestion that they be studied.

Rominger: That was one of the gaps we found in the use of malathion, even though it has been used on large populations for many years. There does not seem to have been epidemiological studies of any consequence done. I'd sure like to second that motion. I'd like to ask another question, going back to the promoters. On the other side of the coin, are there inhibitors and how much research is going on in that area?

Valentine: I was just telling Dr. Lyons I found this aspect of the meeting one of the most exiciting. In fact, there are such compounds. I'm not an expert, but indeed there is a big interest in these areas.

Sugimura: I mentioned at the end of my talk yesterday that anti-mutagenesis is a very important field to be explored. There are very many classes of compounds and different strategies. The first is to destroy the mutagens. The second is to prevent the formation of a mutagen. The third is to prevent the activation of pro-

mutagens. And in addition to that, promotional steps could be
dealt with much more efficiently. Vitamin A definitely is very
active. Retinoic acid, a so-called chemoprevention and a kind of
protease inhibitor, can beautifully inhibit chemopromoting steps.
So there are many, many things that are going to be developed. But
generally speaking, I do not think that these matters are
systematically studied yet. I think bigger steps are needed in the
prevention of, for instance, endogenous formation of a mutagen in
the gut in our body. These things should be very much encouraged
in the future.

A. H. El-Sebae: From the scientific point of view there have been
many constructive suggestions here, and we can expect additional
suggestions, which will enrich the plans for future research. In
the field of genetic toxicology, those chemicals should be considered which pose a human hazard of direct or expected adverse
affect on humans by being introduced into the food chain. This
needs a lot of study by an assigned team, for example of environ-
mentalists, to determine which chemicals are expected to be real
hazards of this type. We are not yet in agreement on those chemicals that pose a problem and to what extent. We need to promote
research in all directions from the environmental point of view.
Ecochemistry, in itself, is a new field. It is a multidisciplinary
science, needing cooperation between the people in biology, chemistry, physics and all other aspects of science. We heard
yesterday that important information about toxaphene has only been
elucidated in the past few years, although it is already
contaminating California, even though the California people don't
know the fate of this chemical being dumped in their state. Is it
reaching the drinking water through the ground water? It was shown
that toxaphene has an appreciable vapor pressure--has this vapor
pressure been a problem to the Canadian people? It is quite clear
that this is not only a concern for the United States. Such problems are a concern on a global scale. This is also illustrated by
one of the natural toxins, aflatoxin. It was beautifully shown, in
yesterday's presentation, that aflatoxin is showing carcinogenic
hazard in many countries, including Africa, Asia and perhaps Latin
America. If we are seeking priorities, we should stress priorities
in advice, in help, and in scientific cooperation with such countries which will also give us an opportunity for epidemiological
studies in humans, because it is there--it is not merely suspected
or expected, it is there. Another dimension is to put together all
the universal scientific activities in one pool for attaining
mutual objectives in this direction. Through the international
genetics organizations or through the international toxicological
organizations a lot of concern should be directed to genetic toxicology as one of the disciplines. I think there is an international toxicology congress to be held in 1983 so perhaps it would
be a good chance to combine the efforts of the American scientists

with scientists from all over the world. I'm sure that the same
ideas are in the minds of scientists all over Europe and in many
other countries all over the world as well. One additional dimension is that all these advances in research need to be supported by
ever deeper basic research. We should go much deeper in genetics,
in ecology, in chemistry, in toxicology. And all of the agencies
which are encouraging and promoting science, like the National
Science Foundation, have a worldwide obligation. They should give
more input in facilities, in cooperation, and in putting together
experiences such as we have enjoyed here, with the team from Japan
and with the team from the United States, and which would be even
stronger if it were an even wider team, putting together the
experience of all of us, for the welfare of the future, because it
is a global environment in which we live.

Raymond Fleck: We've certainly been expanding and prioritizing our
agenda of needed research activities this evening. I'm concerned
with the question that Robert Colton from NSF brought up, namely
the relationship between the universities and industry in the
development of support for research in these areas that we have
been discussing. Looking at it from a university perspective, I
ask myself what kind of reciprocity there might be with industry in
such research. In the symposium program, we have many speakers
from the universities whose interest is prompted perhaps by a personal interest in the subject and the discipline to which they are
committed, as well as their responsibilities in the universities
for teaching and research and service. But what about industry?
Reference was made to the possibility that if we try to solve the
kinds of problems we are talking about, there may be some kind of
guilt by association, that we are partly responsible for the
problem. How can industry bring itself to support research in this
area and justify such support to the stockholders and to the
decision-makers within industry itself? For some years now, NSF
has been addressing itself to the challenge of promoting collaborative research in various areas between university and industry in
areas such as microelectronics, polymer development, and corrosion
control, areas in which there is a research interest from the university point of view and a payoff for industry. But what kind of
positive payoff can industry look to in solving problems of genetic
toxicology? I see this as a problem. How can the universities and
industry really team up, especially in the face of perhaps diminished federal support for research in this area? Is it really
that attractive to industry to take up some of the slack caused by
a decline in federal research funds?

Ray: In the area of toxicology, as you know, the posture of
industry has been to do sufficient research to make sure that the
safety or toxic potential of a chemical is defined. Further, research for this purpose has been done primarily within the confines
of industry. What industry does in large part for safety eval-

uation purposes is to test chemicals. This is very unattractive to
the academician. He has a primary orientation of teaching and
doing basic research to develop new ideas and knowledge and, at the
same time, training students. Therefore, a good deal of what
industry would do in the testing area would probably not be that
attractive to the academician. That's one aspect. Another is that
the only hope industry has in this era of regulation is to utilize
the best science it can in defining the safety and/or toxicity of
potential products. It is totally and utterly dependent upon good
science to do this. Therefore, the way we define toxicity or toxic
potential is a very important problem to industry. For example,
there have been great concerns about the manner in which carcinogenicity studies have been conducted. Research into the development of better models to determine carcinogenic potential and other
types of toxicity could be a focus for a greater association
between universities and industry. For this purpose, perhaps an
association of companies could be formed to interact with universities. You recall that CIIT (Chemical Industry Institute of Toxicology) is funded by a group of companies interested in developing
more knowledge and methods for assessing toxicity of chemicals.
Perhaps there is opportunity for more organizations of that type.
That is, a privately funded organization which was a similar type
of structure to CIIT, but would orient on those basic aspects of
toxicological research which facilitate an association between
academic institutions and industry.

Hollaender: Who would like to express an opinion or make a suggestion about how we could proceed to get industry more involved in
basic academic research? I should mention that this symposium is
well supported by Atlantic Richfield Foundation. In the future, we
will have to count much more on industrial support of these conferences and symposia. Until now, we have not approached industry
in, perhaps, the right way. I think in the future we will have to
learn how to do this and do it in a much better way to show industry how it can profit from such cooperation. I think we will
find a very good reception there - I am quite certain.

Upholt: I would like to make a comment on this, but first I would
like to introduce a guest. Back in 1969, the Secretary of HEW
faced a very serious problem on what the position of the federal
government should be with regard to pesticides, which were becoming
a very critical problem to the nation as a whole. To try to give
him some perspective and handle on this, he appointed a committee
to spend six months in bringing a report to him on what should be
done about pesticides. To find a chairman for this committee he
came to the University of California at Davis and asked the
Chancellor of the University to serve in that position. Just about
that time, Dr. Emil Mrak, the Chancellor of UC Davis was retiring,
and he did, in fact, take on the six-month job, and following that
he became chairman of the Secretary's pesticide advisory

committee. When EPA was formed, he became chairman of the Environmental Protection Agency's Science Advisory Board and served in
that capacity as long as EPA could find legal ways to keep him in
it. I would like to introduce Dr. Mrak and his wife Dr. Vera Mrak.

One of the things that Dr. Mrak helped us promote in 1970-71
was the National Center for Toxicological Research. In the way
that was organized, as suggested at the time, it was to be a collaborative effort between universities, government and industry.
We had representatives from industry. In fact, I had the privilege
of going with a vice president of Dow Chemical Company to meet
before the manufacturing chemical association's governing board, to
ask them if they would be interested in collaborating in the support and financing and carrying out of the center. They gave us a
rather welcome response. But when we went back to the controller
of the Department of HEW, he said there was no possible way that we
could mix government funds with industry funds in an effort of this
sort, and that was absolutely the end of it. So we had to go ahead
with the National Toxicological Center without the benefit of
direct participation by industry. Personally, I think that was a
mistake, but maybe the situation has changed enough now, so maybe
something of that sort might be possible. It certainly was desirable then and it would still be desirable today I believe.

Colton: I might make a suggestion that the conference committee
appoint a committee of industry and university people to explore
this subject and possibly report on it in some period of time. You
have to start the ball rolling somewhere; you might as well start
it here.

Newell: There already exists a good model in the way academia has
interacted with the electronics industry. You have it right close
by here, on the peninsula, but the same thing holds true whether
we're talking about the area of Cambridge, Massachusetts, or in
Texas. There, I think a good share of the success has been the
understanding and the willingess of academia to work with
industry. More typically, there has been reluctance to a great
extent throughout academia to really participate with and try to
assist industry in development and problem-solving. Another
example, which probably is indirect but is functioning very well,
is the Electric Power Research Institute. EPRI has a lot of funds
from industry and those to a great extent go back to academia and
provide support. So I suggest the models are there and they need
to be explored. Incidentally, the Assembly of Life Sciences at the
Academy was discussing this very problem in February of this
year. They already had these concerns and there probably will be
an informal report, and I would be glad to follow up on it and
report back to you.

Hollaender: As I mentioned at the beginning of this evening, the
close cooperation of industry was planned from the start in the
development of studies in genetic toxicology and environmental
mutagenesis. Invariably, there has been excellent success so we
would now like to extend this cooperation into the areas of
straight research. I hope that some kind of pattern can be
developed in this regard to strengthen our mutual productivity.

LIST OF SPEAKERS

ALBERTINI, Richard J.
    University of Vermont
    Burlington, VT
AMES, Bruce N.
    University of California
    Berkeley, CA
BAILEY, George S.
    Oregon State University
    Corvallis, OR
BLAIR, Aaron
    National Cancer Institute
    Bethesda, MD
BORHANI, Nemat O.
    University of California
    Davis, CA
BYARD, James L.
    University of California
    Davis, CA
COLTON, Robert M.
    National Science Foundation
    Washington, D.C.
CONNELLY, Roger R.
    National Cancer Institute
    Bethesda, MD
CROSBY, Donald G.
    University of California
    Davis, CA
EL-SEBAE, A.H.
    University of Alexandria
        Research Center
    Alexandria, Egypt
FLECK, Raymond
    University of California
    Davis, CA
GARDNER, Murray
    University of California
    Davis, CA
GEHRING, Perry J.
    Dow Chemical U.S.A.
    Midland, MI

GENTILE, James M.
    Hope College
    Holland, MI
GRANT, William F.
    McGill University
    Quebec, Canada
HESS, Charles E.
    University of California
    Davis, CA
HOFFMANN, George R.
    College of the Holy Cross
    Worcester, MA
HOLLAENDER, Alexander
    Associated Universities, Inc.
    Washington, D.C.
HSIEH, Dennis P.
    University of California
    Davis, CA
HURLEY, Lucille S.
    University of California
    Davis, CA
KAUFMAN, Donald
    U.S. Department of
        Agriculture
    Beltsville, MD
KILLAM Jr., Keith F.
    University of California
    Davis, CA
KREWSKI, Daniel
    Health & Welfare, Canada
    Ottawa, Canada
LYONS, James
    University of California
    Davis, CA
MENDELSOHN, Mortimer L.
    Lawrence Livermore Lab.
    Livermore, CA
NEWELL, Gordon W.
    Natl. Academy of Sciences
    Washington, D.C.

PLEWA, Michael
   University of Illinois
   Urbana, IL
PRESTON, R. Julian
   Oak Ridge National Lab.
   Oak Ridge, TN
RAY, Verne
   Pfizer, Inc.
   Groton, CT
ROMINGER, Richard E.
   California Department
     of Food and Agriculture
   Sacramento, CA
SEIBER, James N.
   University of California
   Davis, CA
SETLOW, Richard B.
   Brookhaven National Lab.
   Upton, NY
SEVERN, David
   Environmental Protection
    Agency
   Washington, D.C.

STILL, Gerald G.
   U.S. Department of
    Agriculture
   Washington, D.C.
SUGIMURA, Takashi
   National Cancer Center
    Research Institute
   Tokyo, Japan
UPHOLT, William M.
   Silver Spring, MD
VALENTINE, Raymond
   University of California
   Davis, CA
WATERS, Michael D.
   Environmental Protection
    Agency
   Research Triangle Park, NC
WOODHEAD, Avril D.
   Brookhaven National Lab.
   Upton, NY
ZIMMERMAN, Burke
   George Washington University
   Washington, D.C.

LIST OF PARTICIPANTS

ALEXEEFF, George
  Environmental Toxicology
  University of California
  Davis, CA 95616
ALLEN, Jane S.
  American Cyanamid
  East Brunswick, NJ 08816
BADR, Effat A.
  Dept. of Genetics
  Faculty of Agriculture
  University of Alexandria
  Alexandria, Egypt
BATTAGLIA, Gabriella
  Food Science
  University of California
  Davis, CA 95616
BERRY, David L.
  U.S. Department of
    Agriculture
  Western Regional Research
    Center
  Berkeley, CA 94710
BLAZAK, William
  SRI International
  Menlo Park, CA 94025
BODE, Richard
  Dept. of Pharm/Tox
  University of California
  Davis, CA 95616
BOWES, Gerald W.
  Dept. of Environmental
    Toxicology
  University of California
  Davis, CA 95616
BOYNTON, Buck
  Dept. of Genetics
  University of California
  Davis, CA 95616
BROWN, Joseph P.
  Zoecon Corporation
  Palo Alto, CA 94304

BURGE, Wylie D.
  U.S. Department of
    Agriculture
  Silver Spring, MD 20910
CARVER, June H.
  Chevron Env. Health Ctr.
  Richmond, CA 94802
CHAN, David W.
  Air Resources Board
  Sacramento, CA 95812
CHIRIKJIAN, Jack G.
  Dept. of Biochemistry
  Georgetown University
    Medical Center
  Washington, D.C. 20007
COHEN, Rachel
  Dept. of Animal Physiology
  University of California
  Davis, CA 95616
CRAIGMILL, Arthur L.
  Cooperative Extension
  Dept. of Env. Toxicology
  University of California
  Davis, CA 95616
DALEY, Paul F.
  Division of Biological
    Control
  University of California
  Berkeley, CA 94710
DIME, Richard A.
  Dept. of Env. Toxicology
  University of California
  Davis, CA 95616
DI ROSA, Denise
  Vet. Med. Physiological
    Sciences
  University of California
  Davis, CA 95616
DUAFALA, Thomas
  TRICAL
  Morgan Hill, CA 95037

535

DURZAN, Don
  Department of Pomology
  University of California
  Davis, CA 95616
EASTMAN, David
  Vet. Med. Physiological Sci.
  University of Calfornia
  Davis, CA 95616
ELLIGER, Carl A.
  U.S. Department of
    Agriculture
  Albany, CA 94710
FISCHER, Charles
  Department of Environmental
    Toxicology
  University of California
  Davis, CA 95616
FLESSEL, Peter
  California Department
    Health Services
  Berkeley, CA 94704
FORD, Jon E.
  Chevron Env. Health Ctr.
  Richmond, CA 94802
FUKAYAMA, Mark
  Department of Environmental
    Toxicology
  University of California
  Davis, CA 95616
GENTRY, Rodney
  University of Guelph
  Department of Mathematics
  Guelph, Ontario, Canada
  N1G 2W1
GILMORE, Donna R.
  Water Resources Control
    Board
  Atwater, CA 95301
GOODMAN, Jay I.
  Dept. of Pharm. & Toxicology
  Michigan State University
  East Lansing, MI 48824
HAWORTH, Steve
  E G & G Mason Res. Institute
  Rockville, MD 20852
HELFERICH, Bill
  Dept. of Animal Science
  University of California
  Davis, CA 95616

HIXSON, E. Jane
  Mobay Chemical Corp.
  Stilwell, KS 66085
JAWORSKI, Ernest G.
  Monsanto Corp.
  St. Louis, MO 63166
JONES, David C.L.
  SRI International
  Menlo Park, CA 94025
KADO, Norman
  Dept. of Environmental
    Toxicology
  University of California
  Davis, CA 95616
KILLAM, Anne
  Dept. of Pharmacology
  University of California
  Davis, CA 95616
KNADLE, Susan Ann
  Dept. of Environmental
    Toxicology
  University of California
  Davis, CA 95616
KNEZOVICH, John P.
  Dept. of Environmental
    Toxicology
  University of California
  Davis, CA 95616
KRISHNA, Maryala
  SRI International
  Menlo Park, CA 94025
LEE, Marshall
  Dept. of Environmental
    Toxicology
  University of California
  Davis, CA 95616
LINTON, Cathie
  Dept. of Environmental
    Toxicology
  University of California
  Davis, CA 95616
LOONEY, Mary
  Dept. of Animal Science
  University of California
  Davis, CA 95616
LOURY, David
  Dept. of Env. Toxicology
  University of California
  Davis, CA 95616

MA, Paul C.
Hsinchu, Taiwan
Republic of China
MAC GREGOR, James T.
U.S. Department of
Agriculture
Berkeley, CA 94710
MANALE, Andrew
University of California
Berkeley, CA 94720
MARSHACK, Jon B.
Regional Water Quality
Control Board
Sacramento, CA 95816
MARTY, Melanie
Department of Environmental
Toxicology
University of California
Davis, CA 95616
MAST, Terry
Department of Environmental
Toxicology
University of California
Davis, CA 95616
MATHESON, Dale W.
Stauffer Chemical Co.
Farmington, CT 06032
MATSUSHIMA, Taijiro
Dept. of Molecular Oncology
Institute of Medical Science
University of Tokyo
Tokyo 108, Japan
MILAM, Kathryn M.
Department of Environmental
Toxicology
University of California
Davis, CA 95616
MISCHKE, Charles
Department of Botany
University of California
Davis, CA 95616
NGUYEN, Thu-Hong
Department of Environmental
Toxicology
University of California
Davis, CA 95616
NOWELL, Lisa H.
Dept. of Env. Toxicology
University of California
Davis, CA 95616

OLSEN, Hugh
Department of Environmental
Toxicology
University of California
Davis, CA 95616
OSBURN, B.I.
Dean's Office
School of Vet. Med.
University of California
Davis, CA 95616
PARKER, Judith A.
Chevron Env. Health Ctr.
Richmond, CA 94802
PELLEGRINI, Marleen
San Diego, CA 92124
PINKEL, Dan
Lawrence Livermore Lab.
Livermore, CA 94550
POTREPKA, Robert F.
Stauffer Chemical Company
Farmington, CT 06032
PUSEY, John
University of California
Cooperative Extension
Los Angeles, CA 90015
PUTTER, Irving
Merck Sharp & Dohme
Rahway, NJ 07065
RALEIGH, Edward W.
Du Pont Co., Inc.
Wilmington, DE 19898
RICCIO, Ed
SRI International
Menlo Park, CA 94025
RICE, David Warren
Department of Environmental
Toxicology
University of California
Davis, CA 95616
RIGGS, Ralph
Stauffer Chemical Co.
Davis, CA 95616
RUSSELL, G.F.
Food Science & Technology
University of California
Davis, CA 95616
RYAN, Frederick J.
Department of Botany
University of California
Davis, CA 95616

SACKS, L.E.
    U.S. Department of
        Agriculture
    Berkeley, CA 94710
SALOCKS, Charles B.
    Department of Environmental
        Toxicology
    University of California
    Davis, CA 95616
SCHER, Stanley
    School of Public Health
    University of California
    Berkeley, CA 94710
SCHLEGEL, Robert
    University of California
    Berkeley, CA 94710
SCHWASS, Daniel E.
    U.S. Department of
        Agriculture
    Albany, CA 94710
SCIBIENSKI, Carole Davis
    Department of Environmental
        Toxicology·
    University of California
    Davis, CA 95616
SHARMA, Rajendar Kumar
    SRI International
    Menlo Park, CA 94025
SILVA, Marilyn
    Department of Environmental
        Health Science
    University of California
    Berkeley, CA 94710
SINGLETON, Vernon L.
    Viticulture & Enology
    University of California
    Davis, CA 95616
STEWARD, Ruth
    Department of Environmental
        Toxicology
    University of California
    Davis, CA 95616

SUWA, Yoshihide
    National Cancer Center
        Research Institute
    Tokyo, Japan
TAKAYAMA, Shozo
    National Cancer Center
        Research Institute
    Tokyo, Japan
THILAGAR, A.
    E G & G Mason Research
        Institute
    Rockville, MD 20852
VAN GELDER, G.A.
    Shell Development Company
    Westhollow Research
        Center
    Houston, TX 77001
WATT, Dennis
    Department of Environmental
        Toxicology
    University of California
    Davis, CA 95616
WEHR, Carol M.
    U.S. Department of
        Agriculture
    Albany, CA 94706
WILKINSON, Dan
    Pioneer Hi-Bred International
    Johnston, Iowa 50131
WILSON, Dennis W.
    Department of Vet. Pathology
    California Primate Research
        Center
    Davis, CA 94710
YAGER, Jan
    School of Public Health
    University of California
    Berkeley, CA 94710
ZWEIG, Gunter
    School of Public Health
    University of California
    Berkeley, CA 94710